Diagnostic Procedures in Patients with Neck Masses

Jerzy Klijanienko
Beatrix Cochand-Priollet
Olivier Choussy • Wojciech Golusiński
Editors

Diagnostic Procedures in Patients with Neck Masses

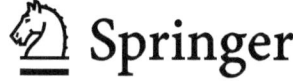 Springer

Editors
Jerzy Klijanienko
Department of Pathology
Institute Curie
Paris, France

Beatrix Cochand-Priollet
Department of Pathology
Cochin AP-HP-Paris Centre, University
Paris-Cité
Paris, France

Olivier Choussy
ENT Department
Institute Curie
Paris, France

Wojciech Golusiński
The Greater Poland Cancer Centre
Head and Neck Surgery, Poznan
University of Medical Sciences
Poznań, Poland

ISBN 978-3-031-67674-1   ISBN 978-3-031-67675-8   (eBook)
https://doi.org/10.1007/978-3-031-67675-8

This Springer imprint is published by the registered company Springer Nature Switzerland AG
The registered company address is: Gewerbestrasse 11, 6330 Cham, Switzerland

If disposing of this product, please recycle the paper.

Introduction

The aim of this book is to bring together authoritative presentations on imaging, biopsy techniques, and both cytopathology and core needle biopsy pathology of the head and neck region in a single text to assist clinicians, radiologists, cytopathologists, and pathologists. Each of these chapters covers its particular topic in detail, and in some cases, there may be some overlap with other sections, which will reinforce and create a holistic review of the head and neck region. Each chapter can be read as a standalone review of its topic and as a guide to managing patients with specific clinical presentations.

Dr. Jerzy Klijanienko was the instigator of this commendable project and has led the editorial team as they brought together an experienced group of writers to cover the wide range of topics. He is to be congratulated on bringing to completion a text with such a broad range of topics written by leading authors in their respective fields of research, authorship, and teaching.

We hope that this text will be of great usefulness to all those practicing medicine in the head and neck region, and that patients will benefit from clinicians, surgeons, and oncologists having a better understanding of the diagnostic workup for lesions of the head and neck.

University of New South Wales, Sydney, Clinical Medical School, Sydney, NSW, Australia
University of Notre Dame, Sydney, Medical School, NSW, Australia
Department of Anatomical Pathology, St Vincent's Hospital, Sydney, NSW, Australia
International Academy of Cytology, Freiburg im Breisgau, Germany
IAC WHO IARC Cytopathology Joint Standing Editorial Board, Lyon Cedex 07, France
WHO Classification of Tumours Standing Editorial Board, Lyon Cedex 07, France

Andrew S. Field

International Academy of Cytology, Freiburg im Breisgau, Germany
Department of Pathology and Oncology, Medical Faculty, University of Porto, Porto, Portugal
RISE (Health Research Network), Porto, Portugal
Molecular Pathology Unit, Institute of Pathology and Molecular Immunology of Porto University, IPATIMUP, Porto, Portugal

Fernando Schmitt

Contents

About the Editors

Klijanienko Jerzy   Professor of pathology at Institut Curie, Paris, France. President of 43rd European Congress of Cytology 2021 in Wroclaw, Poland and past president of European Federation of Cytology Societies 2019–2021. Vice-president of the French Society of Clinical Cytology. Author of around 370 different scientific publications, 4 books, and 30 chapters. Author/co-author/editor of three "WHO blue books" concerning cytology reporting in soft tissue tumors, breast tumors and head and neck tumors including thyroid and salivary glands. Co-author of *The Milan System for Reporting Salivary Gland Cytopathology*.

Cochand-Priollet Beatrix   Pathologist at Cochin Hospital, University Paris Cité, Paris, France. Funding Member of the National Agency for Quality Assurance, responsible for the Pap Smear Committee and later Committee for Cytopathology. Past General Secretary of the European Federation of Cytological Societies and Past president of the French Society of Clinical Cytology. Currently Editor-in-Chief of Eurocytology. Authoring 152 publications; 2 books and some chapters and co-editor for the new version 2023 of *The Bethesda System for Reporting Thyroid Cytology*.

Olivier Choussy   ENT oncology surgeon. Head of Head and Neck Oncological Surgery at the Institut Curie, Paris, France.

Golusiński Wojciech   Professor of ENT and head and neck surgery at University of Medical Sciences at the Greater Poland Cancer Centre. Past president of the European Head and Neck Society (2018–2022). Co-author of European recommendations on diagnosis and treatment of head and neck cancer, prepared by members of three societies: EHNS, ESTRO and ESMO. Author of over 300 papers, reports and lectures. Author and organizer of the National Head and Neck Cancer Prevention Program in Poland.

General Aspects

Jerzy Klijanienko

A neck mass is a common clinical problem and may be of different etiologies including primary lesions of inflammatory and neoplastic origin or metastases from known or unknown cancers (Fig. 1.1).

The clinical presentation may be non-specific and overlap with numerous entities owing to the close proximity of different tissues in a limited tissue space. For example, the epithelial tissues of the aero-digestive tract, the salivary and thyroid glands, the soft and bone tissues, and the lymph nodes may be the source of benign, malignant, and inflammatory tumors. The differential diagnosis may be wide and necessitate a range of investigations.

However, the diagnostic approach may vary according to the experience of a particular institution. Depending upon the initial clinicoradiological evaluations, the subsequent diagnostic protocols are not standardized worldwide. Some institutions use surgical biopsies, others use core-needle or fine-needle aspiration biopsies, and frozen sections may be examined. Many centers have little or no access to molecular studies, which may limit diagnostic evaluation.

Moreover, the performance of the different techniques can vary depending on the experience of a given institution. For example, this is clearly evident from the analysis of the results from cytology or frozen sections. The level of non-significant or false positive results may be elevated in less experienced hands.

At present, histological biopsy examination remains the gold standard for the diagnostic process. It is mandatory for the application of international tumor classifications, to define the prognosis and to ensure the material for various ancillary techniques, molecular analyses, and treatment of patients.

The practice of cytology is also well-established in particular organs and group of tumors. In recent years, the International Academy of Cytology elaborated a series of reporting systems from different organs that have

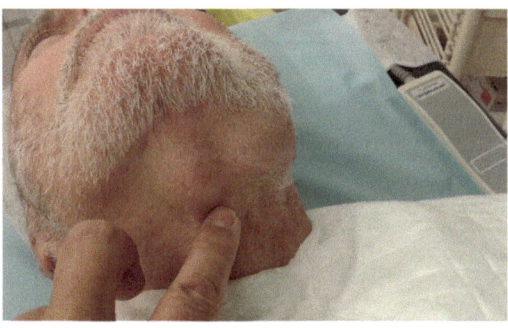

Fig. 1.1 Submandibular tumor, clinically malignant without any apparent primary tumor site. FNA and immediate cytological diagnosis using Rapid On-Site Evaluation technique evidenced metastasis from adenocarcinoma. Primary lung adenocarcinoma was identified on further investigations

J. Klijanienko (✉)
Pathology, Institute Curie, Paris, France
e-mail: jerzy.klijanienko@curie.fr

been designated by the city hosting these cytology congresses—the Yokohama system (1) for breast tumors, the Paris system, (2) for urinary cytology, the Bethesda system, (3) for thyroid cytology and the Milan system, and (4) for salivary cytology.

Moreover, the IAC-IARC-World Health Organization is elaborating a series of fascicles concerning cytological diagnosis in particular tumor localizations. Cytology in lung (5), lymph node, spleen and thymus (6), and pancreaticobiliary system (7) are already published, whereas connective tissue, head and neck, breast and liver cytopathology are under investigation.

These various systems aim to simplify the language of pathologists, i.e., to make diagnostic reporting understandable to oncologists and define the most optimal management. Moreover, the risk of malignancy in each diagnostic category is assessed. This standardization of results has already been introduced into practice, e.g., using cervicovaginal smears (Pap test) with specific diagnostic categories and risks of malignancy.

However, despite growing interest, cytology remains underused and misunderstood. The reasons for this are multiple. It has been repeatedly observed that the problem is partially linked to the imperfect training of pathologists and insufficient demography in this specialization. Another problem may be that pathologists are not always enthusiastic about performing biopsies. In addition, the practice of obtaining good-quality samples has not been sufficiently taught in the training of radiologists. Finally, because of the latter factors, the practice of cytology may remain suboptimal in pathology unless there is greater intellectual investment.

This book aims to present the practical approach about how to manage neck masses by the most experienced specialists in the field. We collected the opinions of all specialties involved in the diagnosis: medical oncologists, head and neck surgeons, nuclear medicine specialists and radiologists, molecular biologists, and pathologists who practice classical surgical pathology and clinical cytology.

Our mission has been to write a book to illustrate the combined experiences of diverse specialties and countries. Every specialist involved in the diagnosis of a neck mass will find his/her discipline represented in this work. All perspectives, even contradictory ones, are presented here. This is the richness of this book. Therefore, some inherent repetition may be present in the various chapters. This is impossible to avoid.

We address ourselves not only to specialists in the field of oncology but also to practitioners in other disciplines, medical students, nurses, and other healthcare providers.

Further Readings

1. Field A, Raymond WA, Schmitt F, editors. The international academy of cytology Yokohama system for reporting breast fine needle aspiration biopsy cytopathology. 1st ed. Springer; 2020.
2. Wojcik EM, Kurtycz DFI, Rosenthal DL, editors. The Paris system for reporting urinary cytology. 2nd ed. Springer; 2022.
3. Ali SZ, Cibas ES, editors. The Bethesda system for reporting thyroid cytopathology: definitions, criteria, and explanatory notes. Springer; 2017.
4. Facquin WC, Rossi ED, Balloch Z, Barkan GA, Foschini MP, Kurtycz DFI, Pustaszeri M, Vielh P, editors. The Milan system for reporting salivary gland cytopathology. Springer; 2018.
5. International Academy of Cytology—International Agency for Research on Cancer—World Health Organization Joint Editorial Board. WHO Reporting System for Lung Cytopathology. Lyon (France): International Agency for Research on Cancer; forthcoming. (IAC-IARC-WHO cytopathology reporting systems series, 1st ed.; vol. 1). https://publications.iarc.fr
6. IAC-IARC-WHO Cytopathology Reporting Systems, 1st Edition: WHO Reporting System for Lymph Node, Spleen, and Thymus Cytopathology.
7. International Academy of Cytology—International Agency for Research on Cancer—World Health Organization Joint Editorial Board. WHO Reporting System for Pancreaticobiliary Cytopathology. (IAC-IARC-WHO cytopathology reporting systems series, 1st ed.; vol. 2). https://tumourclassification.iarc.who.int/chapters/50

Klijanienko Jerzy Professor of pathology at Institut Curie, Paris, France. President of 43rd European Congress of Cytology 2021 in Wroclaw, Poland and past president of European Federation of Cytology Societies 2019-2021. Vice-president of French Society of Clinical Cytology. Author of around 370 publications, 4 books, and 30 chapters. Author/co-author/editor of three "WHO blue books" concerning cytology reporting in soft tissue tumors, head and neck tumors and breast tumors. Co-author of The Milan System for Reporting Salivary Gland Cytopathology

Presentation, Diagnostic Modalities

Olivier Choussy, Guillaume Rougier, and Antoine Dubray-Vautrin

2.1 General Clinical Landscape

Fine-needle aspiration (FNA) is a very important tool in head and neck cancer. Its importance was now well recognized for thyroid pathology.

The aim of this work is to perform the same helpful guide for neck masses.

2.2 Introduction

The lateral neck mass is frequent. The diagnosis is not always challenging. The medical pass, as well as clinical and radiological exams, can help us, but the cytology or histopathology exam allows us to use a better diagnostic approach.

The FNA is superior to the biopsy in different situations:

- To reduce diagnosis delay.
- There is less risk of tumor seeding and local and regional tumor recurrence.
- Its cost-effective test.

- The high sensitivity ($\approx 90\%$) and specificity ($\approx 96\%$).
- The minimal discomfort.
- No modification of imaging results.

But

- There is a risk of nondiagnosis or indeterminate test results.
- And FNA is operator-dependent.

2.3 Anatomical Structures

The lateral part of the neck is rich in anatomical structures.

2.3.1 Lymph Nodes

Lymph nodes are the most common lateral neck masses. They are localized in the whole cervical area from the base to the top of the neck. They are divided into different levels (Robbins) according to the anatomical landmarks (Fig. 2.1).

2.3.2 Salivary Glands

The major salivary glands are three on both sides: parotid, sub-mandibular, and sublingual

O. Choussy (✉) · G. Rougier · Antoine Dubray-Vautrin
ENT department, Institute Curie, Paris, France
e-mail: olivier.choussy@curie.fr;
guillaume.rougier@curie.fr;
Antoine.DubrayVautrin@curie.fr

Fig. 2.1 Robbins classification of laterocervical lymph node levels

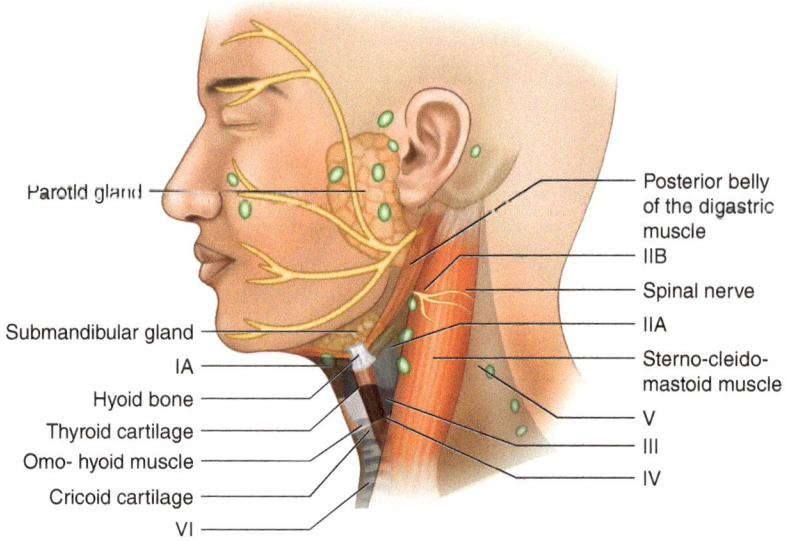

Fig. 2.2 Principals salivary glands

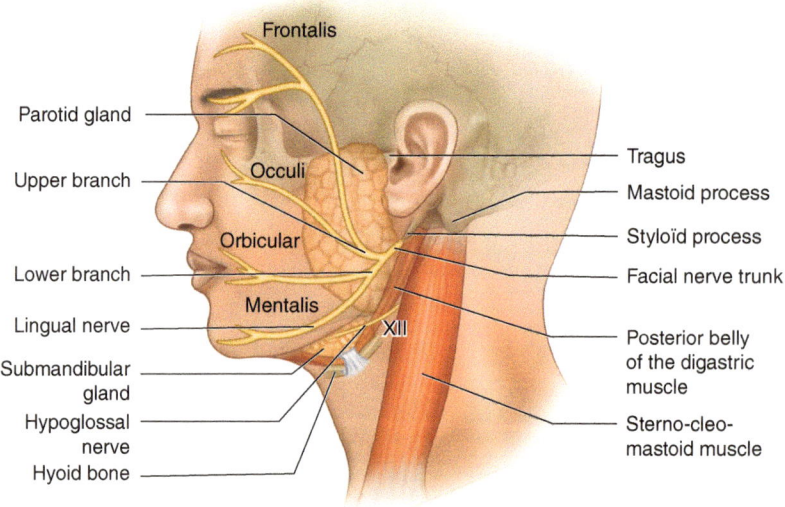

(Fig. 2.2). The parotid area is the higher salivary gland forward and below the ear. In this area, we can find some adenopathy, some benign or malignant salivary tumors but also some soft tissue tumors. The submandibular is just below the mandibular. The same lesions as in the parotid area can be found. The sublingual gland is rarely the origin of the lateral mass. Its situation is more medial and develops less frequently tumor. On physical examina-

tion, the mass are in the mouth and not in the lateral part of the neck.

2.3.3 Soft Tissue Lesions

Several types of anatomical structures are potentially at the origin of neck mass including nerve tracts (sympathic, vagus), carotid artery, muscles, and adipous tissue. Sometimes, due to the

Fig. 2.3 Anatomical origin of different types of branchial cyst

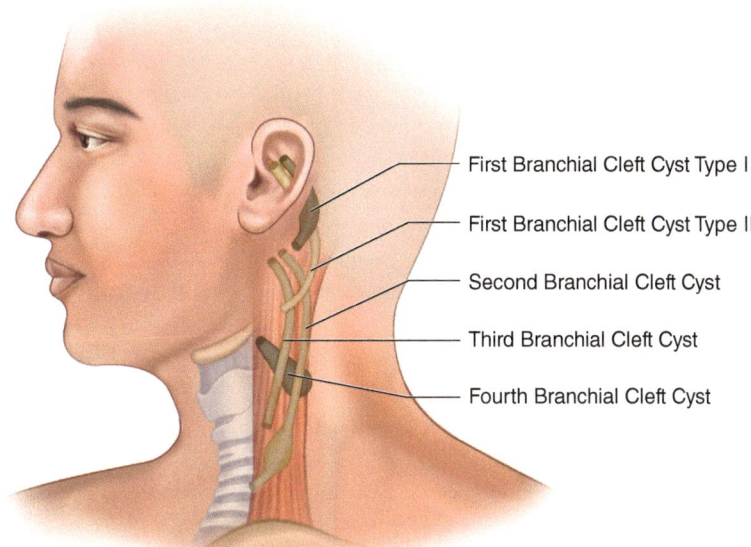

First Branchial Cleft Cyst Type I

First Branchial Cleft Cyst Type II

Second Branchial Cleft Cyst

Third Branchial Cleft Cyst

Fourth Branchial Cleft Cyst

importance of the mass, the diagnosis is not easy without histologic sample. On the other hand, the clinical presentation of branchial cyst can be a lateral neck mass and simulate sarcoma (Fig. 2.3).

2.4   Difficulties in Clinical Differential Diagnosis

The accurate diagnosis may be difficult. The clinical presentation of a branchial cyst and metastatic lymph node of an oropharyngeal cancer HPV positive is quite similar in clinic but also radiologic examination.

In salivary gland tumors, benign and low aggressive malignant lesion are also quite similar in clinical and radiological exams but also in history with low growth.

2.5   Therapeutic Management

The right diagnosis is a very high challenge, but it is necessary to prepare the type of treatment or to avoid surgery in certain cases. The FNA per-

mits the modification of the surgical plan in around 20% [1].

2.5.1   Salivary Gland Lesions may Be Differently Treated

Surgery can be avoided in cases of:

Whartin's tumor
Benign salivary tumor, especially in elderly population

Surgery can be limited in cases of:

Benign salivary tumor (pleomorphic adenoma)
Low-grade malignant salivary tumor

Surgery must be extensive in cases of:

Intermediate-grade malignant salivary tumor
Some types of salivary cancers without lymph node diffusion

Surgery must be extensive with lymph node dissection in cases of:

High-grade malignant salivary tumor
Some types of salivary cancer

2.5.2   Lymph Nodes

The importance of the diagnosis is here more important. Adenopathy is always due to local or general pathology. The total assessment (clinical, radiological exam, and FNA) permits to approach the right diagnosis in around 90%.

The diagnosis can be:

Infectious: tuberculosis or sarcoidosis with treatment by antibiotics
Benign inflammatory conditions like inflammatory or Kikuchi-Fujimoto disease
Malignancies like lymphomas, squamous cell carcinoma, or thyroid and salivary carcinomas

2.5.3   Soft Tissue Tumors

Benign:

Schwannoma: surgery but with consequences for the patient (partial or total palsy)
Glomus tumor: surgery with the possibility of carotid replacement (pre- and per-operative planning)
Branchial cyst: surgery with some surgical particularities for each of them

Malignant:

Sarcoma, the treatment depends on the type of sarcoma. Surgical biopsy can increase the neoplastic progression with less risk when FNA is used.

Reference

1. Eytan DF, Yin LX, Maleki Z, Koch WM, Tufano RP, Eisele DW, Boahene KDO, Fakhry C, Bishop JA, Westra WH, Gourin CG. Utility of preoperative fine needle aspiration in parotid lesions. Laryngoscope. 2018;128(2):398–402. https://doi.org/10.1002/lary.26776. Epub 2017 Aug 7. PMID: 28782105

Olivier Choussy ENT oncology surgeon. Head of Head and Neck Oncological Surgery at the Institut Curie, Paris, France.

Guillaume Rougier Guillaume Rougier is a surgeon of our ENT department with anatomical competence. It's a member of the French ENT cancer society (Société française de chirurgie cervico-faciale).

Antoine Dubray-Vautrin Head and Neck Surgeon and Oncologic Surgeon at Institut Curie, Paris, France. Currently enrolled in a PhD program in Biostatistics at the University of Paris-Saclay. Active administrative and scientific member of the GETTEC (Groupe d'Étude des Tumeurs de la Tête et du Cou).

Gilles Russ and Farida Benoudiba

3.1 Introduction

Ultrasound (US), computed tomography (CT) and magnetic resonance imaging (MRI) have become the cornerstone of the management of cervical lumps. They assist in the diagnosis, the sampling, and for the surveillance after treatments. Dividing the neck into separate anatomic compartments helps to provide limited lists of possible diagnoses. This can be refined by analyzing the specific imaging pattern of masses, their usual frequency and also clinical factors such as the age and sex of the patient, or a smoking habit, for instance. Although it is constantly improving, it is rare that a definite diagnosis can be made with imaging. Thus, guiding a fine-needle aspiration (FNA) or core-needle biopsy (CNB) is usually the next step and purpose of radiological techniques. The correlation between imaging techniques and cytology/histology results is key to providing the most specific possible diagnosis and to decide whether surgery is indicated or not.

G. Russ (✉)
Thyroid and Endocrine Tumors Department,
Pitié-Salpêtrière Hospital, Sorbonne University,
Paris, France

F. Benoudiba
Hôpital Bicêtre, Service de Neuroradiologie,
Le Kremlin-Bicêtre, France
e-mail: farida.benoudiba@aphp.fr

3.2 Techniques

3.2.1 Ultrasound Imaging

US uses high-frequency sound waves to generate an image. To obtain the best resolution, it is recommended to use the highest-frequency transducer that will penetrate to the desired depth. In general, a 10–14-MHz linear probe with a 4–5 cm in length is ideal, and can be supplemented by a small micro-convex probe to image the inferior extent of goiters and the mediastinum. Grayscale real-time two-dimensional, cross-sectional images are the main mode, but other modes, like Doppler and elastography, also have clinical utility. To obtain images of blood flow, color and spectral Doppler are used. Ultrasound elastography measures tissue stiffness by monitoring the response of tissue to acoustic energy. Two methods are at our disposal: quasi-static, or strain-based, and dynamic, or shear wave based.

3.2.2 Computed Tomography and Magnetic Resonance Imaging

CT-scan and MRI are an important part of the diagnostic evaluation of neck masses. They provide tissue discrimination and spatial resolution to identify tumor, help to define the location and extent of the mass, to evaluate the mass effect and the involvement of the surrounding structures.

CT is a practical modality because it provides with excellent discrimination between fat and other soft tissues. It surpasses MRI for the evaluation of calcifications, bone and for cartilaginous extension.

MRI offers a better soft tissue contrast and better discrimination between neck masses and adjacent cervical structures and it allows to evaluate the dynamic enhancement curve of the lesion after contrast media injection.

Usually, CT is used as the first imaging modality (except for the oral cavity, nasopharynx, and salivary glands), with contrast enhancement. If the lesion is not well delineated, MRI should help with providing a more precise diagnosis, using different sequences to evaluate the signal intensity on T1 and T2 weighted images, fat suppression, and the vascularization of the tumor.

3.3   Diagnostic Work-Flow

3.3.1   Thyroid Imaging

US imaging plays a key role with TSH assessment when facing most thyroid pathologies. Its main interests are:

- For goiters: positive diagnosis, volume measurement and presence of a substernal extension. The cause can also be determined or suspected in most cases: simple goiter, nodular goiter, Hashimoto's disease, or suspicion of a malignant mass, such as an anaplastic carcinoma, lymphoma, or a huge thyroid cancer.
- For nodules: positive diagnosis, location, measurement, evolution, and most importantly risk stratification. In 2009, with the first publication of a Thyroid Imaging and Reporting Data System (TI-RADS), thyroid US changed from a simply descriptive tool to a very useful and much more complex one, devised to make the link between US patterns or features with a quantitative appreciation of the risk of malignancy. In this way, TI-RADS is similar to the Bethesda system. Up to now, at least 10 different systems have been pro-

posed, and a universal one is under construction [1]. Most scientifically renowned endocrine or radiology societies have issued such a system: The TI-RADS of The American College of Radiology (ACR)-TIRADS is a point-based system, which means that each US feature is attributed a certain number of points [2]. For each nodule, the number of points is summed, and the total gives the score, which ranges from 1 to 5 (Fig. 3.1, 3.2, 3.3 and 3.4), with an increasing risk of malignancy. The American Thyroid Association Sonographic Pattern System (ATASPS) [3] is a pattern system that consists of recognizing a grouping of US features in a single figure and then classifying the nodule in a category with a specific risk range of malignancy, from benign to high suspicion. The European (EU)-TIRADS [4] and Korean (K)-TIRADS [5] also are pattern-based (Table 3.1).

Practically all systems consider a taller-than-wide shape, microcalcifications, irregular margins, and marked hypoechogenicity to be features of high suspicion. Mildly hypoechoic solid nodules with no features of high suspicion are at intermediate risk and oval-shaped isoechoic nodules with mixed composition are at low risk of malignancy. Simple cysts with no significant solid part and mainly spongiform nodules are practically always benign. In the case of high and intermediate-risk nodules, US imaging will also explore cervical lymph nodes to look for a potential metastatic extension.

In case a thyroid nodule has been asserted with US, TSH assessment is mandatory to detect autonomous nodules. If the TSH is inferior to the normal range, a scintigraphy is advised. Quantitative risk stratification and the size of the nodule are then used to provide guidance regarding the indication for FNA. However, FNA is usually not indicated in autonomous nodules. FNA is advised for high-risk, intermediate-risk, and low-risk nodules measuring at least 10 mm, 15 mm, and 20-25 mm, respectively (Fig. 3.5). However, clinical factors such as age, personal history of cervical irradiation during childhood, genetic factors of susceptibility to thyroid cancer, or a

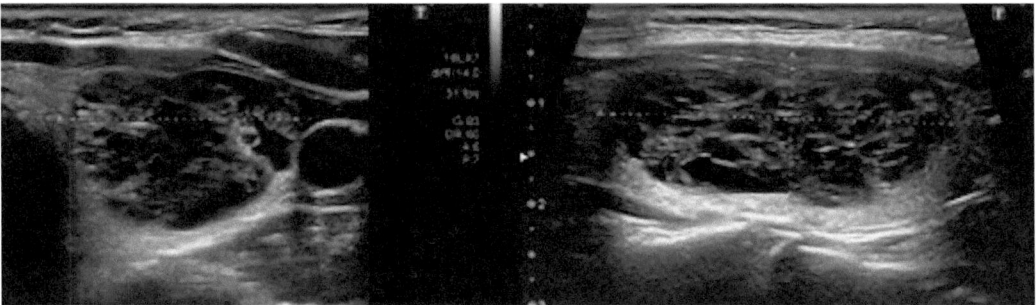

Fig. 3.1 Transverse and longitudinal US planes of a benign spongiform nodule measuring 34 × 21 × 12 mm. Oval regular shape, regular margins, and multiple cystic cavities representing more than 50% of the whole nodule volume

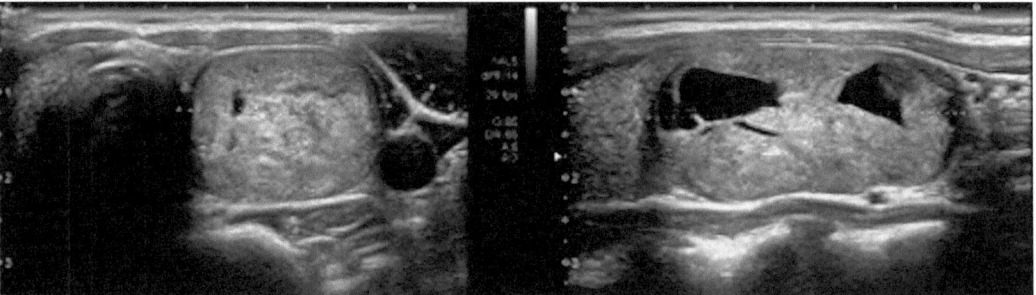

Fig. 3.2 Transverse and longitudinal US planes of a low-risk nodule measuring 38 × 24 × 16 mm. Oval regular shape, regular margins, and mixed composition, mainly solid and isoechoic

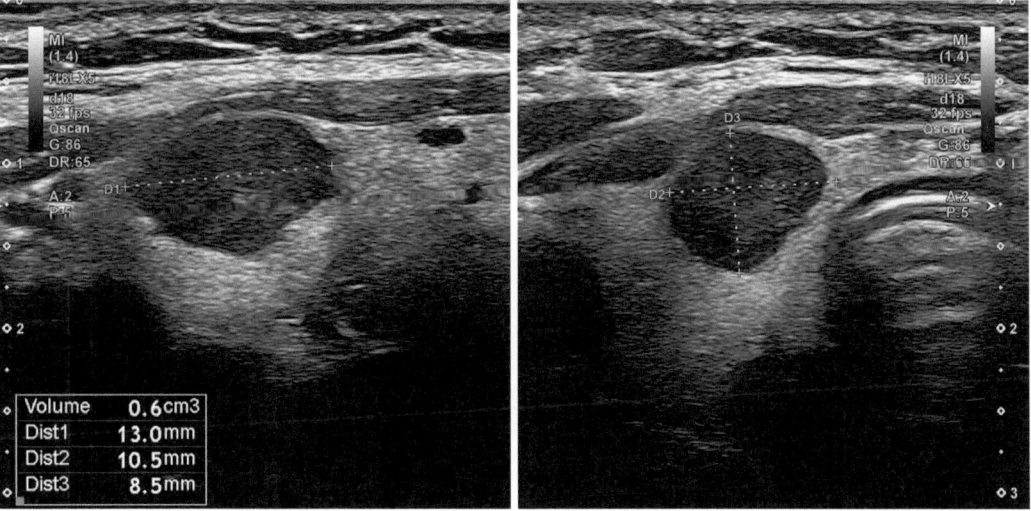

Fig. 3.3 Transverse and longitudinal US planes of an intermediate risk nodule measuring 13 × 11 × 9 mm. Oval regular shape, regular margins, and solid composition, mildly hypoechoic

family history of thyroid cancer must also be taken into account.

Last but not least, thyroid US has also evolved from a diagnostic tool to an interventional one. First, it helps guide FNAs by targeting solid areas, making sure that hypoechoic solid parts or microcalcifications are included. It also allows to avoid large vessels and to evacuate in the most complete possible way compressive cysts. Second, true interventional

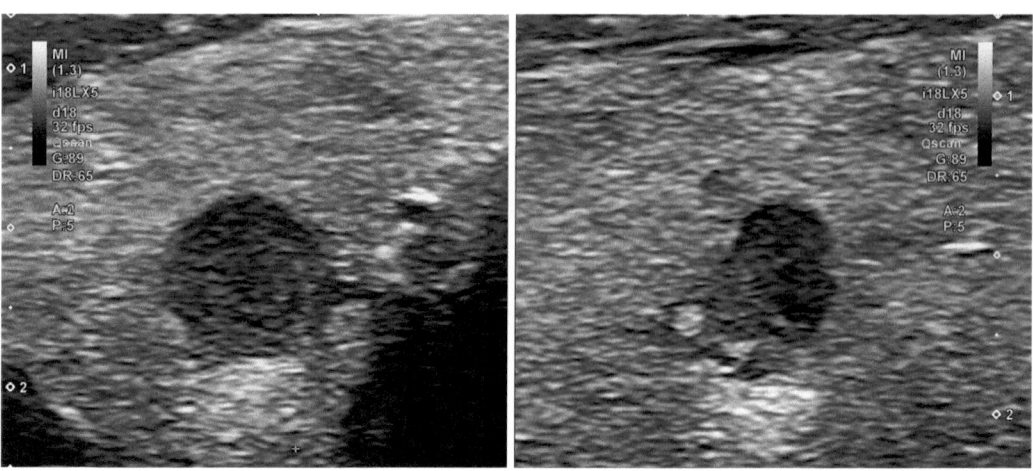

Fig. 3.4 Transverse and longitudinal US planes of a high-risk nodule measuring 5.9 × 5.6 × 5.6 mm. Discretely taller-than-wide shape, irregular spiculated margins, solid composition, mildly hypoechoic

Table 3.1 Comparison of some specificities of existent risk stratification systems (RSSs). Note: *RSS* risk stratification system, *ACR* American College of Radiology, *ATA* American Thyroid Association, *EU* European, *K* Korean, *TIRADS* Thyroid Imaging and Reporting Data System, *FNA* fine-needle aspiration

RSS	Number of Classes	Meaning of TIRADS 1	Pattern or Point-Based RSS	Features of High Suspicion	Indications for FNA
ACR-TIRADS	5	Benign	Point	Marked Hypoechogenicity All punctate Echogenic foci Taller-than-wide Extra-thyroidal Extension	TIRADS 2: No FNA TIRADS 3: ≥25 mm TIRADS 4: ≥15 mm TIRADS 5: ≥10 mm < 10 mm: No FNA
ATA	5	Benign	Pattern	In a solid hypoechoic nodule: Irregular margins microcalcifications Taller than wide Rim calcifications with small extrusive soft tissue component Extra-thyroidal extension	Very low risk: ≥20 mm Or observation Low risk: ≥15 mm Intermediate risk: ≥10 mm High risk: ≥10 mm 5–10 mm: FNA if clinical or US risk factors
EU-TIRADS	5	Absence of significant nodule	Pattern	Marked Hypoechogenicity Irregular margins microcalcifications Taller than wide	TIRADS 2: No FNA TIRADS 3: ≥20 mm TIRADS 4: ≥15 mm TIRADS 5: ≥10 mm < 10 mm: Active surveillance or FNA
K-TIRADS	5	Absence of nodule	Pattern	In a solid hypoechoic nodule: Irregular margins microcalcification nonparallel Orientation	TIRADS 2: 20 mm TIRADS 3: ≥15 mm TIRADS 4: ≥10 mm TIRADS 5: ≥10 mm 5–10 mm: FNA in selected cases

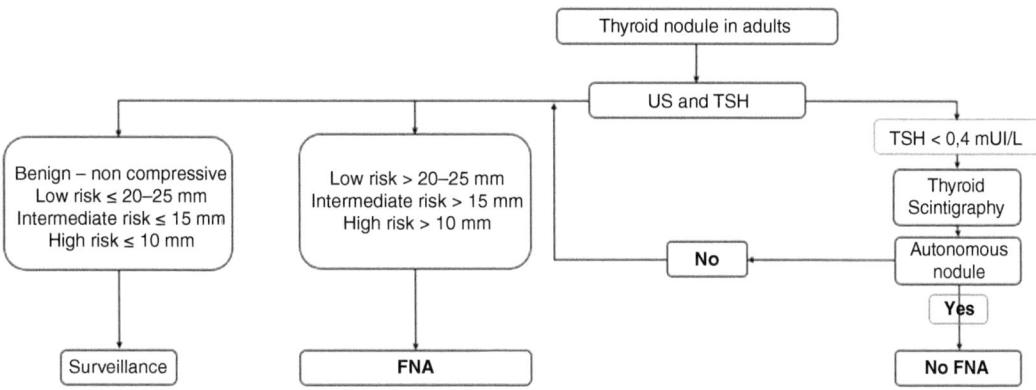

Fig. 3.5 Management algorithm for thyroid nodules

techniques are now directly challenging surgery for treatment. Percutaneous ethanol injection is the first-line tool for thyroid cysts. Thermal ablation techniques, such as radiofrequency, are alternatives in benign mixed or solid nodules [6]. Small carcinomas and recurrences can also be addressed by these [7]. Importantly, once the FNA of a thyroid nodule has been performed, the cytology result should always be compared with the US risk stratification. This is meant to verify the concordance between the two. In case of a benign cytology result and a high-risk pattern on US, a repeat FNA is usually advised to eliminate a false negative cytology result [8]. CT and MRI play little role in the evaluation of thyroid nodules. CT is indicated whenever a mediastinal extension of a goiter is suspected. It can also help during the initial evaluation of an aggressive thyroid carcinoma to give precisions regarding its local extension, for instance, to the trachea. Last, some pathologic lymph nodes cannot be detected with US, especially retropharyngeal ones, where CT or MRI is more performant.

• For auto-immune diseases, biology is the first diagnostic tool. However, in some difficult situations, US can help in diagnosing Hashimoto's and Graves's diseases. Detection of their existence during a US examination is always useful as they can sometimes obscure or mimic thyroid cancer. Notifying the pathologist of this diagnosis

and of the TI-RADS score is also recommended [9].
• Subacute and Riedel's thyroiditis can also be diagnosed with US. Both can be purveyors of false positive US diagnostic of carcinoma, due to their marked hypoechogenicity and sometimes irregular margins.

3.3.2 Cervical Masses (Thyroid Excluded) [10, 11]

Opposite to thyroid imaging, CT and MRI are first-line tools when addressing other cervical masses. US imaging, however, has a very high negative predictive value for lymph nodes and also can be a valuable tool to guide FNA and core-needle biopsies. Neck masses can be divided into two main categories (Fig. 3.6).

• Cystic lesions: they constitute a wide array of congenital and acquired lesions (Fig. 3.7a, b).

The majority of congenital cystic lesions are diagnosed in children and young adult.

• Midline cystic lesions are commonly thyroglossal duct cysts or dermoid cysts. Thymic cysts occur in the lower half of the neck and mediastinum.
• Lateral cysts:
  – Upper lateral cyst: the second branchial cleft cyst is the most common, located

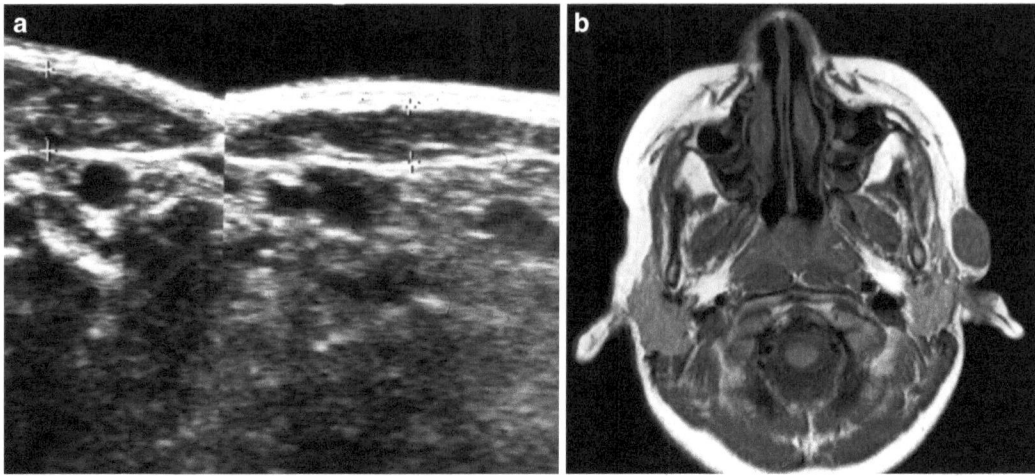

Fig. 3.6 Pseudomass: (**a**) asymmetric muscle (**b**) Subcutaneous lesion: dermoid cyst

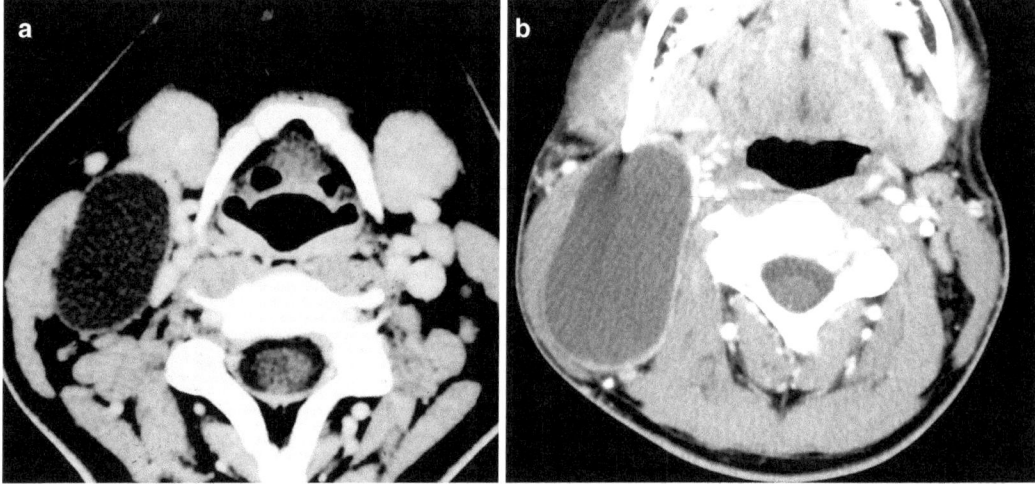

Fig. 3.7 (**a**) Squamous cell carcinoma (60 years old male) (**b**) Second branchial cleft cyst (20 years old girl)

around the mandible, anterior and medial to the sternocleidomastoid muscle. Ranula typically occurs in the sublingual space, in the floor of the mouth, superior to the mylohyoid muscle.

- Lower lateral neck cysts: third and fourth cleft cysts lie superior to the apex of the pyriform sinus next to the larynx, usually on the right for the third one and on the left for the fourth one.
- Lymphangioma are typically transcompartmental multiloculated cystic masses located in the posterior triangle of the neck, but it can occur in the sub lingual, submandibular, or parotid space.

US can be used for the diagnosis of branchial cleft cyst, and CT is useful for the differential diagnosis of an abscess and a necrotic lymph node.

- Solid neck lesions: to evaluate such neck masses, it is fundamental (Table 3.2):
  - To know the anatomy and the content of deep neck spaces (Fig. 3.8a, b).
  - To locate the lesion within these deep neck spaces.
  - To delineate the anatomical extent of the mass.
  - To provide a possible diagnosis.

Table 3.2 Anatomy and differential diagnoses of cervical masses [10, 11]

Carotid space	Carotid artery, jugular vein, cranial nerves (IX, X, XI, XII),Lymph nodes, sympathic plexus	Benign: schwannoma, neurofibroma, meningioma, paraganglioma Malignant: nodal metastasis, lymphoma
Parapharyngeal space	Fat, V3, internal maxillary artery and ascending pharyngial artery, venous plexus	Benign: Abscess, pleomorphic adenoma of salivary gland rest, lipoma Malignant: Adenoid cystic carcinoma, mucoepidermoid carcinoma
Retropharyngeal space	Fat, lymph nodes	Benign: Hemangioma, lymphangioma, abscess, lipoma Malignant: Nodal metastasis (melanoma, non-Hodgkin lymphoma, squamous cell carcinoma)
Masticator space	Muscles of mastication, masticator nerve branches (V3), ramus and posterior body of the mandible, pterygopalatine fossa, fat	Benign: Hemangioma, lymphangioma, odontogenic abscess, osteoblastoma, leiomyoma, neural sheath tumor Malignant: Sarcoma, squamous cell carcinoma non-Hodgkin lymphoma
Parotid space	Parotid gland, facial nerve, retromandibular vein, external carotid artery, intra parotid lymph nodes	Benign: First branchial cleft, hemangioma, lymphangioma, abscess, pleomorphic adenoma, Warthin's tumor, lipoma, oncocytoma, VII schwannoma or neurofibroma Malignant: Primary or metastatic nodes
Sublingual space	Sublingual gland, lingual nerve, IX, XII, lingual artery and vein	Benign: Hemangioma, lymphangioma, epidermoid, dermoid, abcess, ranula, mixed tumor Malignant: Squamous cell carcinoma, sublingual gland malignant tumor
Submandibular space	Submandibular gland, anterior belly of digastric muscle, lymphnode, facial vein and artery, inferior loop of hypoglossal nerve, fat	Benign: Second branchial cleft cyst, suprahyoid thyroglossal duct cyst, hemangioma, lymphangioma, lipoma Malignant: Nodal lymphoma or metastatic, submandibular gland tumor
Prevertebral space	Deep layer of deep cervical fascia	Benign: Schwannoma or neurofibroma (brachial plexus), vertebral body benign bony tumor Malignant: Chordoma, vertebral body malignant tumor

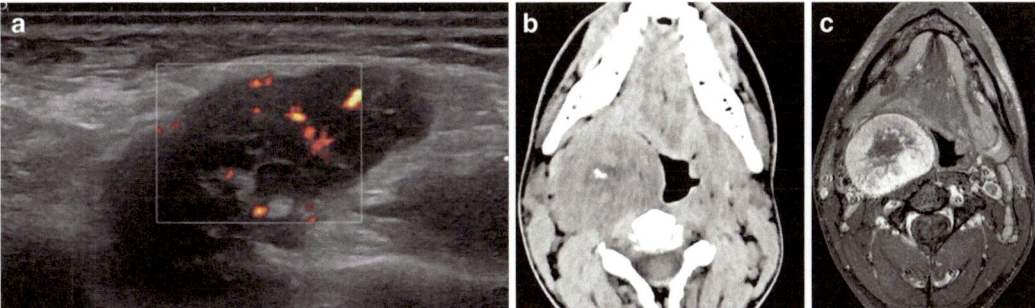

Fig. 3.8 (**a**) longitudinal US planes b) CT scan c) MRI US scan (**a**): Solid hypoechoic mass with regular margin. CT scan (**b**, **c**) Solid mass with calcifications and heterogeneous enhancement. Schwanomma of the vagus nerve

3.4   Recommendations

- In case of suspicion of a thyroid nodule or goiter, a US examination is mandatory.
- Indications for FNA of thyroid nodules are mainly based on US risk stratification and size of the nodule but also on clinical factors and TSH.
- US guidance of FNA is usually advised, if feasible and indicated, on most cervical masses, including thyroid nodules, parotid masses, cystic lesions, and for primary or metastatic nodes without primary tumor detected.

3.5   Framed Text with the Main Messages

Evaluation of Thyroid Nodules

US imaging is the key examination for thyroid nodules and goiters.

It helps in measuring and localizing nodules and providing risk stratification.

Indications for FNA are mainly based on US pattern and nodular size.

US guidance is usually advised when an FNA of a thyroid nodule is indicated.

Evaluation of Other Neck Masses

Locate the lesion within the deep neck spaces and follow a specific algorithm:

First eliminate a pseudomass (Fig. 3.6a, b).

Take patient age into account.

Define whether dealing with a single lesion or multiple lesions.

Determine if the mass is solid or cystic.

Evaluate the extension: trans-compartmental or multi-compartmental.

References

1. Russ G, Trimboli P, Buffet C. The new era of TIRADSs to stratify the risk of malignancy of thyroid nodules: strengths, weaknesses and pitfalls. Cancers (Basel). 2021;13(17):4316. https://doi.org/10.3390/cancers13174316. PMID: 34503125; PMCID: PMC8430750
2. Tessler FN, Middleton WD, Grant EG, Hoang JK, Berland LL, Teefey SA, Cronan JJ, Beland MD, Desser TS, Frates MC, Hammers LW, Hamper UM, Langer JE, Reading CC, Scoutt LM, Stavros AT. ACR thyroid imaging, reporting and data system (TI-RADS): white paper of the ACR TI-RADS Committee. J Am Coll Radiol. 2017;14(5):587–95. https://doi.org/10.1016/j.jacr.2017.01.046. Epub 2017 Apr 2
3. Haugen BR, Alexander EK, Bible KC, Doherty GM, Mandel SJ, Nikiforov YE, Pacini F, Randolph GW, Sawka AM, Schlumberger M, Schuff KG, Sherman SI, Sosa JA, Steward DL, Tuttle RM, Wartofsky L. 2015 American Thyroid Association management guidelines for adult patients with thyroid nodules and differentiated thyroid cancer: the American Thyroid Association guidelines task force on thyroid nodules and differentiated thyroid cancer. Thyroid. 2016;26(1):1–133. https://doi.org/10.1089/thy.2015.0020. PMID: 26462967; PMCID: PMC4739132
4. Russ G, Bonnema SJ, Erdogan MF, Durante C, Ngu R, Leenhardt L. European thyroid association guidelines for ultrasound malignancy risk stratification of thyroid nodules in adults: the EU-TIRADS. Eur Thyroid J. 2017;6(5):225–37. https://doi.org/10.1159/000478927. Epub 2017 Aug 8. PMID: 29167761; PMCID: PMC5652895.
5. Ha EJ, Chung SR, Na DG, Ahn HS, Chung J, Lee JY, Park JS, Yoo RE, Baek JH, Baek SM, Cho SW, Choi YJ, Hahn SY, Jung SL, Kim JH, Kim SK, Kim SJ, Lee CY, Lee HK, Lee JH, Lee YH, Lim HK, Shin JH, Sim JS, Sung JY, Yoon JH, Choi M. 2021 Korean thyroid imaging reporting and data system and imaging-based Management of Thyroid Nodules: Korean Society of Thyroid Radiology Consensus Statement and Recommendations. Korean J Radiol. 2021;22(12):2094–123. https://doi.org/10.3348/kjr.2021.0713. Epub 2021 Oct 26. PMID: 34719893; PMCID: PMC8628155
6. Orloff LA, Noel JE, Stack BC Jr, Russell MD, Angelos P, Baek JH, Brumund KT, Chiang FY, Cunnane MB, Davies L, Frasoldati A, Feng AY, Hegedüs L, Iwata AJ, Kandil E, Kuo J, Lombardi C, Lupo M, Maia AL, McIver B, Na DG, Novizio R, Papini E, Patel KN,

Rangel L, Russell JO, Shin J, Shindo M, Shonka DC Jr, Karcioglu AS, Sinclair C, Singer M, Spiezia S, Steck JH, Steward D, Tae K, Tolley N, Valcavi R, Tufano RP, Tuttle RM, Volpi E, Wu CW, Abdelhamid Ahmed AH, Randolph GW. Radiofrequency ablation and related ultrasound-guided ablation technologies for treatment of benign and malignant thyroid disease: an international multidisciplinary consensus statement of the American head and neck society endocrine surgery section with the Asia Pacific Society of Thyroid Surgery, Associazione Medici Endocrinologi, British Association of Endocrine and Thyroid Surgeons, European thyroid association, Italian Society of Endocrine Surgery Units, Korean Society of Thyroid Radiology, Latin American thyroid society, and thyroid nodules therapies association. Head Neck. 2022;44(3):633–60. https://doi.org/10.1002/hed.26960. Epub 2021 Dec 23

7. Mauri G, Hegedüs L, Bandula S, Cazzato RL, Czarniecka A, Dudeck O, Fugazzola L, Netea-Maier R, Russ G, Wallin G, Papini E. European thyroid association and cardiovascular and interventional radiological Society of Europe 2021 clinical practice guideline for the use of minimally invasive treatments in malignant thyroid lesions. Eur Thyroid J. 2021;10(3):185–97. https://doi.org/10.1159/000516469. Epub 2021 May 25. PMID: 34178704; PMCID: PMC8215982

8. Eloy C, Russ G, Suciu V, Johnson SJ, Rossi ED, Pantanowitz L, Vielh P. Preoperative diagnosis of thyroid nodules: an integrated multidisciplinary approach. Cancer Cytopathol. 2022;130(5):320–5. https://doi.org/10.1002/cncy.22546. Epub 2022 Jan 12

9. Renshaw AA, Gould EW, Russ G, Poller DN. Thyroid FNA: is cytopathologist review of ultrasound features useful? Cancer Cytopathol. 2020;128(8):523–7. https://doi.org/10.1002/cncy.22262. Epub 2020 Mar 10

10. Kansara S, Bell D, Johnson J, Zafereo M. Head and neck inflammatory pseudotumor: case series and review of literature. Neuroradiol J. 2016;29(6):440–6. https://doi.org/10.1177/1971400916665377. Epub 2016 Sep 20.PMID: 27650653

11. Chorath K, Rajasekaran K. Evaluation and Management of a Neck Mass. Med Clin North Am. 2021;105(5):827–37. https://doi.org/10.1016/j.mcna.2021.05.005. Epub 2021 Jul 12.PMID: 34391536 Review

Russ Gilles Radiologist at La Pitie-Salpetriere Hospital and Centre de Pathologie et d'Imagerie, Paris, France. Expert in thyroid diagnostic and interventional imaging. Leader in developing the European-Thyroid Imaging and Reporting Data System (EU-TIRADS). Member of the European Thyroid Association and US Board and American Thyroid Association. Faculty member of the French US Imaging Diploma and the Hungarian Papillon US Course.

Bataille-Benoudiba Farida is a Radiologist. She served as the Chief Clinician at the Department of Neuroradiology at Bicetre Hospital from 1997 to 2000. She has been a Radiologist/Hospital Practitioner in the Department of Neuroradiology at Bicetre Hospital since 2005 and served as Deputy Head of the Department and Head of the Neuroradiology Diagnostic Imaging Department since 2019. She is the Past General Secretary of Head and Neck French Imaging from 2014 to 2020 and President of Head and Neck French Imaging since 2020.

Isotopic Imaging

4

Hubert Tissot

4.1 Introduction

2-[(18)F]fluoro-2-deoxy-D-glucose positron emission tomography/computed tomography (FDG-PET/CT) is currently the main nuclear medicine imaging technique used to investigate cervical masses. It is a combination of a CT and a FDG-PET acquisition. It is most often used to assess the extension of an avid FDG tumor of known origin [1]. However, FDG-PET/CT is also recommended for the exploration of a cervical mass of unknown primary after conventional workup. It allows to guide biopsies, the search for a primary tumor and the assessment of extension [2–4]. Other PET radiotracers are available for staging or localization of primary site of certain ENT tumors such as Somatostatin Receptor (SSTR) radiotracers for paragangliomas.

4.2 FDG-PET/CT: Overview and Procedure

2-[(18)F]fluoro-2-deoxy-D-glucose (FDG) is a glucose analog that allows the evaluation of tissue metabolism. It is taken up by cells via cell membrane glucose transporters, phosphorylated and is trapped into the glycolytic pathway. It is a non-specific radiotracer. Many tumors of benign or malignant origin show an important uptake of FDG as well as many inflammatory or infectious pathologies. In addition, some malignant tumors are not FDG avid. It is therefore particularly important to know the physiological uptake of FDG, main artifacts and pitfalls of FDG-PET/CT and main differential diagnosis of an FDG avid or non-avid cervical mass. In the clinical routine, this is particularly true in the context of a cervical mass of unknown primary, an incidentaloma, or when FDG-PET/CT has been performed before conventional workup.

The CT acquisition coupled to the PET scan allows anatomical localization the FDG uptake sites. It also allows to correct the attenuation of the PET signal by tissue structures.

4.2.1 Patient Preparation and Image Acquisition

The European Association of Nuclear Medicine (EANM) and the Society of Nuclear Medicine and Molecular Imaging (SNMMI) have provided detailed procedure guidelines for the performance of FDG-PET/CT [5, 6]. We recall the main preparation steps as well as the specific points for the exploration of the head and neck region:

H. Tissot (✉)
Department of Nuclear Medicine, Institut Curie, Paris, France
e-mail: hubert.tissot@curie.fr

© The Author(s), under exclusive license to Springer Nature Switzerland AG 2024
J. Klijanienko et al. (eds.), *Diagnostic Procedures in Patients with Neck Masses*,
https://doi.org/10.1007/978-3-031-67675-8_4

- Patients should fast for at least 4 hours before FDG injection. During this period, the patient can only consume plain water. Parenteral nutrition and intravenous fluids containing glucose should be discontinued.
- A capillary blood glucose test is performed upon the patient's arrival in the imaging department and must be less than 200 mg/dl. If the blood glucose level is higher than 200 mg/dl, the nuclear medicine physician is contacted for further instructions.
- The interval between FDG injection and the start of acquisition is 60 min. During this one-hour waiting period, the patient should be at rest, sitting or lying down and keeping warm. This avoids muscular and brown fat FDG uptake, which can considerably hamper the interpretation of the images, particularly in the head and neck region (see Sect. 4.3 below).
- In the case of exploration of a cervical mass, the acquisitions usually extend from the top of the skull to mid-thigh. It can be performed in one step with arms along the body or in two successive steps (with a first acquisition of the head and neck performed arms-down and a second acquisition from the thorax to mid-thigh with arms placed above the head).
- Administered FDG activity and PET acquisition duration vary according to local protocols and machines used. Specific charts and guidelines are provided by the EANM and SNMMI for pediatric populations [7, 8].

The nuclear medicine physician should inquire about certain conditions such as claustrophobia, diabetes and its treatments, and pain management when making the appointment. This allows for a possible pre-medication and an adaptation of the treatments and the date of the examination, in accordance with the recommendations.

Kidney failure does not contraindicate FDG-PET/CT.

The nuclear medicine physician or the technologist assesses the risk of pregnancy before FDG administration in women of childbearing age. A pregnancy test is performed if necessary.

In case of doubt or proven pregnancy, the benefit-risk ratio of FDG-PET/CT is discussed on a case-by-case basis. The physician postpone or cancel the examination if necessary.

4.2.2 Injection of Intravenous Contrast Agent

Contrast-enhanced diagnostic CT scan of the head and neck is possible while performing FDG-PET/CT. It is then necessary to verify the absence of contraindication and to organize the preparation and injection of the contrast agent according to local protocols. The EANM recommends performing the contrast-enhanced CT scan after a low-dose non-enhanced CT and the PET acquisition in order to avoid biases in the CT attenuation map and therefore in the measurement of quantitative PET parameters such as the standard uptake value [6]. However, the use of a contrast-enhanced CT scan for attenuation correction would have little impact on PET image quality and little clinical impact [9–11].

The benefit of contrast-enhanced FDG-PET/CT for head and neck exploration is still debated. Intravenous contrast administration provides better delineation of primary sites and better localization of the lesions. For the nodal and metastatic staging, some studies show that the impact of contrast injection would be low [12, 13]. However, contrast-enhanced FDG-PET/CT would be superior in differentiating between N0 and N+ in tumors with a significant prevalence of necrotic lymph node metastases like human papillomavirus (HPV)-associated tonsillar squamous cell carcinoma. Necrotic tissues are indeed not FDG avid and cystic-necrotic lymph node metastases may be missed, leading to false-negative (Fig. 4.1) [14].

Intravenous contrast administration while performing FDG-PET/CT should be discussed according to the clinical history and the existence of previous diagnostic morphological imaging, in accordance with local protocols and national regulations.

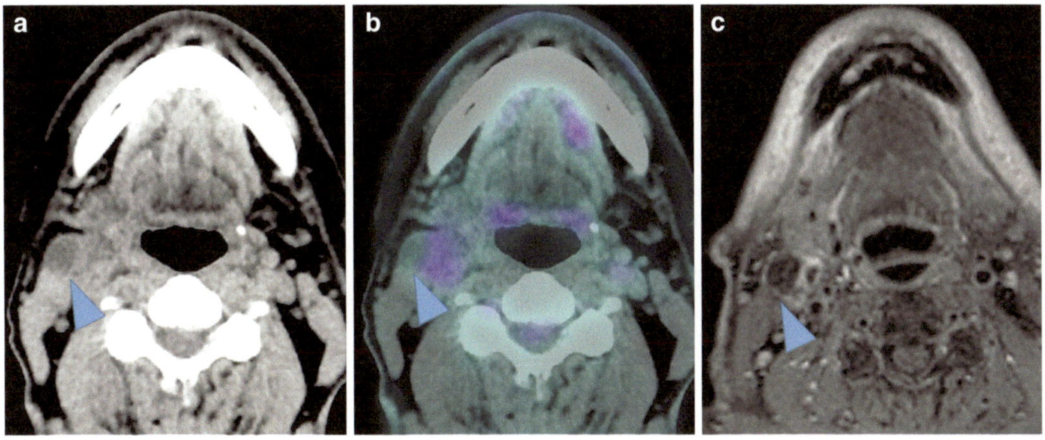

Fig. 4.1 Axial CT (**a**) and axial fused FDG-PET/CT (**b**) images demonstrating low FDG uptake within an HPV-associated squamous cell carcinoma cystic cervical lymph node metastasis (arrows). Contrast-enhanced T1 MRI (**c**) demonstrated a suspicious peripheral enhancement of this lymph node

4.3   Common FDG-PET/CT Pitfalls

4.3.1   Waldeyer's Ring

Intense and symmetrical physiological FDG uptake is frequently observed within the lymphoid tissues of Waldeyer's ring. It is more frequent in young patients but can also occur in adults. An asymmetric uptake is more suspicious of malignancy, especially in case of search for a primary (Fig. 4.2). However, it remains a potential source of false positives, and incidental uptakes without the context of suspected oropharyngeal cancer or lymphoma are rarely of malignant origin when explored [15, 16]. Reactive lymphoid hyperplasia, multiple benign inflammatory, infectious, or granulomatous pathologies are possible causes of symmetric or asymmetric uptake in the Waldeyer's ring.

4.3.2   Brown Fat Uptake

Brown fat's primary function is to produce heat, which is activated by sympathetic nervous stimulation. When brown fat is activated, FDG accumulates symmetrically in it overall. Its usual distribution includes the neck, the supraclavicular areas, paravertebral and retroperitoneal areas. The CT correlation between FDG uptake and fat can theoretically distinguish brown fat activation from pathological uptake (Fig. 4.3). However, due to its extent, intensity, and proximity to lymph nodes, brown fat uptake may interfere with the interpretation of FDG-PET/CT (especially if there is a shift between PET and CT acquisitions).

Brown fat activation is observed more frequently in children, young adults, women, patients with low BMI, and patients at low ambient temperatures. The EANM and SNMMI guidelines provide several recommendations to limit brown fat uptake:

- Advise the patient to stay warm during the hours before the examination. Maintain a sufficiently high temperature in the waiting room and in the resting area during the FDG injection and during the one-hour uptake phase.
- Administration of 20 to 80 mg of propranolol given orally 1 h to 2 h before FDG administration. In children over 10 years of age, the recommended dosage is 1 mg/kg with a maximum of 40 mg [5, 6, 8].

4.3.3 Muscular FDG Uptake

Increased uptake of cervical muscles due to movements or contractures can be a source of misinterpretation by mimicking adenopathy or preventing the interpretation of adjacent lymph node structures. During the injection and the uptake phase, the patient must be comfortably seated or lying down to limit muscle contractures and movements. According to the SNMMI guidelines, oral alprazolam 0.5 mg given immediately after FDG injection can reduce skeletal muscle uptake. Sufficient analgesia pre-medication should be considered for patients with pain [5, 6].

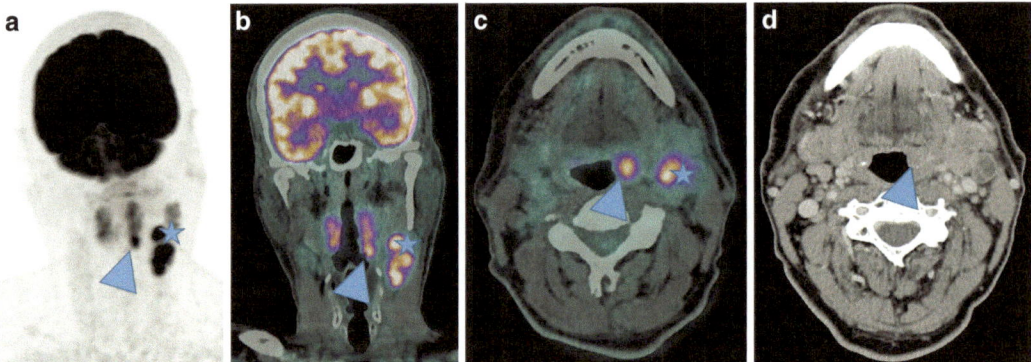

Fig. 4.2 Cervical lymph node metastases of squamous cell carcinoma with unknown primary after conventional imaging by ENT contrast-enhanced CT and MRI. FDG-PET MIP (**a**), coronal and axial fused FDG-PET/CT images (**b**, **c**) demonstrate high FDG uptake of cervical lymph node metastases (asterisks) and an asymmetric and focal suspicious FDG uptake in the lower pole of the left tonsil (arrows). Contrast-enhanced CT (**d**) shows no corresponding enhancement of the left tonsil. Endoscopy with biopsy confirmed the diagnosis of squamous cell carcinoma of the left tonsil

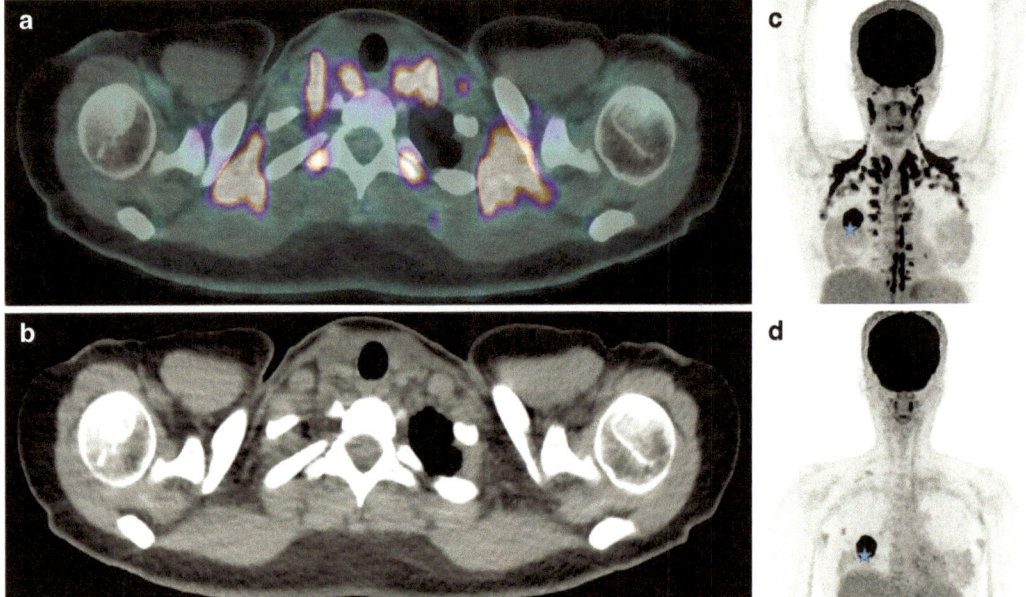

Fig. 4.3 A 33-year-old woman with a newly diagnosed right breast tumor. FDG-PET MIP (**a**), axial fused FDG-PET/CT (**b**) and axial CT (**c**) images of the PET-FDG/CT performed without pre-medication demonstrate FDG uptake of the breast tumor (asterisks) and intense, diffuse, and globally symmetrical brown fat FDG uptake of cervical, supraclavicular and paravertebral areas. FDG-PET/CT was repeated 2 weeks later, with propanolol administration 1 hour before FDG injection. The FDG-PET MIP image of the second FDG-PET/CT (**d**) demonstrates a near disappearance of brown fat uptake

Muscle FDG uptake due to muscle activity is usually linear, diffuse, and homogeneous along the involved muscle, without obvious underlying lesions on the coupled CT scan (Fig. 4.4).

It is also not advisable to talk or read during the uptake phase. Talking may cause intense hypermetabolism of the phonatory muscles and vocal cords (Fig. 4.5). The eye movements may cause intense uptake of the extraocular muscles.

Fig. 4.4 Coronal fused FDG-PET/CT images (**a**) showing increased cervical muscular FDG uptake due to muscle activity during the uptake phase. No corresponding suspicious mass on coronal CT images (**b**) (arrows)

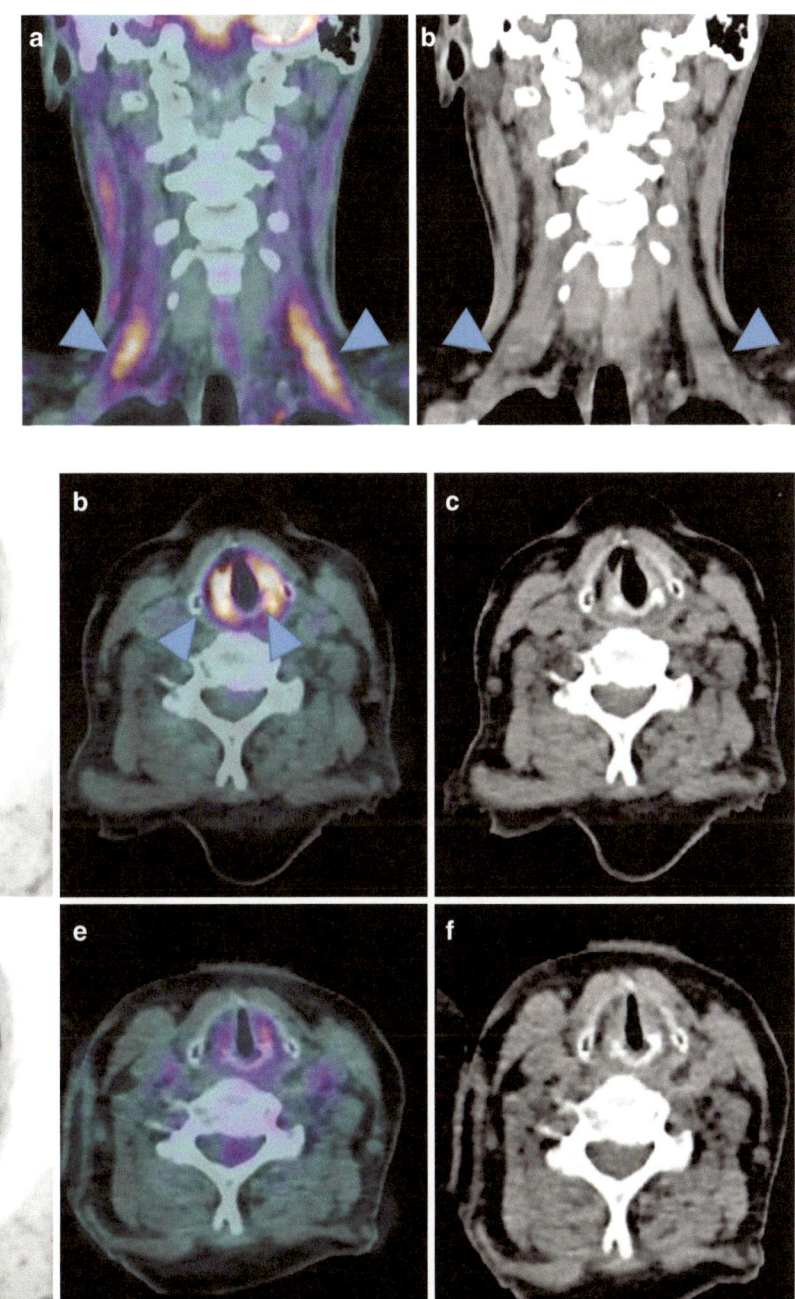

Fig. 4.5 FDG-PET MIP (**a**) and axial fused FDG-PET/CT (**b**) images demonstrating intense and symmetrical FDG uptake of the vocal cords (arrows), with no obvious lesion on axial CT (**c**). The patient had made a phone call during the FDG uptake phase. FDG-PET/CT was repeated a few months later with better compliance during the uptake phase. No particular FDG uptake or CT abnormality of the vocal cords was observed (**d-f**)

Unilateral palsy of a vocal cord results in compensatory functional FDG uptake of the contralateral vocal cord. This uptake can be confused with a tumor fixation and must be correlated with the rest of the workup. Furthermore, if an unknown vocal cord palsy is suspected on FDG-PET/CT, a tumor lesion along the curse of the ipsilateral vagus or recurrent laryngeal nerve should be searched for [17, 18].

A diffuse muscular FDG accumulation with a decrease of the physiological uptake of the other organs and a low uptake of the suspected pathological lesions is observed in case of insulin injection or incorrect fasting before the FDG injection. It is a cause of false negative and decreased sensitivity of PET-FDG/CT (Fig. 4.6).

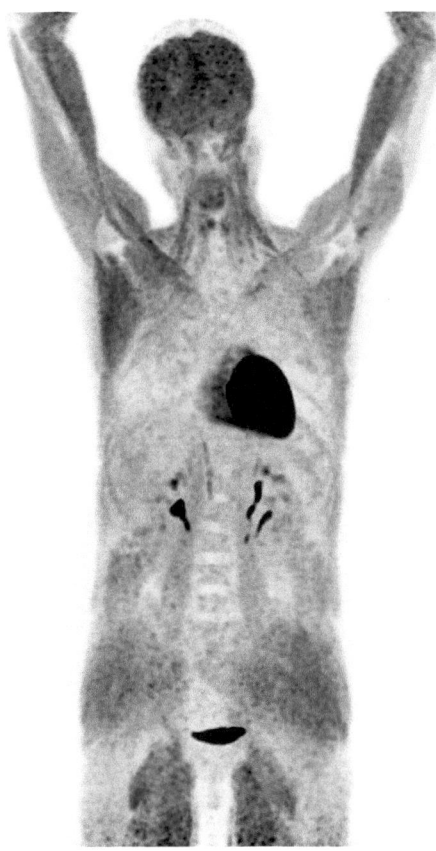

Fig. 4.6 FDG-PET MIP Image. It shows diffuse muscular hypermetabolism due to a lack of fasting before the FDG injection. It also demonstrates a decrease in the physiological uptake of other organs such as the liver, the spleen, or the brain. This FDG-PET is to be considered as uninterpretable

4.3.4 Movements During FDG/CT PET Acquisitions

During the examination, CT and PET acquisitions are performed in sequence without moving the patient. If the patient changes position between the scan and the PET scan, this will result in a poor correlation between the two acquisitions, which may lead to interpretation errors.

The duration of PET acquisitions varies according to local protocols and the machines used. Blurred PET images may be due to motion during PET acquisition.

A good explanation of the examination, comfortable patient positioning and the use of rigid positioning aids reduce the risk of head and neck movements [19]. Sedatives and the use of relaxation techniques may be considered in claustrophobic patients.

4.3.5 Semi-Quantitative Parameters

Interpretation of FDG-PET/CT images for initial diagnostic workup remains essentially visual. The use of semi-quantitative parameters such as SUV is subject to multiple sources of variability and should be interpreted with caution. Efforts to standardize image acquisition and reconstruction techniques are underway.

4.4 Interpretation and Indication of FDG-PET/CT in Different Tumors and Clinical Scenarios

4.4.1 Cervical Lymph Node Metastases of Unknown Primary in the Head and Neck

Nasopharyngeal carcinoma and squamous cell carcinoma of the oral cavity, larynx, oropharynx and hypopharynx are FDG avid tumors. When the location of the primary tumor is known after the conventional workup, FDG-PET/CT is useful to assess the presence of distant metastases or to refine the local staging.

However, during the diagnostic phase, FDG-PET/CT has an important role in the exploration of cervical lymph node metastases of unknown primary. According to the joint clinical practice guidelines of the European Head and Neck Society (EMNS), the European Society for Medical Oncology (ESMO) and the European Society for Radiotherapy & Oncology, and also according to the guidelines of the American Society of Clinical Oncology (ASCO), FDG-PET/CT is indicated for the evaluation of head and neck carcinomas of unknown origin to direct mucosal biopsies after clinical examination and morphological imaging [2, 3] (Figs. 4.2 and 4.7). If possible, FDG-PET/CT should be performed before any pharyngeal biopsy in order to limit the risk of a false positive due to an inflammatory reaction. FDG-PET/CT is also useful to complete the extension workup in search of distant metastasis or another synchronous primary (Fig. 4.8).

In several literature reviews and meta-analyses, the detection rate of primary sites by FDG-PET after conventional workup ranged from 24,5% to 44% with a specificity of 68% to 74,9% and a sensitivity of 88,3% to 97% [16, 20, 21]. In the literature review by Rusthoven et al., the detection rate of unknown primary tumors was 24.5% after a conventional workup including panendoscopy and cervical imaging by CT or MRI [16]. In the same review by Rusthoven et al., FDG-PET altered the management approach in 24,7% of patients [16].

In studies comparing head and neck CT and MRI with FDG-PET/CT, FDG-PET/CT had better sensitivity for detection of primary sites, with no significant difference in specificity. In the prospective study by Lee et al. including patients with cervical metastases of squamous cell carcinoma of unknown primary, the sensitivity of FDG-PET/CT (69%) for primary site detection was significantly higher than that of contrast-enhanced/CT (16%)(p > 0.001) and MRI (41%) (p = 0.039). The specificity of FDG-PET/CT was 88% vs 76% and 59% for CT and MRI (p > 0.4) [22, 23].

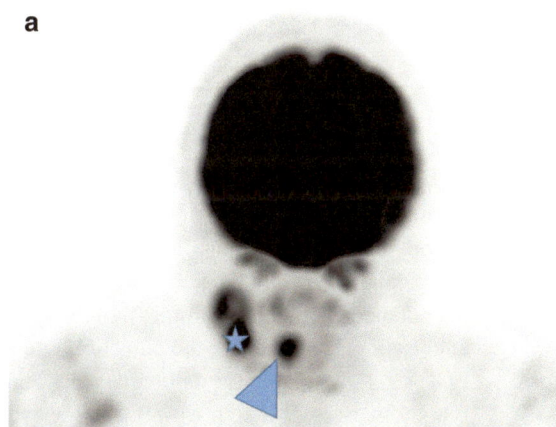
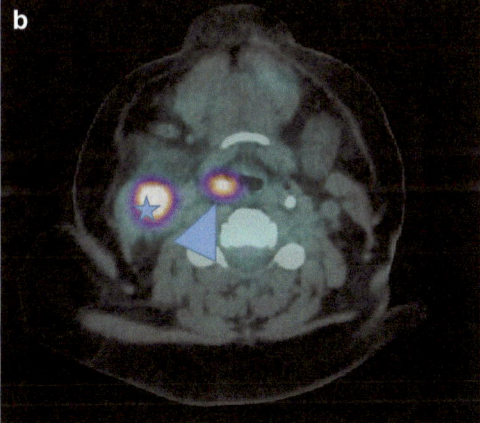
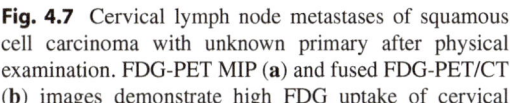

Fig. 4.7 Cervical lymph node metastases of squamous cell carcinoma with unknown primary after physical examination. FDG-PET MIP (**a**) and fused FDG-PET/CT (**b**) images demonstrate high FDG uptake of cervical lymph node metastases (asterisks) and focal suspicious FDG uptake in the right pyriform sinus (arrows). Endoscopy with biopsy confirmed right piriform sinus as the primary site

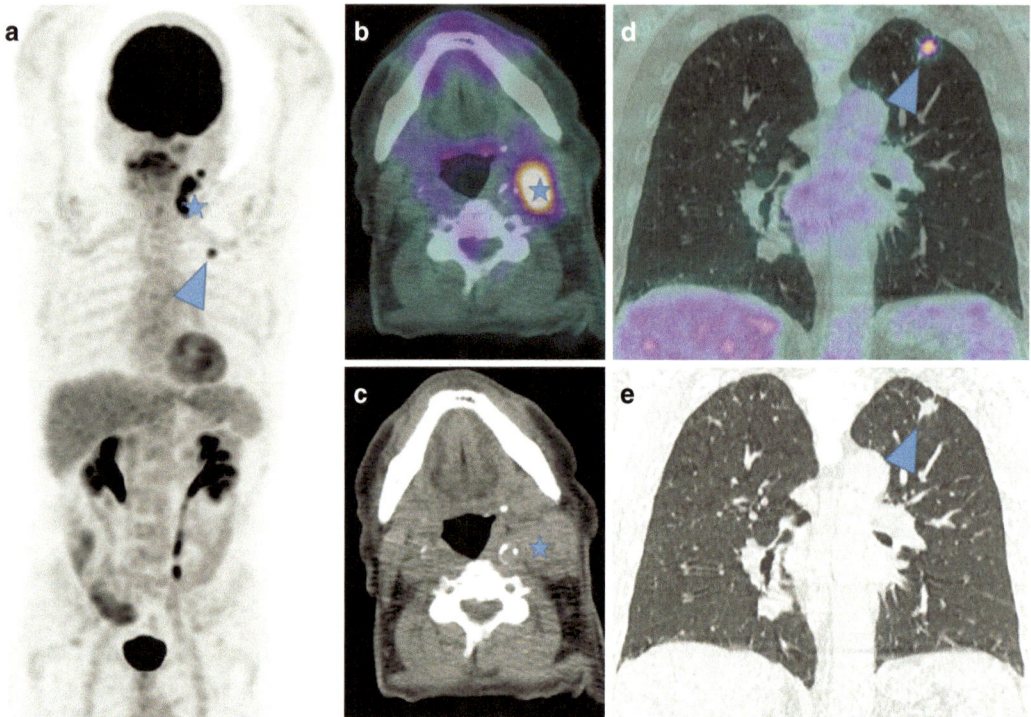

Fig. 4.8 A 69-year-old patient with cervical lymph node metastases of squamous cell carcinoma and synchronous lung adenocarcinoma discovered incidentally on FDG-PET/CT. **Images A, B, and C**: FDG-PET MIP, axial fused FDG-PET/CT, and axial CT images showing high FDG uptake of cervical lymph node metastases (asterisks), without obvious head and neck primary site. **Images A, D, and E**: FDG-PET MIP, coronal fused FDG-PET/CT, and coronal CT images showing the incidentally discovered FDG avid left upper lobe lung adenocarcinoma (arrows)

4.4.2 Lymphomas

Most lymphomas are FDG avid. A lymphoma is generally considered FDG avid if its uptake is higher than in normal liver. This avidity is, however, different according to the histological type, and some histological types of lymphomas show lower or more variable FDG uptake (Fig. 4.9). FDG uptake intensity is higher in aggressive lymphomas compared to indolent lymphomas [24].

The PRoLoG (PINTaD RespOnse criteria in Lymphoma wOrking Group) consensus initiative has classified lymphomas into three main groups [25]:

- Routinely FDG-avid lymphoma (Hodgkin lymphoma, diffuse large B-cell lymphomas (DLBCL), follicular lymphoma, mantle cell lymphoma, nodal peripheral T-cell lymphoma, lymphoblastic and Burkitt lymphoma). Nearly 100% of these lymphomas are FDG avid [26].

- Generally not FDG-avid lymphoma (small lymphocytic lymphoma, chronic lymphocytic leukemia).
- Other lymphomas, with inter-patient or inter-lesion variability in their FDG uptake (some marginal-zone lymphoma, some T-cell notably cutaneous T-cell lymphomas). In the meta-analysis by Treglia et al., the detection rate of FDG-PET in patients with marginal-zone lymphoma was 71% (CI: 61–80%). However, this rate appeared to be better in head and neck MALT lymphomas (90%, CI: 78–98%) [27].

FDG-PET is mostly recommended for initial staging, assessment of therapeutic response and assessment of end-of-treatment response of FDG-avid lymphomas. However, in the diagnostic phase, FDG-PET is recommended to guide biopsy to the site with the highest FDG uptake, particularly when a transformation of indolent lymphoma to aggressive lymphoma is sought [28–30].

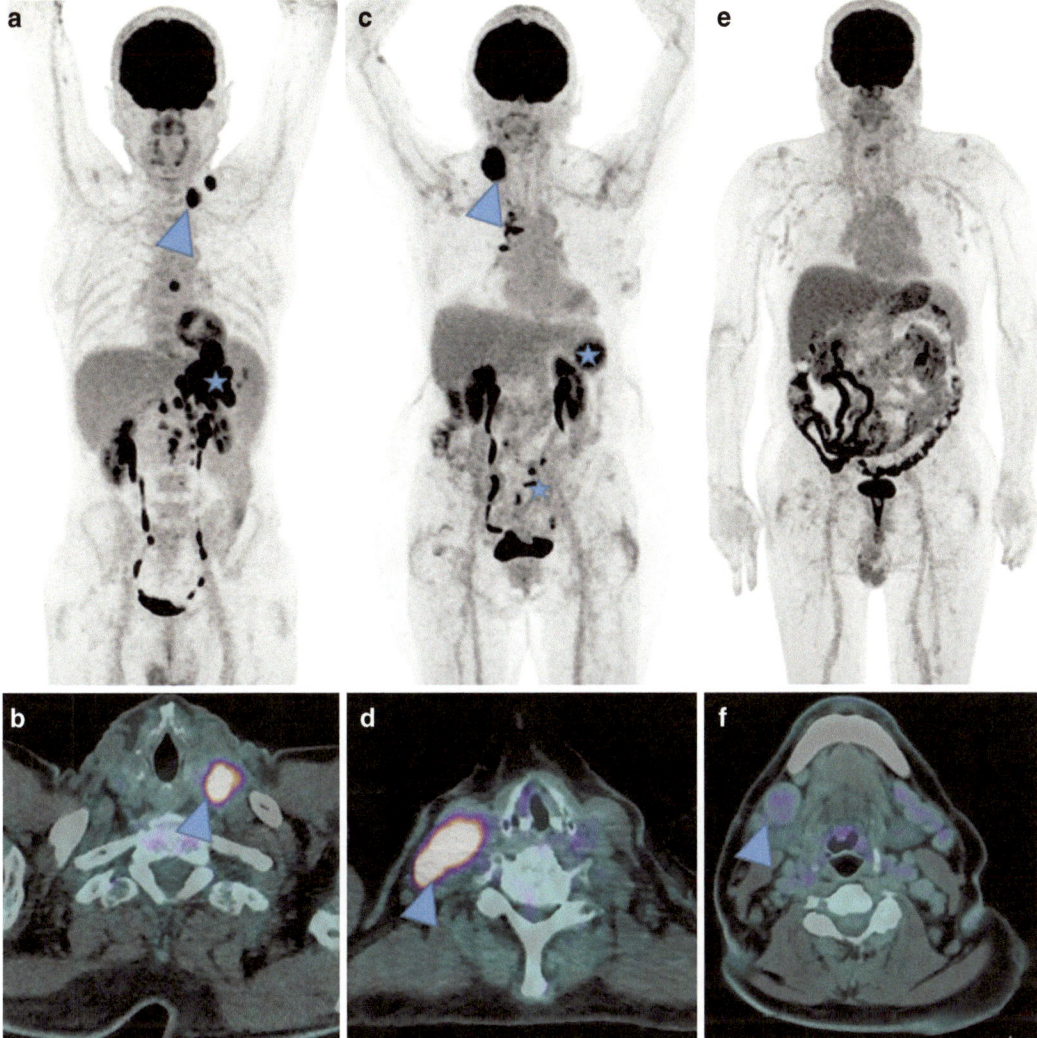

Fig. 4.9 Three cases of lymphoma with cervical lymph node involvement. (**a, b**): diffuse large B-cell lymphoma. FDG-PET MIP (**a**) and axial fused FDG-PET/CT (**b**) images demonstrate intense FDG uptake of left cervical lymphadenopathies (arrows) and involvement on both sides of the diaphragm (asterisk). (**c, d**): follicular lymphoma. FDG-PET MIP (**c**) and axial fused FDG-PET/CT (**d**) images demonstrate intense FDG uptake of right cervical lymphadenopathies (arrows), involvement on both sides of the diaphragm and splenic involvement (asterisks). (**e, f**): chronic lymphocytic leukemia. Cervical lymphadenopathies have little or no FDG uptake on axial fused FDG-PET/CT (**f**) (arrow). The MIP image (**e**) shows no lymphadenopathies with intense FDG uptake suspicious of transformation to an aggressive lymphoma

4.4.3 Salivary Gland Tumors

Primary salivary gland carcinomas, intraparotid localizations of lymphoma, and intraparotid metastases of other malignancies (facial skin tumors, distant primary malignancies) are often FDG avid. High-grade tumors generally have a higher SUVmax than low- or intermediate-grade tumors [31].

However, benign salivary gland tumors such as pleomorphic adenomas and papillary cystadenoma lymphomatosum (Warthin's tumor) are also FDG avid with uptakes that may be similar to those of malignant tumors (Fig. 4.10). Inflammatory diseases such as granulomatosis or Sjögren's syndrome and infection can also result in increased parotid FDG uptake. Finally, symmetrical low to high physiological FDG uptake in the parotid and

Fig. 4.10 MIP FDG-PET and axial fused FDG-PET/CT images of two FDG avid right parotid tumors of similar size and FDG uptake (arrows). FNA led to the diagnosis of a parotid adenocarcinoma in the first patient (**a**, **b**) and of a papillary cystadenoma lymphomatosum (Warthin's tumor) in the second patient (**c**, **d**)

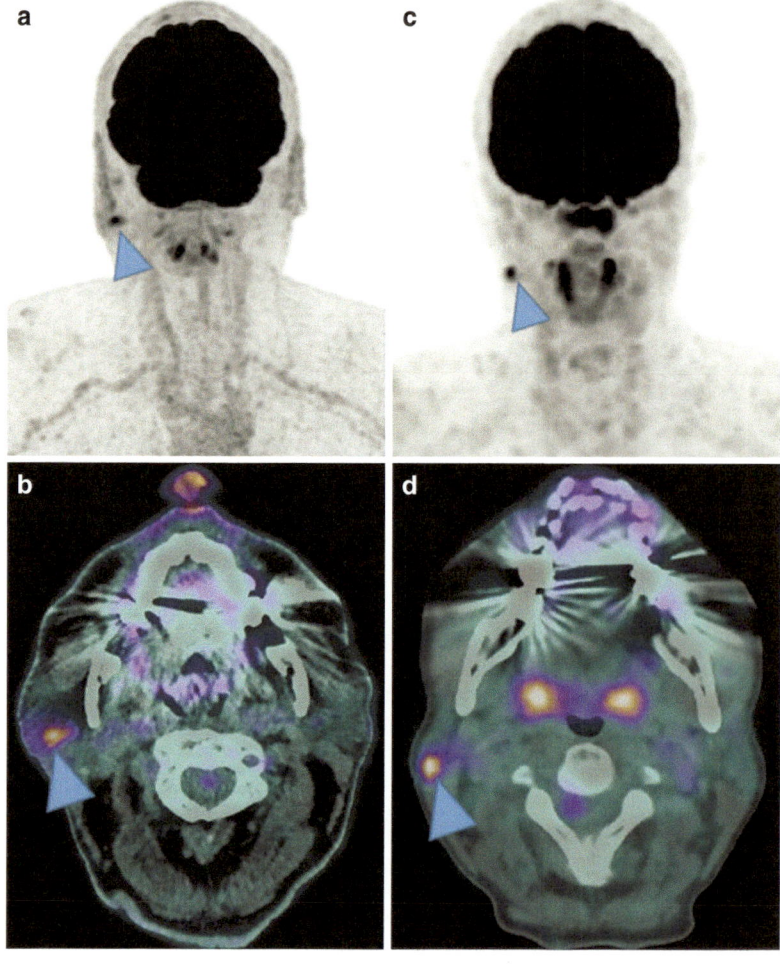

Fig. 4.11 (**a**) Intense FDG uptake of an abscess of the right submandibular gland on axial fused FDG-PET/CT images (arrow). (**b**) Symmetrical physiological FDG uptake of the parotid glands on axial fused FDG-PET/CT images (asterisks)

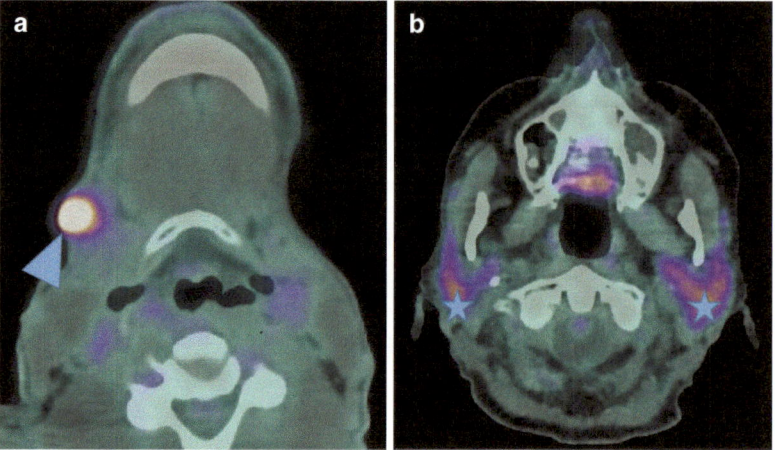

submandibular glands is often observed due to FDG excretion in saliva (Fig. 4.11).

Most metabolic FDG-PET/CT parameters used in clinical routine such as SUVmax, SUVmean or total lesion glycolysis (TLG), or metabolic tumor volume (MTV) do not enable to differentiate lesions of benign or malignant origin of the salivary glands [32, 33]. FDG-PET/CT is therefore not currently recommended for the characterization of salivary gland tumors [4].

4.4.4 Cervical Lymphadenopathies of Benign Origin

Reactive lymphadenopathies of infectious or inflammatory origin are a common cause of focal FDG uptake in the head and neck region [6].

In clinical routine, semi-quantitative FDG-PET parameters like SUVmax are not a good indicator to differentiate malignant lymph node metastasis from benign inflammatory or infectious lymphadenopathy [34]. Hypermetabolic cervical lymph nodes of uncertain origin should lead to the search on FDG-PET/CT for an infection in the corresponding area that may explain the lymphadenopathies (dental infections, sinusitis, Waldeyer's ring infections, jaw osteoradionecrosis, etc.). Finally, these findings should be assessed in conjunction with the clinical examination to increase the specificity of FDG-PET/CT (Fig. 4.12).

4.5 Thyroid Incidentalomas in FDG-PET/CT and Isotopic Evaluation of Thyroid Nodules

4.5.1 Evaluation of Thyroid Nodules

Thyroid ultrasound (US) is the main examination for the exploration of thyroid nodules, and the European Thyroid Association (ETA) provided guidelines for ultrasound malignancy risk stratification of thyroid nodules in adults (EU-TIRADS).

However, thyroid scintigraphy is the only examination that addresses the functional status of thyroid nodules. It can be performed using 123I-natrium (sodium) iodide (123I) or 99mTc-natrium (sodium) pertechnetate (the latter being a pharmacologic mimic of iodine and the most used radiotracers of the two). Hyperfunctioning nodule have increased radiotracer uptake and are often referred as "hot" nodules in literature. Hot nodules are rarely malignant, and therefore, integration of thyroid

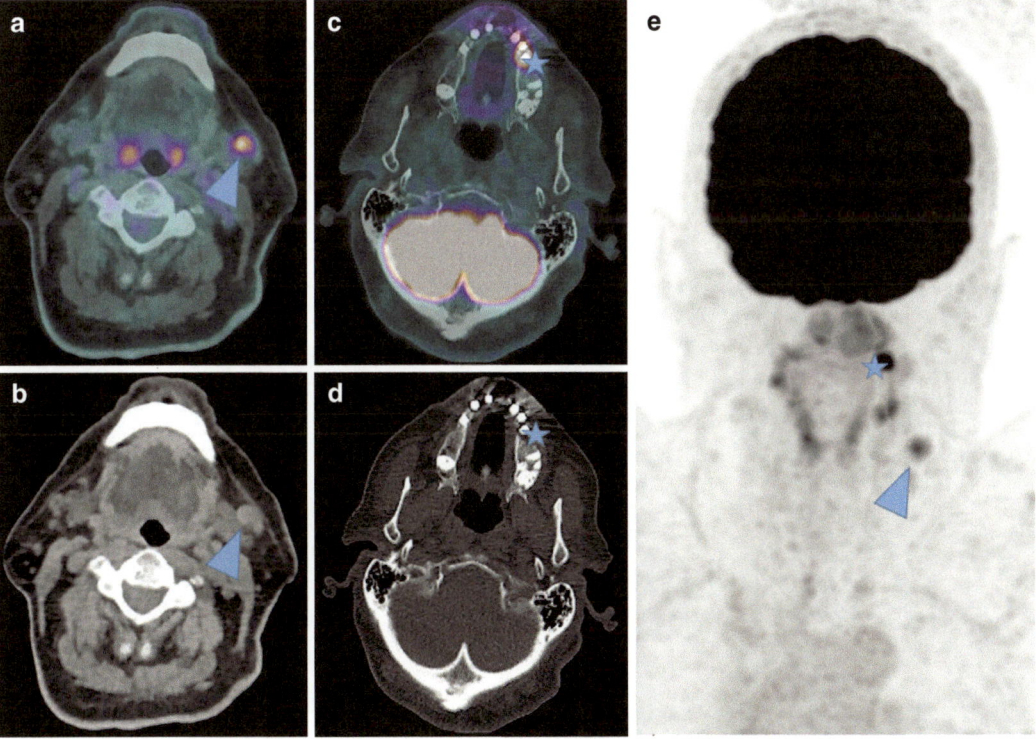

Fig. 4.12 Axial fused FDG-PET/CT (**a, c**), axial CT (**b, d**) and MIP images (**e**) demonstrating FDG uptake in an enlarged left cervical reactive lymph node (arrows) in association with a homolateral maxillary dental infection site (asterisks)

scintigraphy into the EU-TIRADS model is considered essential by the EANM and SNMMI to avoid unnecessary fine-needle aspiration (FNA) of autonomously functioning nodules [35]. ETA and the American Thyroid Association (ATA) recommend performing a thyroid scintigraphy in case of low or subnormal TSH, in order to distinguish a "hot" autonomous nodule and to orientate the FNA toward iso or nonfunctioning sonographically suspicious nodules [36, 37].

FDG-PET/CT is not widely used in the assessment of thyroid nodules. It appears that FDG-PET/CT may have a high negative predictive value for characterizing nodules with fine-needle aspiration with indeterminate cytology. However, ATA does not recommend FDG-PET for this indication [36].

FDG-PET/CT in the preoperative workup of differentiated thyroid cancers is also not recommended [36].

4.5.2 Incidental FDG-PET/CT Uptake in the Thyroid Gland

Thyroid incidentalomas detected by FDG-PET/CT are not rare and should be systematically reported. In case of discovery of an incidental thyroid FDG uptake, two main patterns can be observed:

- A diffuse uptake in the thyroid, which has a low risk of malignancy and points to thyroiditis. It does not require FNA (Fig. 4.13).
- A focal thyroid uptake, which points to a nodular thyroid lesion with an increased risk of malignancy. In the systematic review by Soelberg and al and in the meta-analysis by Treglia and Al, the prevalence of focal thyroid incidental uptake was approximately 2%. Among these incidentally found thyroid FDG-positive nodule, the prevalence of cancer was approximately 35% [38, 39]. Given this prevalence, ATA in its 2015 guidelines recommends FNA of FDG-PET/CT positive and sonographically confirmed thyroid nodules ≥1 cm (Fig. 4.14) [36].

4.5.3 Medullary Thyroid Carcinoma

According to EANM recommendations, no PET-CT is indicated for the initial workup and staging of medullary thyroid cancer (MTC). Fluorine-18 dihydroxyphenylalanine (FDOPA) is an effective way of restaging medullary thyroid cancer with elevated markers and has better performance than other PET radiotracers. However, at the diagnostic phase, in case of suspicion or initial staging of MTC, the lack of data does not allow to recommend FDOPA-PET/CT according to the EANM [40].

Fig. 4.13 FDG-PET MIP (**a**) and fused FDG-PET/CT (**b**) demonstrating diffuse FDG uptake in the thyroid (arrows), suggestive of thyroiditis and not requiring FNA

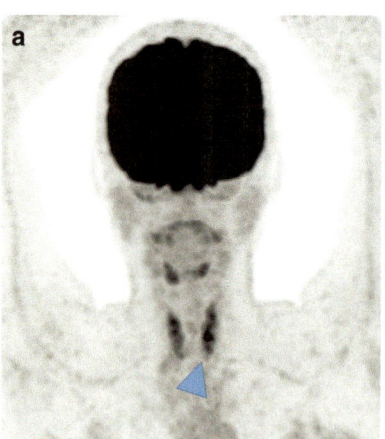
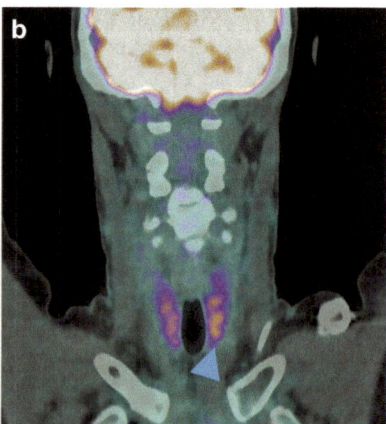

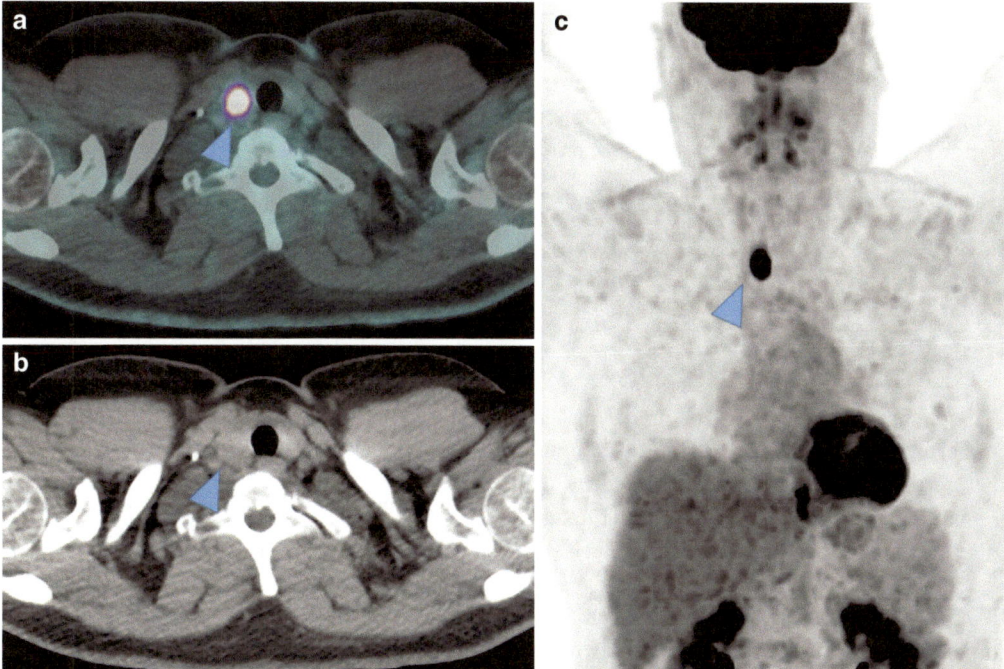

Fig. 4.14 Axial fused FDG-PET/CT (**a**), axial CT (**b**), and FDG-PET MIP images (**c**) demonstrating an incidental FDG uptake in the right thyroid lobe in a 44-year-old woman (arrows). Nodule FNA cytology was "suspicious for malignancy," according to the Bethesda system. Surgery subsequently confirmed the diagnosis of papillary carcinoma

4.6   Head and Neck Paragangliomas

The EANM recommends functional isotopic imaging to confirm the diagnosis, location, and staging of paragangliomas (PGLs), especially when an extra-adrenal location is suspected (high normetanephrine level, risk factor for metastasis, etc.) [41]. Isotopic imaging is also useful in confirming the diagnosis and stage in cases of suspected PGLs without high circulating catecholamine levels (which is often the case for head and neck paragangliomas (HNPGLs)).

4.6.1   Which Radiotracer to Inject for the Assessment of HNPGLs?

Somatostatin Receptor (SSTR) PET/CT is the first-line isotopic imaging for the diagnosis and initial workup of HNPGLs. Several SSTR-PET radiotracers radiolabeled with 68Ga exist like DOTATOC (edotreotide) or DOTATATE (oxodotreotide) [41, 42]. To perform SSTR-PET/CT, no fasting is required and acquisitions start 45 to 90 min after intravenous injection of the radiotracer.

[(18)F]labeled fluorodihydroxyphenylalanine (FDOPA)-PET/CT (if SSTR-PET/CT is not available) is also very sensitive for the detection of HNPGLs. 11In-pentetreotide scintigraphy and FDG-PET/CT are now recommended as second or third line imaging [41, 42].

4.7   Conclusion-Keys Points

FDG-PET/CT is currently the main nuclear medicine imaging technique used to investigate cervical masses. It has an important role in guiding the workup and in assessing the extension of head and neck tumors. Many pitfalls can lead to misinterpretation of FDG-PET/CT, particularly in the cervical region (brown fat uptake, muscular FDG uptake, movements during the acquisitions, etc.). It is therefore important to be familiar with these artifacts, the physiological variations of the normal and to keep in mind that some ENT benign tumors and many ENT inflammatory and infectious pathologies can be FDG avid.

4.7.1 Keys Points

- Compliance with the steps for preparing and performing FDG-PET/CT (fasting for 4 hours before the examination, prevention of brown fat uptake, rest during the 1-hour FDG uptake phase, possible pre-medication,etc.) is essential.
- FDG-PET/CT is indicated for the evaluation of head and neck carcinomas of unknown origin after conventional workup. It should be performed before any pharyngeal biopsy.
- In the diagnostic phase of lymphomas, FDG-PET is recommended for initial staging and to guide biopsy, particularly when a transformation from indolent lymphoma to aggressive lymphoma is suspected.
- Some benign salivary gland tumors such as pleomorphic adenomas and Warthin's tumor are FDG avid with uptakes that may be similar to those of malignant tumors. FDG-PET/CT is not currently recommended for the characterization of salivary gland tumors.
- A diffuse FDG uptake in the thyroid points to thyroiditis and does not require FNA.
- In case of discovery of an incidental thyroid FDG uptake, FNA of FDG avid and sonographically confirmed thyroid nodules ≥1 cm is recommended.
- Thyroid scintigraphy in case of low or subnormal TSH enables to distinguish "hot" autonomous nodules, which are rarely malignant.
- Somatostatin Receptor (SSTR) PET/CT is the first-line isotopic imaging for the diagnosis and initial workup of HNPGLs.

References

1. Pynnonen MA, Gillespie MB, Roman B, Rosenfeld RM, Tunkel DE, Bontempo L, Brook I, Chick DA, Colandrea M, Finestone SA, Fowler JC, Griffith CC, Henson Z, Levine C, Mehta V, Salama A, Scharpf J, Shatzkes DR, Stern WB, Youngerman JS, Corrigan MD. Clinical practice guideline: evaluation of the neck mass in adults. Otolaryngol Head Neck Surg. 2017;157:S1–S30. https://doi.org/10.1177/0194599817722550.
2. Machiels J-P, René Leemans C, Golusinski W, Grau C, Licitra L, Gregoire V. Reprint of "squamous cell carcinoma of the oral cavity, larynx, oropharynx and hypopharynx: EHNS-ESMO-ESTRO clinical practice guidelines for diagnosis, treatment and follow-up.". Oral Oncol. 2021;113:105042. https://doi.org/10.1016/j.oraloncology.2020.105042.
3. Maghami E, Ismaila N, Alvarez A, Chernock R, Duvvuri U, Geiger J, Gross N, Haughey B, Paul D, Rodriguez C, Sher D, Stambuk HE, Waldron J, Witek M, Caudell J. Diagnosis and Management of Squamous Cell Carcinoma of unknown primary in the head and neck: ASCO guideline. JCO. 2020;38:2570–96. https://doi.org/10.1200/JCO.20.00275.
4. Salaün P-Y, Abgral R, Malard O, Querellou-Lefranc S, Quere G, Wartski M, Coriat R, Hindie E, Taieb D, Tabarin A, Girard A, Grellier J-F, Brenot-Rossi I, Groheux D, Rousseau C, Deandreis D, Alberini J-L, Bodet-Milin C, Itti E, Casasnovas O, Kraeber-Bodere F, Moreau P, Philip A, Balleyguier C, Luciani A, Cachin F. Good clinical practice recommendations for the use of PET/CT in oncology. Eur J Nucl Med Mol Imaging. 2020;47:28–50. https://doi.org/10.1007/s00259-019-04553-8.
5. ACR–ACNM–SNMMI–SPR (2022) ACR–ACNM–SNMMI–SPR practice parameter for performing FDG-pet/CT in oncology.
6. Boellaard R, Delgado-Bolton R, Oyen WJG, Giammarile F, Tatsch K, Eschner W, Verzijlbergen FJ, Barrington SF, Pike LC, Weber WA, Stroobants S, Delbeke D, Donohoe KJ, Holbrook S, Graham MM, Testanera G, Hoekstra OS, Zijlstra J, Visser E, Hoekstra CJ, Pruim J, Willemsen A, Arends B, Kotzerke J, Bockisch A, Beyer T, Chiti A, Krause BJ. FDG PET/CT: EANM procedure guidelines for tumour imaging: version 2.0. Eur J Nucl Med Mol Imaging. 2015;42:328–54. https://doi.org/10.1007/s00259-014-2961-x.
7. EANM. European Association of Nuclear Medicine (EANM). Dosage card (version 5.7.2016). EANM website.pdf; 2016.
8. Vali R, Alessio A, Balza R, Borgwardt L, Bar-Sever Z, Czachowski M, Jehanno N, Kurch L, Pandit-Taskar N, Parisi M, Piccardo A, Seghers V, Shulkin BL, Zucchetta P, Lim R. SNMMI procedure standard/

EANM practice guideline on Pediatric ^{18}F-FDG PET/CT for oncology 1.0. J Nucl Med. 2021;62:99–110. https://doi.org/10.2967/jnumed.120.254110.

9. Berthelsen AK, Holm S, Loft A, Klausen TL, Andersen F, Højgaard L. PET/CT with intravenous contrast can be used for PET attenuation correction in cancer patients. Eur J Nucl Med Mol Imaging. 2005;32:1167–75. https://doi.org/10.1007/s00259-005-1784-1.

10. Rebière M, Verburg FA, Palmowski M, Krohn T, Pietsch H, Kuhl CK, Mottaghy FM, Behrendt FF. Multiphase CT scanning and different intravenous contrast media concentrations in combined F-18-FDG PET/CT: effect on quantitative and clinical assessment. Eur J Radiol. 2012;81:e862–9. https://doi.org/10.1016/j.ejrad.2012.04.007.

11. Yau Y-Y, Chan W-S, Tam Y-M, Vernon P, Wong S, Coel M, Chu SK-F. Application of intravenous contrast in PET/CT: does it really introduce significant attenuation correction error? J Nucl Med. 2005;46:283–91.

12. Barai S, Ora M, Gambhir S, Singh A. Does intravenous contrast improve the diagnostic yield of Fluorodeoxyglucose positron-emission tomography/computed tomography in patients with head-and-neck malignancy. Indian J Nucl Med. 2020;35:13–6. https://doi.org/10.4103/ijnm.IJNM_119_19.

13. Yoshida K, Suzuki A, Nagashima T, Lee J, Horiuchi C, Tsukuda M, Inoue T. Staging primary head and neck cancers with (18)F-FDG PET/CT: is intravenous contrast administration really necessary? Eur J Nucl Med Mol Imaging. 2009;36:1417–24. https://doi.org/10.1007/s00259-009-1127-8.

14. Haerle SK, Strobel K, Ahmad N, Soltermann A, Schmid DT, Stoeckli SJ. Contrast-enhanced ^{18}F-FDG-PET/CT for the assessment of necrotic lymph node metastases. Head Neck. 2011;33:324–9. https://doi.org/10.1002/hed.21447.

15. Bujoreanu I, Gujral D, Wallitt K, Awad Z. Incidental uptake of fluorodeoxyglucose in the Waldeyer's ring and risk of oropharyngeal malignancy. Eur Arch Otorrinolaringol. 2022;279:2657–64. https://doi.org/10.1007/s00405-021-07089-6.

16. Rusthoven KE, Koshy M, Paulino AC. The role of fluorodeoxyglucose positron emission tomography in cervical lymph node metastases from an unknown primary tumor. Cancer. 2004;101:2641–9. https://doi.org/10.1002/cncr.20687.

17. Mihailovic J, Killeen RP, Duignan JA. PET/CT variants and pitfalls in head and neck cancers including thyroid cancer. Semin Nucl Med. 2021;51:419–40. https://doi.org/10.1053/j.semnuclmed.2021.03.002.

18. Paquette CM, Manos DC, Psooy BJ. Unilateral vocal cord paralysis: a review of CT findings, mediastinal causes, and the course of the recurrent laryngeal nerves. Radiographics. 2012;32:721–40. https://doi.org/10.1148/rg.323115129.

19. Beyer T, Tellmann L, Nickel I, Pietrzyk U. On the use of positioning aids to reduce Misregistration in the head and neck in whole-body PET/CT studies. J Nucl Med. 2005;46:596–602.

20. Al-Ibraheem A, Buck A, Krause BJ, Scheidhauer K, Schwaiger M. Clinical applications of FDG PET and PET/CT in head and neck cancer. J Oncol. 2009;2009:208725. https://doi.org/10.1155/2009/208725.

21. Zhu L, Wang N. 18F-fluorodeoxyglucose positron emission tomography-computed tomography as a diagnostic tool in patients with cervical nodal metastases of unknown primary site: a meta-analysis. Surg Oncol. 2013;22:190–4. https://doi.org/10.1016/j.suronc.2013.06.002.

22. Lee JR, Kim JS, Roh J-L, Lee JH, Baek JH, Cho K-J, Choi S-H, Nam SY, Kim SY. Detection of occult primary tumors in patients with cervical metastases of unknown primary tumors: comparison of (18)F FDG PET/CT with contrast-enhanced CT or CT/MR imaging-prospective study. Radiology. 2015;274:764–71. https://doi.org/10.1148/radiol.14141073.

23. Roh J-L, Kim JS, Lee JH, Cho K-J, Choi S-H, Nam SY, Kim SY. Utility of combined (18)F-fluorodeoxyglucose-positron emission tomography and computed tomography in patients with cervical metastases from unknown primary tumors. Oral Oncol. 2009;45:218–24. https://doi.org/10.1016/j.oraloncology.2008.05.010.

24. Schöder H, Noy A, Gönen M, Weng L, Green D, Erdi YE, Larson SM, Yeung HWD. Intensity of 18fluorodeoxyglucose uptake in positron emission tomography distinguishes between indolent and aggressive non-Hodgkin's lymphoma. J Clin Oncol. 2005;23:4643–51. https://doi.org/10.1200/JCO.2005.12.072.

25. Ricard F, Cheson B, Barrington S, Trotman J, Schmid A, Brueggenwerth G, Salles G, Schwartz L, Goldmacher G, Jarecha R, Broussais F, Narang J, Galette P, Liu M, Bajpai S, Perlman E, Gillis J, Smalberg I, Terve P, Zahlmann G, Korn R (2022) Application of the LUGANO CLASSIFICATION for initial evaluation, staging, and response assessment of HODGKIN and non-HODGKIN lymphoma: the PROLOG consensus initiative (part 1- clinical). J Nucl Med jnumed.122.264106. https://doi.org/10.2967/jnumed.122.264106.

26. Barrington SF, Mikhaeel NG, Kostakoglu L, Meignan M, Hutchings M, Müeller SP, Schwartz LH, Zucca E, Fisher RI, Trotman J, Hoekstra OS, Hicks RJ, O'Doherty MJ, Hustinx R, Biggi A, Cheson BD. Role of imaging in the staging and response assessment of lymphoma: consensus of the international conference on malignant lymphomas imaging working group.

JCO. 2014;32:3048–58. https://doi.org/10.1200/JCO.2013.53.5229.

27. Treglia G, Zucca E, Sadeghi R, Cavalli F, Giovanella L, Ceriani L. Detection rate of fluorine-18-fluorodeoxyglucose positron emission tomography in patients with marginal zone lymphoma of MALT type: a meta-analysis. Hematol Oncol. 2015;33:113–24. https://doi.org/10.1002/hon.2152.

28. Bodet-Milin C, Kraeber-Bodéré F, Moreau P, Campion L, Dupas B, Le Gouill S. Investigation of FDG-PET/CT imaging to guide biopsies in the detection of histological transformation of indolent lymphoma. Haematologica. 2008;93:471–2. https://doi.org/10.3324/haematol.12013.

29. Bruzzi JF, Macapinlac H, Tsimberidou AM, Truong MT, Keating MJ, Marom EM, Munden RF. Detection of Richter's transformation of chronic lymphocytic leukemia by PET/CT. J Nucl Med. 2006;47:1267–73.

30. Rajamäki A, Kuitunen H, Sorigue M, Kokkonen S-M, Kuittinen O, Sunela K. FDG-PET/CT-guided rebiopsy may find clinically unsuspicious transformation of follicular lymphoma. Cancer Med. 2023;12:407–11. https://doi.org/10.1002/cam4.4924.

31. Roh J-L, Ryu CH, Choi S-H, Kim JS, Lee JH, Cho K-J, Nam SY, Kim SY. Clinical utility of 18F-FDG PET for patients with salivary gland malignancies. J Nucl Med. 2007;48:240–6.

32. Bertagna F, Nicolai P, Maroldi R, Mattavelli D, Bertoli M, Giubbini R, Lombardi D, Treglia G. Diagnostic role of (18)F-FDG-PET or PET/CT in salivary gland tumors: a systematic review. Rev Esp Med Nucl Imagen Mol. 2015;34:295–302.

33. Kendi ATK, Magliocca KR, Corey A, Galt JR, Switchenko J, Wadsworth JT, El-Deiry MW, Schuster DM, Saba NF, Hudgins PA. Is there a role for PET/CT parameters to characterize benign, malignant, and metastatic parotid Tumors? Am J Roentgenol. 2016;207:635–40. https://doi.org/10.2214/AJR.15.15590.

34. Pijl JP, Nienhuis PH, Kwee TC, Glaudemans AWJM, Slart RHJA, Gormsen LC. Limitations and pitfalls of FDG-PET/CT in infection and inflammation. Semin Nucl Med. 2021;51:633–45. https://doi.org/10.1053/j.semnuclmed.2021.06.008.

35. Giovanella L, Avram AM, Iakovou I, Kwak J, Lawson SA, Lulaj E, Luster M, Piccardo A, Schmidt M, Tulchinsky M, Verburg FA, Wolin E. EANM practice guideline/SNMMI procedure standard for RAIU and thyroid scintigraphy. Eur J Nucl Med Mol Imaging. 2019;46:2514–25. https://doi.org/10.1007/s00259-019-04472-8.

36. Haugen BR, Alexander EK, Bible KC, Doherty GM, Mandel SJ, Nikiforov YE, Pacini F, Randolph GW, Sawka AM, Schlumberger M, Schuff KG, Sherman SI, Sosa JA, Steward DL, Tuttle RM, Wartofsky L. 2015 American Thyroid Association management guidelines for adult patients with thyroid nodules and differentiated thyroid cancer: the American Thyroid Association guidelines task force on thyroid nodules and differentiated thyroid cancer. Thyroid. 2016;26:1–133. https://doi.org/10.1089/thy.2015.0020.

37. Russ G, Bonnema SJ, Erdogan MF, Durante C, Ngu R, Leenhardt L. European thyroid association guidelines for ultrasound malignancy risk stratification of thyroid nodules in adults: the EU-TIRADS. Eur Thyroid J. 2017;6:225–37. https://doi.org/10.1159/000478927.

38. Soelberg KK, Bonnema SJ, Brix TH, Hegedüs L. Risk of malignancy in thyroid incidentalomas detected by 18F-fluorodeoxyglucose positron emission tomography: a systematic review. Thyroid. 2012;22:918–25. https://doi.org/10.1089/thy.2012.0005.

39. Treglia G, Bertagna F, Sadeghi R, Verburg FA, Ceriani L, Giovanella L. Focal thyroid incidental uptake detected by 18F-fluorodeoxyglucose positron emission tomography. Meta-analysis on prevalence and malignancy risk. Nuklearmedizin. 2013;52:130–6. https://doi.org/10.3413/Nukmed-0568-13-03.

40. Giovanella L, Treglia G, Iakovou I, Mihailovic J, Verburg FA, Luster M. EANM practice guideline for PET/CT imaging in medullary thyroid carcinoma. Eur J Nucl Med Mol Imaging. 2020;47:61–77. https://doi.org/10.1007/s00259-019-04458-6.

41. Taïeb D, Hicks RJ, Hindié E, Guillet BA, Avram A, Ghedini P, Timmers HJ, Scott AT, Elojeimy S, Rubello D, Virgolini IJ, Fanti S, Balogova S, Pandit-Taskar N, Pacak K. European Association of Nuclear Medicine Practice Guideline/Society of Nuclear Medicine and Molecular Imaging procedure standard 2019 for radionuclide imaging of phaeochromocytoma and paraganglioma. Eur J Nucl Med Mol Imaging. 2019;46:2112–37. https://doi.org/10.1007/s00259-019-04398-1.

42. Lin EP, Chin BB, Fishbein L, Moritani T, Montoya SP, Ellika S, Newlands S. Head and neck Paragangliomas: an update on the molecular Classification, state-of-the-art imaging, and management recommendations. Radiol Imaging Cancer. 2022;4:e210088. https://doi.org/10.1148/rycan.210088.

Hubert Tissot is a nuclear medicine physician at the Institut Curie, Paris, France. His areas of interest include molecular imaging of ENT tumors, radioligand therapy, and molecular imaging of prostate cancer.

Fine-Needle Aspiration and Rapid on-Site Examination (ROSE)

5

Zahra Maleki

5.1 Introduction

Fine-needle aspiration (FNA) is a method of tissue biopsy to investigate the underlying pathologic conditions of a lesion by microscopic evaluation of the aspirated material using a small-gauge needle [1, 2]. Aspiration cytology is considered a separate field from exfoliative cytology [3]. In the era of modern medicine, the utility of needle aspiration goes back to 1833 when Baron Dupuytren and Stanley separately reported the diagnosis of echinococcal cyst by puncture aspiration [2, 4, 5]. In 1846, Kun published his experience with the use of needle biopsy for the diagnosis of cancer entitled "A new instrument for the diagnosis of tumors," which was a pivotal point for modern fine-needle aspiration cytology [2, 6]. Later on, Lebert (1851), Menetrier (1886), and Kroning (1887) reported the application of needle biopsy for cancer diagnosis [2, 7–9]. The application of needle aspiration for diagnostic purposes was expanded to different organs, solid and cystic lesions, and even for infectious conditions [2]. In 1912, Hirschfeld published a paper about needle aspiration on lymph nodes [10]. In 1921, at Johns Hopkins Hospital, Guthrie performed lymph node FNA using a 21-gauge needle. He smeared the material on glass slides that were air-dried and stained with Romanowsky staining. He reported that he diagnosed conditions like syphilis, tuberculosis, lymphoma, and metastatic carcinoma with that method [11]. In the UK, at St Thomas' Hospital in London, Dudgeon and Patrick described the use of fine-needle aspiration techniques and proposed the utility of needle aspiration of tumors as a tool for rapid microscopic diagnosis in 1927 [12]. They also described touch imprints of surgical specimens. The same year, Arinkin published his experience on bone marrow biopsy [13]. In the USA, Martin and Ellis advocated needle aspiration at the Memorial Sloan Kettering in 1930 [14]. Their procedure consisted of a small incision over the lesion using a scalpel, followed by aspiration with an 18-gauge needle [2].

In Germany, Ernest Mannheim published his work entitled "Die Bedeutung der Tumorpunktion für die Tumordiagnose" ("The significance of tumor punctures for tumor diagnosis") in 1931. His paper should be considered as the first paper on modern FNA technique using 22-gauge needle, which did not require any incision prior to FNA [2, 15]. Martin and Stewart published their observation on the advantages and limitations of aspiration cytology in 1936 [16].

It was in Sweden in 1950s that the modern era of FNA flourished and quickly expanded in Europe. Soderstrom and Franzen in Sweden, Lopes Cardozo in Holland, and Zajdela in France

Z. Maleki (✉)
Department of Pathology Division of Cytopathology,
Johns Hopkins Hospital Pathology,
Baltimore, MD, USA
e-mail: zmaleki1@jhmi.edu

at the Institut Curie, were pioneers of FNA of the new era, studying thousands of FNA cases [17–22]. Zajicek [23, 24] and Franzen, at the Karolinska Hospital, published a collaborative work on diagnostic criteria and diagnostic accuracy [19]. Later on, Koss in the USA and Osborn in the UK, established diagnostic cytology and its histological correlation [2, 25, 26]. Certainly, the collaborative work of Papanicolaou and Traut on exfoliative samples of uterine cervix for the detection of cervical cancer cells as a screening test played a significant role in flourishing FNA cytology globally [3]. The most significant contribution of FNA from the clinical standpoint is providing information about the aspirated lesion without surgical intervention.

Currently, FNA is widely utilized to investigate head and neck lesions [1]. Neck masses are common in adults. A neck mass can be the initial presentation of variable conditions such as HPV (human papillomavirus)-related squamous cell carcinoma [27].

Fine-needle aspiration (FNA) is a method of choice for initial evaluation of neck lesions. FNA is a minimally invasive, rapid to perform, cost-effective, well-accepted by patients with minimal morbidity and rare complications [1] [28, 29]. Moreover, FNA services are cost-effective in a dedicated head and neck clinic [30]. FNA is an accurate, highly sensitive, and specific procedure that avoids open biopsies and its associated potential complications or delays in treatment [31].

It has high accuracy when the FNA performer is well-trained and experienced. A meta-analysis of FNA performance on all head and neck masses showed an 89.6% sensitivity, 96.5% specificity, 93.1% accuracy, 96.2% positive predictive value (PPV), and 90.3% negative predictive value (NPV) [32, 33]. The rate of false negative FNA results is relatively low (5.9%), leading by thyroid FNA followed by lymph nodes and salivary glands [34]. Repeat FNA is suggested if the aspirated material is scant precluding a diagnosis [34]. Inadequate sampling, sampling errors, lack of experience of FNA performers, and misinterpretation are factors resulting in misdiagnosis [35, 36]. FNA is performed to evaluate both solid and cystic lesions of the neck [28, 37, 38].

Thyroid, salivary glands, lymph nodes, cervical masses, mesenchymal lesions, and paraspinal masses are all amenable to FNA procedures [1, 39]. Each one of these sites are associated with a range of differential diagnoses and its own diagnostic challenges. Neck masses can be the clinical presentation of diverse pathologic conditions. By definition, a neck mass is a distinct abnormal lesion that is palpable or visible by examination or imaging studies. It is located above the clavicle, below the mandible, and deep to the skin. While a neck mass is most likely due to an infectious process in children, a neck mass is mainly due to a malignant process in adults. An asymptomatic neck mass can be the initial clinical presentation of a malignant process such as head and neck squamous cell carcinoma, thyroid and salivary gland cancers, or lymphoma or even a metastasis of an unknown primary [27, 31]. In general, a neck mass in adults should be considered malignant until it is proven otherwise. FNA is highly sensitive (83% to 97%) and specific (91% to 100%) to detect metastatic disease in cervical lymph nodes [28]. The most common metastatic neoplasms involving the cervical lymph nodes include squamous cell carcinoma, papillary thyroid carcinoma, nasopharyngeal carcinoma, and malignant melanoma. The underlying cause of the mass lesions can be inflammatory, infectious, congenital/developmental, or neoplastic including benign tumors with uncertain behavior and malignant [28]. Reactive lymph node hyperplasia, metastatic carcinoma, and lymphoma were the most common findings in FNA of head and neck masses [36].

Initial evaluation of a patient with a neck mass includes taking a thorough clinical history and physical examination.

A detailed clinical history is very valuable including the duration of the mass. A prior history of malignancy, even remote history of malignancy, and type of malignancy and the primary site is of paramount importance. Considering the fact that squamous cell carcinoma is the most common malignant neoplasm of the neck, history plays particularly an important role in differential diagnosis of squamous lesions in both enlarged lymph nodes and cystic lesions [27, 37].

A delay in diagnosis of metastatic cancer, particularly head and neck squamous cell carcinoma including mucosal squamous cell carcinoma is associated with worse prognosis and tumor stage [31]. Delay in diagnosis of head and neck squamous cell carcinoma is common, which in turn leads to cancer recurrence, lower quality of life, and death [31].

In the absence of an infectious etiology, a neck mass can be associated with increased risk of malignancy if a neck mass has persisted for two weeks or more or a neck mass is manifested with one these characteristics including size greater than 1.5 cm in diameter, firm to palpation, fixation to adjacent tissues, or ulceration of overlying skin [31]. A clinician should advise the patient to follow-up to reassess a neck mass if the findings favor a benign process. In patients with a neck mass suspicious for a malignant process, the neck should be further examined including visualizing the mucosa of the larynx, base of tongue, and pharynx. A cystic neck mass also requires further work up with imaging studies or FNA and the clinician should not assume that a cystic neck mass is benign. For instance, a cystic neck mass can be the initial clinical presentation of HPV (human papillomavirus) related head and neck squamous cell carcinoma, which can be mistaken for branchial cleft cyst [37]. Overall, in patients older than 40 years of age, a solitary lateral neck cyst should be presumed malignant until it is proven otherwise [37] [40]. Based upon clinical findings and history, a patient's upper aerodigestive tract may be evaluated under anesthesia during a workup process. FNA is indicated in all neck masses with an increased risk of malignancy. FNA is a cost-effective procedure compared to open biopsy [29].

FNA can be performed on both superficial and deeply located lesions. FNA decreases the days of hospital stay by providing rapid diagnosis and preventing the cost associated with surgery, operating room staff, anesthetists, and the operating room. FNA can be performed in the office, outpatient center, and in radiology. It is well-tolerated, and it can be done on patients with multiple comorbidities. It can be repeated and multiple lesions can be aspirated at the same office visit. It does not leave any scar and the patient can resume daily activities very quickly. Major complications such as hemorrhage, sepsis, and disseminate tumor cells along the needle tack are rare. Seeding along the needle track after FNA procedure is estimated 0.00012% while it is estimated 0.0011% for needle core biopsy [41]. However, these rare complications do not diminish the clinical value of FNA. FNA can be associated with post procedure changes of the aspiration site including infarction, hematoma, reactive changes, and capsular pseudoinvasion. FNA is limited by the fact that architecture is missing. There are instances that despite adequate material, a definitive diagnosis cannot be rendered.

5.1.1 Reporting Systems

Reporting the FNA findings play an important role in-patient management. The FNA findings may result in a definitive diagnosis, including benign and malignant diagnoses. Occasionally, the specimen is inadequate. There are circumstances that regardless of the experience of the pathologist, the diagnosis is indeterminant. In addition, the pathologists may use different formats for reporting an entity and FNA reports may differ from one institution to the other, causing misunderstanding among clinicians. Moreover, the patients may choose to receive treatment in a facility different from the place that FNA has been performed. To standardize pathology reports and to improve pathologist-clinician communication, international efforts have been made and reporting systems have been created to address these issues. In head and neck, the Bethesda System for reporting thyroid cytology and the Milan System for reporting salivary gland cytology have been universally accepted [42, 43]. The reporting systems are created to uniform the pathology reports and to improve communication between the pathologist and the clinician. More importantly, each diagnostic category provides associated risk of malignancy and a recommendation for clinicians.

5.1.2 Clinical Guidelines and FNA

Different specialty disciplines consist of experts collect and evaluate the clinical data, management modalities and the clinical outcomes and provide clinical guidelines. The guidelines include recommendations that are based on observational studies with a preponderance of benefits over harm. The guidelines aim to promote the efficient, effective, and accurate diagnostic workup of neck mass and to ensure that patients with neck masses suspicious for malignancy are diagnosed and treated promptly. The specific goal of the guidelines is to avoid delay in diagnosis of head and neck cancers by recommending appropriate targeted examination, imaging studies, pathology evaluation, and empiric medical therapies in patients older than 18 years of age with a neck mass [31].

The role of patient in clinical decision making is very important. FNA provides information about the lesion in most instances, which let the patient and the clinician have better understanding about the clinical condition before making any decisions. This is true about both conservative and surgical approaches. Factors to be considered by patients are the benefits, adverse effects, costs, frequency and duration of treatment, and quality of life [31].

Neck remains one of the most challenging body sites for FNA cytology due to a wide spectrum of entities that can occur in this anatomic site. The number of pathologists that are performing FNA is increasing and more clinicians are requesting FNA on mass lesions with unknown etiology. It is expected to provide a diagnosis, preferably a definitive diagnosis, and collect adequate material for ancillary studies such as molecular studies. The broad range of differential diagnoses for each anatomic site in the neck, variable techniques in performing FNA, using or not using ROSE, different preferences in stains, different clinical settings, and variable access to resources are encountered for writing this book.

The aim of the book is to provide a practical approach to neck FNA cytology. This book targets practicing pathologists, pathologists in training, and cytotechnologists. It covers different practicing pathology settings, different FNA procedures, slide preparation methods, and different stains. The book discusses the essential role of medical history, clinical and imaging findings, and laboratory data in rendering a diagnosis on FNA samples. Various techniques are included to improve specimen adequacy and to collect additional material for ancillary studies. Special circumstances requiring specimen triage have been explained. The common, uncommon, and rare entities in the neck are covered along with their diagnostic criteria, differential diagnosis, and diagnostic pitfalls. Ancillary studies associated with different cytomorphology or clinical and imaging findings are discussed such as flow cytometry in the presence of atypical lymphocytes. Doing more with less specimen is commonly referred to FNA samples, which puts pathologist under compelling pressure. The aim of this book is to provide adequate information to a practicing pathologist to the point that the pathologist feels comfortable to handle variable neck FNAs with confidence, knowing the limitations of a neck FNA and how to address those in the report, and communicate effectively with clinicians. The chapters cover imaging studies in different pathologic conditions, FNA techniques, specimen collection, preparation, staining, and diagnostic entities related to each anatomic site. In conclusion, the aim of this book is to provide comprehensive information on the neck FNA cytology to assist pathologists in handling each case exclusively, using their judgment to ensure best practice for each patient.

5.2 Techniques

By definition, a neck mass is a discrete lesion from its surrounding tissue found by palpation or imaging modalities. FNA is a procedure that allows a small portion of a lesion is obtained through a small needle. FNA can be conducted in different settings. The procedure can be performed by palpation, or under image- guidance [44]. Image-guided FNA is often requested for nonpalpable lesions or palpation guided FNA biopsies with non-diagnostic results [45]. In cases suspected of infection, image-guided FNA is useful in identifying microorganisms and subsequent treatment with appropriate antibiotics. In cases suspicious for a neoplastic process, image-guided FNA is helpful in planning surgery including the extent of surgery and possible nodal dissection, possible preoperative chemo-radiation, or non-operative treatments (i.e. lymphoma) [45]. FNA can safely performed in an outpatient clinic, ultrasound unit, CT area, magnetic resonance image (MRI) facility or even on bedside for in-patient cases. Ultrasound-guided fine-needle aspiration is done by radiologists, endocrinologists, and pathologists [46].

Important clinical findings include age greater than 40 years, non-tender neck mass, alcohol or tobacco use, prior head and neck malignancy, prior head and neck irradiation, dysphagia, pharyngitis, ulceration of oral cavity, pharynx and neck area, recent voice change, ipsilateral otalgia related to a mass, tonsillar asymmetry, recent ipsilateral hearing loss, epistaxis, nasal obstruction, unintended weight loss, and skin lesions [31].

The ultrasound-guided FNA can be "freehand" using a syringe holder (Cameco, Tayby, Sweden), a 23 gauge or 25 gauge noncutting needle equipped with 10 or 20 ml aspiration syringe [47]. After antiseptic preparation, the needle is advanced 0.5 to 1 cm from the middle of the long axis of the transducer applying suction. After visualization of the needle tip in the lesion, needle should be moved back and forth gently but rapidly through the mass. If the aspirate is bloody, the sample can be obtained through capillary action also called "French" or "Zajdela" technique or "fine-needle non-aspiration" [31]. Capillary action allows cells to move into the needle as it is moved in a back and forth excursion within the mass [47]. Compared to FNA by palpation, ultrasound guidance of FNA improves the sensitivity, specificity, PPV and NPV. Ultrasound guidance allows real-time visualization of the lesion and its adjacent tissue and FNA of smaller, nonpalpable, or complex lesions [48, 49]. Studies reveal that ultrasound-guided FNA resulted in a lower rate of non-diagnostic

cases compared to FNA by palpation (6.7%–12% vs 20.7%–34%) [50, 51]. Ultrasound-guided FNA was 92% sensitive and 90% specific in non-thyroid head and neck FNA cases [51]. In detecting malignant lesions, ultrasound-guided FNA displayed higher accuracy than ultrasound or FNA alone (97% vs. 86% and 92%, respectively) [52]. Ultrasound-guided FNA is considered the first line of evaluation of head and neck masses [52]. Ultrasound guidance confirms the target lesion and occasionally identifies "pseudotumor" or normal anatomy that does not require FNA procedures [53]. An example of ultrasound-guided FNA is shown (Fig. 5.1a-c).

The final diagnosis may remain the same as ROSE in large number of cases (Fig. 5.2).

Performing FNA procedure under palpation is still commonly practiced. It is mostly performed by otolaryngologists, endocrinologists, and pathologists in the outpatient setting [54]. The FNA by palpation is done on both solid and cystic masses measuring 1.0 cm or larger. The setup for the fine-needle aspiration procedure in an Otolaryngology clinical setting also includes a syringe filled with lidocaine (Fig. 5.3). Thyroid nodules, salivary gland masses, lymph nodes, cystic lesions, and any palpable masses are amenable to FNA procedure. A 22-gauge needle is used attached to a disposable 10 ml or 20 ml plastic syringe, which is held in a metal syringe holder (Fig. 5.4).

The operator holds the syringe in one hand while using the other hand to stabilize the mass [1]. The needle is inserted into the mass, vacuum is applied and the needle is moved back and forth quickly and gently. It is allowed the pressure in the syringe to equalize before removing the needle from the mass. Then the syringe is withdrawn from the mass, the needle is detached and air is introduced to into the syringe. The needle is reattached and one drop of the aspirate is expressed onto a glass slide with gentle advancement of the plunger of the syringe [1].

FNAs performed by palpation are associated with a low false negative rate (4%–6.1%) [1, 36] and a small rate of false positive (2%) [36]. There is no delay in diagnosis, no associated complications, and no evidence of tumor seeding in the

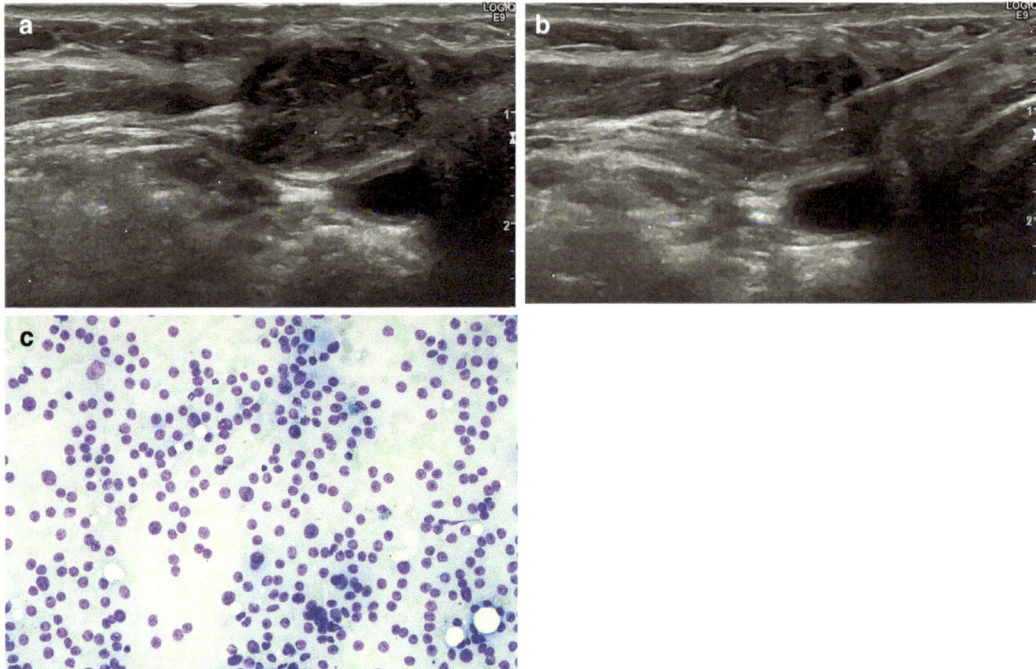

Fig. 5.1 (a-c) is an example of ultrasound-guided FNA with rapid on-site evolution. (a) Ultrasound of an enlarged right level VI lymph node was suspicious for involvement with a malignant process. (b) Ultrasound-guided FNA was performed by a radiologist. Needle track is seen within the lymph node. (c) Rapid on-site evaluation was performed. A Diff-Quik stained slide showed involvement of the lymph node with patient's known Hurthle/onco-cytic cell carcinoma of the thyroid (Diff-Quik stain, smear)

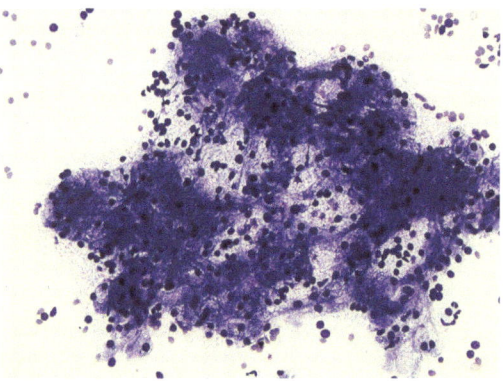

Fig. 5.2 Acinic cell carcinoma is characterized by clus-ters and fragments of relatively uniform round nuclei, abundant finely granular delicate cytoplasm, and rich cap-illary vasculature (Diff-Quik, smear)

needle tract following aspiration of malignant lesions [1]. Ultrasound-guided FNA has the advantage of providing information about the lesion; however, ultrasound increases the cost compared to FNA by palpation.

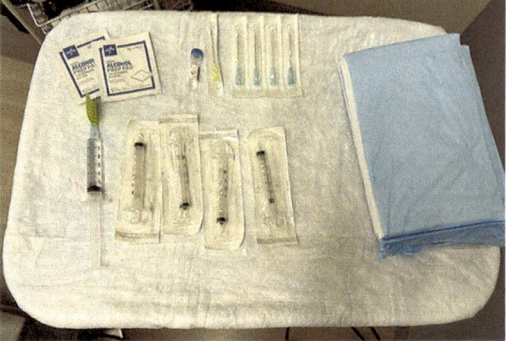

Fig. 5.3 The set up for fine-needle aspiration procedure in Otolaryngology clinical setting includes a syringe filled with lidocaine. In this tray, there is a small container with trans-port medium used for collection of two dedicated passes of thyroid FNA for molecular testing (Courtesy of Dr. Jonathon O. Russell, Otolaryngologist at the Johns Hopkins Hospital; the picture is taken by Dr. Dipan Desai)

Transoral ultrasound-guided FNA is used to evaluate oral lesions and more importantly retro-pharyngeal masses. Transoral ultrasound-guided

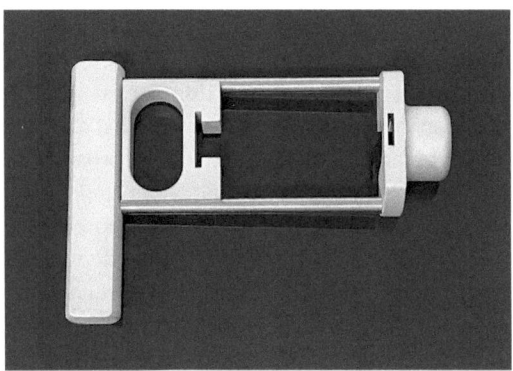

Fig. 5.4 A metal, reusable, aspiration biopsy syringe gun can be used for FNA of palpable masses

FNA is utilized to evaluate retropharyngeal lymph nodes or Rouviere lymph nodes. This technique is occasionally used for intraoperative evaluation of lymph nodes [55, 56].

CT-guided FNA is an accurate, well-tolerated, and safe procedure for the diagnosis of head and neck lesions. CT-guided FNA is an imaging technique of choice for biopsy of deep-seated or poorly localized head and neck lesions when ultrasound is inadequate [45]. CT-guided FNA is occasionally used on nonpalpable lesions, lesions in regions adjacent to critical structures such as carotid arteries, vertebral arteries, or cranial nerves, or postoperative or post-irradiation areas suspicious for recurrence [57]. Most CT-guided head and neck FNA procedures are performed by neuroradiologists due to their more experience of head and neck FNA procedures compared with body imaging radiologists. The growing quantity of cross-sectional imaging studies has led to the detection of nonpalpable head and neck masses, mostly asymptomatic, and found incidentally during imaging studies for other conditions. CT-guided FNA has the advantage of less image degradation by the air-containing aerodigestive system structures, the bony content of the head and neck, and an accurate assessment of adjacent anatomy. In one study, all 216 patients had prior contrast-enhanced CT or MR imaging, which was reviewed to determine appropriate landmarks for tissue sampling. Local anesthesia was administered for all cases. In most cases, a 19-gauge introducer needle was passed to the margin of the lesion, and the aspiration was performed using 22-gauge lumbar puncture spinal needles (Becton Dickinson, Franklin Lakes, NJ). A cytopathologist was present during the procedure to assess the specimen adequacy on site and to determine the number of passes for each case. The aspirated material was processed as air-dried direct smears for Giemsa stain for immediate evaluation and as ethanol fixed for subsequent Papanicolaou staining. The FNA procedure was repeated until adequate diagnostic material was obtained for diagnosis and ancillary studies if requested by the cytopathologist. If a core biopsy was required for diagnosis, a 20-gauge device was used. The FNA sites were labeled as parapharyngeal space, skull base, paraspinal location, thyroid, parotid, and other locations such as the oral cavity, supraglottic larynx, carotid space, paraoesophageal and paratracheal regions, masticator space, supraclavicular space, brachial plexus, and sternocleidomastoid muscle. The majority (90.3%) of cases were adequate for diagnosis, and only 9.7% of the cases were inadequate. A correct diagnosis was made in 88.4% of the cases. The final FNA diagnosis was discordant in 1.9% of the cases, mainly of the parapharyngeal space and parotid gland. The number of passes varied from one to six passes. The most common malignant neoplasms were squamous cell carcinoma, papillary thyroid carcinoma, and adenocarcinoma. Multinodular goiter and pleomorphic adenoma were the most common benign conditions. CT-guided thyroid FNA cases are mostly referral cases by otolaryngologists. The possible minor side effects are pain, minor hemorrhage, vasovagal reaction, and minor infection [58]. Rare severe complications are reported in 0.003–0.031% of patients including pneumothorax, severe hemorrhage, and death [59].

Paramaxillary CT-guided FNA uses a different approach, advancing the needle through the infrazygomatic buccal space in between the maxilla and mandible. A study demonstrated diagnostic material for FNA diagnosis in 85.0% (17/20), all concordant with histology diagnosis [60].

Magnetic resonance image (MRI)-guided FNA in the head and neck is a feasible, safe, well-tolerated procedure by patients and time effective.

It uses different approaches depends on site of the lesion and it can be used in both superficial and deep lesions. Mucosal lesions, parapharyngeal space, skull base, parotid space, submandibular space, cervical vertebral column/paraspinal tissues, larynx/ hypopharynx, and infrahyoid area are among anatomic sites that performed MRI guided FNA has been reported. MRI-compatible 18- to 22-gauge needles (E-Z-EM, Westbury, NY) are utilized for FNA biopsy. The advantages of MRI imaging are excellent tissue contrast and multiplanar imaging capability, no X-ray use, and minimal or no complication. MRI-guided FNA application is limited by the fact that it requires the performer's experience, the facility, and the MRI machine. Moreover, a basic understanding of MRI-guided FNA and its related parameters is essential for a safe, successful, and time-efficient procedure [61].

5.2.1 FNA in Under-Resourced Countries

Fine-needle aspiration is a diagnostic procedure requiring minimal laboratory infrastructure and cost. It is rapid, minimally invasive, well-tolerated by patients, and an inexpensive biopsy technique with a high accuracy rate. It can provide diagnosis in infectious conditions and non-infectious conditions including cancer cases. FNA can be integrated as a diagnostic modality in low-income and middle-income countries to improve health care. This can be made possible by using well-established protocols, and specific training in the technique and interpretation of FNA specimens. Establishing FNA services requires rapid increase in the training of cytopathologists and cytotechnologists, increase education and awareness of clinicians in the diagnostic utility of FNA and commitments from governments, specialists, training groups, and funding [62–64]. Moreover, FNA specimens are utilized for ancillary studies including flow cytometry and molecular studies in high-income countries in the era of personalized medicine, which is gradually spreading to low-income and middle-income countries [63].

5.2.2 Rapid on-Site Evaluation

Rapid on-site evaluation (ROSE) is specimen assessment in real time by a cytologist during an FNA procedure and or core biopsy procedure in order to enhance diagnostic yield and prevent diagnostic delays. The primary purpose of performing ROSE is to enhance the likelihood of an accurate diagnosis by improving adequate sampling of the targeted lesion, thereby preventing inadequate specimens and the need for repeat biopsy [65]. ROSE has been proven to improve specimen adequacy up to 12% [66]. The rate of improvement in specimen adequacy after ROSE depends on the rate of specimen adequacy before ROSE [66]. ROSE allows adequate material is properly collected and allocated for ancillary studies based on the initial cytologic impression. ROSE also allows specimen triage at the site for instance the presence of atypical lymphocytes warrants flow cytometry or a dedicated pass may be collected for thyroglobulin level (TG) assessment in an enlarged lymph node suspicious for metastatic papillary thyroid carcinoma. In routine practice of ROSE and when a cytologist assists a clinician, two passes are performed and then there is a pause for slide preparation and ROSE. An immediate assessment of the aspirated material provides feedback to the FNA performer if the needle of the first pass targets the lesion and if so what is the quantity of the aspirated material. In challenging cases when the lesion is hard to reach due to its anatomic site, small size, being ill-defined, necrotic, or proximity to large vessels or nerves, one pass may be performed for ROSE and then there is a pause for slide preparation. Occasionally, the aspiration site might be adjusted or a different size needle is used to improve the FNA specimen for example if the first pass shows abundant necrosis with few malignant cells on ROSE. In the operating room, ROSE has been reported as a helpful approach of head and neck lesions with 100% specificity, which means no false-positive cases [67].

Specimen adequacy for an accurate diagnosis is determined by cytologist and the number of subsequent passes is usually at the discretion of cytologist. ROSE is a process that a small portion of the aspirated material is used to make direct smears for in real time assessment. In the setting of ROSE, the FNA performer expresses a drop of aspirated material on one slide. A cytotechnologist or a pathologist makes a direct smear and stains it. The slide is examined microscopically for specimen adequacy and a preliminary diagnosis. The preliminary diagnosis may play a major role in treatment of patient in critical conditions. The pathologist can be physically present in the procedure room to examine the slide or remotely can assess the slide [68, 69]. Limited studies claim that telecytology is cost-effective, improves patient care, and provides a more efficient use of the pathologists' time [68]. Studies suggest that ROSE improves quality of cell block [70]. Rose is utilized to evaluate touch imprints of core biopsies in some practices.

ROSE allows specimen triage for ancillary studies. Occasionally dedicated passes are requested by pathologists or cytotechnologist. Needle rinses and remaining material are collected and allocated for cell block preparation and ancillary studies. ROSE with cytomorphologic features concerning for mesenchymal neoplasms demands additional material for molecular and cytogenetic studies (t(X;18) in synovial sarcoma) [28].

ROSE plays an important role in specimen triage of enlarged lymph nodes. Small core biopsy or cell block preparation can be conducted if metastatic carcinoma is the initial impression. TG level assessment can be requested if the lymph node is cystic and metastatic papillary thyroid carcinoma is suspected. FNA can be followed by additional passes for flow cytometry and core biopsies in enlarged lymph nodes suspicious for lymphoma whenever it is feasible. In cases of initial impression of abscess or granulomas on the ROSE, a dedicate pass is triaged for microbiology studies.

ROSE is performed by pathologists or cytotechnologists and there is no difference in their performance regardless of imaging modality used [71]. Considering a limited amount of time for assessment of the specimen, ROSE can be very stressful for the pathologists and cytotechnologists.

Lack of cytology personnel, time-consuming process, inadequate reimbursement, and travel distance between pathology to procedure sites are some factors for not doing ROSE [72].

Depending on the practice setting and the preference of each laboratory, the aspirated material of each pass can be smeared on two slides in the manner of making a blood smear, one can be air-dried and stained with Diff-Quik or methachrome B stain, and the other slide can be immediately fixed by fixing spray or immersing in 95% ethyl alcohol or wet-fixed (Papanicolaou stain, and hematoxylin and eosin stain) staining techniques are used. Both techniques have advantages and disadvantages for instance matrix and cytoplasmic details are better visualized with Diff-Quik stain and nuclear details are better seen with Papanicolaou stain [73].

5.2.3 Steps for FNA Biopsy

The pathologist or the clinician should assess the feasibility of FNA procedure before performing FNA by reviewing the clinical and imaging findings and obtaining clinical history and a targeted physical exam. After completion of assessment and if the lesion is amenable for FNA biopsy, the FNA performer should explain the FNA procedure to the patient along with its benefits and risks. The clinician should communicate with the patient about possible FNA results.

A consent form should be prepared prior to starting FNA biopsy including patient's demographic, the date and time, the biopsy site, and a written list of possible complications. The clinician should proceed to FNA procedure after the consent form is signed by both patient and the clinician. The biopsy site can be marked with a skin marker if it is available.

A set of equipment is needed for performing FNA procedure, which is essentially similar for both by palpation FNA in office setting and by imaging guidance in imaging suits.

Disposable needles 25 to 27 gauge are used for FNA by palpation. The smaller gauge needles yield more cellular and less bloody samples.

Disposable 5–20 ml syringes are needed to produce negative pressure. Syringe holders are commonly used to secure the syringe and allow better precision of targeting the lesion. Cameco syringe holder (Cameco AB, Taby, Sweden) is a model using 10 ml syringes [73].

Glass slides are used for immediate smearing. Slides with frosted ends are commonly used. All slides need to be labeled with at least two patient identifiers. The self-adhesive labels can be created and printed for use or the slides can be handwritten.

The smeared slides can be air-dried and stained with Diff-Quik stain. Fixatives are used to preserve cellular morphology, for instance 95% ethanol in Coplin jars is used for smears that are subsequently stained with Papanicolaou stain [73].

Sterile containers are used for specimen transportation and Hank's balanced salt solution is used for needle rinses. Dedicated passes can be collected for ancillary studies such as microbiology studies or flow cytometry.

Transport medium is used for carrying needle rinses. Hank's balanced salt solution is an example of transport medium.

ThinPrep or PreservCyt vial or CytoLyt or sterile containers can be used for specimen collection for liquid-based collection and ThinPrep preparation methods.

Stains such as Diff-Quik stain or rapid Papanicolaou stain and a microscope are needed if the pathologist does ROSE during the procedure.

Slider holder keeps the slides separate.

Disinfectant agents such as rubbing alcohol wipes, sterile gloves, band-aid, sterile gauze, and a basket are other equipment needed for each FNA procedure. Plastic bags labeled with the patient's identification can be used to store different parts of a specimen in high volume facilities. It is recommended that the aspirator examine the patient and locate the target area before proceeding any further.

Patient either lays down supine on an exam bed or sits on an exam chair. After signing the consent form and timeout (a process to verify the patient identification and the biopsy site), the biopsy site is cleaned with alcohol wipes in a clockwise fashion and from center to periphery for three times or until the surface is clean. It is advised to explain the procedure to the patient at

each step so the patient would have a clear sense of the process.

Local anesthesia is not needed for superficial FNAs performed by palpation since the injection of anesthetists can cause more pain and discomfort for the patient.

The aspirator stabilizes the mass with one hand and secure the lesion between two fingers and inserts the needle that is already mounted in a syringe and syringe-holder with the other hand. When the needle is in the lesion and negative pressure maintained, the needle should be moved back and forth vigorously in order to obtain a cellular material. The negative pressure should be released before the needle is withdrawn. The specimen can be collected without negative pressure in some cases. The cyst fluid should be completely drained if a lesion is cystic. The more passes, the higher probability to have a sufficient specimen. However, the procedure stops after six passes regardless of the specimen adequacy. The needle should be removed immediately and relocated if the patient experiences sharp pain. The procedure will be stopped if that is the patient's wish.

After completion of FNA biopsy, pressure should be applied over the biopsy site and is covered by a band-aid. Patients are advised to avoid vigorous exercise and immersing in water for 24 hours after FNA biopsy. Small bruise of the biopsy site is expected [73].

Safety precautions are mandatory for all FNA cases and all specimens should be considered contaminated.

FNA supply cart or FNA shelf is used for storage of items necessary for FNA procedure (Fig. 5.5a-d). Maintenance of the FNA cart or FNA shelf is essential for smooth operation of FNA clinic. It is imperative to (1) sort out the items in FNA cart or shelf and arrange necessary items in an orderly fashion, (2) remove all unnecessary items, (3) clean the cart and workplace completely, (4) maintain the inventory and checking them every morning [74]. A study has proposed smart FNA cart using lean methods such as value stream mapping (VSM), the 5S method (Sort, Set in order, Shine, Standardize, Sustain), and Kanban improves patient flow [74].

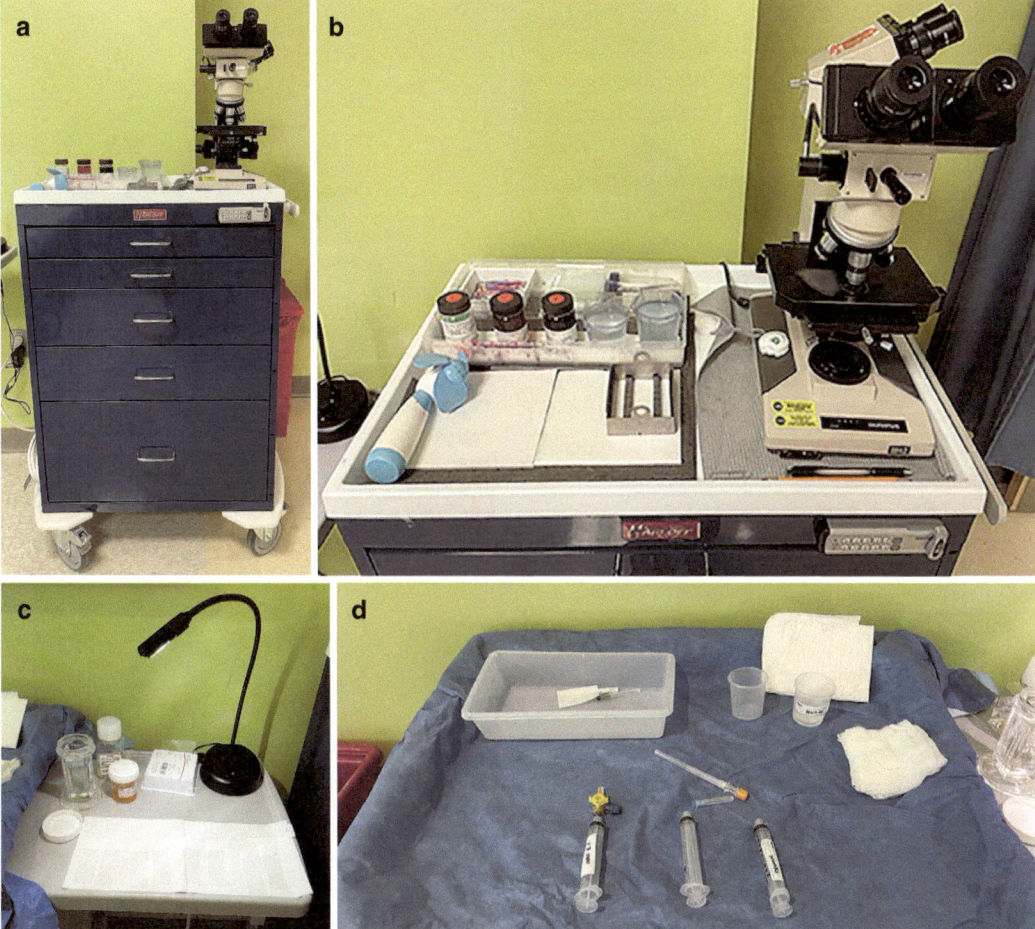

Fig. 5.5 (**a**-**d**) show the equipment and the set up used for fine-needle aspiration in ultrasound biopsy unit. (**a**) The ROSE cart is used for rapid on-site evaluation in ultrasound biopsy suit. The cart has several drawers for storage of equipment needed for ROSE, transport medium, and packaging. (**b**) The top part of the ROSE cart is used for staining the slides and rapid on-site evolution. It contains a bi-headed microscope, Diff-Quik staining setup, and a slide holder. (**c**) A stage that is used for slide preparation. The slides are numbered and then labeled with transparent two identifier labels prior to the procedure (the slides in this picture do not have labels yet for patient's privacy protection for imaging purposes only, and labels were placed after taking the picture). Koplan jar containing 95% ethanol alcohol is used for alcohol fixation of slides to be stained with Papanicolaou stain, and 10% formalin is used for fixation of small core biopsies later to be stained with H&E stain in the Prep laboratory. (**d**) The radiology cart is mainly used for storage of different types of needles. The top part of the ultrasound cart is sterile area used for placement of the FNA procedure equipment such as anesthetic and different needles.

5.2.4 Specimen Processing

The specimen is smeared directly on glass slides or transported in liquid biopsy medium [75]. For direct smears, carefully exert one drop of the sample on the first-third of two slides, starting from the frosted end. Use the third slide (smearing slide) and rapidly but evenly slide on top of the specimen from the frosty end to the opposite side. One slide can be air-dried for Diff-Quik staining and the second smear can be immersed in 95% ethanol for Papanicolaou staining. The residual material in the needle hob is rinsed with Hank's balanced salt solution and collected for further processing in the lab. The final result of a correct smear should be flame shape. Uneven pressure, being too fast or too slow may result in compromise in morphology. ThinPrep is an indirect smearing technique in that the slides are prepared from the aspirated material transferred in the liquid. The cells are more evenly distributed, and the morphology compromise due to suboptimal smearing does not exist; however, ThinPrep preparation is costlier. Needle rinses transported in Hank's balanced salt solution can be processed for cell block creation [76]. A cell block is stained with H&E stain, and similar to histology slides, it can be utilized for ancillary studies such as immunohistochemistry and molecular studies (Fig. 5.6, 5.7, 5.8, 5.9, 5.10 and 5.11).

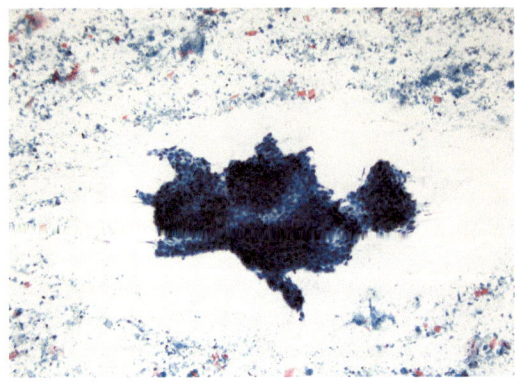

Fig. 5.7 Papanicolaou stain, smear: Metastatic squamous cell carcinoma to the supraclavicular lymph node shows a large fragment of cohesive malignant squamous cells, keratin, with high nuclear to cytoplasmic ratio and hyperchromatic nuclei. Scattered keratinized and non-keratinized squamous cells and necrotic debris are seen in the background

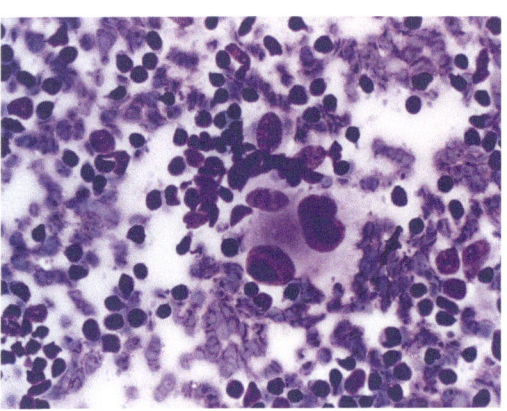

Fig. 5.6 Diff-Quik stain, smear; Hodgkin Lymphoma is characterized by a large Reed- Sternberg cell in the center, surrounded by small lymphocytes. The material was aspirated from an enlarged neck lymph node. Dedicated passes are collated for flow cytometry studies when there is a suspicion of lymphoma, although it might not be helpful in Hodgkin's disease

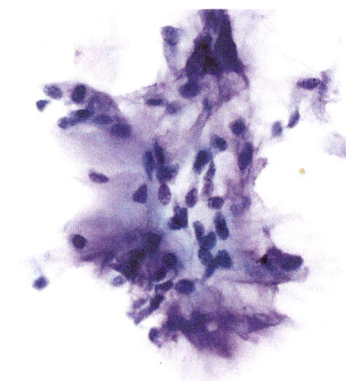

Fig. 5.8 Papanicolaou stain, ThinPrep; Pleomorphic adenoma is characterized by fibrillary matrix, embedded myoepithelial cells, and few epithelial cells at the edge. The FNA was performed by an otolaryngologist at the clinic, and the aspirated material was collected in ThinPrep transport medium

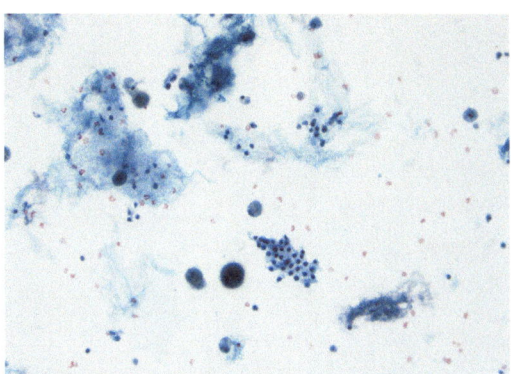

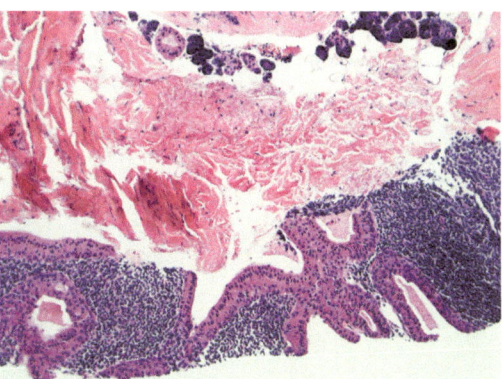

Fig. 5.9 Papanicolaou stain, SurePath; Adenomatoid nodule of the thyroid shows a fragment of follicular cells, a few scattered follicular cells, hemosiderin-laden macrophages (large round cells with abundant cytoplasm and small nuclei), and colloid in strings

Fig. 5.11 H&E stain, formalin-fixed paraffin-embedded; Warthin tumor on a small core biopsy performed subsequently after FNA of the parotid gland comprised of large aggregates of mature small lymphocytes and bilayer oncocytes characterized by abundant eosinophilic cytoplasm. The small core biopsy was performed by a radiologist in an ultrasound biopsy suit, and the specimen was directly placed in formalin

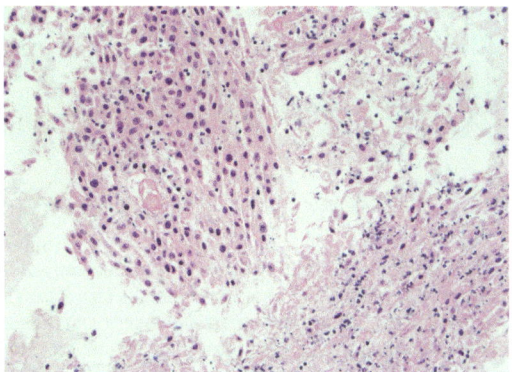

Fig. 5.10 H&E stain, cell block; Metastatic squamous cell carcinoma was presented as a cystic neck mass. The cystic content was collected, and a cell block was prepared. The slide shows a fragment, clusters, and individual malignant squamous cells, keratin, and necrotic debris

5.2.5 Special Studies

Aspirated material can be sent to the microbiology lab if FNA material is suspicious of an infectious process. Aspiration of pus and the presence of numerous neutrophils are suggestive of a bacterial infection, while granulomatous inflammation warrants mycobacterial and fungal studies. Atypical lymphocytes are further investigated by

sending aspirated material for flow cytometry. Histochemical stains can be applied on cell blocks similar to histology blocks. Dedicated passes can be collected and submitted to clinical laboratory for measurement of the TGB level of aspirated material in lymph node specimens suspicious of metastatic papillary thyroid carcinoma or PTH (parathyroid hormone) level of aspirated material can be measured if there is suspicion of parathyroid tissue. Dedicated passes of thyroid nodules can be collected for molecular testing such as Afirma testing in a designated container. It is crucial to do a final check of the paper work of a specimen for proper labeling and special attention should be paid to correct labeling of pair organs (right or left) before leaving the procedure room.

An effective communication between the aspirator and the clinician prior to FNA procedure is the key element in specimen triage. It prevents delay in patient's diagnosis and treatment and avoids repeat FNA for specimen collection for ancillary studies. In addition, there should be instructions available to the staff on how and where to send the specimen for special studies (Fig. 5.12a–d).

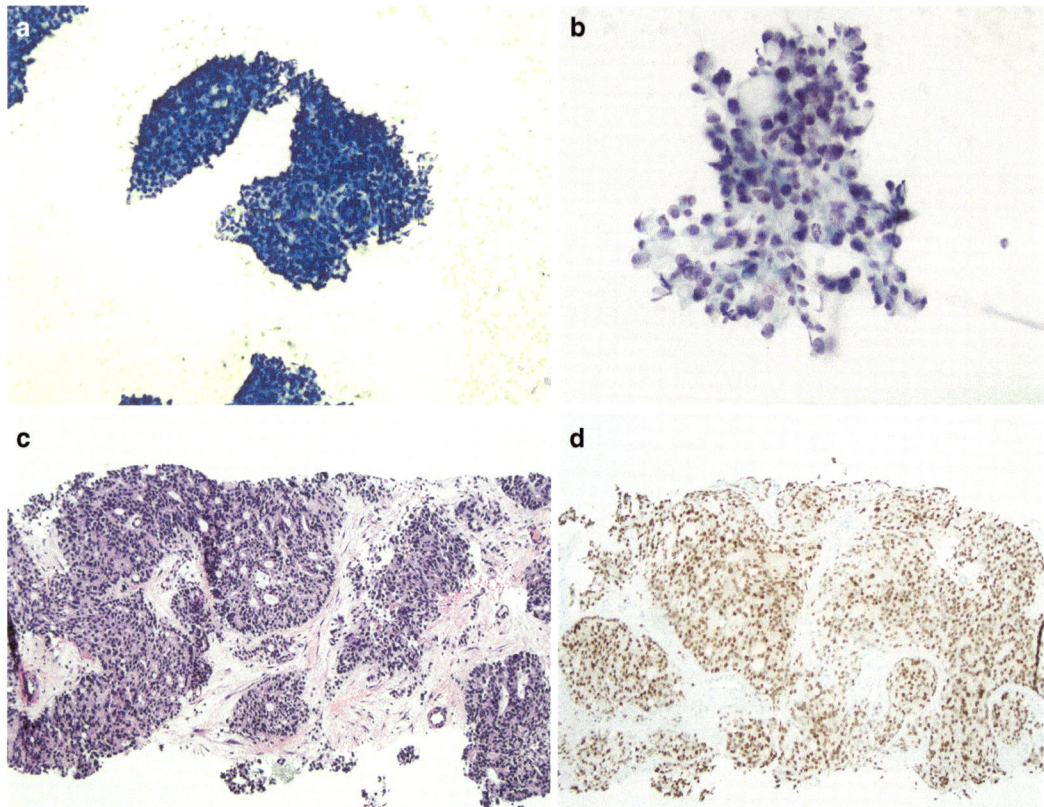

Fig. 5.12 (**a-d**) Metastatic adenocarcinoma consistent with patient's known prostate primary involving a neck lymph node. (**a**) Large fragments of malignant cells are comprised of cohesive cells with focal glandular formation (Diff-Quik, smear). (**b**) A fragment of malignant cells display nuclei with mild to moderate anisonucleosis, coarse chromatin and small nucleoli. The cytoplasm is finely vacuolated. Note: a mitotic figure and a few large intracytoplasmic vacuoles (Papanicolaou stain, smear). (**c**) Metastatic adenocarcinoma is characterized by glandular and cribriform arrangement of malignant cells containing relatively uniform nuclei and moderate to abundant cytoplasm (H&E stain, small core biopsy). (**d**) Nuclear expression of NKX3.1 confirms the diagnosis of prostatic adenocarcinoma (immunostaining, small core biopsy)

5.3 Diagnostic Work-Flow

5.3.1 Accessioning

When the specimen arrives in the cytology laboratory, the specimen should be accessioned. During accessioning process, the paper work and the specimen parts are checked. The staff in accessioning area check all identification data, parts of the specimen, number of slides, and the labels. The possible discrepancies should be resolved before accessioning the case, and the aspirator should be contacted for clarification and solving the issues. The specimen is accessioned and is given a cytol-ogy number when all given information is correct and matches with the specimen. The patient demographic, the biopsy site, the specimen parts, and the details about the FNA process are recorded.

5.3.2 Rush Cases

There are circumstances that which clinicians request the specimen processing gets expedited such as in-patients with deteriorating conditions, or rapidly enlarging masses. These cases can be marked on site for rushing the process so the processing is prioritized.

5.3.3 Processing

The specimen is processed accordingly. The slides stained with Diff-Quik stain are covered with a coverslip. The alcohol-fixed smears are stained with Papanicolaou stain, either manually or automatically. The needle rinses are spun, and a cell block is made if there is a visible pallet at the bottom of the tube. The pallet is fixed is buffered formalin, and it is processed like tissue biopsies and stained with H&E stains. The last step is putting the slides of one case all in one tray and sticking the permanent label on the slides.

5.3.4 Previewing

The stained slides and H&E slide of cell blocks are delivered to cytotechnologists to screen the cases. The cytotechnologists screen the cases. They mark important findings of each slide such as malignant cells, markedly atypical cells and matrix. Cytotechnologists keep a record of cases that they screen including case number, the number of slides, and the diagnosis.

5.3.5 Signing out

The pathologist receives the screened slides. She/he reviews pertinent clinical information, imaging studies, and laboratory tests for each specimen. The pathologist may order ancillary studies such as immunostains or molecular studies. Immunostains are usually ordered and reviewed before releasing a final diagnosis in order to assist the pathologist to further characterize the suspicious cells. Molecular studies are ordered when the diagnosis is final or per the request of the clinician. The diagnosis is entered in the electronic system and the final diagnosis is released.

5.3.6 Quality Assurance

All first-time malignant diagnosis must be reviewed by at least one more pathologist. It is recommended that cases with rare diagnosis or unusual presentations or morphology are reviewed at least by another pathologist. The result of QA must be recorded in the final report.

5.3.7 Filing the Slides

The last step is to file the slides. The slides can be filed based on their accession number, dates, or patient's last name.

5.4 Recommendations

All neck masses warrant further investigation.

Fine-needle aspiration should be performed on neck masses to identify the underlying conditions, differentiate an inflammatory/infectious or a developmental condition from a neoplastic process, and distinguish between benign and malignant neoplasms.

Adequate material should be collected for diagnosis and potential ancillary studies whenever possible, to avoid repeat biopsies and delay in patient care.

Providing a brief explanation in FNA cases without a definitive diagnosis is the key for further work up of the patient.

5.5 Framed Text with the Main Message

Neck masses in adults should be carefully evaluated. Any neck masses, solid, cystic, or solid and cystic, in individuals older than age 40 should be considered malignant until it is proven otherwise.

A detailed history, physical examination including specific exams, and imaging can provide valuable information about the mass.

FNA procedure and aiming for obtaining adequate material for diagnosis and potential ancillary studies is crucial in patient care, and it can prevent repeat biopsies and delays in treatment.

FNA in conjuction with medical history, clinical information, imaging studies, and laboratory findings, plays an important role in clinical decision-making.

In diagnostically challenging FNA cases, the cytopathologist should at least provide information about concerning cytologic findings, limitations of the specimen, and recommend appropriate further follow-up.

References

1. Frable WJ, Frable MA. Thin-needle aspiration biopsy in the diagnosis of head and neck tumors. Laryngoscope. 1974;84(7):1069–77.
2. Diamantis A, Magiorkinis E, Koutselini H. Fine-needle aspiration (FNA) biopsy: historical aspects. Folia Histochem Cytobiol. 2009;47(2):191–7.
3. Naylor B. The century for cytopathology. Acta Cytol. 2000;44(5):709–25.
4. Dupuytren G. On hydatic tumor s developed within muscles and the viscera. Lancet. 1832–33;I:737.
5. Stanley E. Abcess of the liver with hydatids. Lancet. 1833;34I:189–90.
6. Kün M. A new instrument for the diagnosis of tumors. 1846;7:853–4.
7. Lebert H. Physiologie Pathologique. Paris: Balliere; 1847.
8. Ménétrier P. Cancer primitif au poumon. Bull. Soc. Anat. Paris. 1886;61:643–7.
9. Krönig G. Diagnostischer Beitrag zur Hertz-Und Lungenpathologie. Berlin Klin Wschr. 1887;24:961–7.
10. Hirschfeld H. Über isolierte aleukämische Lymphadenose der Haut. Z Krebsforsch. 1912;11:397–407.
11. Guthrie C. Gland puncture as a diagnostic measure. Bull Johns Hopkins Hospital. 1921;32:266–9.
12. Dudgeon L, Patrick S. A new method for the rapid microscopical diagnosis of tumors: with an account of 200 cases so examined. Br J Surg. 1927;15:250–61.
13. Arinkin M. Die intravitale Untersuchungsmethodik des Knochenmarks. Folia Haematol. 1927;38:233–40.
14. Martin H, Ellis E. Aspiration biopsy. Surg Gynecol Obstet. 1934;59:578–89.
15. Mannheim E. Die Bedeutung der Tumorpunktion für die Tumordiagnose. Z. Krebsforsch. 1931;34:572–93.
16. Martin H, Stewart F. The advantages and limitations of aspiration biopsy. Am J Roentgenol. 1936;35:245–7.
17. Söderström N. Puncture of goiters for aspiration biopsy. A preliminary report. Acta Med Scand. 1952;144:237–44.
18. Söderström N. Identification of normal tissues and tumor s by cytologic aspiration biopsy. Acta Soc Med Uppsala. 1958;63:53–87.
19. Franzen S, Giertz G, Zajicek J. Cytological diagnosis of prostatic tumor s by transrectal aspiration biopsy. A preliminary report. Brit J Urol. 1960;32:193–6.
20. Lopes-Cardozo P. Clinical cytology. Leiden: Stafleu; 1954.
21. Lopes-Cardozo P. Atlas of clinical cytology. Leiden; 1978.
22. Zajdela A. Valeur et intérèt du diagnostic cytologique dans les tumeurs du sein par ponction. Etude de 600 cas confrontés cytologiquement et histologiquement. Arch. Ana. Path. 1963;11:85–7.
23. Zajicek J. Aspiration biopsy cytology: part I: cytology of Supradiaphragmatic organs (monographs in clinical cytology), vol. 4. Basel: Karger; 1974.
24. Zajicek J. Aspiration biopsy cytology: part II: Cytology of Infradiaphragmatic organs (monographs in clinical cytology), vol. 7. Basel: Karger; 1979.
25. Koss L. Diagnostic cytology and its histopathologic bases, vol. 242. Philadelphia: Lippincott company; 1961. p. 790.
26. Osborn G. Applied cytology. London: Butterworths; 1953.
27. Allison DB, Miller JA, Coquia SF, Maleki Z. Ultrasonography-guided fine-needle aspiration with concurrent small core biopsy of neck masses and lymph nodes yields adequate material for HPV testing in head and neck squamous cell carcinomas. J Am Soc Cytopathol. 2016;5(1):22–30.
28. Layfield LJ. Fine-needle aspiration in the diagnosis of head and neck lesions: a review and discussion of problems in differential diagnosis. Diagn Cytopathol. 2007;35(12):798–805.
29. Layfield LJ, Gopez E, Hirschowitz S. Cost efficiency analysis for fine-needle aspiration in the workup of parotid and submandibular gland nodules. Diagn Cytopathol. 2006;34(11):734–8.
30. O'Donnell ME, Salem A, Badger SA, Sharif MA, Kamalapurkar D, Lieo T, Spence RA. Fine needle aspiration at a regional head and neck clinic: a clinically beneficial and cost-effective service. Cytopathology. 2009;20(2):81–6.
31. Pynnonen MA, Gillespie MB, Roman B, Rosenfeld RM, Tunkel DE, Bontempo L, Brook I, Chick DA, Colandrea M, Finestone SA, Fowler JC, Griffith CC, Henson Z, Levine C, Mehta V, Salama A, Scharpf J, Shatzkes DR, Stern WB, Youngerman JS, Corrigan MD. Clinical practice guideline: evaluation of the neck mass in adults. Otolaryngol Head Neck Surg. 2017;157(2_suppl):S1–S30.
32. Tandon S, Shahab R, Benton JI, Ghosh SK, Sheard J, Jones TM. Fine-needle aspiration cytology in a regional head and neck cancer center: comparison with a systematic review and meta-analysis. Head Neck. 2008;30(9):1246–52.
33. Gonzalez M, Blanc JM, Pardo J, Bosch R, Vinuela JA. Head and neck fine-needle aspiration: cytohistological correlation. Acta Otorrinolaringol Esp. 2008;59(5):205–11.
34. Hosokawa S, Takebayashi S, Sasaki Y, Nakamura Y, Shinmura K, Takahashi G, Mineta H. Clinical analysis of false-negative fine needle aspiration cytology of head and neck cancers. Postgrad Med. 2019;131(2):151–5.
35. Paker IO, Kulacoglu S, Eruyar T, Ergul G. Fine needle aspiration cytology of head and neck masses: a

cytohistopathological correlation study with emphasis on false positives and false negatives. Kulak Burun Bogaz Ihtis Derg. 2013;23(3):163–72.

36. Tatomirovic Z, Skuletic V, Bokun R, Trimcev J, Radic O, Cerovic S, Strbac M, Zolotarevski L, Tukic L, Stamatovic D, Tarabar O. Fine needle aspiration cytology in the diagnosis of head and neck masses: accuracy and diagnostic problems. J BUON. 2009;14(4):653–9.

37. Vazquez Salas S, Pedro K, Balram A, Syed S, Kotaka K, Kadivar A, Eke BO, McFarland M, Sung M, Behera N, Dubner BG, Maleki Z. Head and neck cystic lesions: a cytology review of common and uncommon entities. Acta Cytol. 2022;66(5):359–70.

38. Allison DB, McCuiston AM, Kawamoto S, Eisele DW, Bishop JA, Maleki Z. Cystic major salivary gland lesions: utilizing fine needle aspiration to optimize the clinical management of a broad and diverse differential diagnosis. Diagn Cytopathol. 2017;45(9):800–7.

39. Lee J, Kazmi S, VandenBussche CJ, Ali SZ. Mesenchymal neoplasms of the head and neck: a cytopathologic analysis on fine needle aspiration. J Am Soc Cytopathol. 2017;6(3):105–13.

40. Gourin CG, Johnson JT. Incidence of unsuspected metastases in lateral cervical cysts. Laryngoscope. 2000;110(10 Pt 1):1637–41.

41. Shah KS, Ethunandan M. Tumour seeding after fine-needle aspiration and core biopsy of the head and neck–a systematic review, Br J Oral Maxillofac Surg. 2016;54(3):260–5.

42. Ali SZ, Cibas ES. The Bethesda system for reporting thyroid cytopathology. Definitions, Criteria and Explanatory Notes. New York, Springer; 2010.

43. Rossi ED, Faquin WC, Baloch Z, Barkan GA, Foschini MP, Kurtycz DF, Pusztaszeri M, Vielh P, editors. The Milan system for reporting salivary gland cytopathology. Springer International Publishing AG.

44. Heslop G, Oliver CL. Modern approach to the neck mass. Surg Clin North Am. 2022;102(2S):c1–6.

45. Hutchins T. Image guided head and neck biopsies: from superficial to deep. Tech Vasc Interv Radiol. 2021;24(3):100769.

46. Robitschek J, Straub M, Wirtz E, Klem C, Sniezek J. Diagnostic efficacy of surgeon-performed ultrasound-guided fine needle aspiration: a randomized controlled trial. Otolaryngol Head Neck Surg. 2010;142(3):306–9.

47. Som PM, Curtin HD. Head and neck imaging. St. Louis: Mosby; 2011.

48. Lieu D. Cytopathologist-performed ultrasound-guided fine-needle aspiration and core-needle biopsy: a prospective study of 500 consecutive cases. Diagn Cytopathol. 2008;36(5):317–24.

49. Wu M. A comparative study of 200 head and neck FNAs performed by a cytopathologist with versus without ultrasound guidance: evidence for improved diagnostic value with ultrasound guidance. Diagn Cytopathol. 2011;39(10):743–51.

50. Conrad R, Yang SE, Chang S, Bhasin M, Sullivan PS, Moatamed NA, Lu DY. Comparison of Cytopathologist-performed ultrasound-guided fine-needle aspiration with Cytopathologist-performed palpation-guided fine-needle aspiration: a single institutional experience. Arch Pathol Lab Med. 2018;142(10):1260–7.

51. Addams-Williams J, Watkins D, Owen S, Williams N, Fielder C. Non-thyroid neck lumps: appraisal of the role of fine needle aspiration cytology. Eur Arch Otorrinolaringol. 2009;266(3):411–5.

52. Horvath L, Kraft M. Evaluation of ultrasound and fine-needle aspiration in the assessment of head and neck lesions. Eur Arch Otorrinolaringol. 2019;276(10):2903–11.

53. Jakowski JD, DiNardo LJ. Advances in head and neck fine-needle aspiration and ultrasound technique for the pathologist. Semin Diagn Pathol. 2015;32(4):284–95.

54. DiMaggio PJ, Kutler DI, Cohen MA, Chen Z, Hoda RS. Cytopathologist-performed ultrasonography-guided fine-needle aspiration of head and neck lesions: the Weill Cornell experience. J Am Soc Cytopathol. 2015;4(6):313–20.

55. Vu TH, Kwon M, Ahmed S, Gule-Monroe M, Chen MM, Sun J, Fornage BD, Debnam JM, Edeiken-Monroe B. Diagnostic accuracy and scope of intraoperative Transoral ultrasound and Transoral ultrasound-guided fine-needle aspiration of retropharyngeal masses. AJNR Am J Neuroradiol. 2019;40(11):1960–4.

56. Shah SB, Singer MI, Liberman E, Ljung BM. Transmucosal fine-needle aspiration diagnosis of intraoral and intrapharyngeal lesions. Laryngoscope. 1999;109(8):1232–7.

57. Sherman PM, Yousem DM, Loevner LA. CT-guided aspirations in the head and neck: assessment of the first 216 cases. AJNR Am J Neuroradiol. 2004;25(9):1603–7.

58. Charboneau JW, Reading CC, Welch TJ. CT and sonographically guided needle biopsy: current techniques and new innovations. AJR Am J Roentgenol. 1990;154(1):1–10.

59. Welch TJ, Sheedy PF 2nd, Johnson CD, Johnson CM, Stephens DH. CT-guided biopsy: prospective analysis of 1,000 procedures. Radiology. 1989;171(2):493–6.

60. Wang D, Chazen JL, Kutler DI, Tassler AB, Phillips CD, Strauss SB. Paramaxillary CT-guided fine needle aspiration of head and neck lesions: technique, diagnostic yield, and safety profile. Neuroradiology. 2022;64(11):2207–11.

61. Merkle EM, Lewin JS, Aschoff AJ, Stepnick DW, Duerk JL, Lanzieri CF, Strauss M. Percutaneous magnetic resonance image-guided biopsy and aspiration in the head and neck. Laryngoscope. 2000;110(3 Pt 1):382–5.

62. Field AS. Training for cytotechnologists and cytopathologists in the developing world. Cytopathology. 2016;27(5):313–6.

63. Field AS. Cytopathology in low medical infrastructure countries: why and how to integrate to capacitate health care. Clin Lab Med. 2018;38(1):175–82.

64. Field AS, Geddie W, Zarka M, Sayed S, Kalebi A, Wright CA, Banjo A, Desai M, Kaaya E. Assisting cytopathology training in medically under-resourced countries: defining the problems and establishing solutions. Diagn Cytopathol. 2012;40(3):273–81.

65. da Cunha Santos G, Ko HM, Saieg MA, Geddie WR. "The petals and thorns" of ROSE (rapid on-site evaluation). Cancer Cytopathol. 2013;121(1):4–8.

66. Schmidt RL, Witt BL, Lopez-Calderon LE, Layfield LJ. The influence of rapid onsite evaluation on the adequacy rate of fine-needle aspiration cytology: a systematic review and meta-analysis. Am J Clin Pathol. 2013;139(3):300–8.

67. Arabi H, Yousef N, Bandyopadhyay S, Feng J, Yoo GH, Al-Abbadi MA. Fine needle aspiration of head and neck masses in the operating room: accuracy and potential benefits. Diagn Cytopathol. 2008;36(6):369–74.

68. Lin O, Rudomina D, Feratovic R, Sirintrapun SJ. Rapid on-site evaluation using telecytology: a major cancer center experience. Diagn Cytopathol. 2019;47(1):15–9.

69. Xing J, Monaco SE, Cuda J, Pantanowitz L. Telecytology rapid on-site evaluation: diagnostic challenges, technical issues and lessons learned. Cytopathology. 2020;31(5):402–10.

70. Collins BT, Garcia TC, Hudson JB. Rapid on-site evaluation improves fine-needle aspiration biopsy cell block quality. J Am Soc Cytopathol. 2016;5(1):37–42.

71. Burlingame OO, Kesse KO, Silverman SG, Cibas ES. On-site adequacy evaluations performed by cytotechnologists: correlation with final interpretations of 5241 image-guided fine-needle aspiration biopsies. Cancer Cytopathol. 2012;120(3):177–84.

72. Sauter JL, Chen Y, Alex D, Balassanian R, Cuda J, Flanagan MB, Griffith CC, Illei P, Johnson DN, McGrath CM, Randolph ML, Reynolds JP, Spiczka AJ, van Zante A, VanderLaan PA, C. American Society of Cytopathology Clinical Practice. Results from the 2019 American Society of Cytopathology survey on rapid onsite evaluation (ROSE)-part 2: subjective views among the cytopathology community. J Am Soc Cytopathol. 2020;9(6):570–8.

73. Orell SR, Sterrett GF, Whitaker D. Fine needle aspiration cytology. 5th ed. London: Elsevier Churchhill Livingstone; 2011.

74. Haghighi M, Nair V, Mashiana SS, Oza T, Zakowski MF. Building a smart FNA cart: when Google meets cytology. Cancer Cytopathol. 2020;128(12):948–61.

75. Robinson I. A diagnostic head and neck fine needle aspiration service can be provided using liquid-based cytology only. Cytopathology. 2017;28(1):24–30.

76. Carter MD, Moore DP, MacIntosh RF, Bullock MJ. Impact of routine cell block preparation on results of head and neck fine needle aspirates. Diagn Cytopathol. 2016;44(11):880–7.

Maleki Zahra Associate Professor of pathology at the Johns Hopkins University School of Medicine, at the Johns Hopkins Hospital, Division of Cytopathology, Baltimore, MD, USA. Director of the Johns Hopkins Medical School Scientific Foundations of Medicine, Histology and Pathobiology course. Member of Cancer Registry Committee, co-chair of the Membership Committee at the American Society of Cytopathology and an active committee member at the American Society of Cytopathology and the USA and Canadian Academy of Pathology.

Chien-Chin Chen

6.1 Introduction

Head and neck anatomy is intricate due to the proximity of numerous functioning systems. Head and neck lesions encompass a vast array of pathologic conditions. These lesions may result from developmental abnormalities or benign or malignant neoplastic alteration of normal tissue. Deficiencies in the relevant structures' organogenesis, histogenesis, or functional maturity can lead to developmental issues. Therefore, these lesions can manifest at any stage during life, typically due to the interplay of environmental and hereditary variables.

This chapter highlights and examines the general principles for processing and interpreting histological specimens and the most critical diagnostic characteristics of epithelial and mesenchymal neoplasms of the head and neck. Histological patterns and/or subpatterns are distinctive of specific tumors or groups of tumors [1]; hence, these specific patterns are essential for histopathological diagnosis. The understanding of numerous patterns and subpatterns in various malignancies aids in the diagnosis and administration of the most effective treatment.

6.2 Techniques

Any symptomatic head and neck mass should prompt referral to a head and neck specialist who will thoroughly evaluate and perform a proper examination. For example, a flexible fiberoptic laryngoscopy examination evaluates the larynx and pharynx.

A tissue-based examination is essential for further management. For a neck mass, fine-needle aspiration (FNA) is utilized; it is well tolerated, accurate, and, unlike an open biopsy, does not affect future treatment. Oral lesions are usually assessed with incisional biopsy or brush biopsy. Endoscopic biopsies of lesions in the nasopharynx, oropharynx, and larynx are preferable.

Nevertheless, a core needle biopsy (CNB) for histological evaluation or minimally invasive FNA cytology may be debated for the initial tissue evidence. Meta-analyses for head and neck lesions [2], salivary gland neoplasms [3], and thyroid gland [4] demonstrated CNB yielded fewer nondiagnostic results compared with FNA. Compared to FNA, CNB had higher diagnostic efficacy in detecting salivary gland cancers [3]. However, a higher incidence of architectural

C.-C. Chen (✉)
Department of Pathology, Ditmanson Medical Foundation Chia-Yi Christian Hospital, Chiayi, Taiwan

Department of Biotechnology and Bioindustry Sciences, College of Bioscience and Biotechnology, National Cheng Kung University, Tainan, Taiwan

Department of Cosmetic Science, Chia Nan University of Pharmacy and Science, Tainan, Taiwan

Ph.D. Programin Translational Medicine, National Chung Hsing University, Taichung, Taiwan

atypia and follicular neoplasm occurred in thyroid CNB [4]. Herein, FNA combined with ultrasound imaging should continue to be the investigational technique of choice, saving CNB for patients with repeated failures of FNA or considering conservative treatment. Further, while ultrasound-guided FNA is simple and reliable enough to be widely applied for head and neck masses and thyroid nodules, there was no difference in the diagnostic rates, adverse events, or number of passes, whether advanced practice providers or interventional radiologists performed the procedure [8]. The general pipeline for diagnosing head and neck tumors is illustrated in Fig. 6.1.

In addition, ultrasound-guided biopsies are more routinely requested and used for most superficial targets. CT-guided biopsies are often reserved for deeper sites, most commonly around the skull base or in parapharyngeal or retropharyngeal areas that are inaccessible through ultrasonography. Regarding the needle, CNB needles are either side-cutting or end-cutting [6, 7]. The side-cutting needles comprise the outer cutting shaft and inner stylet with a specimen notch. Under ultrasound guidance, the needle tip is introduced to the edge of the target tissue, and the inner stylet is advanced into it with a portion of the tissue prolapsing into the specimen notch.

The outer cutting shaft advances to resheath the inner stylet and cut out the specimen core. Then, remove the specimen from the specimen notch. However, side-cutting needles have two primary drawbacks. The first is that the part of the stylet (usually around 0.5 cm) projecting beyond the specimen notch and outer shaft may have to protrude outside the target to accommodate the specimen notch in the best position for minor lesions, putting surrounding structures in danger. Herein, it may make biopsy difficult if neck lesions are near major vessels. Second, the specimen notch limits the sample obtained with each pass; therefore, numerous punctures and passes are needed to get enough tissue samples. This is common when histology, microbiological, and biochemical specimen testing are expected.

Comparably, the end-cutting needles are composed of an outer trochar and an inner stylet [7]. The needle is inserted under ultrasound guidance so that the needle tip is located within the center of the target. The trochar is then connected to a syringe via a connection tube once the inner stylet has been removed. Under real-time ultrasound guidance, the stylet is moved back and forth and rotated while applying suction with a syringe to retrieve the specimen. Reintroducing trochar or saline flush into the specimen bottle will remove the sample from the needle. The use of the end-

Diagnostic algorithm for head and neck tumors

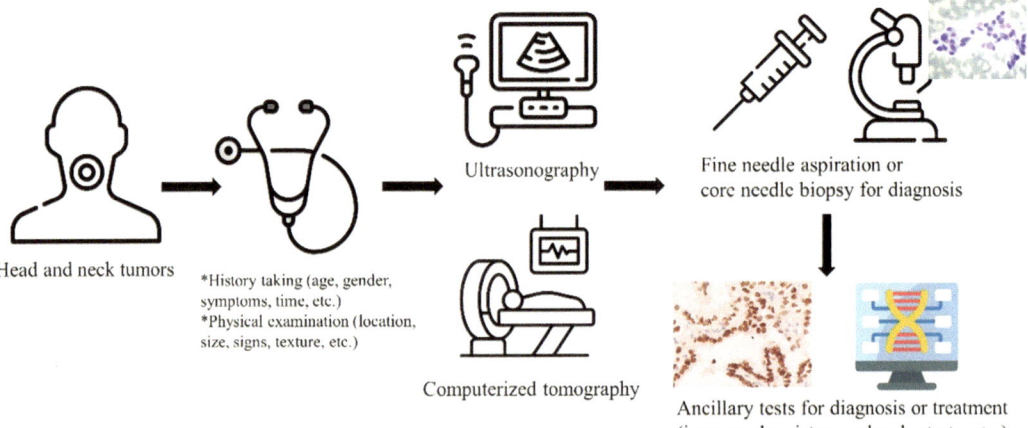

Head and neck tumors *History taking (age, gender, symptoms, time, etc.) *Physical examination (location, size, signs, texture, etc.)

Ultrasonography

Computerized tomography

Fine needle aspiration or core needle biopsy for diagnosis

Ancillary tests for diagnosis or treatment (immunochemistry, molecular tests, etc.)

Fig. 6.1 The general approaches for diagnosing head and neck tumors

cutting needle is simple and comparable to the employment of fine needles for cytology aspiration. Therefore, it is safe to be used on lesions near vital structures regardless of the size as long as the needle tract is clear and the cutting needle tip is kept inside the target tissue [7]. In addition, the end-cutting needle can typically gather adequate tissue samples in a single pass, as lengthy cores of tissue are returned into the needle lumen by the cutting and suction mechanism, as opposed to side-cutting needles, which are limited by the size of the specimen notch [7].

Deep head and neck masses are challenging to approach securely and accurately due to the critical anatomy. In terms of deep soft tissue masses in the head and neck that are difficult to reach using palpation, sonography, or laryngoscopy, computerized tomography (CT)-guided percutaneous core biopsy can be a safe and effective method, eliminating the need for open biopsies and the associated risks in those locations [5]. To limit the risk of vascular injury, it also outlines the use of CT angiography for vessel localization and mapping prior to needle placement after patient positioning on the procedural table [5].

Tumor excision is still the gold standard for a definitive diagnosis in the head and neck because the tissue architecture is retained, and sufficient tissue is available for any supplementary investigation. However, excisional biopsy often requires general anesthesia and a relatively stable, tolerant body condition, given the burdens of invasive procedures and surgical risks.

6.3 Diagnostic Workflow

Despite the varying locations of origin and complex anatomy that result in the different types of resections in the head and neck neoplasm, there are general principles for the histological evaluation technique [10] [11]. The histopathological assessment and diagnostic roadmap for head and neck lesions primarily depend on the location and morphological patterns. Dive et al. aimed to diagnose head and neck tumors based on the six major histological patterns: glandular/pseudo-glandular, nonglandular epithelial/epithelioid pattern, round cell pattern, spindle cell pattern, biphasic pattern, surface epithelial patterns associated with or affected by neoplastic process [1]. Based on their patterns, Table 6.1 provides the modified results with updated information. For example, sinonasal tract angiofibroma is histologically constituted of various-sized vasculature and cellular fibrotic stroma containing bipolar or stellate fibroblasts, affecting exclusively young men (Fig. 6.2). In addition, sclerosing microcystic adenocarcinoma, a new entity, is characterized by ducts/tubules, strands/cords, and nests that heavily infiltrate the surrounding collagenous stroma (Fig. 6.3). Two types of cells coexist in

Table 6.1 Major histological patterns and corresponding tumors

Growth patterns	Head and neck neoplasms
1. Glandular/pseudoglandular	
1.1 Tubular pattern	Adenoid cystic carcinoma, polymorphous adenocarcinoma, basal cell adenocarcinoma, basal cell adenoma, striated duct adenoma
1.2 Acinar/microacinar pattern	Acinic cell carcinoma, polymorphous adenocarcinoma
1.3 Cribriform pattern	Adenoid cystic carcinoma, intraductal carcinoma, polymorphous adenocarcinoma (cribriform subtype)
1.4 Follicular pattern	Acinic cell carcinoma, clear cell carcinoma, follicular ameloblastoma, secretory carcinoma
1.5 Microcystic pattern	Acinic cell carcinoma, sclerosing microcystic adenocarcinoma, microsecretory adenocarcinoma, secretory carcinoma, polymorphous adenocarcinoma
1.6 Mucinous cell pattern	Mucinous adenocarcinoma,
1.7 Canalicular pattern	Canalicular adenoma, pleomorphic adenoma, basal cell adenoma, polymorphous adenocarcinoma, adenoid cystic carcinoma

(continued)

Table 6.1 (continued)

Growth patterns	Head and neck neoplasms
1.8 Oncocytic cell pattern	Mucoepidermoid carcinoma (oncocytic variant), intraductal carcinoma (oncocytic type), Warthin tumor, oncocytoma, cystadenoma of salivary gland (papillary oncocytic subtype)
1.9 Pseudoglandular pattern	Adenoid basal cell carcinoma, squamous cell carcinoma, myxoid liposarcoma
2. Nonglandular/epithelial/epithelioid pattern	
2.1 Basaloid pattern	Basal cell carcinoma, cylindroma, sialoblastoma, basal cell adenoma, basal cell hyperplasia, basal cell ameloblastoma
2.2 Comedo pattern	Salivary duct carcinoma
2.3 Alveolar pattern	Rhabdomyosarcoma, melanoma, intradermal nevus with pseudovascular spaces
2.4 Packeted pattern	Melanoma, desmoplastic small round cell tumor
2.5 Palisading pattern	Basal cell carcinoma, schwannoma, palisaded encapsulated neuroma, keratocystic odontogenic tumor
2.6 Reticular/lattice pattern	Acinic cell tumor, pleomorphic adenoma, myoepithelioma
2.7 Squamoid pattern	Squamous cell carcinoma, adenosquamous carcinoma, mucoepidermoid carcinoma, nasopharyngeal carcinoma, hyalinizing clear cell carcinoma
2.8 Trabecular pattern	Myoepithelial carcinoma, Merkel cell tumors, smooth muscle tumors, basal cell adenoma
2.9 Desmoplastic/scirrhous pattern	Basal cell carcinoma, fibrosarcoma, sclerosing polycystic adenoma, hyalinizing clear cell carcinoma
2.10 Solid nested pattern	Sebaceous adenocarcinoma, melanoma, Spitz nevus
3. Round cell pattern	
3.1 Diffuse pattern	Lymphoma, leukemia, small-cell carcinoma, undifferentiated carcinoma, Ewing's Sarcoma, Merkel cell tumor, melanoma
3.2 Septate/lobulated pattern	Ewing's sarcoma, alveolar rhabdomyosarcoma
3.3 Alveolar/pseudoalveolar pattern	Alveolar rhabdomyosarcoma
3.4 Round cell pattern with rosettes	Primitive neuroectodermal tumor, adenomatoid odontogenic tumor, neuroblastoma
3.5 Hobnail pattern	Hemangioendothelioma, angiosarcoma
3.6 Slit-like pattern	Angiosarcoma
4. Spindle cell pattern	
4.1 Diffuse monomorphic bland pattern	Fibromatosis, nodular fasciitis, salivary gland myoepithelioma, neurofibroma, schwannoma, smooth muscle tumors
4.2 Diffuse monomorphic highly cellular pattern	Malignant peripheral nerve sheath tumor, melanoma, myoepithelial carcinoma
4.3 Pleomorphic spindle cell pattern	Undifferentiated/unclassified sarcoma, spindle cell squamous cell carcinoma, lymphoepithelial carcinoma
4.4 Spindle cell pattern with prominent sclerosis	Sclerosing liposarcoma, desmoplastic melanoma, epithelioid sarcoma, sclerosing fibrosarcoma
4.5 Whorled/storiform pattern	Dermatofibrosarcoma protuberans, benign fibrous histiocytoma, soft tissue perineurioma
4.6 Hemangiopericytomatous pattern	Solitary fibrous tumor, mesenchymal chondrosarcoma, sinonasal glomangiopericytoma
5. Biphasic pattern	Adenoid cystic carcinoma, epithelial-myoepithelial carcinoma, malignant peripheral nerve sheath tumor, perivascular epithelioid cell tumor, sclerosing microcystic adenocarcinoma, carcinosarcoma, basal cell adenocarcinoma, basal cell adenoma, pleomorphic adenoma, intercalated duct lesions, myopericytoma/myofibroma, sinonasal tract angiofibroma

Table 6.1 (continued)

Growth patterns	Head and neck neoplasms
6. Surface epithelial patterns	
6.1 Lichenoid reaction pattern	Intraepidermal carcinoma, lichen planus-like keratosis, lichenoid reaction, seborrheic keratosis, flat wart
6.2 Psoriasiform pattern	Mycosis fungiodes, clear cell acanthoma
6.3 Clear cells within epidermis	Verrucous carcinoma, clear cell variant of squamous cell carcinoma, clear cell acanthoma
6.4 Dysplastic changes of epithelium	Carcinoma in situ, hyperkeratosis complex, actinic keratosis,
6.5 Pseudoepitheliomatous hyperplastic pattern	Melanoma, Spitz nevus, granular cell tumor
6.6 Pattern with cup-shaped/ inverted lobules of squamous epithelium	Follicular keratosis, keratoacanthoma, warty dyskeratoma, molluscum contagiosum
6.7 Nesting/clonal proliferation (Borst-Jadassohn pattern)	Intraepidermal basal cell carcinoma, intraepidermal squamous cell carcinoma, melanoma, clonal seborrheic keratosis
6.8 Pagetoid pattern	Pagetoid Bowen disease, superficial spreading of melanoma, extramammary Paget disease
6.9 Elongated anastomosing strands	Fibroepithelial variant of basal cell carcinoma, reticulated seborrheic keratosis
6.10 Verrucous pattern	Verrucous carcinoma, verrucous xanthoma, seborrheic keratosis, condyloma acuminatum, viral wart

Note: The table was modified from the reference Dive AM et al. and the fifth edition of the World Health Organization Classification of Head and Neck Tumors

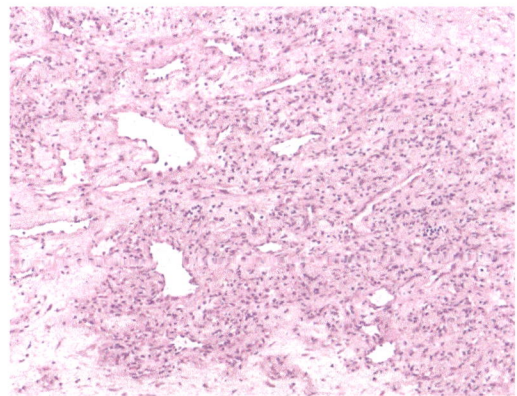

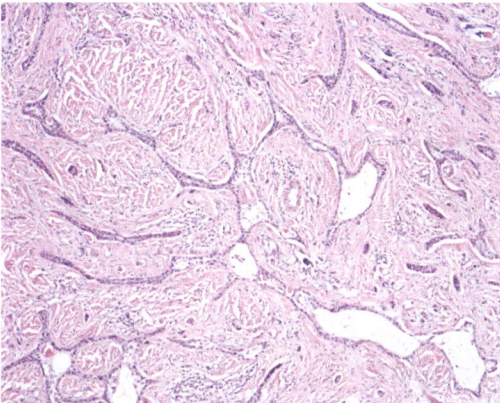

Fig. 6.2 Sinonasal tract angiofibroma comprises proliferative slit-like capillaries to irregularly dilated and branching blood channels. Stromal cellularity ranges from loose and edematous to heavily collagenized with bipolar or stellate fibroblastic cells bearing plump, vesicular, spindled nuclei and inconspicuous nucleoli. Mitoses are rare. (HE stain, 100×)

Fig. 6.3 Sclerosing microcystic adenocarcinoma is characterized by significantly infiltrative ducts/tubules, strands/cords, and nests in densely collagenous stroma and has a biphasic cell population made up of flattened myoepithelial cells and luminal ductal cells with monotonous nuclei and uniformly dispersed chromatin. (HE stain, 100×)

the epithelium: the flattened myoepithelial cells and the round to oval luminal cells whose nuclei are uniformly dispersed [12].

Over 90% of all malignant neoplasms affecting the head and neck are squamous cell carcinomas (SqCC), making this cancer extremely significant and frequent [13]. In particular, in the oral cavity, tongue, oropharynx, hypopharynx, larynx, trachea, and parapharyngeal space, SqCC and its variants are unquestionably the most prevalent malignancies at these sites, yet novel information is scarce [14] [15] [16].

In the oral cavity and tongue, most malignancies are typical keratinizing SqCC. However, carcinoma cuniculatum and verrucous carcinoma are distinct entities frequent in the area with unique clinical and pathologic features than ordinary squamous cell carcinoma [14]. Carcinoma cuniculatum is extremely well-differentiated, devoid of cytological malignancy, and has a burrowing invasion pattern and destructive bone invasion without metastases. Comparably, verrucous carcinoma is a surface carcinoma with verrucous architecture that lacks atypia and demonstrates pushing cohesive invasion with a good prognosis, sluggish behavior, and predominantly laterally spreading carcinoma that poses a long-term risk of squamous carcinoma development.

Regarding the hypopharynx, larynx, trachea, and parapharyngeal space, since SqCC is the most prevalent cancer, precancerous lesions are important to recognize. They can be divided into two classifications using either a two-tiered system with low-grade dysplasia/squamous intraepithelial lesions (SIL) and high-grade dysplasia/SIL or a three-tiered system with an extra category, carcinoma in situ (CIS) [16]. Table 6.2 demonstrates the differences between two- and three-tiered systems. The subtypes of SqCC include lymphoepi-

thelial carcinoma, verrucous carcinoma, basaloid SqCC, papillary SqCC, spindle cell squamous carcinoma, and adenosquamous carcinoma with different prognostic significance.

About 80% of salivary tumors are found in the main salivary glands (parotid and submandibular), while 20% originate in minor salivary glands, frequently in odd sites [9]. However, due to their rarity and widespread anatomical distribution, diagnostic techniques, prognoses, and treatment strategies are frequently distinct and less established. For instance, the increased frequency of incisional biopsies in minor salivary tumors usually has complex repercussions.

Salivary gland tumors exhibit a variety of histological and clinical characteristics. Due to the rarity of these tumors and their heterogeneous histology, there is insufficient research that can be used to offer solid recommendations for each unique salivary gland tumor. Besides the morphological diversity and diagnostic difficulties, new distinguishing genetic changes have been identified in several salivary gland cancers. Specifically, they consist of gene fusions, which have been demonstrated to be highly tumor-type specific and, hence, advantageous in diagnostically problematic instances. In addition, recurrent molecular changes were incorporated into the definitions of mucoepidermoid carcinoma, adenoid cystic carcinoma, secretory carcinoma, polymorphous adenocarcinoma, hyalinizing clear cell carcinoma, mucinous adenocarcinoma, and microsecretory adenocarcinoma [17].

In terms of head and neck neuroendocrine neoplasms, the updated classification contains epithelial neuroendocrine neoplasms (neuroendocrine tumors and neuroendocrine carcinomas) arising from the upper aerodigestive tract and salivary glands, as well as unique neuroendocrine

Table 6.2 Two- and three-tiered systems for grading laryngeal and hypophayrngeal epithelial dysplasia

Clinical relevance	Extension of epithelial abnormalities	2-tiered grading system	3-tiered grading system
Low-risk	The lower half of the epithelium	Low-grade dysplasia/ SIL	Low-grade dysplasia/ SIL
High-risk	More than the lower half of the epithelium	High-grade dysplasia/ SIL	High-grade dysplasia/ SIL
	Whole thickness		CIS

SIL squamous intraepithelial lesions, *CIS* carcinoma in situ

neoplasms such as middle ear neuroendocrine tumors (MeNET), ectopic or invasive pituitary neuroendocrine tumors (PitNET), Merkel cell carcinoma, and non-epithelial neuroendocrine neoplasms (paragangliomas) [18]. In this classification, well-differentiated epithelial neuroendocrine neoplasms are referred to as neuroendocrine tumors (NETs), which are categorized as G1 NET (no necrosis and < 2 mitoses per 2 mm^2; Ki67 < 20%), G2 NET (necrosis or 2–10 mitoses per 2 mm^2; Ki67 < 20%), and G3 NET (> 10 mitoses per 2 mm^2 or Ki67 > 20%, and absence of poorly differentiated cytomorphology) (Table 6.3). Based on cytomorphological features, neuroendocrine carcinomas (> 10 mitoses per 2 mm^2, Ki67 > 20%) are further subtyped as small-cell and large-cell neuroendocrine carcinomas. In contrast to neuroendocrine carcinomas, head and neck NETs often lack abnormal p53 expression and RB loss.

6.4 Recommendations

Before surgery, a clinically suspected cancer should be confirmed by biopsy or cytology. To maximize the information received from each mode of study, cytopathological and histological findings should be addressed with surgeons and radiologists. Surgeons and oncologists must comprehend the extent and limitations of cellular pathology in order to contribute to interprofessional conversations. Pathological examinations are the foundation of appropriate cancer staging and outcome classification. Therefore, accurately diagnosing cancer is essential for appropriate treatment. The recommendations for pathology practice and histological diagnosis should be established on published data with essential references determined by the updated World Health Organization (WHO) Classification of Tumors.

Table 6.3 The 2022 World Health Organization (WHO) classification for epithelial neuroendocrine neoplasms of the upper aerodigestive tract and salivary glands

Morphological difference	Neoplasms	Criteria
Well-differentiated neuroendocrine neoplasm (neuroendocrine tumor, NET)	Well-differentiated neuroendocrine tumor, grade 1. (NET, G1)	No necrosis and < 2 mitoses/2 mm^2 Ki67 < 20%
	Well-differentiated neuroendocrine tumor, grade 2. (NET, G2)	Necrosis and/or 2–10 mitoses/2 mm^2 Ki67 < 20%
	Well-differentiated neuroendocrine tumor, grade 3. (NET, G3)	>10 mitoses/2 mm^2 Ki67 > 20% Without poorly differentiated cytomorphology
Poorly differentiated neuroendocrine neoplasm (neuroendocrine carcinoma, NEC)	Small-cell neuroendocrine carcinoma	>10 mitoses/2 mm^2 Ki67 > 20% (often >70%) Small-cell NEC cytomorphology[*]
	Large-cell neuroendocrine carcinoma	>10 mitoses/2 mm^2 Ki67 > 20% (often >50%) Large-cell NEC cytomorphology[**]

[*]Small-cell NEC cytomorphology: Cell size less than the width of three lymphocytes, hyperchromatic nuclei, finely granular chromatin, imperceptible nucleoli, significant apoptotic bodies, and necrosis
[**]Large-cell NEC cytomorphology: Nested, organoid, or trabecular growth accompanied by abundant cytoplasm, spherical nuclei with conspicuous nucleoli, peripheral palisading, rosette formation, and comedo necrosis

References

1. Dive AM, Bodhade AS, Mishra MS, Upadhyaya N. Histological patterns of head and neck tumors: an insight to tumor histology. J Oral Maxillofac Pathol. 2014;18:58–68. https://doi.org/10.4103/0973-029x.131912.
2. Novoa E, Gürtler N, Arnoux A, Kraft M. Role of ultra-sound-guided core-needle biopsy in the assessment of head and neck lesions: a meta-analysis and systematic review of the literature. Head Neck. 2011;34:1497–503. https://doi.org/10.1002/hed.21821.
3. Cho J, Kim J, Lee JS, et al. Comparison of core needle biopsy and fine-needle aspiration in diagnosis of malignant salivary gland neoplasm: systematic review and meta-analysis. Head Neck. 2020;42:3041–50. https://doi.org/10.1002/hed.26377.
4. Ahn S-H. Usage and diagnostic yield of fine-needle aspiration cytology and Core needle biopsy in thyroid nodules: a systematic review and meta-analysis of literature published by Korean authors. Clin Exp Otorhinolaryngol. 2021;14:116–30. https://doi.org/10.21053/ceo.2020.00199.
5. Hillen TJ, Baker JC, Long JR, et al. Percutaneous CT-guided Core needle biopsies of head and neck masses: technique, histopathologic yield, and safety at a single academic institution. Am J Neuroradiol. 2020;41:2117–22. https://doi.org/10.3174/ajnr.a6784.
6. Yamashita Y, Kurokawa H, Takeda S, et al. Preoperative histologic assessment of head and neck lesions using cutting needle biopsy. Oral Surg Oral Med Oral Pathol Oral Radiol Endod. 2002;93:528–33. https://doi.org/10.1067/moe.2002.123867.
7. Yuen HY, Lee Y, Bhatia K, et al. Use of end-cutting needles in ultrasound-guided biopsy of neck lesions. Eur Radiol. 2011;22:832–6. https://doi.org/10.1007/s00330-011-2323-z.
8. Paez SN, Zawacki W, Nolan T, Wicky van Doyer S. Performance of advanced practice providers compared with that of physician providers in ultrasound-guided fine-needle aspiration of thyroid nodules and superficial neck masses. J Vasc Interv Radiol. 2022; https://doi.org/10.1016/j.jvir.2022.08.029.
9. Ihrler S, Agaimy A, Guntinas-Lichius O, et al. Why is the histomorphological diagnosis of tumours of minor salivary glands much more difficult? Histopathology. 2021;79:779–90. https://doi.org/10.1111/his.14421.
10. Helliwell TR, Giles TE. Pathological aspects of the assessment of head and neck cancers: United Kingdom National Multidisciplinary Guidelines. The Journal of Laryngology & Otology. 2016;130:S59–65. https://doi.org/10.1017/s0022215116000451.
11. López F, Mäkitie A, de Bree R, et al. Qualitative and quantitative diagnosis in head and neck cancer. Diagnostics. 2021;11:1526. https://doi.org/10.3390/diagnostics11091526.
12. Lee Y-Y, Hwang T-Z, Jin Y-T, Chen C-C. Sclerosing microcystic adenocarcinoma arising from the tongue: a case report and literature review. Diagnostics. 2022;12:1288. https://doi.org/10.3390/diagnostics12051288.
13. Thompson LDR. Squamous cell carcinoma variants of the head and neck. Curr Diagn Pathol. 2003;9:384–96. https://doi.org/10.1016/s0968-6053(03)00069-3.
14. Muller S, Tilakaratne WM. Update from the 5th edition of the World Health Organization classification of head and neck Tumors: tumours of the Oral cavity and Mobile tongue. Head Neck Pathol. 2022;16:54–62. https://doi.org/10.1007/s12105-021-01402-9.
15. Badoual C. Update from the 5th edition of the World Health Organization classification of head and neck Tumors: oropharynx and nasopharynx. Head Neck Pathol. 2022;16:19–30. https://doi.org/10.1007/s12105-022-01449-2.
16. Zidar N, Gale N. Update from the 5th edition of the World Health Organization classification of head and neck Tumors: hypopharynx, larynx, trachea and Parapharyngeal space. Head Neck Pathol. 2022;16:31–9. https://doi.org/10.1007/s12105-021-01405-6.
17. Skálová A, Hyrcza MD, Leivo I. Update from the 5th edition of the World Health Organization classification of head and neck Tumors: salivary glands. Head Neck Pathol. 2022;16:40–53. https://doi.org/10.1007/s12105-022-01420-1.
18. Mete O, Wenig BM. Update from the 5th edition of the World Health Organization classification of head and neck Tumors: overview of the 2022 WHO classification of head and neck neuroendocrine neoplasms. Head Neck Pathol. 2022;16:123–42. https://doi.org/10.1007/s12105-022-01435-8.

Chien-Chin Chen President of the Taiwan Society of Clinical Cytology, Associate Professor at National Chung Hsing University (Taiwan) and Chia Nan University of Pharmacy and Science (Taiwan), Editorial Board of "Cancer Cytopathology" and "Cytopathology," and pathologist at Ditmanson Medical Foundation Chia-Yi Christian Hospital (Taiwan).

Immunohistochemistry of the Head and Neck Masses

Jan Klos

7.1 Introduction

The basic requirement for successful immunohistochemistry, like for any other test, is a sufficient amount of properly preserved representative material. There is a quite wide tolerance regarding the amount of the material (from the cell blocks with the few diagnostic cells to large operation specimens), but compromising the quality of the material may often lead to confusion and erroneous conclusions.

7.2 Immunohistochemical Method

The main principle of immunohistochemistry is a specific binding of the primary antibody to the epitopes (usually in the size of 10–15 amino acids or equivalent). The primary antibody bound to the epitope is identified with the secondary antibody which is often labeled with the enzyme (most often peroxidase). The enzymatic reaction between labeling enzyme and the substrate (usually DAB) gives an optically detectable product at the structures displaying epitopes to which the primary antibodies can bind. The high sensitivity and specificity of the method have made it one of the most commonly used auxiliary techniques in diagnostic histopathology and cytopathology. The results of IHC staining may be affected by a number of factors including not only the quality of the material but also the quality, quantity and concentration of the reagents, pH, incubation time, temperature just to name the most important. Any deviation from the optimal conditions may lead to false positive or false negative results and erroneous conclusions as a consequence. Immunohistochemistry is a complex multistep diagnostic test where each step is important for the final result, and all parameters have to be strictly controlled under all phases of the process [1–4]. From the practical point of view, the following phases can be distinguished:

I. **Preanalytical phase: covering the period before the arrival of the specimen at the laboratory.** The aim is to secure a sufficient amount and quality of the diagnostic material and secure optimal preservation of the tissue/cell components by proper fixation and transportation. Many variables in this phase are often out of control by the pathology laboratory. The type and concentration of the fixative, temperature, and duration of the fixation (including fixation delay) are essential for the quality of immunohistochemical staining. The most commonly used fixative for tissue material is formalin and most of the commercially available antibod-

J. Klos (✉)
Department of Pathology, Stavanger University Hospital, Stavanger, Norway

J. Klijanienko et al. (eds.), *Diagnostic Procedures in Patients with Neck Masses*,
https://doi.org/10.1007/978-3-031-67675-8_7

ies are standardized for formalin fixed paraffin embedded (FFPE) material and standardization of the staining results seems possible. On the other hand, cytological material is exposed to a great variation of fixatives used for preservation in different laboratories which makes inter-laboratory standardization of immunocytochemical procedures difficult [5, 6].

II. **Analytical phase: from the arrival of the specimen to the laboratory to the examination of the slides by the pathologist.** The success at this stage requires optimal processing of the specimen and optimized staining protocols including carefully selected well-performing antibody clones. The number of variables at this stage is very high and if are not properly controlled, they may lead to suboptimal results of the staining. Each intended-for-use antibody should be carefully tested in the laboratory, and optimal staining protocols should be established. It is worth mentioning that different antibody clones may show varying performance on different automated staining platforms, and this aspect deserves attention when selecting and purchasing the antibodies for diagnostic use [2, 3].

III. **Postanalytical phase: from the first examination of the stained sides to concluding the final diagnosis in the pathology report.** The sufficient experience and knowledge of the laboratory procedures as well as knowledge of morphology and immunohistochemical profiles of the lesions considered in differentials by the pathologist are fundamental at this stage. The above creates the background for the selection of appropriate antibodies for building an optimal diagnostic panel but also is a basis for the interpretation of the staining and arriving at the correct diagnosis in the report [7–9].

7.3   Introducing New Antibodies

Selecting antibodies for diagnostic application is a challenging task since there are hundreds of antibodies capable of identifying different epit-

opes/targets and generating information potentially relevant *to* diagnosis, therapy or prognosis. A careful reading of publications documenting both sensitivity and specificity of the antibody clones as well as checking recommendations from external quality control programs is important before selecting optimal clones. Careful testing of the staining protocol on its own material following international recommendations should always be a part of the validation of a new test [2, 3].

7.4   Building Antibody Panel

A careful morphological study is necessary to define possible differentials or parameters necessary for the final diagnosis before selecting appropriate/relevant antibodies for the diagnostic panel. At this stage, it is important to:

- Be familiar with classic immunohistochemical profiles of the considered differentials and variations of the immunohistochemical profiles within the tumor type.
- Know the spectrum of reactivity of the selected antibody clones.
- Be aware of possible cross-reactivity of selected antibodies, e.g., differentiating small cell carcinoma from B-cell lymphoma, the choice of PAX5 is not optimal since both tumors are expected to be positive unless other Abs in the panel will solve the problem.
- Select antibodies that show maximal differences in reactivity between tumors are considered as differentials. The low percentage of almost all tumors, in addition to anonymous morphology, used to show true positive staining for single/some antibodies, which are otherwise characteristic for other tumor types (aberrant expression). In such cases, the application of a limited panel of antibodies may lead to erroneous classification/diagnosis. Keeping this in mind, the optimal panel should combine the antibodies typically positive for each of the considered diagnoses, which are largely negative for the other diagnosis.

- *For example*, differential diagnosis of primary squamous cell carcinoma and primary adenocarcinoma of the lung should optimally include P40, CK5, or CK5/6 as markers positive in more than 95% of squamous cell carcinoma and positive in less than 10% of lung adenocarcinoma as well as TTF1 or Napsin A as positive in more than 80% of lung adenocarcinoma but positive in less than 10% of squamous cell carcinoma [10].

	P40	P63	CK5	CK5/6	CK14	CK17	CK7	TTF1	Napsin A
Squamous cell carcinoma lung	*>95%*	*>95%*	*>95%*	*>95%*	*>95%*	*>90%*	*>20%*	*<10%*	*<10%*
Adenocarcinoma NOS lung	*<10%*	*>20%*	*<10%*	*<10%*	*>20%*	*>10%*	*>95%*	*>80%*	*>80%*

7.5   Interpretation of Staining

Since immunohistochemistry is a complex procedure and "if anything can go wrong it will" each performed test should have its own positive control. The separate section from the block with external control tissues should always be placed on the same glass as the section from the specimen and stained together with the section from the specimen. The staining should demonstrate an adequate intensity and be localized on appropriate structures of both external and internal control tissues. No staining of the other structures should be present at the control tissues [1–3]. Sometimes, the preanalytical data like type of fixative used may explain unexpected results of staining, e.g., negative staining for CD30 or CD5 in material fixed in mercuric chloride containing fixatives [11].

Typically, IHC staining is qualitatively evaluated by a pathologist as positive or negative. Only sometimes the estimated percentage of positive cells assessed with subjective semi-quantitative manual score (e.g., 0, 1+, 2+, and 3+) or descriptively (e.g., weak, moderate, or strong), which is sufficient in most of the cases. The Allred score developed to quantify estrogen and progesterone receptors in breast cancers summarizes scores for the intensity (0–3) and the proportion of positive cells (0–5) into the final score (0–8). The H-score is calculated by a semi-quantitative assessment of both the intensity of staining graded from 0 (no staining) to 3 (strong staining) and the percentage of positive cells. The H-score captures both the intensity and the proportion of the biomarker of interest from the IHC image and comprises values between 0 and 300, thereby offering a dynamic range to quantify the amount of biomarker [1]. Increasing the use of immunohistochemical markers to guide the therapy will most probably need more sensitive and more objective methods of standardized quantifying based on digital picture analysis.

7.6   Diagnostic Considerations

The complex morphological and clinical pattern, as well as a variety of lesions in the region of head and neck, requires more than a hundred different antibodies to cover a full spectrum of pathological conditions at this location. The detailed description of all diagnosis-relevant antibodies is beyond the scope of this chapter, and other sources are available and recommended. Several tables summarizing the most important elements of immunohistochemical profiles of the most common diagnoses within the region of the head and neck are constructed in order to make a comparison of the immunoprofiles easier.

7.6.1   Squamous Cell Carcinomas and their Differential Diagnoses

The most common malignant tumors in the head and neck region are squamous cell carcinomas. They show a wide spectrum of morphology, and immunohistochemical staining is essential for subtyping. Detection of cytokeratins in the cytoplasm of tumor cells is essential for diagnosing tumors as carcinoma, especially in poorly differentiated cases. Tumor cells react with cytokeratin cocktails covering a wide spectrum of cytokeratins (e.g., AE1/AE3 and OSCAR). Squamous cell tumors, as a rule, are positive for cytokeratins of high molecular weight (CK5, CK5/6, CK14, or CK17). The nuclear expression of p63 or p40 is also present in addition to positive staining for high molecular weight cytokeratins. More than half of these tumors also express p53. The immunohistochemical profile is not specific for squamous differentiation and is also present in myoepithelial tumors and some urothelial tumors. The majority of squamous cell carcinomas in the oropharynx and some carcinomas in other locations at the head and neck are related to infection with oncogenic HPV. Immunohistochemical staining for P16 is considered a surrogate marker of HPV status with a cutoff value of positive nuclear and cytoplasmic staining in >70% of tumor cells, preferably with p40/p63 positivity and negative staining for neuroendocrine markers [12]. Positive staining for p16 does not always equal the presence of HPV infection, and positivity in the absence of HPV is reported in 5–20% of cases of oropharyngeal carcinomas. Some other tumors like sinonasal undifferentiated carcinoma (SNUC) or small cell neuroendocrine lung carcinoma are constantly positive for p16; however, there is no confirmation of HPV presence.

For more information about immunohistochemical profiles of primary squamous cell carcinomas, myoepithelial tumors, and adenocarcinoma of non-intestinal type, see Table 7.1.

7.6.2 Salivary Gland Tumors

Salivary gland cancers are not very common, making up 5% to 8% of all head and neck cancers. Most of the tumors are located in the parotid gland; around 80% are benign, and more than 50% represent pleomorphic adenomas. Morphological similarities can make the diagnosis difficult and the application of immunohistochemistry or molecular tests may be of great value even if many tumors show overlapping immunohistochemical profiles.

Immunohistochemistry can be of help in identifying myoepithelial cells, assessing proliferation rates, or identifying the extension of the tumor including perineural invasion. Tumors of salivary glands may show differentiation toward both the luminal (ductal or acinar) cells, and abluminal (myoepithelial/basal) cells are called biphasic. Monophasic tumors show differentiation toward only the luminal or abluminal cell type. Tumors with varying, often unique cellular differentiation like sebaceous, mucinous, squamous, or lymphoid differentiation are also a part of the spectrum. Ductal/acinar cells are characterized by the expression of CK7, low molecular cytokeratins (CK8, CK18, and CAM 5.2) and EMA. Focal positivity for CK5, CK5/6, and CK14 may be seen. Staining for p40/p63, Smooth Muscle Actin (SMA), Calponin, Smooth Muscle Myosin Heavy Chain (SMMHC), and CK20 is rare and if present is usually focal and weak in ductal/acinar cells. Myoepithelial are usually positive for p40/p63, myoid markers (SMA, SMMHC, and Calponin), vimentin, S100, and CK5, CK5/6, CK14, and CK17. Only rarely show weak expression of low molecular weight cytokeratins (CK8, CK18, and CAM5.2). Expression for EMA is not seen as a rule. Basal cells show some overlapping with myoepithelial cells, being positive for high molecular weight cytokeratins and p63 but weakly positive or negative for CK7, CAM 5.2, and myoid markers (SMA, SMMHC, and Calponin). Staining for CK20, vimentin, S100, and EMA is negative. It is worth mentioning that combined positivity for P40/P63 and high molecular weight cytokeratin is also characteristic of squamous epithelium. The use of the sensitive clone 34BE12 for the detection of high molecular weight cytokeratins is not always the optimal choice since this clone may show cross-reactivity with denatured epitope, possibly of low molecular weight cytokeratin CK19 [10, 26].

SOX10 is a relatively new marker widely applied for melanocytic tumors is also expressed in both luminal, basal, and myoepithelial cells [27, 28]. SOX10 stains nuclei in cells of acinus and intercalated ducts in normal salivary, all cells

Table 7.1 Immunohistochemical profiles of primary squamous cell carcinomas, myoepithelial carcinoma, neuroendocrine carcinoma, and adenocarcinoma of non-intestinal type in Head and Neck[1]

Antibody	KSCC	NKSCC	BSCC	LEC	SNUC	NUTCA	SCSCC	INI1 DefCa	MECA	NECA	ADCA[2]
PanCK							60-75				
CK5/6								60-75	75-92	10-25	40-60
CK7		75-90			25-40	25-40		40-60		10-25	
CK8 (Cam5.2)				---		---		---			
CK14				---		---	10-25	---	60-75	10-25	---
CK18				---	---	---		---			
CK19					40-60	75-90		---		75-90	40-60
CK20				25-40		10-25				3	2
EMA				40-60	10-25	25-40 f	10-25	60-75	---	---	
P63					10-25 f	60-75	75-90	40-60	75-90		25-40
P40			f			60-75	40-60	25-40 f	75-90		---
P16	10-25	60-75	75-90		HPV-	HPV-	10-25	10-25		60-75	---
EBV											
NUT1		10-25		10-25	10-25						
m-CEA	25-40	25-40	40-60	25-40	---			---	10-25	---	40-60
CD34						25-40		---			
CD56[4]			5	---	---	40-60	---	25-40			---
CD117				75-90	75-90			10-25 f		75-90	25-40
S100						10-25			75-90		25-40
INI1/SMARCB1[6]								60-75			
Chromogr. A					75-90	25-40 f				75-90	25-40
Synaptophysin				---	25-40	25-40 f		10-25 f			25-40
TTF1					10-25				---	25-40	---
Other				SATB2+ 89%; CAD17+ 89%; CDX2+ 67%	Vim+ 10-25%	SMA+ <10%	Vim+ >90%; SMA+ 10-25%	SMA+ <10%	SMA+ 75-90%; INSM1<10	SMA+ <10%; INSM1>90%	Vim+ 40-60%; SMA+ <10%

■ 0->10% positive cases, 10-25% positive cases, 25-40% positive cases, 40-60%positive cases, 60-75% positive cases, 75 -90%positive cases, ■ >90% positive cases, f = focal staining, ---= no sufficient data,

Abbreviations: ADCA adenocarcinoma primary non-intestinal type NOS, *BSCC* basaloid SCC, *KSCC* keratinizing SCC, *LEC* lymphoepithelial SCC, *MECA* myoepithelial carcinoma, *NECA* neuroendocrine carcinoma, *NKSCC* non-keratinizing SCC, *SNUC* sinonasal undifferentiated carcinoma, *NUTCA* NUT carcinoma, *INI1DefCA* SMARCB1/INI1 deficient carcinoma, *SCSCC* spindle cell (sarcomatoid) squamous cell carcinoma

[1]Partially based on accumulated data from Refs. [1, 7, 12–25]
[2]Including NOS and ductal but excluding of intestinal-type adenocarcinoma
[3]Excluding Merkel cell carcinoma
[4]Careful interpretations warranted if only CD56 is positive and other neuroendocrine markers are negative
[5]Discrepant results reported (bias from other tumor types can't be excluded)
[6]Additional tumors with loss of INI1/SMARCB1 include malignant rhabdoid tumor of kidney and soft tissue, atypical teratoid/rhabdoid tumor of CNS, conventional and proximal type epithelioid sarcoma, medullary renal carcinoma, poorly differentiated chordoma, epithelioid variant of MPNST, myoepithelial carcinoma and epithelioid schwannoma and other with lower frequency of protein loss

in pleomorphic adenoma and basal cell adenoma, but no other benign tumors. SOX10 positivity is seen in acinic cell carcinoma, adenoid cystic carcinoma, carcinoma ex pleomorphic adenoma, myoepithelial carcinoma, and polymorphous low-grade adenocarcinoma. SOX10 staining is negative in salivary duct carcinoma, mucoepidermoid carcinoma, squamous cell carcinoma, oncocytic tumors, and Warthin tumor [29]. Expression of C-Kit (CD117) commonly found on luminal cells in cases of adenoid cystic carcinoma is also reported in polymorphous low-grade adenocarcinoma, mucoepidermoid carcinoma, and the majority of pleomorphic adenomas as well as in the minority of other salivary gland tumors does not seem to be useful in subtyping of salivary gland tumors.

Table 7.2 summarizes common immunohistochemical profiles of selected malignant salivary gland tumors.

Table 7.2 Immunohistochemistry of selected malignant tumors of salivary glands[1]

Antibody	ACC	AdCC	AdC NOS	AdCa Ductal	BCAC	CCC	ITAC	LEC	MUC[6]	MEC	OCC	PAC (PLGA)	SecCa (MASC)	SCC
PanCK		e + m			e + m									
CK5/6	25-40	m		40-60	75-90[m]									
CK7	75-90	75-90			---		75-90							25-40
CK8 (Cam5.2)			---					---		---	---		---	---
CK20				25-40			75-90				---			---
CD117	25-40	e +2	25-40	25-40	40-60	---			25-40	---	---	60-75 weak	---	
DOG1	5	70 e	---			---					---	25-40	10-25	---
EMA	25-40				60-75	60-75		---	75-90	---	---	---	75-90	---
EPCAM		75-90			40-60						---			
GATA3	10-25	25-40	---	40-60	---		---	---	40-60		40-60	---		
GFAP		10-25		25-40								10-25		
Mammaglobin			---	40-60	---							75-90	4	
Myb			75-90[3]	10-25		---	---			---	---	10-25	---	---
P63		Nᵉ Aᵐ	25-40	25-40										
P40		Nᵉ Aᵐ												
P16			---	---	------	HPV	25-40	---	---	---	---	---	---	---
PLAG[7]					40-60				10-25			10		
S100	10-25	m	25-40	40-60	75-90[m]	25-40		---					4	
SMA		m			---			---				10-25		
SOX10	5	m	10-25	10-25					10-25			75-90	40-60	
AR	10-25	10-25	---	60-75		---	---	---	10-25	---	---	---	10-25	---
Vimentin	75-90	---	40-60	40-60	---			---	25-40					
Other markers		PSA+ PSMA+ LEF1+ 5%	BRAF+30 PSMA+ 30%	CEAm+, CD30+, GCDFP1+, BRAF70% PSMA+, NKX-230% PSA= 7% TTF1= 2%	B-Catenin+ nuclei in adenoma 80% and some carcinomas LEF1+70%	RCC 100 mCEA 100 DD from meta: p63, CK7+/CK20+ EWSR1-ATF1	CDX288 ChgrA 70 CEA-M+ B-Cat+ nucl 30% Her2+15% Synapt-	NUT+ 20	D2-40+ 100 PSA+ 70% BRAF+ 10% ESR+ 10% AR 20% NUT neg		CD10neg		[3]GCDFP15	

■ 0->10% positive cases, 10-25% positive cases, 25-40% positive cases, 40-60% positive cases, 60-75% positive cases, 75-90% positive cases, >90% positive cases, --- = no sufficient data; **e**= epithelial; **m**= myoepithelial

Abbreviations: *ACC* acinic cell carcinoma, *AdCC* adenoid cystic carcinoma, *AdC NOS* adenocarcinoma primary NOS, *BCAC* basal cell adenocarcinoma, *CCC* clear cell carcinoma, *CS* Carcinosarcoma, *ITAC* intestinal-type adenocarcinoma, *LEC* lymphoepithelial carcinoma, *MUC* mucoepidermoid carcinoma, *MEC* myoepithelial carcinoma, *NEC* neuroendocrine carcinoma, *ONC* oncocytic carcinoma, *PAC (former PLGA)* polymorphous (low grade) adenocarcinoma, *SCC* small cell carcinoma, *SDC* salivary duct carcinoma, *SEBAC* sebaceous adenocarcinoma, *SEC (MASC)* secretory carcinoma, *SNUC* sino-nasal undifferentiated carcinoma, *SqCC* squamous cell carcinoma, *e* epithelial component, *m* myoepithelial component, *f* focal staining

[1]Partially based on accumulated data from Refs. [24, 28–50]

[2]Strong, diffuse staining of epithelial elements, but no mutations in the CD117 gene.

[3]Positive staining strongly supports AdCC (~80%) and speaks against pleomorphic adenoma (10–25%); t(6:9) MYB-NFIB translocation alone is not pathognomonic for AdCC and is reported in other tumors [49]

[4]SEC (MASC) is strongly positive for Mammaglobin, focally for GCDFP15 and weak but diffuse for S100. Translocation results in ETV6-NTRK3 fusion

[5]DOG1 and SOX10 strongly positive in most of the cases

[6]Translocation MECT1:MAML2 (t11:19) in 60% of cases

[7]Rearrangements of PLAG1 gene are characteristic for pleomorphic adenoma but are also reported from other tumors.

7.6.3 Thyroid Tumors

Tumors of the thyroid gland are the most common endocrine neoplasms. Most of them are derived from follicular epithelial cells. Few only are derived from calcitonin-secreting C cells, and only exceptionally are composed of both C cells and follicular cells. Major recent developments in the pathology of the thyroid gland are the characterization of well-differentiated thyroid tumors composed of follicular cells and showing follicular morphology. These tumors show cytological features of malignancy but no convincing evidence of invasive growth, and they show a low frequency of metastases. Tumors are named non-invasive follicular tumors with papillary-like nuclear features (NIFT-P) or tumors with uncertain malignant potential (TUMP), and tumors with cells arranged in wide trabeculae, nuclear features of papillary carcinoma, intra-trabecular hyalinization and hyaline material in the cytoplasm (HTT). Immunohistochemistry can contribute to confirmation of follicular thyroid cell origin (thyroglobulin, TTF1, and PAX8). Cross-reactivity with PAX5 of antibodies directed against N-terminal of PAX8 molecule may be annoying [51]. Application of neuroendocrine markers like synaptophysin, Chromogranin A, INSM1, calcitonin together with CEA can confirm the origin of the primary tumors from C-cells (medullary carcinoma). The distinction between primary and metastatic thyroid tumors is also often assisted by immunohistochemistry [1, 52]. Regarding the interpretation of calcitonin staining in tumor biopsy, one should remember that positive staining has been reported among other tumors including paraganglioma, neuroendocrine neoplasms in pancreas and laryngeal neuroendocrine carcinomas, so the antibody alone is not enough specific marker for medullary thyroid carcinoma [53–55]. Only as a part of the panel and in agreement with clinical data will positive calcitonin staining support the diagnosis of medullary thyroid carcinoma. Regarding several variants of papillary carcinoma the classical immunohistochemical profile of thyroid cell is present in all. The exception is cylinder cell variant of papillary carcinoma, showing in more than 50% of cases positive CDX2 nuclear staining in tumor cells [1, 52]. Another special tumor type is cribriform morular variant of thyroid carcinoma associated with mutation of AFP gene. It will show positive nuclear β-Catenin staining, negative staining for thyroglobulin but positive TTF1 staining and formation of squamoid morular structures which stain for CDX2, CD10, and CD5 [52].

Mutation-specific antibodies become more important, providing additional information on the molecular classification of tumors and even if they are often claimed "specific" they may, like many other antibodies, show unexpected reactivity with components of normal or disease-affected tissue [56]. Since aspiration cytology is still commonly used in the diagnosis and management of thyroid lesions, it is important to test the performance of antibodies on own cytological material before using them as reliable diagnostic tools.

Immunohistochemical characteristics of the most common tumors in thyroid are summarized in Table 7.3.

7.6.4 Neuroendocrine Tumors and Paraganglioma

Neuroendocrine neoplasms (NEN) account for around 2% of all tumors worldwide. They are commonest in gastrointestinal tract pancreas (70%) and lungs (25%). Other primary sites are identified only in 5% of cases. Relatively few NENs are localized in the head and neck region. The diagnosis NEN is based on the demonstration of neuroendocrine differentiation in the setting of appropriate morphology. Antibodies against synaptophysin, INSM1, and Chromogranin A are recommended as the first choice for detecting neuroendocrine differentiation. Synaptophysin and INSM1 are very sensitive markers, and simultaneous use is recommended. Both are positive in almost all NENs, with some variation in the percentage of reactivity in different tumors, but they are not fully specific. Although the majority of NETs stain well for all three neuroendocrine markers, the majority of NEC show weak and focal staining for Chromogranin A. Positive synaptophysin staining is reported in non-endocrine neoplasms including adrenal cortex, solid pseudopapillary tumor in the pancreas and a number of other tumors [72]. INSM1 is also reported positive in cases of non-endocrine carcinomas and a few cases of sarcomas [73].

Evaluation of the biological potential of neuroendocrine tumors (NETs) is based on the presence of necrosis and proliferation activity (number of mitoses or percentage of Ki67 positive cells). Proliferation index using Ki-67 staining (Ki-67 labeling index: <2% for NET grade 1, <20% for NET grade 2 and > 20% for NET grade 3). The presently used cut of values for grading is still debated [12, 52]. It is important to distinguish an epithelial NEN from a non-epithelial one using cytokeratin staining. Wide spectrum cytokeratin cocktails are recommended, but good results are achieved with low molecular weight

Table 7.3 Tumors of thyroid gland[1]

Antibody	FTC	PTC	OTC	PDTC	ATC	MTC	HTT[4]	TUMP (FT, WDT)
Thyroglobulin				75-90				
TTF1[2]					10-25			
CK19	40-60	75-90	40-60	25-40	40-60	75-90	0-50	10-25
CD56 (NCAM)	40-60	Varies[3]	75-90		40-60			10-25
BRAF		40-60	---	10-25	10-25			
mCEA				---		75-90	---	---
Synapt.	---[9]	80						---
Chromogr. A							0-25	
Calcitonin				---				
INSM1		---	---	---	---	60-75		
PAX8[8]		---		60-75	75-90	25-40		
Galectin 3	60-75	[7]	60-75	---	75-90	40-60	0-50	10-25
HBME-1	---	[6]	---		---	---	0-50	---
CDX2		0-60[4]	---	---				
S100	25-40	25-40	40-60	---	25-40		---	---
Vimentin		40-60	---			40-60		

■ 0->10%positive cases, **10-25%** positive cases, **25-40**% positive cases, **40-60%**positive cases,

60-75% positive cases, **75-90%** positive cases, ■ **>90%** positive cases, --- = no sufficient data,

Abbreviations: FTC Follicular thyroid carcinoma, *PTC* Papillary thyroid carcinoma, *OTC* oncocytic (Hürthle cell) thyroid carcinoma, *PDTC* Poorly differentiated thyroid carcinoma, *ATC* Anaplastic thyroid carcinoma, *MTC* Medullary thyroid carcinoma, *HTT* Hyalinizing trabecular tumor, *TUMP* Tumors of uncertain malignant potential (*FT* Follicular tumor, *WDT* Well-differentiated tumor).

[1]Partially based on accumulated data from Refs [1, 9, 52, 57–70.]

[2]TTF1 Most sensitive clones are SPT24 and the rmAb SP141. Granular cytoplasmic staining of hepatocytes with clone 8G7G3/1 is a result of cross-reactivity.

[3]CD56 expression is lost in more than 90% of classic, diffuse sclerosing, and infiltrative follicular variants of PTCs. Tall cell variant, Warthin-like variant, and cribriform-morular variant show better preservation of CD56 reactivity than other variants [58].

[4]CDX2 nuclear positivity is common in columnar cell variants and in morular structures of cribriform PTC, which carries risk of confusion with metastatic adenocarcinoma. Rare cribriform variant of PTC with the formation of modular structures is associated with mutation of AFP gene and shows also nuclear staining for Beta-Catenin [1, 52, 57].

[5]HTT shows consistently characteristic membranous/cytoplasmic positivity with the MIB-1 antibody when incubated at room temperature [1].

[6]HBME1 stains conventional variant of PTC but shows lower frequency in follicular variant of PTC [52].

[7]Galectin 3 nuclear and cytoplasmic staining is seen in most conventional PTC but is also reported in benign lesions.

[8]PAX8 mAb clone MRQ-50 and EP331 directed against N-terminal of protein show cross-reactivity with PAX5. Clone MRQ-50 was also shown to react with breast cancer cells. Optimal staining can be obtained with the rmAb clones SP348, ZR-1, BP6157, IHC048, QR016, and the mAb clone BC12 [9, 51, 71].

[9]Single publications [65] report as many as 80% follicular carcinomas being positive for synaptophysin, but these data are not confirmed by others.

cytokeratins too (CAM 5.2). Cytoplasmic positivity of cytokeratin staining can vary from strong and diffuse to focal and quite weak. It often shows a dot-like paranuclear pattern. Only rare cases of NET show negative staining for cytokeratin. Among NETs there is a significant number of tumors with negative staining for both CK7 and CK20. Differential diagnosis between NET grade 3 and neuroendocrine carcinomas (NEC) is based on morphology. In cases of suboptimal biopsy material or borderline features, the possibility of NET grade 3 is supported by negative staining for ATRX (alpha-thalassemia/mental retardation syndrome X-linked), DAXX (death-associated protein), menin (orphan protein encoded on *MEN1* gene and mutated in MEN1 syndrome) or p27, when the expression of SSTR2/5 (somatotropin receptor 2 and 5 proteins) is retained. In favor of NEC will speak the negative staining Rb protein and SSTR2/5. Negative or diffusely positive staining for p53 indicating mutation of *P53* gene will also support NEC, since mutation of p53 is only a rare event in cases of NET [12].

When interpreting staining results it is essential to remember about the spectrum of reactivity of applied antibody clone since different clones may show different affinity to the studied epitopes, e.g., medullary carcinoma of thyroid stains positive for PAX8 with clone SP348 but is consistently negative with clones PAX8R1 and BC12 [66]. The monoclonal BC12 antibody or polyclonal antisera show no or focal weak staining for PAX8 in cribriform morular thyroid carcinoma too [52]. Profiles of common neuroendocrine tumors and paraganglioma are summarized in Table 7.4.

7.6.5 Melanocytic Tumors

Melanocytic tumors are common and only a low percentage of them become malignant. Approximately 10% to 25% of all melanomas have primaries in the head and neck region. The most common sites are the skin of the occipital scalp and the skin of the cheek. Common locations are face (40 to 60%), scalp (14 to 49%),

neck (20 to 29%), and ear (8 to 11%). Mucosal melanomas represent less than 1% of all melanomas and most frequently affect the sinonasal or oral mucosa. Since as many as 50% of sinonasal mucosal melanomas are growing as amelanotic tumors [95] the differential diagnosis in such cases will usually include many tumors of different lineages like sarcomas, lymphomas, and carcinomas. Melanocytic tumors show in general great variation in morphology, and they predominantly spindle cell forms must be differentiated from spindle cell carcinomas and sarcomas. Metastatic melanomas not only have a tendency to lose the expression of typical melanocytic markers during progression but may also express unusual "aberrant" markers like keratins (especially CK8, CK18, MNF-116) more often than primary melanomas. So, the positive staining for cytokeratin in undifferentiated or poorly differentiated neoplasm does not necessarily exclude the diagnosis of melanoma [96]. Among melanocytic tumors is also an emerging group of tumors with intermediate morphology and biological aggressiveness which also should be diagnosed correctly.

Great variation in morphology and immunophenotype makes the subtyping of melanocytic tumors and estimation of the biological potential of many melanocytic proliferations challenging. Pathology-related medical malpractice lawsuits mostly for underdiagnoses of melanoma are the second largest group of malpractice claims in the USA and constitute 13% of the total claims. Malignant melanoma and melanocytic proliferations of intermediate biological behavior (melanocytomas) may show overlapping in morphology and differential diagnosis may require support from immunohistochemical surrogates of molecular changes in many cases. The most important and most commonly used markers for melanocytic tumors are described below as precision in diagnostics may also depend on awareness of advantages and disadvantages of used antibodies.

S100: nuclear and cytoplasmic staining; member of the widely present family of Ca^{++} binding acidic proteins involved in many basal cellular functions [7]. The protein of diagnostic

Table 7.4 Neuroendocrine tumors and paraganglioma[1]

Antibody	Paraganglioma	Lung NET-NEC	Gastro-intestinal NET	Colorectal NET	Pancreas NET-NEC	Thyroid Medullary Carcinoma
PanCK				60-75	70-99	
S100	S-cells	0-30	10-25	40-60	---	
SOX10	S-cells	4-50				
GATA3	75-90				---	
Synapto		70-97				
Chromogr	75-90	50-97	60-75	40-60		
INSM1						
CD56		85-90	40-60	10-25	59-86	
TTF1[2]		50-70		11-25	2-15	0-95
CDX2[6]			40-60	40-60	16-50	
SATB2[4]	10-25	25-71		>90 rectum[7] ~80 appendix		10-25
mCEA		40	---	---	---	75-90
PAX8		---	---	---	60	0-70[3]
Calcitonin[5]		---	10-25	---		

■ 0->10% positive cases, **10-25**% positive cases, **25-40**% positive cases, **40-60**% positive cases, 60-75% positive cases, 75-90% positive cases, ■ >90% positive cases, --- = no sufficient data,

Abbreviations: *NET* neuroendocrine tumor, *NEC* neuroendocrine carcinoma, *S-cells* sustentacular cells

[1]Partially based on accumulated data from Refs. [1, 12, 19, 52, 57, 63, 72–93]

[2]Optimal results are obtained with clone SPT24 or clone SP141 staining with the clone 8G7G3/1 is often false negative. Clone SPT24 stains positive also NET in thymus. TTF1 may be also expressed by NEC from other locations than lung

[3]All polyclonal Abs and mAb clones MRQ-50, C12A32, IHC008, 2774R, and PAX8R1 directed against N-terminus of the PAX8 molecule crossreact with the epitope on PAX2, PAX5, and PAX6, giving positive nuclear staining [51, 63, 81]. Clones directed against C-terminal of PAX8 like BC12, EP298, EP331, SP348, ZR-1, BP6157, and IHC048 do not show this cross-reactivity ([9]). PAX8 staining in medullary thyroid carcinoma using clone MRQ-50 is negative but positive with clones SP348 or EP298 [81]

[4]SATB2, in addition to positivity in NETs arising in large bowel is relatively specific marker of mainly distal colorectal differentiation. It stains also positive circa 80% of Merkel cell carcinomas, almost 100% of osteosarcoma and 90% of phosphaturic mesenchymal tumors, mesenchymal chondrosarcoma, around 10% of epithelioid fibrosarcoma and Ewing sarcoma. It is negative in enteric type of pulmonary adenocarcinoma [80]

[5]Calcitonin staining is positive in other tumors than medullary carcinoma of thyroid (e.g., paraganglioma, neuroendocrine neoplasms in pancreas, and laryngeal neuroendocrine carcinomas) and therefore is recommended to use only in panel [3, 94]

[6]CDX2 is used to stain positive NETs from the gastrointestinal tract but is also positive in the majority of enteric types of pulmonary carcinoma

[7]Hindgut and genitourinary NETs are often positive for PSAP (Prostate Specific Acid Phosphatase)

interest is composed of two subunits α and β which are forming dimers in different combinations (antibodies against β subunit are in common use). It is a sensitive but non-specific marker expressed in normal cells, their benign and malignant counterparts in chondroid and adipose tissue, skin adnexa, salivary glands, myoepithelial cells, melanocytes, a variety of dendritic cells, sustentacular cells and macrophages. Normal Schwann cells and satellite cells in ganglia and their benign tumors are stained positive as a rule, but their malignant counterparts show often focal staining or are negative. A wide variety of adenocarcinomas originating from different organs including thyroid, breast, and endometrium is also positive.

SOX10: nuclear staining; member of the family of transcription factors, important for maturation and cell maintenance of Schwann cells and melanocytes [7]. Sensitive but non-specific marker staining melanocytic tumors (more sensitive than S100 for desmoplastic and spindle cell melanoma), gliomas (astrocytomas, oligodendrogliomas, glioblastomas), clear cell sarcoma,

Schwann cells and their tumors, sustentacular cells, myoepithelial cells and their tumors, and some salivary gland tumors as well as triple-negative breast carcinomas (~70% are positive).

Melan A/MART1: cytoplasmic staining; the antigen is localized to the endoplasmic reticulum and melanosomes [7]. There are two different antibody clones against the same antigen generated by two independent research groups (Melan A and MART1). Both are highly sensitive and specific markers of melanogenesis staining melanocytes and their benign and malignant tumors (both show low sensitivity 20%—30% in desmoplastic melanomas) as well as PECOMA, t(6;11) translocation kidney carcinoma, clear cell sarcoma and melanotic schwannoma. Only Melan A clone A-103 cross-reacts with an unknown epitope in cells producing steroid hormones and gives strong staining of the adrenal gland and sex cord-stromal tumors.

HMB45: cytoplasmic staining; a sensitive and highly specific marker of melanosomes at the early stage of differentiation [7] but not melanocytes as cells. The distribution of staining in benign melanocytic tumors varies. In benign nevi staining is positive in the junctional component and subepidermal zone of melanocytes, but staining in the deeper dermal parts is negative. The proportion of positive melanoma cases is usually high at the primary location (approaching 90%) with the exception of desmoplastic melanoma, where percentage of positive cases approach 20%. The frequency of positive staining is lower in the metastatic setting. Positive staining is seen in pigmented tumors like adrenal pheochromocytoma, melanotic progonoma, some translocation carcinomas of kidney and others. The cells containing premelanosomes in angiomyolipoma and other PEComas are also positive as a rule.

PRAME: nuclear staining; relatively new, sensitive but not specific marker [97–99] expressed in 90% of malignant melanomas and around 95% of metastatic melanomas A good correlation with the cut of 75% of positive tumor cells is reported. Around 1/3 of desmoplastic melanomas and Spitzoid melanomas are positive. A high percentage of positive cases is reported in squamous cell carcinoma of the thymus, subtypes

of liposarcomas and osteosarcoma. Between 20% and 40% of breast carcinomas, myeloid and lymphoid leukemias, and renal cell carcinoma are also positive. Around 10% of benign melanocytic tumors are also positive usually in the minority of nuclei. Clear cell sarcoma gives consistently negative staining in contrast to malignant melanomas.

Tyrosinase: cytoplasmic staining; a key enzyme in the synthesis of melanin; a highly specific and sensitive marker of melanin-producing cells. It stains >80% of metastatic malignant melanomas. The positive rate of staining in desmoplastic variants of melanoma is only 20–30% of cases. Positivity is also reported in clear cell sarcoma, PECOMAs, and pigmented nerve sheath tumors.

BRAF: cytoplasmic staining; serine/threonine kinase, which is often mutated in a number of tumors. Antibody (BRAF VE1) is sensitive and quite specific for *BRAF* V600E mutation and reliably detects mutated protein correlating well with mutation status. Positive staining is reported in ~60–70% of melanocytic nevi, some melanocytomas, ~50% of cutaneous melanomas, 50% of papillary thyroid carcinomas, 15% of poorly differentiated thyroid carcinomas, 20–60% of anaplastic thyroid carcinomas, 10% colorectal adenocarcinomas, 90% serrated lesions, 70% of borderline serous ovarian tumors, 10–20% of low-grade serous carcinoma, > 90% of hairy cell leukemia, 50% Erdheim-Chester disease, 65% Langerhans histiocytosis, 60% of ameloblastoma, metanephric adenoma and 95% papillary craniopharyngeoma, 60% of pleomorphic xanthoastrocytomas, 4% frequency in non-small cell lung carcinomas. The publication of Jones [56] described that the monoclonal BRAF VE1 antibody cross-reacts with the protein component of normal cilia in ciliated epithelial cells, ACTH-producing cells in pituitary adenomas and cells in the zona fasciculata, and the zona reticularis of the adrenal cortex. Cross-reactivity with unknown epitopes in the nuclei of spermatids and Leydig cells is also described. Additional cross-reactivity for this antibody is described in the cells with ganglionic features that frequently bind VE1 but are not associated with $BRAF^{V600E}$ mutation

[100]. Both mentioned situations may lead to diagnostic misinterpretation with therapeutic consequences.

P16 (p16 INK4a): nuclear and cytoplasmic staining; Tumor suppressor protein encoded by *CDKN2A* gene involved in regulating the progression of the cell cycle by inhibiting CDK4 and CDK6, which keeps Retinoblastoma protein (Rb) hypophosphorylated preventing dissociation of Rb from E2F and entry into S-phase as a consequence. Total loss of nuclear expression of P16 supports the diagnosis of malignant melanocytic tumor, but reported data show a good deal of variation, and p16 staining is generally considered of limited use differentiating benign from malignant lesions. Staining for p16 may be of help in distinguishing nodal nevi from metastatic melanoma and subtyping melanocytic tumors especially if used in a panel. A number of tumors may have silenced P16 protein due to genetic or epigenetic changes (e.g., breast carcinoma, colon carcinoma, pancreatic carcinoma, head and neck carcinoma related to smoking), with negative staining as a result. On the other hand, overexpression is considered often as a surrogate marker for oncogenic HPV infection in many tumors (oropharyngeal carcinoma and anogenital lesions). Many other lesions harboring dysregulated Rb pathway due to other mechanisms than HPV infection also show positive staining (e.g., liposarcoma, gastric adenocarcinoma, pulmonary adenocarcinoma, neuroendocrine carcinoma, and serous carcinoma of the ovary). Immunohistochemistry correlates quite well with P16 status in tumors.

Ki67: (nuclear staining); Marker of cell proliferation. It is a non-histone nuclear protein expressed in G1, S, G2, and M phases of the cell cycle, then rapidly catabolized at end of the M phase and not detectable in G0 and early G1 cells.

Surrogates of molecular changes: Detecting fusion proteins (ALK, ROS1, and NTRK) often seen in Spitzoid melanocytomas, as well as staining for BAP1, PKAR1A, β-Catenin, and LEF1 is often of diagnostic help in difficult cases. The use of genetic profiling for detecting abnormalities characteristic for different tumors (melanoma vs. melanocytoma) can also effectively support the final classification and prediction of the biological behavior.

Immunohistochemical profiles of melanocytic tumors are summarized in Table 7.5.

7.6.6 Hematolymphoid Proliferations

The second most common primary malignancy in the head and neck region is hematolymphoid tumors. The peak incidence is the 6-seventh decade of life but young patients are also affected. There is some variation in the geographical distribution of different subtypes of lymphoma but the absolute majority are B-cell non-Hodgkin lymphomas (around 80%) followed by Hodgkin lymphoma (10–15%) and the remaining 5% are NK/T-cell lymphomas.

About one-third of non-Hodgkin lymphomas manifest in extranodal locations in the head and neck region and the majority are found in oral cavity. Hodgkin lymphoma both classic (cHL) and nodular lymphocyte predominant (NLPHL) most commonly involve cervical lymph nodes while primary extranodal involvement is rarely seen [12, 127].

Immunohistochemistry is essential for the diagnosis and subtyping of lymphomas since the type of lymphoma is the basis for a therapeutic decision and prognosis. Results of immunohistochemical tests can also have a predictive value (e.g., treatment with anti-CD20 antibodies in case of B-cell malignancy).

Among non-Hodgkin lymphomas of NK/T-cell type, the most common in the head and neck region are extranodal NK/T-cell lymphoma nasal type, anaplastic large-cell lymphoma (ALCL), angioimmunoblastic T-cell lymphoma, peripheral T-cell lymphoma (NOS) and T-cell lymphoblastic lymphoma.

The simplified practical approach presented in Table 7.6 with a basic panel of four antibodies is helpful in the identification of lymphomas and their classification into one of the larger groups [128]. Tables 7.7, 7.8 and 7.9 present the most important immunohistochemical characteristics

Table 7.5 Melanocytic tumors[1]

Antibody	MelNOS	MelDes	MelMet	DPN[6]	aSpitz	PEM[5]	aBNLike	MelBN
S100				variable		variable	variable	variable
SOX10								
MelanA/MART1	75-90	20-30 12	75-90[4]		75-90		variable	f
HMB45	75-90	10-25	60-75[4]	diffuse	75-90		f	f
PRAME		25-40			27-100	---	---	---
BRAFV600E	40-60		40-60	variable	10-25	variable		
P16	40-60	75-90	75-90		40-90		10-25	variable
B-Cateninnucl.								
LEF1(nuclear)	75							
Cyclin D1	60-75	---	---		60-75			---
BAP1			---				---	25-40
PRKAR1A			---	2	---	3		
Ki67	high	high	high	low	intermediate	low	intermediate	high
Other					ALK, ROS1, NTRK1/3 RET, MET		NRAS	

🟥 0->10% positive cases, 10-25% positive cases, 25-40% positive cases, 40-60% positive cases, 60-75% positive cases, 75-90% positive cases, 🟩 >90% positive cases, f = focal staining, --- = no sufficient data,

Abbreviations: *MelNOS* Malignant melanoma (except desmoplastic) Not Otherwise Specified, *MelDes* Melanoma desmoplastic, *MelMet* Melanoma metastatic, *DPN* Deep penetrating nevus, *aSpitz* Spitz tumor (atypical, Spitzoid melanoma), *PEM* Pigmented epithelioid melanocytoma, *aBNLike* atypical blue nevus-like (cellular), *MelBN* Melanoma arising in blue nevus.
[1]Partially based on accumulated data from Refs. [27, 56, 95–126]
[2]May be negative in a subset of tumors.
[3]Sporadic PEM and Carney complex-associated PEM are histologically indistinguishable but cases of Carney complex show negative immunohistochemical staining for PRKAR1A.
[4]Percentage of positive cells in metastatic melanoma is usually lower than in primary tumors [116].
[5]PEMs are indolent melanocytic tumors with metastatic potential limited to regional lymph nodes and otherwise rare distant metastasis. Immunostaining shows expression of melanocytic markers, including Melana, S100 protein, HMB45 antigen, and SOX10. A subset of PEMs shows loss of expression PRKAR1A (gene mutated in around 60% of families with Carney complex [125].
[6]DPNs express S100 protein and SOX10, as well as the melanocyte differentiation antigens HMB45 antigen, Melan A (MART1), tyrosinase, and MITF. Diffuse HMB45 staining is characteristic for DPN. Nuclear β-catenin staining is useful in identifying DPNs and distinguishing them other nevi and melanoma [109].

of common lymphomas of B-cell type, NK/T-cell type, and Hodgkin, respectively.

It is worth remembering that diagnosis of rare lymphoid tumors or variants of T-cell lymphomas requires not only additional immunohistochemical tests but additional information, molecular tests and often some special competence. In such situations, it is often wise to consider a consultation. Table 7.9 also includes the recently recognized important entity EBV+ mucocutaneous ulceration (EBV+CMU) often developing in the oral cavity and pharynx including tonsils. This is a reactive, ulcerating lesion with a proliferation of EBV-positive, variable-sized atypical B-cells, morphologically mimicking cHL, affecting immunocompromised patients and showing spontaneous regression when the patient's immune status returns to normal [127, 129].

Myeloid (Granulocytic) Sarcoma is a rare tumor in general and only exceptionally reported in the head and neck region, which, because of its rarity, may represent a diagnostic challenge. It consists of myeloblasts at extramedullary location distorting the architecture of surround-

Table 7.6 Algorithmic approach to lymphomas (basic panel with CD20[2], CD5[3], CD3[4] and optional CD138[5])[1]

Diagnostic group	Phenotype	Diagnoses	Additional markers	Comments
B-cell non-Hodgkin lymphomas CD5 positive	CD20+/ CD5+/CD3−/CD138-	B-CLL, MCL, 10% DLBCL	CyclinD1/SOX11, CD23, Bcl2, Bcl6, CD10, MUM1, Ki67,	See Table 7.7
B-cell non-Hodgkin lymphomas CD5 negative	CD20+/ CD5-/CD3−/CD138-	Burkitt, LPL, MZL, HCL, FCL, DLBCL, and all other types of mature B-cell lymphomas	Bcl2, Bcl6, CD10, MUM1, Ki67, EBV, ALK	See Table 7.7
Plasma cell proliferations Plasmablastic Lymphomas B-ALL	CD20−/+ CD5-/CD3−/CD138+	Myeloma, Plasmacytoma, Plasmablastic lymphoma B-ALL	Kappa, lambda, CD56, PAX5, TdT, CD10	See Table 7.7
T/NK cell lymphomas	CD20−/ CD5+/−/CD3+/CD138-	All T/NK cell lymphomas	CD2, CD7, CD4,CD8, CD10, CD30, PD1, cytotoxic proteins, EBV, CD56, ALK	See Table 7.8
Hodgkin lymphoma	HRS cells: CD20−/+/ PAX5 weak/CD30+/ CD138−/+/ Background dominated by CD3+/CD5+ T-cells and scattered B-cells and CD138+ plasma cells	Classic Hodgkin lymphoma (cHL), EBV+ mucocutaneous ulceration (polymorphous type)	CD15, BOB1/OCT2, LMP, EBER Eber	See Table 7.9
	LP cells: CD20+/PAX5+ strong/CD30−/+/CD138- Background dominated by CD20+ B-cells, scattered CD3+/CD5+ T-cells and CD138+ plasma cells	Nodular lymphocytic predominant Hodgkin lymphoma (NLPHL)	EMA, CD56, J-chain	
Non-lymphoid	CD20-/CD5-/CD3-/ CD138−/+	Myeloid, Histiocytoid, Plasmacytoid, Carcinoma/sarcoma	MPO, CD43, CD68, CD45, etc. Kappa/lambda PANCK, S100	

Abbreviations: *B-CLL* B-Cell Chronic lymphatic leukemia/small lymphocytic lymphoma, *MCL* Mantle cell lymphoma, *DLBCL* Diffuse large B-cell lymphoma, *Burkitt* Burkitt lymphoma, *LPL* lymphoplasmacytic lymphoma, *MZL* Marginal zone lymphoma, *HCL* Hairy cell leukemia, *FL* Follicular lymphoma

[1]Data in Tables 7.6, 7.7, 7.8 and 7.9 are partially based on accumulated data from Refs. [12, 127–165]

[2]**CD20:** highly specific marker of B-cells, rarely weakly expressed on a few neoplastic T-cells.—Weak expression or absence of membranous expression is seen in immature B-cells.—Cells differentiating toward plasma cells are losing expression of this antigen.—Neoplastic plasma cell proliferations with translocation t(11;14) are expressing this antigen.—Treatment with anti-CD20 antibodies leads to transitional suppression of the expression

[3]**CD5:** marker expressed on T-lymphocytes and a subpopulation of B-lymphocytes

[4]**CD3:** highly specific marker of T-lymphocytes present in their cytoplasm and cell membranes but expressed also only in the cytoplasm by NK-cells

[5]**CD138:** sensitive but not specific marker of plasma cells, stains positive many other cell types including precursor B-cells, confirms plasma cells when used in combination with light chain staining

Pay special attention to morphology of germinal centers including presence of phagocytizing macrophages. Staining for Bcl2 is recommended when follicular lymphoma is suspected

Table 7.7   Immunophenotyping of selected B-cell lymphomas[1]

Antibody	B-ALL	B-CLL/SLL	LPL	ENMZL (MALT)	NMZL	MCL	HCL	Burkitt	FL	DLBCL	PCN PBL[9]
CD45	10-25										
CD20	10-25		[2]								[3]
PAX5											[4]
CD3											
TdT										[5]	
CD5					10-25					10-25	
CD10						[6]	10-25		75-90	40-60	
CD23					25-40				25-40		
CD30										10-25	
CD34	25-40										
CD43	60-75	60-75	10-25	40-60	25-75	75-90		75-90		10-25	25-40
Cycl. D1							75-90				[7]
Bcl2			25-40							40-60	
Bcl6		25-40				[8]				60-75	
MUM1		40-60	40-60	25-40	40-60	40-60			10-25	10-25	40-60
CD138			25-40		10-25						
Other	SOX11+ 50%, CD99+ 50%	SOX11+ <10% LEF1+ 100%,	CD25+ EMA- 60-75%	IgM+	IgD-	SOX11+ 95%,	CD25+, Annexin + >95%, BRAF+ TRAP+ >90%, Cycl D1+ 75%, SOX11+ 60%, TIA+ 50%	MYC+ 90% EBER+ 20%, EBNA1+ 100%,	SOX11+ 10-25%, P63+ in 10-25%	P63+ in 70%, FLI-1+ in 30%	Lambda+ or Kappa+, CD117+ in 30%,

◼ *0->10% positive cases, 10-25% positive cases, 25-40% positive cases, 40-60% positive cases, 60-75%*

positive cases, 75-90% positive cases, ◼ >90% positive cases, F = focal staining, --- = no sufficient data,

Abbreviations: B-ALL B-cell acute lymphatic leukemia, *B-CLL/SLL* B-cell chronic lymphatic leukemia/small lymphocytic lymphoma, *LPL* lymphoplasmacytic lymphoma, *ENMZL (MALT)* extranodal marginal zone lymphoma (mucosa-associated lymphoid tissue lymphoma), *NMZL* nodal marginal zone lymphoma, *MCL* mantle cell lymphoma, *HCL* hairy cell leukemia, *Burkitt* Burkitt lymphoma, *FL* follicular lymphoma, *DLBCL* diffuse large B-cell lymphoma, *PCN* plasma cell neoplasm, *PBL* plasmablastic lymphoma

[1]Data is partially based on accumulated data from references in Table 7.6

[2]CD20 is weaker as compared with B-lymphocytes on cells undergoing plasmacytic transformation

[3]Cells with translocation t(11;14) retain expression of CD20 [127, 130]

[4]Nuclear expression of PAX5 of often retained in cases with translocation t(11;14) [127, 130]

[5]Few cases of TdT-positive lymphomas with otherwise DLBCL profile are described [131]

[6]Blastoid variants of mantle cell lymphoma may express CD10

[7]Nuclear staining for Cyclin D1 is often present in cases with t(11;14) [127, 130]

[8]Expression of Bcl6 may be present in mantle cell lymphoma under blastoid transformation

[9]CD56 positivity in neoplastic plasma cells speaks in favor of primary location in bone marrow [127, 130]

ing normal tissues. It can occur as an isolated tumor, sometimes preceding or more often being synchronous with acute myeloid leukemia in the bone marrow. The diagnosis of myeloid sarcoma is considered equivalent to the diagnosis of acute myeloid leukemia (AML). Tumor cells are as a rule positive for vimentin and in more than 90% positive for CD43. Myeloid markers that are positive in more than 2/3 of cases are lysozyme, MPO, CD117, CD68 and ERG. Part of the diagnostic challenge is that the typical marker of blasts CD34 is positive only in about half of the cases and common leukocyte antigen CD45 is positive only in circa 60%. Expression of other

Table 7.8 Immunohistochemical profiles of selected NK/T-cell lymphomas[1]

Antibody	T-ALL	ETP-ALL[9]	ENKTL	ALCL-ALK-	ALCL-ALK+	nTFHL-AI[6]	PTCL[7,8]
CD45	75-90	---		40-60	40-60		75-90
CD20							
PAX5							
CD79a							
CD3	75-90 c	c	c	75-90	10-25		
CD2	40-60	---		40-60	10-25		75-90
CD5		3	10-25	10-25	25-40		40-60
CD7			25-40	---	---	variable	---
CD4		3	10-25	60-75	40-60		40-60
CD8	2		10-25	10-25			10-25
CD10	25-40	40-60		---	---		
CD30	10-25	---	40-60				10-25
TIA/GRNZB	---	---		40-60	75-90		25-40
CD34	25-40	25-40		---	---		
CD43	75-90	75-90		40-60	60-75		
CD56			75-90				25-40
CD99		---	---				
CD33	25-40	25-40					
CD1a	25-40						
EMA			---	40-60		---	10-25
MUM1			40-60	60-75	60-75	25-40	25-40
TdT							
P63	---		10-25	10-25			
Other	SOX11+ 10-25		S100+[4] EBER+[4]	P63+[5]			Bcl6+ 20% CD20+20% CD10+12%

▬ *0->10% positive cases, 10-25% positive cases, 25-40% positive cases, 40-60% positive cases, 60-75% positive cases, 75-90% positive cases,* ▬ *>90% positive cases, f= focal staining, --- = no data, c= cytoplasmic staining only*

Abbreviations: *T-ALL* T-cell lymphoblastic leukemia/lymphoma, *ETP-ALL* early precursor lymphoblastic leukemia, *ENKTL* extranodal NK/T-cell lymphoma nasal type, *ALCL* anaplastic large-cell lymphoma **ALK+** and **ALK-**, *nTFHL-AI* nodal T-follicular cell lymphoma (angioimmunoblastic T-cell lymphoma), *PTCL* peripheral T-cell lymphoma (NOS)

[1]Data is partially based on accumulated data from references in Table 7.6
[2]In ~50% is coexpressed with CD4 [12, 127]
[3]Negative or weak expression [12, 127]
[4]Viable tumor cells are positive for EBER and S100 [12, 127]
[5]Positive of p63 staining may indicate genetic abnormalities associated with worse prognosis [132]
[6]In addition to CD4+/CD8- phenotype a positive staining for at least two of follicular T helper markers (PD1, ICOS, CXCL13, CD10, BCL6, CXCR5, SAP, c-MAF, and CD200) including PD1 are required [12, 127]
[7]GATA3 positivity in a subset of T-cell lymphomas (30–45%) and is usually associated with worse prognosis [55]
[8]TTF1 positivity is reported in 10–25% of cases, usually more often with clone SPT24 than clone 8G7G3/1 [104]
[9]More than 25% of ETP-ALL cases are positive for myeloid antigens including CD117, but negative for MPO [12, 127].

Table 7.9 Immunophenotyping of Hodgkin lymphoma and EBV+MCU[1]

Antibody	Classic Hodgkin lymphoma Hodgkin/Reed-Sternberg cells	Nodular lymphocytic predominant Hodgkin lymphoma L&H (popcorn) cells	EBV+ mucocutaneous ulceration (cHL-like)[2]
CD30		10-25	
CD15	75-90	10-25	~40
EMA	-	40-60	
CD20	10-40 variable data		~60
CD79a	-		>90
CD138	1-40 variable data		---
MUM1		25-40	
J-chain (and κ/λ)			
CD45		75-90	0-50%
PAX-5	Usually weaker than B-cells	Strong as other B-cells	Variable intensity of expression
EBV-EBER	20-60 Depending on subtype		
EBV-LMP1	25-40		80-90
Fascin			
OCT2 / BOB.1	Both negative in 80% one negative in 20%	Both positive	Positive for OCT2 /variable BOB.1
BCL6	10-25		Negative or focal
Background	CD3+ lymphocytes, plasma cells, histiocytes, eosinophils	CD20+ lymphocytes (Usually arranged in nodular pattern)	CD3+ lymphocytes, plasma cells, histiocytes, eosinophils

■ 0->10% positive cases, 10-25% positive cases, 25-40% positive cases, 40-60% positive cases, 60-75% positive cases, 75-90% positive cases, ▬ >90% positive cases, F = focal staining, --- = no data,

[1]Data is partially based on accumulated data from references in Table 7.6
[2]EBV+MCU is similar to classic Hodgkin Lymphoma by immunoprofile and morphology

hematolymphoid markers associated with T- or B-cells is reported in 10–30% of cases [127].

Some histiocytic and dendritic cell proliferations are included in the newest WHO classification as neoplastic, since they have a number of genetic abnormalities which have been recently documented. They may also manifest in the head and neck region, often affecting lymph nodes or as extranodal lesions, but because of their rarity, they are not described in this chapter. A number of immunohistochemical markers like CD1a, CD21, CD23, CD35, CD68, CD123, CD163, S100, and langerin are useful in their diagnostic work up [127].

7.6.7 Small Round Blue Cell Tumors

Malignant tumors included in this group typically offer a diagnostic challenge since biopsy material is often limited, and tumors show a good deal of overlapping morphology and immunophenotype. This group is very heterogeneous and includes poorly differentiated carcinomas, lymphomas, sarcomas, neuroblastoma, and even poorly differentiated mucosal melanoma, especially since mucosal melanomas are often poorly pigmented. Immunoprofiles of poorly differentiated carcinomas in this region are presented in Table 7.1, malignant lymphomas are included in Tables 7.7, and 7.8, and the remaining tumor types are included in Tables. 7.10 and 7.11.

7.6.8 Soft Tissue Tumors

Soft tissue sarcomas are rare at the head and neck. Prevalence is estimated to be less than 1% of all malignant tumors in adults. Head and neck are primary locations for circa 5–10% of all sarcomas. There is no significant geographical variation in frequency, but distribution varies depending on age. Soft tissue tumors comprise numerous different tumor types that are classified according to the type of mesenchymal tissue that they resemble. The most common are adipocytic tumors, followed by MPNST in adults and rhabdomyosarcomas (RMS) among pediatric patients. About 40% of RMS is localized to the head and neck, affecting the orbit, sinonasal tract, ear, and oral cavity most commonly. Finding features of rhabdomyoblastic differentiation, especially in the biopsy one should keep in mind that some other sarcomas may also show minor components of rhabdomyoblastic differentiation. Up to 15% of MPNST may show focal heterologous differentiation, most frequently rhabdomyoblastic (malignant Triton tumor). The focal presence of muscle markers and often foci of S100-positive tumor cells should indicate the diagnosis in such cases. Diagnosis may, however, get complicated by the fact that embryonal RMS may sometimes show a focal presence of S100+ cells. Cases of sarcomatoid carcinoma may also show a 7–15%

presence of heterologous elements, including rare foci of skeletal muscle differentiation. An additional confusing fact is that expression of cytokeratin may be found in up to 7% of RMS, sometimes with the presence of p63+/p40- cells. On the other hand, sarcomatoid carcinoma may be negative for cytokeratins. Rare cases of carcinosarcoma of the salivary glands may show differentiation toward chondrosarcoma, osteosarcoma, leiomyosarcoma, and fibrosarcoma. Olfactory neuroblastoma may show expression of cytokeratin and EMA, but cases with rhabdomyoblastic differentiation or pigmentation due to the presence of melanin-like pigment are described. Malignant melanoma may also show the presence of heterologous mesenchymal elements.

Identification of the direction of differentiation in the neoplastic cells is rather simple in tumors that morphologically are similar to normal tissue types but much more complex and challenging for tumors showing multidirectional differentiation. Tumors are characterized by specific chromosomal changes since they often represent novel lineages with the expression of specific antigens in some cases. The most rational in many cases seems to be the two steps approach.

An initial panel of antibodies is often required in order to establish the broad lineage of the tumor at step one and a subsequent, more focused panel is to allow precise classification at step two. It is important to remember that immunohistochemical evaluation must be correlated with the clinical picture and the morphology, and, when necessary, with other ancillary techniques such as molecular genetics and cytogenetics.

Immunohistochemical profiles for a heterogeneous group of tumors known as small blues round cell tumors are summarized in Table 7.10, and selected soft tissue tumors are in Table 7.11.

7.6.9 Approach to Unknown Primary Tumor (CUP)

Defining the type of metastatic tumor and indicating the most probable location of the primary

Table 7.10 Selected small round blue tumors in head and neck region[1]

Antibody	SCCSal	SCCM lung	MCC	NUTCA	B-ALL/LBL	T-ALL/LBL	EWS[2]	RMS	ONBL[9]	MESCH
PanCK							10-25	40-60	---	
CK7		25-40		40-60						
CK20	40-60									
P40	---			60-75					---	
P63	---	10-25	40-60	60-75			40-60		25-40	
Synapt		60-75					26-40	25-40[3]		
Chromog								10-25[3]		
CD99	---	10-25	25-40	10-25	41-60					40-60
ALK			---				10-25	6	40-60	
TTF1		75-90		11-25					25-40 f	
CD56	25-40			40-60		4	25-40			
CD45					25-40	75-90			10-25	
PAX5	---	80	80	---				60-75		---
CD3										
CD20					10-25					
CD45					10-25	75-90				
TdT	---		60-75			75-90				
SMA								7		
S100				10-25			10-25	10-25	S-cells	40-60
MSA/HHF35									9	
Desmin									9	25-40
MyoD1									9	
Myogenin								8	9	
ERG						60-75	60-75[5]			10-25
FLI1	---		40-60		75-90	---	60-75			
NKX2.2		25-40							75-90	60-75
Other			CDX2 30%, SATB2+ and MCPyV+ 80%				PAX8+ 43% SATB2 og EMA 10%	Biphenot hypic sinonsasal sarcoma APLAP 100% Sox10-7%	PHOX2B	INSM1+ 90%

▬ 0->10% positive cases, 10-25% positive cases, 25-40% positive cases, 40-60% positive cases, 60-75% positive cases, 75-90% positive cases, ▬ >90% positive cases, F = focal staining, --- = no sufficient data,

Abbreviations: SCCSal small cell carcinoma of salivary gland, *SCCM lung* small cell lung carcinoma metastatic, *MCC* Merkel cell carcinoma (metastatic and primary), *B-ALL/LBL* B-cell acute lymphoblastic leukemia/lymphoma, *T-ALL/LBL* T-cell acute lymphoblastic leukemia/lymphoma, *EWS* Ewing sarcoma, *ONBL* neuroblastoma (including olfactory), *RMS* rhabdomyosarcoma (embryonal), *MESCH* mesenchymal chondrosarcoma, *S-cells* sustentacular cells only, *PCPyW* Merkel Cell Polyoma Virus

[1]Data is partially based on accumulated data from Refs. [26, 135, 162, 166–192]
[2]Ewing sarcoma adamantinoma-like subtype is positive as a rule for PANCK, CD99, P40 (positivity for P63 is much lower).
[3]Positive staining for neuroendocrine markers is reported in alveolar type of RMS [167].
[4]Variable reactivity depending on type of lymphoma from 0–100%.
[5]ERG is also commonly positive in blastic extramedullary myeloid tumors—possible pitfall [181].
[6]ALK expression varies between types of RMS 70% in alveolar and 15% embryonal and none pleomorphic or sclerosing type.
[7]Smooth Muscle Actin (SMA) is differently expressed in subtypes of RMS—negative in alveolar, almost always positive in embryonal and around half of the cases of pleomorphic types.
[8]Myogenin is expressed differently being positive almost all cases of embryonal and alveolar type RMS and stains slightly more than half of cases of pleomorphic type.
[9]Neuroblastoma may contain areas of rhabdomyoblastic differentiation.

Table 7.11 Selected soft tissue tumors[1]

Antibody	ARMS	ERMS[9]	MPNST	SS[7]	LMS	EHE	ASA	SFT	IMF	WD-LS/DD–LS[8]	MLS	DSRCT[10]	LGMFS
PanCK	40-60		10-25		10-25	40-60	60-75f		40-60				10-25
CK7		---		70	---	25-40	10-25						---
CD31			25-40										
CD34						60-75	40-60			40-60	25-40		60-75
ERG											40-60		
Actin SMA				10-25		25-40	25-40	10-25	75-90	40-60[3]	10-25	10-25	75-90
MSA/HHF35			40-60		75-90		40-60	10-25	60-75		10-25		75-90
B-Cat (nucl)						25-40	10-25	10-25				40-60	10-25
MUC4[6]				25-40									
Desmin				---	60-75					40-60	25-40*	25-40	40-60
H-Caldes.	---	---	---		60-75			---	10-25		---	---	10-25f
Myogenin													
MyoD1				10-25				---		---			25-40
PRAME	---	---	25-40	10-25			25-40	25-40	---		75-90	---	---
H3K27me3[2]			25-40	25-40			75-90			25-40	---	---	
S100	---		40-60[3]	24							10-25	10-25	
SOX10			60-75[3]	75									
TFE3[11]	---	---	---		---	60-75	25-40				---		
ALK	60-75	10-25							50-70	40-60	60-75		60-75
MDM2[4]		40-60	25-40	28	---				---	75-90		25	---
CDK4[4]		10-25	---		---				---	75-90			---
P16	---	---	25-40	40-60	90	---	40-60		---		10-25	---	
DDIT3		?						25-40			10-25	5	---
Other	PLAP+, CD56+ 97%, Syp 30%, Chromo 20%,	Syp+, ALK+ in spindle cell type	CD56 20% Epithelioid lost SMARCB1,	CK5/6+ in epithelioid	Rb lost in 50%	CAMTA 1+ often, rare TFE3+ fusion	Podoplanin+/- Claudin + INSM1 25%	STAT6+ nuclear reactivity 96%, Bcl2+	ALK+ 50-70, ROS+ Calpo+			Syp 20% CKLMW 90% CD56-80 PLAP+52	Calp, + H-cald+

◼ 0->10% positive cases, **10-25%** positive cases, **25-40%** positive cases, **40-60%** positive cases, **60-75%** positive cases, **75-90%** positive cases ◼ **>90%** positive /cases, --- = no data, f= focal

Abbreviations: *ARMS* alveolar rhabdomyosarcoma, *ERMS* embryonal rhabdomyosarcoma, *MPNST* malignant peripheral nerve sheath tumor, *SS* synovial sarcoma NOS, *LMS* leiomyosarcoma, *EHE* epithelioid hemangioendothelioma, *ASA* angiosarcoma NOS, *SFT* solitary fibrous tumor, *IMF* inflammatory myofibroblastic tumor, *ALT/WD-LS* atypical lipomatous tumor/well-differentiated liposarcoma, *MLS* myxoid liposarcoma, *DSRCT* desmoplastic small round cell tumor, *LGMFS* low grade myofibroblastic sarcoma

[1]Data is partially based on accumulated data from Refs. [12, 94, 118, 167, 193–204]

[2]Loss of expression is more frequent in high-grade and radiation-induced MPNST. Negative staining is also seen in some other tumors [200]

[3]Epithelioid variant of MPNST shows diffuse positivity for S-100, SOX10 and loss of SMARCB1/INI1 (50%) but retains nuclear expression of H3K27me3 in 90%

[4]MDM2 and CDK4 can stain endothelial cells, macrophages and multinucleated giant cells—possible interpretation pitfall. MDM2 stains positive also cases of intimal sarcoma

[5]Positive in 100% of myxoid liposarcoma, 15% of dedifferentiated and 7% of pleomorphic liposarcoma

[6]MUC4 stains also 78% of Sclerosing Epithelioid Fibrosarcoma, 33% Malignant Ossifying Fibromyxoid Tumor of Soft Parts, and 26% Sarcoma CIC-arranged and a number of carcinomas from different organs

[7]SS18-SSX fusion-specific and SSX C-terminus antibodies show high sensitivity and specificity and have a potential to replace molecular testing in cases with this genetic aberration (4)

[8]Myoblastic differentiation often in cases of dedifferentiated liposarcomas

[9]Around 10% of cases show positivity for p63 but p40 is negative as a rule

[10]Reactivity with WT1 antigen is only for C-terminal directed antibodies. Staining with antibodies against N-terminal is negative

[11]Positive staining for TFE3 seen in tumors with gene translocation (alveolar soft part sarcoma and translocation-associated renal cell carcinoma), is also present in some tumors without this translocation [201]

tumor are clinically relevant data. It may take a good deal of resources to answer these questions, especially in cases with limited and or not fully representative biopsy material. Around 3% of all metastatic tumors are today treated without recognition of their primary location and belong to the CUP category. Around 80% of CUP cases represent spread from tumors with the morphology of adenocarcinoma. The remaining 20% represent tumors with other or uncertain lines of differentiation. There are many publications addressing optimal approach to CUP [1, 36, 205–208]. The most rational seems to start the investigation with a careful morphological study of the tumor without any clinical bias. Next is to get as much as possible clinical information including sex, age, and make a careful correlation between clinical data and the morphological impression. At this level, the decision to order or not to order the auxiliary tests is taken. It is important to remember at the early stage of an investigation **to secure** a sufficient amount of material for more extended analysis (e.g., by planning a number of additional unstained slides or dividing material into more paraffin blocks), especially when the primary panel will not give straightforward answers. It is usually better and safer to plan auxiliary tests in at least two steps. It happens that tumor biopsy contains mostly necrotic tissue, but even in such cases may immunohistochemical test generate important however often limited information. Positive staining in necrotic tissue should always be interpreted with caution, but it may be useful in planning the next phase of care; e.g., positivity for cytokeratin may suggest carcinoma, positivity for CD20 may support suspicion of B-cell lymphoma or positivity for markers of melanogenesis like Melan A/MART1 or HMB45 may indicate melanocytic tumor in proper clinical and morphological context [116].

The primary panel in cases with uncertain morphological features should focus on a wide spectrum of antibodies helpful in identifying the line of differentiation of tumor cells (CD45, PanCytokeratin, S100 or SOX10, and optionally vimentin). Replacing S100 with SOX10 may have rational arguments, but one has to be aware of differences in the spectrum of reactivity of both antibodies. There are also rational arguments for using SALL4 in a primary panel in an appropriate morphological context. In case the morphology is enough characteristic for a certain type of tumor (e.g., adenocarcinoma, squamous cell carcinoma, melanoma, or germ cell tumor), the most likely positive antibodies are the first priority, e.g. selected transcription factors, ISNM1 and synaptophysin, p40/p63 and CK5/6, Melan A and HMB45 or SALL4/OCT4/CD30/CD117/D2–40, etc. When the biopsy material is scanty, it is often wise and usually cheaper to wait for the results of the first round of staining and then apply the extended panel of antibodies at the second step.

The secondary panel should include the selection of antibodies, further narrowing the diagnostic possibilities, e.g., transcription factors or other characteristic markers like SMAD4/DPC4. It is important to report the results of staining for prognostic markers (e.g., p16, p53, and Ki-67). The final report should also include information about potential targets for therapy (predictive markers) and here the selection will often depend on tumor type, e.g., cases of breast carcinoma will require reporting of receptor status (estrogen, progesterone, and Her-2), melanoma will require the result of BRAF staining, B-cell malignant lymphoma will call for CD20 and lung adenocarcinoma will need information about staining for ALK, ROS1, NTRK, reporting PDL1 status, etc.

7.6.9.1 Tumor with "Uncharacteristic" Morphology

Analyzing the results of the wide spectrum panel (Table 7.12), is worth remembering that:

1. **PanCytokeratin +** is not always equal to the epithelial origin of the tumor, since many other tumor types are also positive.
2. **S100+** is not only seen in melanocytes, neural, chondroid, and lipomatous tissues but is also present in some other tumor types including carcinomas, many myoepithelial tumors, and some lymphomas. Other markers may vary **PanCK−/+; CD45-,** and **Vimentin+/−.**
3. **CD45+** indicates hematolymphoid origin, but it is often negative in most plasma cell proliferations, some cases of anaplastic large cell lymphoma (ALCL), as well as in acute leukemia with lymphoid or myeloid differentiation. Slightly less than half of dendritic cell sarcomas are also negative. Other markers may vary **PANCK−/+, S100−/+,** and **Vim+/−).**
4. **Vimentin +** is considered a non-specific marker, but in combination with other mark-

ers may sometimes be useful in limiting the spectrum of diagnoses. Other markers may vary **PanCK+/−, CD45+/−,** and **S100+/−.**

5. **PanCytokeratin+/S100+/CD45−/ Vimentin −/+** profile is common in carcinomas of the ovary, thyroid, kidney, poorly differentiated breast carcinoma, and myoepithelial tumors.
6. **PanCytokeratin+/CD45+/**profile indicates usually the aberrant expression of cytokeratins in hematolymphoid tumor (often plasma cell tumor). Only exceptional cases of other tumors will show aberrant expression of **CD45**. Other markers may vary **S100−/+** and **Vim−/+.**
7. **PanCytokeratin+/Vimentin +** characterizes quite heterogeneous group of tumors including carcinomas (most commonly thyroid, endometrium, kidney, poorly differentiated tumors, and sarcomatoid types), mesothelioma, myoepithelial tumors, chordoma, and some sarcomas (e.g., epithelioid sarcoma, synovial sarcoma, and leiomyosarcoma).
8. **PanCytokeratin+/Vimentin-** profile is seen in most carcinomas, particularly pancreas, prostate, breast, small cell carcinoma, NUT midline carcinoma, but also in epithelioid sarcoma.
9. **PanCytokeratin-/Vim+** profile speaks in favor of non-epithelial tumors as a first choice but some types of epithelial tumors including adrenal cortical carcinoma, epithelial-myoepithelial and sarcomatoid/spindle cell carcinoma of ENT origin, solid pseudopapillary tumor of the pancreas may also be in this group.
10. **CD45+/S100+** profile is often associated with dendritic cell tumors and T-cell lymphomas. Other markers may vary **PanCK−/+** and **Vim +/−.**

7.6.9.2 Adenocarcinoma of Unknown Origin

Tumors showing more or less a characteristic morphologic pattern of adenocarcinoma used to show variable expression of Cytokeratin 7 and Cytokeratin 20. Staining for these cytokeratins

Table 7.12 Flow chart for unknown primary tumor (CUP) with common tumors for different results from the basic panel

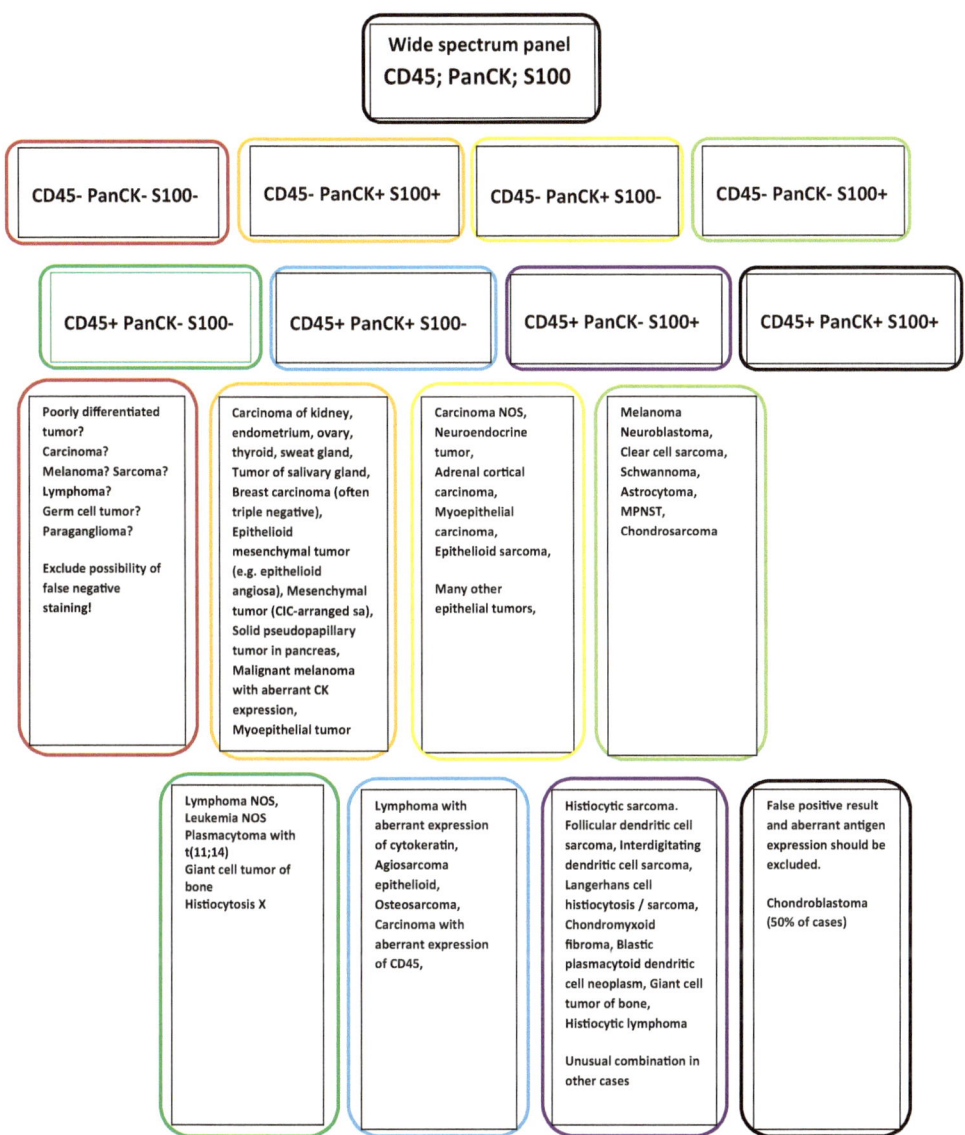

helps to subgroup primary carcinomas into one of four following expression patterns: **CK7−/CK20−, CK7+/CK20−, CK7+/CK20+** and **CK7−/CK20+** reflecting the most common combination of the expression of both cytokeratins in adenocarcinomas of different organs (see Table 7.13). Each major group also contains a varying percentage of adenocarcinomas which differ in this paired cytokeratin expression from the dominating pattern. One should keep in mind that some mesenchymal tumors with epithelioid morphology (i.e., synovial sarcoma and epithelioid sarcoma) in addition to deceptive morphology can also express CK7 or/and CK20. Search for the primary location of adenocarcinoma usually benefits from additional staining for selected more specific organ/tissue markers (e.g., PSA, Thyroglobulin, S100, or synaptophysin) or lineage markers including selected transcription factors (e.g., CDX2, SATB2, GATA3, PAX8, BAP1, or TTF1).

Table 7.13 Distribution of reactivity CK7 and CK20 among adenocarcinomas (Based partially on Refs. [1] and [205])

	CK20+	CK20-
CK7+	Esophageal adenocarcinoma Extrahepatic cholangiocarcinoma Gastric adenocarcinoma (subset) Lung adenocarcinoma with enteric differentiation (subset) MMR-deficient colon adenocarcinoma Mucinous ovarian carcinoma Pancreas adenocarcinoma (ductal) Peritoneal pseudomyxoma Small intestinal adenocarcinoma Urothelial adenocarcinoma (subset) Yolk sac tumor	Breast adenocarcinoma NOS Cholangiocarcinoma NOS Endometrioid adenocarcinoma Endocervical adenocarcinoma Gastric adenocarcinoma (subset) Lung adenocarcinoma NOS Mesothelioma (non-sarcomatous) Ovarian (non-mucinous) adenocarcinoma Pancreas adenocarcinoma (subset) Thyroid carcinoma (non-medullary) Thyroid carcinoma medullary
CK7-	Colorectal adenocarcinoma Merkel cell carcinoma Small cell carcinoma of salivary glands	Adrenal cortical carcinoma Hepatocellular carcinoma Neuroendocrine carcinoma prostate adenocarcinoma Renal cell carcinoma,

7.6.10 Perspectives in Immunohistochemistry and Molecular Testing

A rapidly expanding class of antibodies detecting specific products of molecular changes ("mutation-specific antibodies") in different tumors follows the development in molecular biology of neoplasia and becomes increasingly important in verifying diagnosis and predicting response to therapy. Certain antibodies/tests may be used alone but more often are used as effective screening tools in connection with specific molecular testing done to confirm the result of immunohistochemical tests. It should be remembered that these important new products have to be thoroughly tested regarding their sensitivity and specificity and possible cross-reactivity with non-intended targets to avoid serious pitfalls [56, 209–211]. The rapidly growing knowledge about cancer immunology will certainly generate new drugs and new tests helping to choose the optimal treatment for the patient and more exactly predict the tumor response, especially in the field of immunotherapy. The tendency within immunohistochemistry toward multiplexing the targets will increase our ability to extract more information from a single section of tissue but will also demand high standards of quality control and high-quality automation.

7.7 Essentials of Immunohistochemistry

Immunohistochemistry is a complex, multistep procedure with many variables where each step is important and where high standards of quality are essential for optimal results.

- Absolutely essential in diagnostic work is ability to integrate morphology and immuno-profiles with demographic and clinical data.
- Algorithms are useful but many exceptions from the standard immunohistochemical profiles of tumors make pathology a diagnostic art.
- Application of antibodies with overlapping spectrum of reactivity often means a waste of resources.
- Awareness of spectrum of reactivity of antibodies and reactivity of their different clones is essential for correct interpretation.
- BRAFV600E positive staining is not compatible with neither thyroid tumors of uncertain malignant potential (UMP) nor non-invasive follicular thyroid neoplasm with papillary-like nuclear features (NIFTP)—it indicates papillary thyroid carcinomas (PTC).
- CD56 (NCAM) has a wide distribution and is detected in a number of different cell types including neuroendocrine cells as well as in

their tumors. If used as a marker of neuroendocrine differentiation, it should be applied and interpreted in a panel because of its low specificity.

- Carcinoma is usually characterized by uniform, strong expression of cytokeratins, and true negative cytokeratin staining practically rules out carcinoma. Focal staining for cytokeratins usually speaks for their aberrant expression.
- Carcinomas negative for both CK7 and CK20 are often positive for neuroendocrine markers.
- Chromogranin A is an integral part neuroendocrine granules and is a specific marker of neuroendocrine differentiation, but the sensitivity of staining is low in some tumors.
- CD56 is a sensitive antibody but is not recommended alone as a neuroendocrine marker due to poor specificity.
- Cytokeratins are the most important markers for diagnosis of epithelial neoplasms and a number of robust anti-cytokeratin antibodies (both wide and narrow spectrum) with verified sensitivity and minimal cross-reactivity should be available in the stock.
- Cytokeratin-low tumors include adrenal cortical carcinoma, spindle cell carcinomas, and neuroendocrine carcinomas.
- Diagnostic power of any immunohistochemical test is never greater than the wisdom of the pathologist interpreting it (by Allen Gown).
- Dot-like pattern of cytokeratin staining is characteristic for neuroendocrine tumors/carcinomas.
- Keeping up with published information is essential, but referring also to own judgments and experience often critical.
- Magic bullets do not exist in immunohistochemistry, and there are neither 100% specific nor 100% sensitive antibodies.
- Malignant melanocytic tumors are genetically unstable and in addition to great morphological variation often show aberrant expression of different markers (e.g., cytokeratin, neuroendocrine markers, and CD117) in addition to typical melanoma markers or on the contrary they can lose expression of melanocytic markers during the progression of the tumor.
- Myoepithelial cells show a combination of positive staining for high molecular weight cytokeratin (CK5, CK5/6, CK14, and CK17) with the presence of smooth muscle-related contractile proteins (SMA, Calponin, and SMMHC). Other sensitive but non-specific markers include P63, P40, S100, SOX10, CD10, GFAP, Maspin, and Podoplanin. Myoepithelial tumors often show variation in their immunophenotype.
- Quality of staining of internal and external controls should always be evaluated before the interpretation of diagnostic staining.
- S100+/CD34+/SOX10- profile in spindle cell mesenchymal tumors is not specific but is often seen in association with NTRK fusions.
- Selecting the most sensitive and most specific antibodies to address considered differential diagnoses is a part of the rational use of resources.
- In B5 fixed material the staining for CD5, CD30, and Synaptophysin is often false negative, and staining for ALK, Ulex, and GFAP is often clearly weakened [11].
- Staining for S100 has low specificity and should be used and interpreted in the panel. Cases with strong and diffuse staining for S100 should always have malignant melanoma among differentials.
- Synaptophysin is present in presynaptic vesicles of neurons, neuroendocrine cells, and adrenal gland (cortex and medulla) and their tumors—it is considered sensitive but not a fully specific marker of neuroendocrine differentiation since some non-endocrine tumors (e.g., Ewing sarcoma and alveolar rhabdomyosarcoma) are also positive. It is recommended to be used in tandem with new highly sensitive and specific marker of neuroendocrine cells (INSM1).
- Type of fixative and the time when fixation has started should always be recorded on the request form.
- Unexpected results with false negative or false positive staining are a part of everyday work.

- Unexpected or morphologically unusual staining should always be verified with other antibodies (e.g., positive granular cytoplasmic staining for CD31 in histiocyte-like cells should be verified with staining, e.g., ERG to prevent erroneous classification of the lesion as vascular tumor).

7.8   Microphotographic images

Selection of microphotographs from different types of biopsy materials, tissues and tumors illustrating variation of immunohistochemical patterns and possible pitfalls is presented below (Figs. 7.1, 7.2, 7.3, 7.4, 7.5, 7.6, 7.7, 7.8, 7.9, 7.10, 7.11, 7.12, 7.13, 7.14, 7.15, 7.16, 7.17, 7.18, 7.19, 7.20, 7.21, 7.22, 7.23 and 7.24).

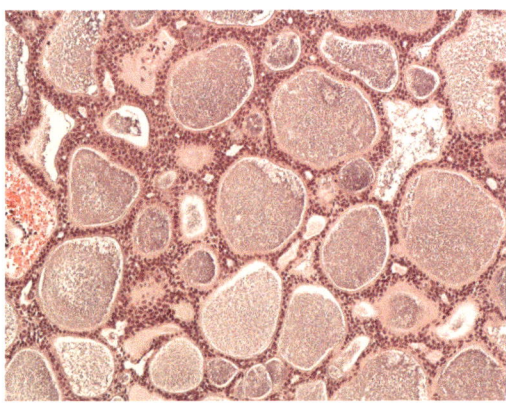

Fig. 7.1 Adenoid cystic carcinoma of epipharynx. FFPE material. 10x. HE

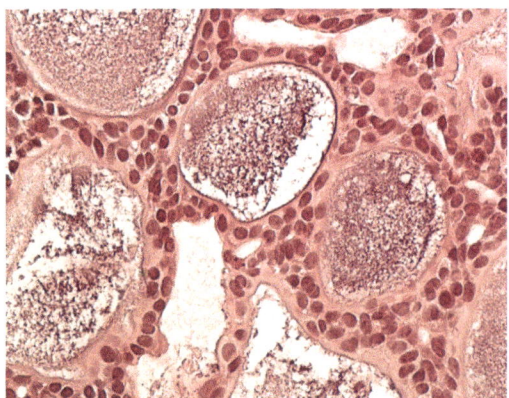

Fig. 7.2 Adenoid cystic carcinoma of epipharynx. FFPE material. 40x. HE

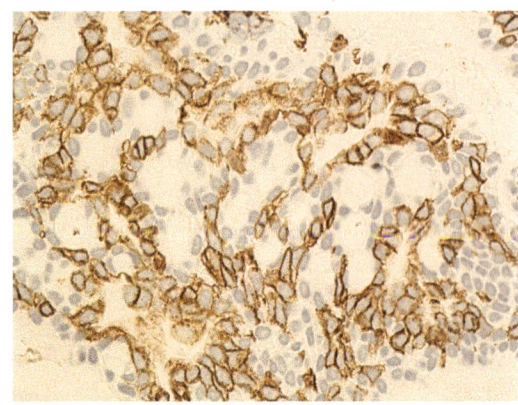

Fig. 7.3 Adenoid cystic carcinoma of epipharynx. FFPE material. CD117 positive membranous staining of luminal cells

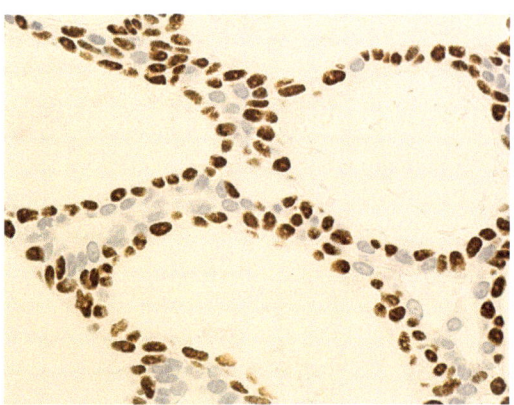

Fig. 7.4 Adenoid cystic carcinoma of epipharynx. P63 positive staining of nuclei of myoepithelial cells

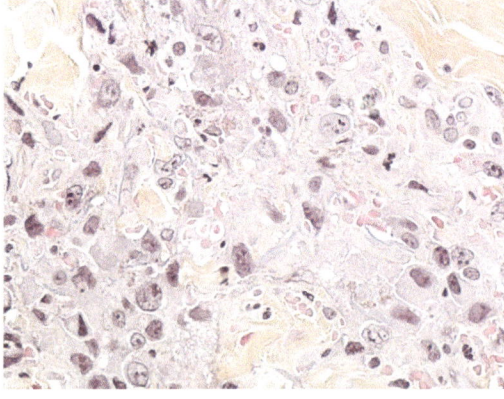

Fig. 7.5 Epithelioid angiosarcoma. FFPE material. Epithelioid cells with formation of vascular spaces with single erythrocytes. HE

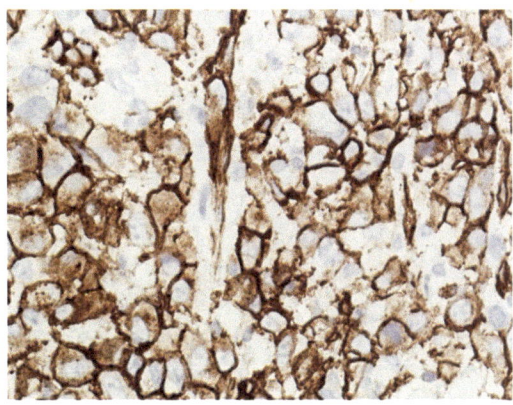

Fig. 7.6 Epithelioid angiosarcoma. FFPE material. Membranous staining of tumor cells with endothelial cell marker CD31

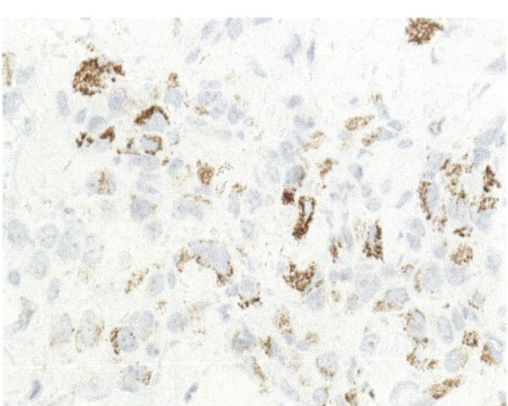

Fig. 7.9 Epithelioid angiosarcoma. FFPE material. MelanA (clone A103) aberrant cytoplasmic staining of varying intensity. Potential pitfall

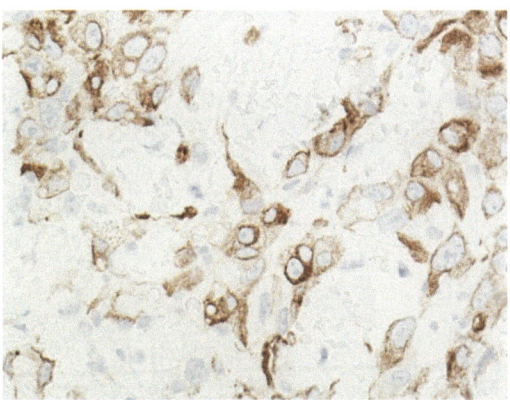

Fig. 7.7 Epithelioid angiosarcoma. FFPE material. Pancytokeratin (A1/A3/5D3) staining in the cytoplasm of tumor cells. Potential pitfall

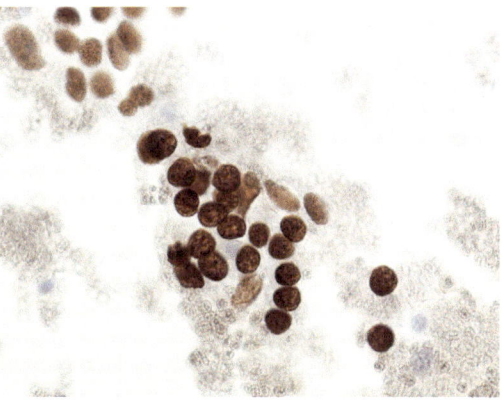

Fig. 7.10 Medullary thyroid carcinoma. FNAC. Fixed smear. Positive nuclear staining of tumor cells for TTF1 (clone SP24)

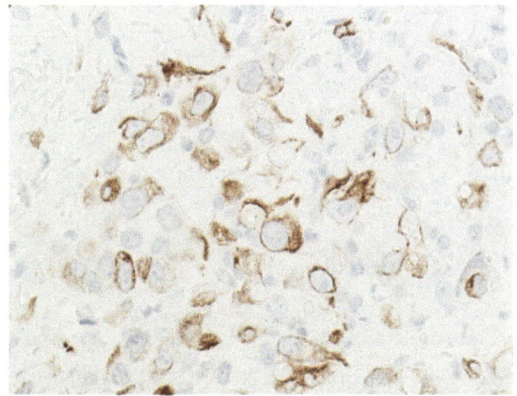

Fig. 7.8 Epitelioid angiosarcoma. FFPE material. Cytoplasmic staining for CK7. Potential pitfall

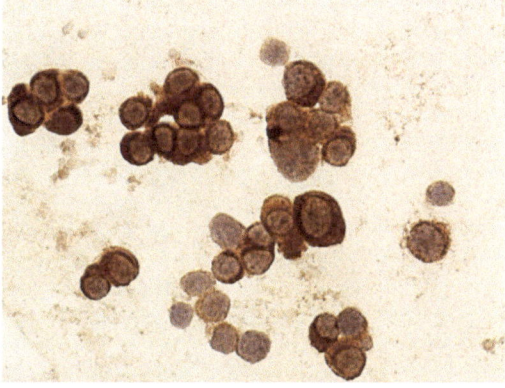

Fig. 7.11 Medullary thyroid carcinoma. FNAC. Fixed smear. Calcitonin staining. Preservation of the positively stained cytoplasm overlaying nucleus may give false impression of nuclear positivity in this case

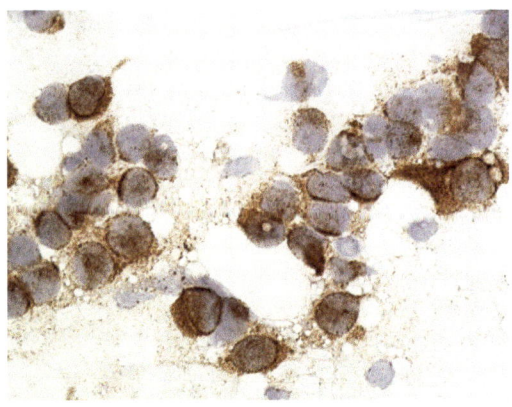

Fig. 7.12 Metastatic melanoma. FNAC. Fixed smear. Melan A (clone 103)

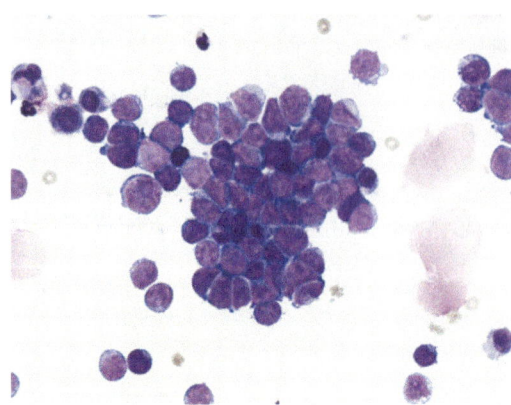

Fig. 7.15 Metastatic Merkel cell carcinoma. Smear from pleural fluid. HC

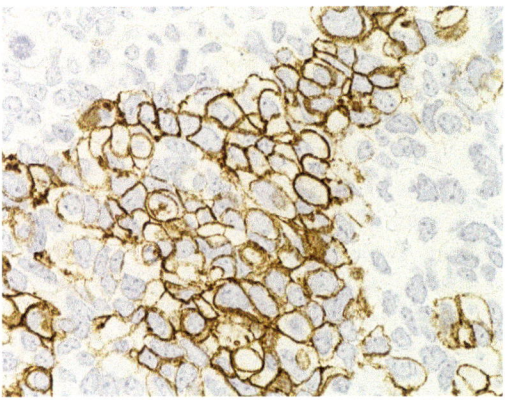

Fig. 7.13 Metastatic melanoma. FFPE material. Focus of tumor cells with aberrant membranous positive staining for CD45 (Common Leukocyte Antigen)

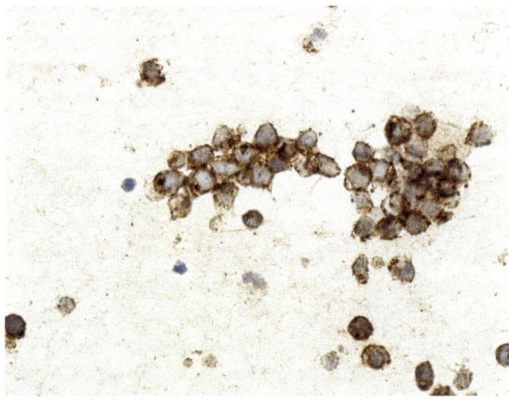

Fig. 7.16 Metastatic Merkel cell carcinoma. Fixed smear from pleural fluid. ALK (clone D5F3) shows positive cytoplasmic staining in tumor cells

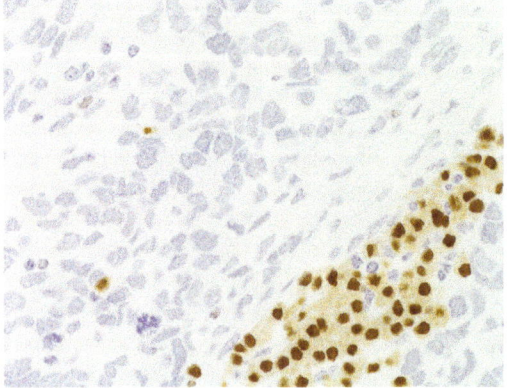

Fig. 7.14 Metastatic melanoma. FFPE material. MUM1 positive plasma cells close to focus of melanoma cells from Fig. 7.13

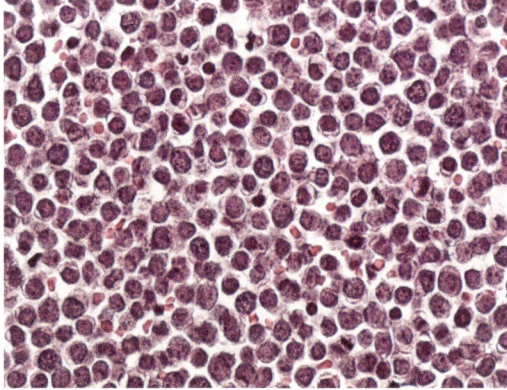

Fig. 7.17 Metastatic Merkel cell carcinoma. FFPE cell block from pleural fluid. HE

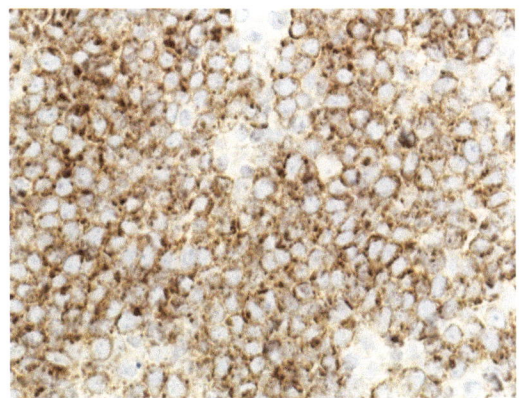

Fig. 7.18 Metastatic Merkel cell carcinoma. FFPE cell block from pleural fluid. Positive cytoplasmic staining for neuroendocrine marker Synaptophysin

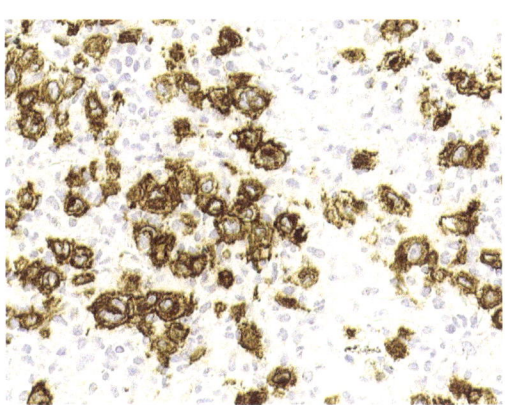

Fig. 7.21 EBV+ mucocutaneous ulceration. FFPE biopsy. Large atypical Reed-Sternberg-like cells show the characteristic positive pattern of staining for CD30

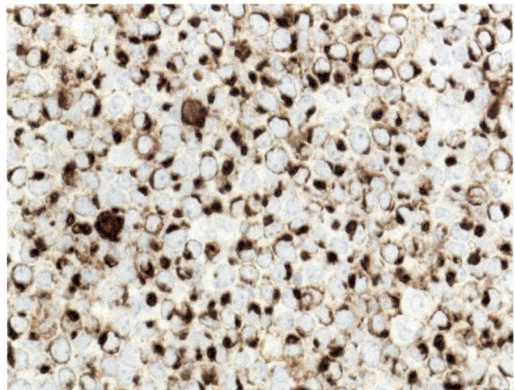

Fig. 7.19 Metastatic Merkel cell carcinoma. FFPE cell block from pleural fluid. Positive dot-like cytoplasmic staining for CK20 in tumor cells

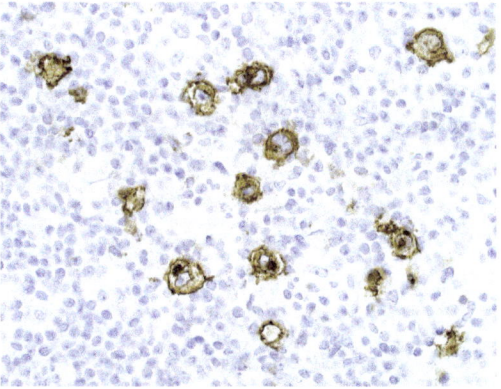

Fig. 7.22 Classic Hodgkin lymphoma. FFPE biopsy of the lymph node. Characteristic positive CD30 staining of Reed-Sternberg cells. Compare with Fig 7.21

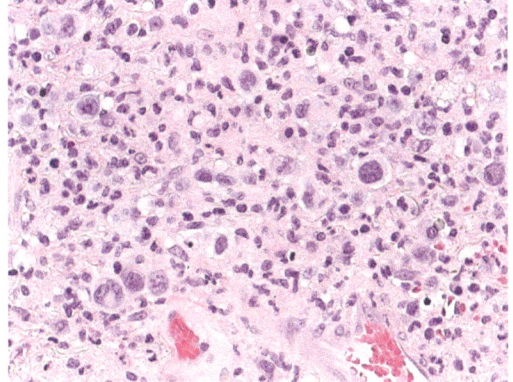

Fig. 7.20 EBV+ mucocutaneous ulceration. FFPE biopsy. Large atypical Reed-Sternberg-like cells present. HE

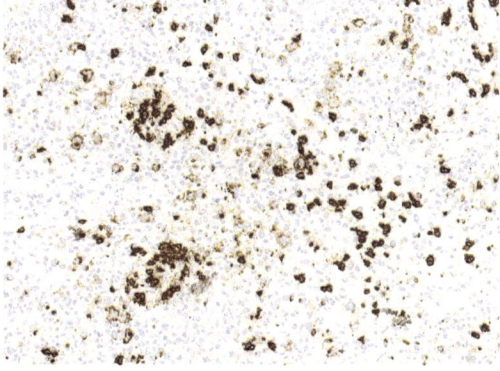

Fig. 7.23 EBV+ mucocutaneous ulceration. Large atypical Reed-Sternberg-like cells and granulocytes stained with CD15

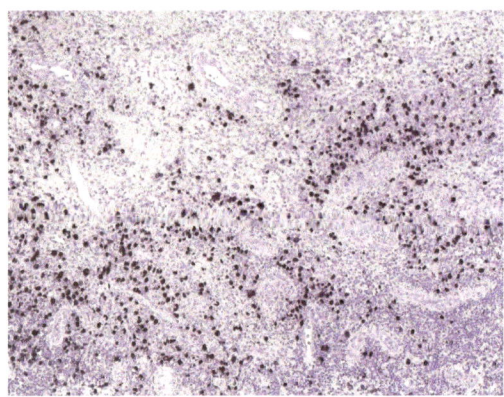

Fig. 7.24 EBV+ mucocutaneous ulceration with large atypical Reed-Sternberg-like cells. Positive EBER staining confirms the presence of EBV

References

1. Dabbs DJ. Diagnostic immunohistochemistry. Theranostic and genomic applications. 6th ed. Elsevier; 2022. ISBN-13: 978-0-323-72172-1
2. Torlakovic EE, Nielsen S, Vyberg M, et al. Getting controls under control: the time is now for immunohistochemistry. Rev J Clin Pathol. 2015;68(11):879–82. Epub 2015 Aug 18
3. Torlakovic EE. Fit-for-purpose Immunohistochemical biomarkers. Endocr Pathol. 2018;29(2):199–205. Review
4. Vyberg M. Anvendt immunhistokjemi. 7th ed; 2007. ISBN: 87-89579-25-9
5. Kirbis IS, Maxwell P, Fležar MS, et al. External quality control for immunocytochemistry on cytology samples: a review of UK NEQAS ICC (cytology module) results. Cytopathology. 2011;22(4):230–7. Epub 2011 Apr 25
6. Srebotnik Kirbiš I, Rodrigues Roque R, Bongiovanni M, et al. Immunocytochemistry practices in European cytopathology laboratories-Review of European Federation of Cytology Societies (EFCS) online survey results with best practice recommendations. Cancer Cytopathol. 2020;128(10):757–66. Epub 2020 Jun 29
7. Chetty R, Cooper K, Gown AM. Leong's manual of diagnostic antibodies for immunohistochemistry. 3rd ed. Cambridge University Press; 2016. ISBN 978-1-107-07778-2
8. www.ihc-academy.patomorfologia-cmuj.pl annual courses of academy of immunohistochemistry, Krakow 2014–2019.
9. www.nordiqc.org; https://nordiqc.org/downloads/assessments/158_64.pdf
10. Rekhtman N, Ang DC, Sima CS, et al. Immunohistochemical algorithm for differentiation of lung adenocarcinoma and squamous cell carcinoma based on large series of whole-tissue sections with validation in small specimens. Mod Pathol. 2011;24(10):1348–59. Epub 2011 May 27
11. Wan X, Cochran G, GreinerTC. Removal of mercuric chloride deposits from B5-fixed tissue will affect the performance of immunoperoxidase staining of selected antibodies. Appl Immunohistochem Mol Morphol. 2003;11(1):92–5.
12. WHO Classification of Tumours Editorial Board. Head and neck tumours [Internet; beta version ahead of print]. Lyon (France): International Agency for Research on Cancer; 2022 [cited 2023.01.09]. (WHO classification of tumours series, 5th ed.; vol. 9). Available from: https://tumourclassification.iarc.who.int/chapters/52
13. Bishop JA. Ne   cribed tumor entities in sinonasal tract pathology. Head Neck Pathol. 2016;10(1):23–31. Epub 2016 Feb 1
14. Bishop JA, Antonescu CR, Westra WH. SMARCB1 (INI-1)-deficient carcinomas of the sinonasal tract. Am J Surg Pathol. 2014;38(9):1282–9.
15. Bishop JA, Westra WH. NUT midline carcinomas of the sinonasal tract. Am J Surg Pathol. 2012;36(8):1216–21.
16. Chernock RD, Perry A, Pfeifer JD, et al. Receptor tyrosine kinases in sinonasal undifferentiated carcinomas--evaluation for EGFR, c-KIT, and HER2/neu expression. Head Neck. 2009;31(7):919–27.
17. Hung YP, Chen AL, Taylor MS, et al. Thoracic nuclear protein in testis (NUT) carcinoma: expanded pathological spectrum with expression of thyroid transcription factor-1 and neuroendocrine markers. Histopathology. 2021;78(6):896–904. Epub 2021 Mar 12
18. Lewis JS Jr, Chernock RD, Bishop JA. Squamous and neuroendocrine specific Immunohistochemical markers in head and neck squamous cell carcinoma: a tissue microarray study. Head Neck Pathol. 2018;12(1):62–70. Epub 2017 May 20
19. Montone KT. The Differential Diagnosis of Sinonasal/Nasopharyngeal Neuroendocrine/Neuroectodermally Derived Tumors. Arch Pathol Lab Med. 2015;139(12):1498–507.
20. Stelow EB, Bellizzi AM, Taneja K, et al. NUT rearrangement in undifferentiated carcinomas of the upper aerodigestive tract. Am J Surg Pathol. 2008;32(6):828–34.
21. Stelow EB, Bishop JA. Update from the 4th edition of the World Health Organization classification of head and neck Tumours: tumors of the nasal cavity, paranasal sinuses and Skull Base. Head Neck Pathol. 2017;11(1):3–15.
22. Thompson LDR, Franchi A. New tumor entities in the 4th edition of the World Health Organization classification of head and neck tumors: nasal cavity, paranasal sinuses and skull base. Virchows Arch. 2018;472(3):315–30.
23. Wadsworth B, Bumpous JM, Martin AW, et al. Expression of p16 in sinonasal undifferentiated carcinoma (SNUC) without associated human papilloma-

virus (HPV). Head Neck Pathol. 2011;5(4):349–54. Epub 2011 Jul 30

24. Xu B, Katabi N. Myoepithelial Carcinoma. Surg Pathol Clin. 2021;14(1):67–73.

25. Zhou L, Yong X, Zhou J, et al. Clinicopathological analysis of five cases of NUT midline carcinoma, including one with the gingiva. Biomed Res Int. 2020; eCollection 2020

26. Mukhopadhyay S, Katzenstein A-LA. Subclassification of non-small cell lung carcinomas lacking morphologic differentiation on biopsy specimens: utility of an immunohisto-chemical panel containing TTF-1, napsin a, p63, and CK5/6. Am J Surg Pathol. 2011;35(1):15–25.

27. Nonaka D, Chiriboga L, Rubin BP. Sox10: a pan-schwannian and melanocytic marker. Am J Surg Pathol. 2008;32(9):1291–8.

28. Ohtomo R, Mori T, Shibata S, et al. SOX10 is a novel marker of acinus and intercalated duct dif-ferentiation in salivary gland tumors: a clue to the histogenesis for tumor diagnosis. Mod Pathol. 2013;26(8):1041–50.

29. Lee JH, Kang HJ, Yoo CW, et al. PLAG1, SOX10, and Myb expression in benign and malignant salivary gland neoplasms. J Pathol Transl Med. 2019;53(1):23–30. Epub 2018 Nov 14

30. Agaimy A, Hartmann A, Antonescu CR, et al. SMARCB1 (INI-1)- deficient Sinonasal carcinoma: a series of 39 cases expanding the morphologic and Clinicopathologic Spectrum of a recently described entity. Am J Surg Pathol. 2017;41(4):458–71.

31. Antony VM, Kakkar A, Sikka K, et al. p16 Immunoexpression in sinonasal and nasopharyn-geal adenoid cystic carcinomas: a potential pitfall in ruling out HPV-related multiphenotypic sinona-sal carcinoma. Histopathology. 2020;77(6):989–93. Epub 2020 Sep 20

32. Bilodeau EA, Acquafondata M, Barnes EL, et al. A comparative analysis of LEF-1 in odontogenic and salivary tumors. Hum Pathol. 2015;46(2):255–9. Epub 2014 Nov 12

33. Bishop JA, Rooper LM, Chiosea SI, et al. Clear cell carcinoma of salivary glands is frequently p16 posi-tive: a pitfall in the interpretation of oropharyngeal biopsies. Am J Surg Pathol. 2018;42(3):367–71.

34. Hsieh M-S, Lee Y-H, Chang Y-L. SOX10-positive salivary gland tumors: a growing list, including mammary analogue secretory carcinoma of the sali-vary gland, sialoblastoma, low-grade salivary duct carcinoma, basal cell adenoma/adenocarcinoma, and a subgroup of mucoepidermoid carcinoma. Hum Pathol. 2016;56:134–42. Epub 2016 Jun 17

35. Li W, Chastain K. NUT midline carcinoma with leu-kemic presentation mimicking CD34-positive acute leukemia. Blood. 2018;132(4):456.

36. Meer S, Altini M. CK7+/CK20- immunoexpres-sion profile is typical of salivary gland neoplasia. Histopathology. 2007;51(1):26–32.

37. Nagao T, Gaffey TA, Olsen KD, et al. Small cell carcinoma of the major salivary glands: clinico-pathologic study with emphasis on cytokeratin 20 immunoreactivity and clinical outcome. Am J Surg Pathol. 2004;28(6):762–70.

38. Nagao T, Sato E, Inoue R, et al. Immunohistochemical analysis of salivary gland tumors: application for surgical pathology practice. Acta Histochem Cytochem. 2012;45(5):269–82.

39. Nikitakis NG, Tosios KI, Papanikolaou VI, et al. Immunohistochemical expression of cytokeratins 7 and 20 in malignant salivary gland tumors. Mod Pathol. 2004;17(4):407–15.

40. Patel KR, Solomon IH, El-Mofty SK, et al. Mammaglobin and S-100 immunoreactivity in salivary gland carcinomas other than mam-mary analogue secretory carcinoma. Hum Pathol. 2013;44(11):2501–8. Epub 2013 Sep 10

41. Rezende RB, Drachenberg CB, Kumar D, et al. Differential diagnosis between monomorphic clear cell adenocarcinoma of salivary glands and renal (clear) cell carcinoma. The American Journal of Surgical Pathology. 1999;23(12):1532.

42. Ronen S, Aguilera-Barrantes I, Giorgadze T, et al. Polymorphous sweat gland carcinoma: an Immunohistochemical and molecular study. Am J Dermatopathol. 2018;40(8):5.

43. Rooney SL, Robinson RA. Immunohistochemical expression of MYB in salivary gland basal cell ade-nocarcinoma and basal cell adenoma. J Oral Pathol Med. 2017;46(9):798–802. Epub 2017 Aug 8

44. Schwartz LE, Begum S, Westra WH, et al. GATA3 immunohistochemical expression in salivary gland neoplasms. Head Neck Pathol. 2013;7(4):311–5. Epub 2013 Apr 20

45. Seethala RR, Stenman G. Update from the 4th edi-tion of the World Health Organization classification of head and neck tumours: tumors of the salivary gland. Head Neck Pathol. 2017;11(1):55–67.

46. Shah AA, Jain D, Ababneh E, et al. SMARCB1 (INI-1)-deficient adenocarcinoma of the Sinonasal tract: a potentially under-recognized form of Sinonasal adenocarcinoma with occasional yolk sac tumor-like features. Head Neck Pathol. 2020;14(2):465–72. Epub 2019 Aug 29

47. Sun T, Akalin A, Dresser K, et al. The utility of MYB immunohistochemistry (IHC) in fine needle aspira-tion (FNA) diagnosis of adenoid cystic carcinoma (AdCC). Head Neck Pathol. 2021;15(2):389–94. Epub 2020 Jul 13

48. Takada N, Nishida H, Oyama Y, et al. Immunohistochemical reactivity of prostate-specific markers for salivary duct carcinoma. Pathobiology. 2020;87(1):30–6.

49. West RB, Kong C, Clarke N, et al. MYB expression and translocation in adenoid cystic carcinomas and other salivary gland tumors with clinicopathologic correlation. Am J Surg Pathol. 2011;35(1):92.

50. Zhu S, Schuerch C, Hunt J. Review and updates of immunohistochemistry in selected salivary gland and head and neck tumors. Arch Pathol Lab Med. 2015;139(1):55–66.

51. Moretti L, Medeiros LJ, Kunkalla K, et al. N-terminal PAX8 polyclonal antibody shows cross-reactivity with N-terminal region of PAX5 and is responsible for reports of PAX8 positivity in malignant lymphomas. Mod Pathol. 2012;25(2):231–6.

52. WHO Classification of Tumours Editorial Board. Endocrine and neuroendocrine tumours [internet]. Lyon: International Agency for Research on Cancer; 2022 [cited 2023 Jan 20]. (WHO classification of tumours series, 5th ed.; vol. 10). Available from: https://tumourclassification.iarc.who.int/chapters/53

53. Kiriakopoulos A, Giannakis P, Menenakos E. Calcitonin: current concepts and differential diagnosis. Ther Adv Endocrinol Metab. 2022; eCollection 2022

54. Llewellyn DC, Srirajaskanthan R, Vincent RP, et al. Calcitonin-secreting neuroendocrine neoplasms of the lung: a systematic review and narrative synthesis. Endocr Connect. 2021;10(4):447–61.

55. Uccella S, Blank A, Maragliano R, et al. Calcitonin-producing neuroendocrine neoplasms of the pancreas: clinicopathological study of 25 cases and review of the literature. Endocr Pathol. 2017;28(4):351–61.

56. Jones RT, Abedalthagafi MS, Brahmandam M, et al. Cross-reactivity of the BRAF VE1 antibody with epitopes in axonemal dyneins leads to staining of cilia. Mod Pathol. 2015;28(4):596–606. Epub 2014 Nov 21

57. Baloch Z, Mete O, Asa SL. Immunohistochemical biomarkers in thyroid pathology. Endocr Pathol. 2018;29(2):91–112.

58. Cho U, Kim Y, Jeon S, et al. CD56 expression in papillary thyroid carcinoma is highly dependent on the histologic subtype: a potential diagnostic pitfall. Appl Immunohistochem Mol Morphol. 2022;30(5):389–96. Epub 2022 Mar 1

59. Hirsch SM, Faquin WC, Krane JF. Thyroid transcription factor-1, but not p53, is helpful in distinguishing moderately differentiated neuroendocrine carcinoma of the larynx from medullary carcinoma of the thyroid. Mod Pathol. 2004;17(6):631–6.

60. Kebebew E, Weng J, Bauer J, et al. The prevalence and prognostic value of BRAF mutation in thyroid cancer. Ann Surg. 2007;246(3):466–70; discussion 470–1

61. Liu Y, Huang X, Hu Y, et al. Hyalinizing trabecular tumor of the thyroid: a clinicopathological analysis of four cases and review of the literature. Int J Clin Exp Pathol. 2017;10(7):7616–26. eCollection 2017

62. Muthusamy S, Azhar Sha S, Abdullah Suhaimi SN, et al. CD56 expression in benign and malignant thyroid lesions. Malays J Pathol. 2018;40(2):111–9. PMID: 30173227

63. Ordóñez NG. Value of PAX 8 immunostaining in tumor diagnosis: a review and update. Adv Anat Pathol. 2012;19(3):140–51.

64. Pyo J-S, Kim D-H, Yang J. Diagnostic value of CD56 immunohistochemistry in thyroid lesions. Int J Biol Markers. 2018;33(2):161–7.

65. Satoh F, Umemura S, Yasuda M, et al. Neuroendocrine marker expression in thyroid epithelial tumors. Endocr Pathol. 2001;12(3):291–9.

66. Singh K, Hanley LC, Sung CJ, et al. Comparison of PAX8 expression in breast carcinoma using MRQ50 and BC12 monoclonal antibodies. Appl Immunohistochem Mol Morphol. 2020;28(7):558–61.

67. Tastekin E, Keskin E, Can N, et al. CD56, CD57, HBME1, CK19, Galectin-3 and p63 immunohistochemical stains in differentiating diagnosis of thyroid benign/malign lesions and NIFTP. Pol J Pathol. 2019;70(4):286–94.

68. Walczyk A, Kopczyński J, Gąsior-Perczak D, et al. Histopathology and immunohistochemistry as prognostic factors for poorly differentiated thyroid cancer in a series of polish patients. PLoS One. 2020; eCollection 2020

69. www.nordiqc.org; https://nordiqc.org/epitope.php?id=75

70. www.nordiqc.org; https://nordiqc.org/epitope.php?id=64

71. www.nordiqc.org

72. Mete O, Asa SL, Gill AJ, et al. Overview of the 2022 WHO classification of Paragangliomas and Pheochromocytomas. Endocr Pathol. 2022;33(1):90–114. Epub 2022 Mar 13

73. Rooper LM, Bishop JA, Westra WH. INSM1 is a sensitive and specific marker of neuroendocrine differentiation in head and neck tumors. Am J Surg Pathol. 2018;42(5):665–71.

74. Alos L, Hakim S, Larque A-B, et al. p16 overexpression in high-grade neuroendocrine carcinomas of the head and neck: potential diagnostic pitfall with HPV-related carcinomas. Virchows Arch. 2016;469(3):277–84. Epub 2016 Jul 8

75. Bell D, Hanna E-Y, Weber RS, et al. Neuroendocrine neoplasms of the sinonasal region. Head Neck. 2016;38(Suppl 1):E2259–66. Epub 2015 Jul 18

76. Bellizzi AM. SATB2 in neuroendocrine neoplasms: strong expression is restricted to well-differentiated tumours of lower gastrointestinal tract origin and is most frequent in Merkel cell carcinoma among poorly differentiated carcinomas. Histopathology. 2020;76(2):251–64. Epub 2019 Nov 15

77. Berg KB, Schaeffer DF. SATB2 as an immunohistochemical marker for colorectal adenocarcinoma: a concise review of benefits and pitfalls. Arch Pathol Lab Med. 2017;141(10):1428–33.

78. Dabir PD, Svanholm H, Christiansen JJ. SATB2 is a supplementary immunohistochemical marker to CDX2 in the diagnosis of colorectal carcinoma metastasis in an unknown primary. APMIS. 2018;126(6):494–500.

79. Delfin L, Asa SL. Paraganglioma. PathologyOutlines.com website. https://www.pathologyoutlines.com/topic/adrenalparaganglioma.html. Accessed 9 Nov 2022.

80. De Michele S, Remotti HE. Special AT-rich sequence-binding protein 2 (SATB2). PathologyOutlines.com

website. https://www.pathologyoutlines.com/topic/stainssatb2.html. Accessed 16 Jan 2023.

81. Gucer H, Caliskan S, Kefeli M, et al. Do you know the details of your PAX8 antibody? Monoclonal PAX8 (MRQ-50) is not expressed in a series of 45 medullary thyroid carcinomas. Endocr Pathol. 2020;31(1):33–8.

82. Hakim AS, Raboh MAN. The diagnostic utility of INSM1 and GATA3 in discriminating problematic medullary thyroid carcinoma, thyroid and parathyroid lesions. Pol J Pathol. 2021;72(1):11–22.

83. Hoskoppal D, Epstein JI, Gown AM, et al. SATB2 protein expression by immunohistochemistry is a sensitive and specific marker of appendiceal and rectosigmoid well differentiated neuroendocrine tumours. Histopathology. 2020;76(4):550–9. Epub 2020 Jan 24

84. Inoue H, Matsushima J, Kobayashi S, et al. Expression of SATB2 in neuroendocrine carcinomas of the lung: frequent immunopositivity of large cell neuroendocrine carcinoma with a diagnostic pitfall. Int J Surg Pathol. 2022;30(2):151–9. Epub 2021 Dec 16

85. Lin F, Shi J, Zhu S, et al. Cadherin-17 and SATB2 are sensitive and specific immunomarkers for medullary carcinoma of the large intestine. Arch Pathol Lab Med. 2014;138(8):1015–26. Epub 2014 Jan 17

86. Machado I, Navarro S, Picci P, et al. The utility of SATB2 immunohistochemical expression in distinguishing between osteosarcomas and their malignant bone tumor mimickers, such as Ewing sarcomas and chondrosarcomas. Pathol Res Pract. 2016;212(9):811–6. Epub 2016 Jun 26

87. Mamilla D, Manukyan I, Fetsch PA, et al. Immunohistochemical distinction of paragangliomas from epithelial neuroendocrine tumors-gangliocytic duodenal and cauda equina paragangliomas align with epithelial neuroendocrine tumors. Hum Pathol. 2020;103:72–82. Epub 2020 Jul 12

88. Miettinen M, McCue PA, Sarlomo-Rikala M, et al. GATA3: a multispecific but potentially useful marker in surgical pathology: a systematic analysis of 2500 epithelial and nonepithelial tumors. Am J Surg Pathol. 2014;38(1):13–22.

89. Rindi G, Mete O, Uccella S, et al. Overview of the 2022 WHO classification of neuroendocrine neoplasms. Endocr Pathol. 2022;33(1):115–54. Epub 2022 Mar 16

90. Rosenbaum JN, Guo Z, Baus RM, et al. INSM1: novel Immunohistochemical and molecular marker for neuroendocrine and Neuroepithelial neoplasms. Am J Clin Pathol. 2015;144(4):579–91.

91. Skalova A, Sar A, Laco J, et al. The role of SATB2 as a diagnostic marker of sinonasal intestinal-type adenocarcinoma. Appl Immunohistochem Mol Morphol. 2018;26(2):140–6.

92. Warmke LM, Tinkham EG, Ingram DR, et al. INSM1 Expression in Angiosarcoma. Am J Clin Pathol. 2021;155(4):575–80.

93. Zou Q, Zhang L, Cheng Z, et al. INSM1 is less sensitive but more specific than Synaptophysin in gynecologic high-grade neuroendocrine carcinomas: an Immunohistochemical study of 75 cases with specificity test and literature review. Am J Surg Pathol. 2021;45(2):147–59.

94. Li XQ, Hisaoka M, Shi DR, et al. Expression of anaplastic lymphoma kinase in soft tissue tumors: an immunohistochemical and molecular study of 249 cases. Hum Pathol. 2004;35(6):711–21.

95. Prasad ML, Williams MD, Helliwell T, et al. Melanocytic tumours. Mucosal melanoma. In: WHO Classification of Tumours Editorial Board. Head and neck tumours [Internet; beta version ahead of print]. Lyon (France): International Agency for Research on Cancer; 2022 [cited 2023 Jan 21]. (WHO classification of tumours series, 5th ed.; vol. 9). https://tumourclassification.iarc.who.int/chapters/52

96. Safadi RA, Bader DH, Abdullah NI, et al. Immunohistochemical expression of keratins 6, 7, 8, 14, 16, 18, 19, and MNF-116 pancytokeratin in primary and metastatic melanoma of the head and neck. Oral Surg Oral Med Oral Pathol Oral Radiol. 2016;121(5):510–9. Epub 2015 Dec 19

97. Kaczorowski M, Chłopek M, Kruczak A, et al. PRAME expression in cancer. A systematic immunohistochemical study of >5800 epithelial and nonepithelial tumors. Am J Surg Pathol. 2022;46(11):1467–76.

98. Lezcano C, Jungbluth AA, Nehal KS, et al. PRAME expression in melanocytic tumors. Am J Surg Pathol. 2018;42(11):1456–65.

99. Raghavan SS, Wang JY, Kwok S, et al. PRAME expression in melanocytic proliferations with intermediate histopathologic or spitzoid features. J Cutan Pathol. 2020;47(12):1123–31. Epub 2020 Sep 10

100. Tan CL, Lian DWQ, Kuick CH, et al. Cells with ganglionic differentiation frequently stain for VE1 antibody: a potential pitfall. Brain Tumor Pathol. 2020;37(1):14–21. Epub 2019 Dec 9

101. Al Dhaybi R, Agoumi M, Gagné I, et al. p16 expression: a marker of differentiation between childhood malignant melanomas and Spitz nevi. J Am Acad Dermatol. 2011;65(2):357–63. Epub 2011 May 6

102. Alomari AK, Tharp AW, Umphress B. The utility of PRAME immunohistochemistry in the evaluation of challenging melanocytic tumors. J Cutan Pathol. 2021;48(9):1115–23.

103. Beck EM, Bauman TM, Rosman IS. A tale of two clones: Caldesmon staining in the differentiation of cutaneous spindle cell neoplasms. J Cutan Pathol. 2018;45(8):581–7. Epub 2018 May 22

104. Chang LM, Cassarino DS. p16 expression is lost in severely atypical cellular blue nevi and melanoma compared to conventional, mildly, and moderately atypical cellular blue nevi. ISRN Dermatol. 2014; eCollection 2014

105. Cho WC, Prieto VG, Aung PP. Melanocytic lesions with blue naevus-like (dendritic) morphology: an update with an emphasis on histopathologi-

cal, immunophenotypic, and molecular features. Histopathology. 2021;79(3):291–305. Epub 2021 May 27

106. Choi JH, Ro JY. Cutaneous spindle cell neoplasms: pattern-based diagnostic approach. Arch Pathol Lab Med. 2018;142(8):958–72.

107. Cohen JN, Joseph NM, North JP, et al. Genomic analysis of pigmented epithelioid Melanocytomas reveals recurrent alterations in PRKAR1A, and PRKCA genes. Am J Surg Pathol. 2017;41(10):1333–46.

108. Couts KL, Bemis J, Turner JA, et al. ALK inhibitor response in melanomas expressing *EML4-ALK* fusions and alternate *ALK* isoforms. Mol Cancer Ther. 2018;17(1):222–31.Epub 2017 Oct 20

109. de la Fouchardière A, Caillot C, Jacquemus J, et al. β-Catenin nuclear expression discriminates deep penetrating nevi from other cutaneous melanocytic tumors. Virchows Arch. 2019;474(5):539–50. Epub 2019 Feb 12

110. Elder DE, Bastian BC, Cree JA, et al. The 2018 World Health Organization classification of cutaneous, mucosal, and uveal melanoma: detailed analysis of 9 distinct subtypes defined by their evolutionary pathway. Arch Pathol Lab Med. 2020;144(4):500–22. Epub 2020 Feb 14

111. Garrido-Ruiz MC, Requena L, Ortiz P, et al. The immunohistochemical profile of Spitz nevi and conventional (non-Spitzoid) melanomas: a baseline study. Mod Pathol. 2010;23(9):1215–24. Epub 2010 Jun 11

112. Helbig D, Mauch C, Buettner R, et al. Immunohistochemical expression of melanocytic and myofibroblastic markers and their molecular correlation in atypical fibroxanthomas and pleomorphic dermal sarcomas. J Cutan Pathol. 2018;45(12):880–5.

113. Hilliard NJ, Krahl D, Sellheyer K. p16 expression differentiates between desmoplastic Spitz nevus and desmoplastic melanoma. J Cutan Pathol. 2009;36(7):753–9.

114. Koh SS, Cassarino DS. Immunohistochemical expression of p16 in melanocytic lesions: an updated review and meta-analysis. Arch Pathol Lab Med. 2018;142(7):815–28.

115. López F, Rodrigo JP, Cardesa A, et al. Update on primary head and neck mucosal melanoma. Head Neck. 2016;38(1):147–55. Epub 2015 May 22

116. Nonaka D, Laser J, Tucker R, et al. Immunohistochemical evaluation of necrotic malignant melanomas. Am J Clin Pathol. 2007;127(5):787–91.

117. Oaxaca G, Billings SD, Ko JS. p16 Range of expression in dermal predominant benign epithelioid and spindled nevi and melanoma. J Cutan Pathol. 2020;47(9):815–23. Epub 2020 Jul 6

118. Ordóñez NG. Value of SOX10 immunostaining in tumor diagnosis. Adv Anat Pathol. 2013;20(4):275–83.

119. Piris A, Mihm MC Jr, Hoang MP. BAP1 and BRAFV600E expression in benign and malignant melanocytic proliferations. Hum Pathol. 2015;46(2):239–45. https://doi.org/10.1016/j.humpath.2014.10.015. Epub 2014 Nov 4.PMID: 25479927

120. Raghavan SS, Saleem A, Wang JY, et al. Diagnostic utility of LEF1 immunohistochemistry in differentiating deep penetrating nevi from histologic mimics. Am J Surg Pathol. 2020;44(10):1413–8.

121. Saleem A, Narala S, Raghavan SS. Immunohistochemistry in melanocytic lesions: updates with a practical review for pathologists. Semin Diagn Pathol. 2022;39(4):239–47. Epub 2022 Jan 1

122. Tacha D, Qi W, Ra S, et al. A newly developed mouse monoclonal SOX10 antibody is a highly sensitive and specific marker for malignant melanoma, including spindle cell and desmoplastic melanomas. Arch Pathol Lab Med. 2015;139(4):530–6.

123. Torres-Cabala C, Li-Ning-Tapia E, Hwu WJ. Pathology-based biomarkers useful for clinical decisions in melanoma. Arch Med Res. 2020;51(8):827–38. Epub 2020 Sep 16

124. Troxel DB. Pitfalls in the diagnosis of malignant melanoma: findings of a risk management panel study. Am J Surg Pathol. 2003;27(9):1278–83.

125. Zembowicz A, Knoepp SM, Bei T, et al. Loss of expression of protein kinase a regulatory subunit 1alpha in pigmented epithelioid melanocytoma but not in melanoma or other melanocytic lesions. Am J Surg Pathol. 2007;31(11):1764–75.

126. Zubovits J, Buzney E, Yu L, et al. HMB-45, S-100, NK1/C3, and MART-1 in metastatic melanoma. Hum Pathol. 2004 Feb;35(2):217–23.

127. WHO Classification of Tumours Editorial Board. Haematolymphoid tumours [Internet; beta version ahead of print]. Lyon (France): International Agency for Research on Cancer; 2022 [cited 2023 Feb 10]. (WHO classification of tumours series, 5th ed.; vol. 11). Available from: https://tumourclassification.iarc.who.int/chapters/63

128. Garcia CF, Swerdlow SH. Best practices in contemporary diagnostic immunohistochemistry: panel approach to hematolymphoid proliferations. Arch Pathol Lab Med. 2009;133(5):756–65.

129. Dojcinov SD, Venkataraman G, Raffeld M, et al. EBV positive mucocutaneous ulcer—a study of 26 cases associated with various sources of immunosuppression. Am J Surg Pathol. 2010;34(3):405–17.

130. Ferry JA. Update from the 5th edition of the world health organization classification of head and neck tumors: hematolymphoid proliferations and neoplasia. Head Neck Pathol. 2022;16(1):101–9.

131. Ok CY, Medeiros LJ, Thakral B, et al. High-grade B-cell lymphomas with TdT expression: a diagnostic and classification dilemma. Mod Pathol. 2019;32(1):48–58. Epub 2018 Sep 4

132. Tzankov A, Zimpfer A, Pehrs AC, et al. Expression of B-cell markers in classical hodgkin lymphoma: a tissue microarray analysis of 330 cases. Mod Pathol. 2003;16(11):1141–7.

133. Adams H, Schmid P, Dirnhofer S, et al. Cytokeratin expression in hematological neoplasms: a tissue microarray study on 866 lymphoma and leukemia cases. Pathol Res Pract. 2008;204(8):569–73. Epub 2008 Apr 23

134. Bai M, Panoulas V, Papoudou-Bai A, et al. B-cell differentiation immunophenotypes in classical Hodgkin lymphomas. Leuk Lymphoma. 2006;47(3):495–501.

135. Bourne TD, Bellizzi AM, Stelow EB, et al. p63 expression in olfactory neuroblastoma and other small cell tumors of the sinonasal tract. Am J Clin Pathol. 2008;130(2):213–8.

136. Buettner M, Greiner A, Avramidou A, et al. Evidence of abortive plasma cell differentiation in Hodgkin and Reed-Sternberg cells of classical Hodgkin lymphoma. Hematol Oncol. 2005;23(3–4):127–32.

137. Chang S-T, Chen S-W, Chen B-J, et al. Aberrant TTF-1 expression in peripheral T-cell lymphomas: a diagnostic pitfall. Int J Surg Pathol. 2021;29(2):165–8. Epub 2020 Aug 10

138. Chen BJ, Chiang WF, Chen TS, et al. EBV positive mucocutaneous ulcer with plasmacytic/plasmablastic differentiation and MYC rearrangement: a diagnostic challenge and a mimic of plasmablastic lymphoma. Pathology. 2019;51(6):648–50.

139. Cho Y-R, Seo J-W, Oh S-Y, et al. The expressions of MUM-1 and Bcl-6 in ALK-negative systemic anaplastic large cell lymphoma with skin involvement and primary cutaneous anaplastic large cell lymphoma. Int J Clin Exp Pathol. 2020;13(7):1682–7.

140. Costes V, Magen V, Legouffe E, et al. The Mi15 monoclonal antibody (anti-syndecan-1) is a reliable marker for quantifying plasma cells in paraffin-embedded bone marrow biopsy specimens. Hum Pathol. 1999;30(12):1405–11.

141. Crane GM, Duffield AS. Hematolymphoid lesions of the sinonasal tract. Semin Diagn Pathol. 2016;33(2):71–80.

142. Gualco G, Weiss LM, Bacchi CE. MUM1/IRF4: a review. Appl Immunohistochem Mol Morphol. 2010;18(4):301–10.

143. Hapgood G, Savage KJ. The biology and management of systemic anaplastic large cell lymphoma. Blood. 2015;126(1):17–25. Epub 2015 Apr 13

144. Hsi ED, Said J, Macon WR, et al. Diagnostic accuracy of a defined immunophenotypic and molecular genetic approach for peripheral T/NK-cell lymphomas. A North American PTCL study group project. Am J Surg Pathol. 2014;38(6):768–75.

145. Huang W, Ma W, Qiu T, et al. Histological type distribution and expression of nm23, VEGF, TOP2A and MUM-1 in peripheral T-cell and NK-cell lymphomas in Chinese: analysis of 313 cases. Int J Clin Exp Pathol. 2018;11(10):5086–93. eCollection 2018

146. Huang W, Zhang W, Zeng L, et al. ERG expression is helpful in differentiating T-lymphoblastic lymphoma from thymoma. Int J Surg Pathol. 2022;

147. Huettl KS, Staiger AM, Horn H, et al. Cytokeratin expression in plasmablastic lymphoma—a possible diagnostic pitfall in the routine work-up of tumours.

Histopathology. 2021;78(6):831–7. Epub 2020 Dec 25

148. Ikeda T, Gion Y, Nishimura Y, et al. Epstein-barr virus-positive mucocutaneous ulcer: a unique and curious disease entity. Int J Mol Sci. 2021;22(3):1053.

149. Menter T, Trivedi P, Ahmad R, et al. Diagnostic utility of lymphoid enhancer binding factor 1 immunohistochemistry in small B-cell lymphomas. Am J Clin Pathol. 2017;147(3):292–300.

150. Moran NR, Webster B, Lee KM, et al. Epstein Barr virus-positive mucocutaneous ulcer of the colon associated Hodgkin lymphoma in Crohn's disease. World J Gastroenterol. 2015;21(19):6072–6.

151. O'Connell FP, Pinkus JL, Pinkus GS. CD138 (syndecan-1), a plasma cell marker immunohistochemical profile in hematopoietic and nonhematopoietic neoplasms. Am J Clin Pathol. 2004;121(2):254–63.

152. Plocharczyk E, Wakely PE Jr. CD31 expression in plasmacytic/plasmablastic lesions. Ann Diagn Pathol. 2013;17(6):498–501. Epub 2013 Sep 24

153. Pu Q, Qiao J, Liu Y, et al. Differential diagnosis and identification of prognostic markers for peripheral T-cell lymphoma subtypes based on flow cytometry immunophenotype profiles. Front Immunol. 2022; eCollection 2022

154. Rangan A, Reinig E, McPhail ED, et al. Immunohistochemistry for LEF1 and SOX11 adds diagnostic specificity in small B-cell lymphomas. Hum Pathol. 2022;121:29–35. Epub 2022 Jan 20

155. Satou A, Nakamura S. EBV-positive B-cell lymphomas and lymphoproliferative disorders: review from the perspective of immune escape and immunodeficiency. Cancer Med. 2021;(10, 19):6777–85. Epub 2021 Aug 13

156. Thakral B, Zhou J, Medeiros LJ. Extranodal hematopoietic neoplasms and mimics in the head and neck: an update. Hum Pathol. 2015;46(8):1079–100.

157. Uppal G, Ly V, Wang ZX, et al. The utility of BRAF V600E mutation-specific antibody VE1 for the diagnosis of hairy cell leukemia. Am J Clin Pathol. 2015;143(1):120–5.

158. Wang DZ, Liu P, Yao L, et al. Aberrant expression of thyroid transcription factor-1 in schwannomas. Hum Pathol. 2018;71:84–90. Epub 2017 Dec 5

159. Wang T, Feldman AL, Wada DA, et al. GATA-3 expression identifies a high-risk subset of PTCL, NOS with distinct molecular and clinical features. Blood. 2014;123(19):3007–15. Epub 2014 Feb 4

160. Wang X, Boddicker RL, Dasari S, et al. Expression of p63 protein in anaplastic large cell lymphoma: implications for genetic subtyping. Hum Pathol. 2017;64:19–27. Epub 2017 Jan 30

161. Willemze R, Cerroni L, Kempf W, et al. The 2018 update of the WHO-EORTC classification for primary cutaneous lymphomas. Blood. 2019;133(16):1703–14. Epub 2019 Jan 11

162. Wooff JC, Weinreb I, Perez-Ordonez B, et al. Calretinin staining facilitates differentiation of olfactory neuroblastoma from other small round

blue cell tumors in the sinonasal tract. Am J Surg Pathol. 2011;35(12):1786–93.

163. Wotherspoon AC, Norton AJ, Isaacson PG. Immunoreactive cytokeratins in plasmacytomas. Histopathology. 1989;14(2):141–50.

164. Wu H, Du J, Li H, et al. Aberrant expression of thyroid transcription factor-1 in meningeal solitary fibrous tumor/hemangiopericytoma. Brain Tumor Pathol. 2021;38(2):122–31. Epub 2021 Mar 5

165. Zheng W, Medeiros JL, Young KH, et al. CD30 expression in acute lymphoblastic leukemia as assessed by flow cytometry analysis. Leuk Lymphoma. 2014;55(3):624–7. Epub 2013 Aug 13

166. Ashraf M, Beigomi L, Azarpira N, et al. The small round blue cell tumors of the sinonasal area: histological and immunohistochemical findings. Iran Red Crescent Med J. 2013;15(6):455–61. Epub 2013 Jun 5

167. Bahrami A, Gown AM, Baird GS, et al. Aberrant expression of epithelial and neuroendocrine markers in alveolar rhabdomyosarcoma: a potentially serious diagnostic pitfall. Mod Pathol. 2008;21(7):795–806. Epub 2008 May 16

168. Bishop JA, Thompson LD, Cardesa A, et al. Rhabdomyoblastic differentiation in head and neck malignancies other than rhabdomyosarcoma. Head Neck Pathol. 2015;9(4):507–18. Epub 2015 Mar 11

169. Botiralieva GK, Sharlai AS, Roshchin VY, et al. Rhabdomyosarcomas: structural distribution and analysis of an immunohistochemical profile [article in Russian]. Arkh Patol. 2020;82(5):33–41.

170. Cortelazzo S, Ponzoni M, Ferreri AJ, et al. Lymphoblastic lymphoma. Crit Rev Oncol Hematol. 2011;79(3):330–43. Epub 2011 Jan 26. Review

171. Czapiewski P, Gorczyński A, Haybaeck J, et al. Expression pattern of ISL-1, TTF-1 and PAX5 in olfactory neuroblastoma. Pol J Pathol. 2016;67(2):130–5.

172. Czapiewski P, Kunc M, Gorczyński A, et al. Frequent expression of somatostatin receptor 2a in olfactory neuroblastomas: a new and distinctive feature. Hum Pathol. 2018;79:144–50. Epub 2018 May 25

173. Faragalla H, Weinreb I. Olfactory neuroblastoma: a review and update. Adv Anat Pathol. 2009;16(5):322–31.

174. Folpe AL, Hill CE, Parham DM, et al. Immunohistochemical detection of FLI-1 protein expression: a study of 132 round cell tumors with emphasis on CD99-positive mimics of Ewing's sarcoma/primitive neuroectodermal tumor. Am J Surg Pathol. 2000;24(12):1657–62.

175. Filtenborg-Barnkob BE, Bzorek M. Expression of anaplastic lymphoma kinase in Merkel cell carcinomas. Hum Pathol. 2013;44(8):1656–64. Epub 2013 Apr 8

176. Fukuhara M, Agnarsdóttir M, Edqvist P-H, et al. SATB2 is expressed in Merkel cell carcinoma. Arch Dermatol Res. 2016;308(6):449–54. Epub 2016 Jun 4

177. Hung YP, Fletcher CD, Hornick JL. Evaluation of NKX2-2 expression in round cell sarcomas and other tumors with EWSR1 rearrangement: imperfect specificity for Ewing sarcoma. Mod Pathol. 2016;29(4):370–80. Epub 2016 Feb 5

178. Hung YP, Lee JP, Bellizzi AM, et al. PHOX2B reliably distinguishes neuroblastoma among small round blue cell tumours. Histopathology. 2017;71(5):786–94. Epub 2017 Sep 6

179. Jo VY, Fletcher CD. p63 immunohistochemical staining is limited in soft tissue tumors. Am J Clin Pathol. 2011;136(5):762–6.

180. Karamchandani JR, Nielsen TO, van de Rijn M, et al. Sox10 and S100 in the diagnosis of soft-tissue neoplasms. Appl Immunohistochem Mol Morphol. 2012;20(5):445–50.

181. Koo M, Natkunam Y. ERG Immunoreactivity in Blastic Hematolymphoid neoplasms: diagnostic pitfall in the workup of undifferentiated malignant neoplasms. Appl Immunohistochem Mol Morphol. 2022;30(1):42–8.

182. McCuiston A, Bishop JA. Usefulness of NKX2.2 immunohistochemistry for distinguishing Ewing sarcoma from other Sinonasal small round blue cell tumors. Head Neck Pathol. 2018;12(1):89–94. Epub 2017 Jun 14

183. Miettinen M. Immunohistochemistry of soft tissue tumours—review with emphasis on 10 markers. Histopathology. 2014;64(1):101–18. Epub 2013 Nov 28

184. Miettinen M, Wang Z, Sarlomo-Rikala M, et al. ERG expression in epithelioid sarcoma: a diagnostic pitfall. Am J Surg Pathol. 2013;7(10):1580–5.

185. Ptaszyński K, Szumera-Ciećkiewicz A, Pekul M, et al. Differential diagnosis of small round cell tumours (SRCT), fluorescence in situ hybridization (FISH) and immunohistochemical (IHC) study. Pol J Pathol. 2009;60(4):151–62.

186. Shah K, Perez-Ordóñez B. Neuroendocrine neoplasms of the sinonasal tract: neuroendocrine carcinomas and olfactory neuroblastoma. Head Neck Pathol. 2016;10(1):85–94.

187. Simons SA, Bridge JA, Leon ME. Sinonasal small round blue cell tumors: An approach to diagnosis. Semin Diagn Pathol. 2016;33(2):91–103. Epub 2015 Sep 10

188. Sullivan LM, Atkins KA, LeGallo RD. PAX immunoreactivity identifies alveolar rhabdomyosarcoma. Am J Surg Pathol. 2009;33(5):775–80.

189. Thompson LD. Small round blue cell tumors of the sinonasal tract: a differential diagnosis approach. Mod Pathol. 2017;30(s1):S1–S26.

190. Tilson MP, Bishop JA. Utility of p40 in the differential diagnosis of small round blue cell tumors of the Sinonasal tract. Head Neck Pathol. 2014;8(2):141–5.

191. Tomlins SA, Palanisamy N, Brenner JC, et al. Usefulness of a monoclonal ERG/FLI1 antibody for immunohistochemical discrimination of Ewing family tumors. Am J Clin Pathol. 2013;139(6):771–9.

192. Yoshida A, Makise N, Wakai S, et al. INSM1 expression and its diagnostic significance in extraskeletal myxoid chondrosarcoma. Mod Pathol. 2018;31(5):744–52. Epub 2018 Jan 12

193. Baranov E, McBride MJ, Bellizzi AM, et al. A novel SS18-SSX fusion-specific antibody for the diagnosis of synovial sarcoma. Am J Surg Pathol. 2020;44(7):922–33.

194. Bishop JA, Alaggio R, Zhang L, et al. Adamantinoma-like Ewing family tumors of the head and neck: a pitfall in the differential diagnosis of basaloid and myoepithelial carcinomas. Am J Surg Pathol. 2015;39(9):1267–74.

195. Carlson JW, Fletcher CD. Immunohistochemistry for beta-catenin in the differential diagnosis of spindle cell lesions: analysis of a series and review of the literature. Histopathology. 2007;51(4):509–14. Epub 2007 Aug 17

196. Clay M. Atypical lipomatous tumor/well differentiated liposarcoma. PathologyOutlines.com website. https://www.pathologyoutlines.com/topic/softtissuewdliposarcoma.html. Accessed 12 Jan 2023.

197. Liu L, Kakiuchi-Kiyota S, Arnold LL, et al. Pathogenesis of human hemangiosarcomas and hemangiomas. Hum Pathol. 2013;44(10):2302–11.

198. Makise N, Sekimizu M, Kubo T, et al. Clarifying the distinction between malignant peripheral nerve sheath tumor and dedifferentiated liposarcoma: a critical reappraisal of the diagnostic utility of MDM2 and H3K27me3 status. Am J Surg Pathol. 2018;42(5):656–64.

199. Miettinen M. Modern soft tissue pathology. Tumours and non-neoplastic conditions. 1st ed. Cambridge University Press; 2010. ISBN-13: 978-0521874090

200. Panse G, Mito JK, Ingram DR, et al. Radiation-associated sarcomas other than malignant peripheral nerve sheath tumours demonstrate loss of histone H3K27 trimethylation†. Histopathology. 2021;78(2):321–6.

201. Sharain RF, Gown AM, Greipp PT, et al. Immunohistochemistry for TFE3 lacks specificity and sensitivity in the diagnosis of TFE3-rearranged neoplasms: a comparative, 2-laboratory study. Hum Pathol. 2019;87:65–74.

202. Suurmeijer AJH, Dickson BC, Swanson D, et al. A novel group of spindle cell tumors defined by S100 and CD34 co-expression shows recurrent fusions involving RAF1, BRAF, and NTRK1/2 genes.

Genes Chromosomes Cancer. 2018;57(12):611–21. Epub 2018 Oct 1

203. Thway K, Flora R, Shah C, et al. Diagnostic utility of p16, CDK4, and MDM2 as an immunohistochemical panel in distinguishing well-differentiated and dedifferentiated liposarcomas from other adipocytic tumors. Am J Surg Pathol. 2012;36(3):462–9.

204. Xu B, Suurmeijer AJH, Agaram NP, et al. Head and neck mesenchymal tumors with kinase fusions: a report of 15 cases with emphasis on wide anatomic distribution and diverse histologic appearance. Am J Surg Pathol. 2023;47(2):248–58. Epub 2022 Oct 21

205. Bellizzi AM. An algorithmic immunohistochemical approach to define tumor type and assign site of origin. Adv Anat Pathol. 2020;27(3):114–63.

206. Kandukuri SR, Lin F, Gui L, et al. Application of immunohistochemistry in undifferentiated neoplasms: a practical approach. Arch Pathol Lab Med. 2017;141(8):1014–32.

207. Kennel T, Garrel R, Costes V, et al. Head and neck carcinoma of unknown primary. Eur Ann Otorhinolaryngol Head Neck Dis. 2019;136(3):185–92. Epub 2019 Apr 17

208. Laprovitera N, Riefolo M, Ambrosini E, et al. Cancer of unknown primary: challenges and progress in clinical management. Cancers (Basel). 2021;13(3):451.

209. Swanson PE. Immunohistochemistry as a surrogate for molecular testing: a review. Appl Immunohistochem Mol Morphol. 2015;23(2):81–96.

210. Troxell ML, Fulton RS, Swanson PE, et al. Predictive markers require thorough analytic validation. Arch Pathol Lab Med. 2019;143(8):907–9.

211. Tsao MS, Yatabe Y. Old soldiers never die: is there still a role for immunohistochemistry in the era of next-generation sequencing panel testing? J Thorac Oncol. 2019;14(12):2035–8.

212. www.pathologyoutlines.com

Klos Jan Pathologist, Department of Pathology, Stavanger University Hospital, Norway. Actively engaged in teaching immunohistochemistry. Member of the core group and assessor in Nordic Immunohistochemistry Quality Control (NordiQC) since 2008, founding member of International Society of Immunohistochemistry and Molecular Morphology, international member of Australasian Immunohistochemistry Society.

HPV Testing

Adam Kowalewski and Stamatios Theocharis

8.1 Introduction

Human papillomavirus (HPV) infection holds the distinction of being the most common worldwide. The International Agency for Research on Cancer (IARC) classifies HPV as a carcinogenic infectious agent, attributing it to approximately 4.5% of all cancers. While over 200 HPV genotypes have been identified, a select few possess carcinogenic properties [1, 2]. These genotypes fall into two categories: low-risk HPVs (LR-HPVs), responsible for skin warts on the hands, feet, genitals, and anus, and high-risk HPVs (HR-HPVs), linked to anogenital cancers (such as cervical, anal, vulvar, vaginal, and penile) as well as head and neck cancers [2]. Among the HR-HPV types reported (HPV types 16, 18, 31, 33, 35, 39, 45, 51, 52, 56, 58, 59, 68, 73, and 82), HPV 16 is the most frequently observed oncogenic variant [2, 3].

Head and neck squamous cell carcinoma (HNSCC), ranking as the sixth most common malignancy globally, incorporates a heterogeneous group of cancers primarily attributed to tobacco smoking and alcohol consumption [3–6]. While the decline in tobacco use has led to a reduction in overall HNSCC incidence, there has been an observed increase in the prevalence of oropharyngeal squamous cell carcinoma (OPSCC) due to HPV infection [4].

HPV infection is prevalent in 20–60% of OPSCCs [7], with the highest incidence rates observed in Western Europe and North America [8–10]. While earlier studies primarily associated HPV induced OPSCCs with younger patients, recent findings suggest that these malignancies also manifest in older individuals under specific geographic and sociosexual circumstances [11–13].

HPV-driven OPSCC exhibits distinct clinical characteristics, such as a favorable response to radiotherapy and improved overall survival rates [14]. In a study involving 323 patients with OPSCC, those with HPV-positive tumors exhibited superior 3-year overall survival rates (82.4% compared to 57.1%). Adjusting for factors like age, race, tumor and nodal stage, tobacco exposure, and treatment assignment, these patients experienced a remarkable 58% reduction in the risk of death [15]. Similarly, a study conducted

A. Kowalewski (✉)
Center of Medical Sciences, University of Science and Technology, Bydgoszcz, Poland

Department of Tumor Pathology, Oncology Center - Prof. Franciszek Łukaszczyk Memorial Hospital, Bydgoszcz, Poland
e-mail: adam.kowalewski@pbs.edu.pl

S. Theocharis
First Department of Pathology, Medical School, National and Kapodistrian University of Athens, Athens, Greece

© The Author(s), under exclusive license to Springer Nature Switzerland AG 2024
J. Klijanienko et al. (eds.), *Diagnostic Procedures in Patients with Neck Masses*,
https://doi.org/10.1007/978-3-031-67675-8_8

on a larger cohort of 21,627 OPSCC patients revealed that the 5-year overall survival rates for those with HPV-positive status and HPV-negative status were 77.6% and 50.7%, respectively [16]. Recognizing these distinctions, the eighth edition of the UICC TNM classification (Union for International Cancer Control) and the AJCC eighth edition staging system have established a specific classification system dedicated to HPV-positive OPSCCs [17, 18]. Consequently, the determination of the HPV status in OPSCCs has become a mandatory aspect of clinical assessment. In line with this, the College of American Pathologists (CAP) has recently issued guidelines that primarily focus on HPV testing in OPSCCs, emphasizing the importance of HPV testing for all tumors in routine clinical practice [19].

High-risk HPV testing is also useful in the workup and management of cancers of unknown primary in the neck. When a malignant cervical lymph node is suspected, the preferred diagnostic procedure is fine needle aspiration (FNA), and in cases of squamous cell carcinoma and undifferentiated epithelial cancer, HPV testing is recommended [20–22]. This is because a positive HPV result strongly suggests a primary cancer in the oropharynx, particularly in the palatine tonsil or base of the tongue [23]. If metastasis is detected within the lymph node, FNA remains the favored diagnostic approach to examine areas of mucosal abnormalities that raise suspicions about the primary site. Notably, biopsies of normal-appearing mucosa in potential primary sites often reveal a primary cancer. Even if the primary site cannot be found, the strong link between HPV positivity and primary cancer in the oropharynx leads to these patients being staged according to the classification for HPV-positive oropharyngeal cancer and becoming eligible for radiotherapy targeting the palatine tonsils and base of the tongue regions [24, 25].

In this chapter, we aim to elucidate the various tests presently utilized for HPV detection while also providing insights into novel diagnostic approaches currently being explored in research.

These emerging methods hold the potential to extend beyond the realm of scientific investigation and find practical application in routine clinical practice. Finally, there is a noteworthy occurrence of HR-HPV in different nonoropharyngeal HNSCCs [2], which is substantiated by our investigations at the Institut Curie. Our findings demonstrate that 66% of nasal fossae carcinomas, 10% of nasopharyngeal carcinomas, and 10% of oral cavity carcinomas exhibit HPV positivity. Consequently, there is an anticipation for the revision of guidelines specific to these distinct tumor types to incorporate the emerging insights in this field.

8.2   Techniques

Different tissue and cytology liquid-based direct HPV and other molecular tests have been standardized and are commonly used in HNSCC patients. HPV in HNSCC is commonly diagnosed by p16 INK4a immunohistochemistry (IHC) or by RT-qPCR of HPV-16 E6 and E7 oncoproteins. The CAP and American Society of Clinical Oncology (ASCO) recommend HPV testing exclusively for OPSCC using p16 IHC as the most cost-effective method [19]. In the majority of tumor cells in OPSCC, p16 exhibits a robust and widespread staining pattern, both in the cytoplasm and the nucleus. Its sensitivity ranges from 94% to 97%, indicating its effectiveness in identifying positive cases. However, the specificity of p16 testing is relatively modest, ranging from 83% to 84% [26]. Given the significance of precise and reliable test results, there is an anticipation that alternative molecular techniques will surpass the limitations associated with p16 testing, offering enhanced specificity and accuracy in HPV detection.

RNA in situ hybridization for HR-HPV is a clinically available test for tissue specimens and cytology cell block preparations or cellular aspirate specimens. These detection options are in combination more effective to detect transcriptionally active HR-HPV cases, although they do not individually support HPV genotyping. Droplet digital polymerase chain reaction (ddPCR) shows promise for minimally invasive HPV detection, allowing for precise and reproducible quantification of target nucleic acids [27, 28]. Using quantitative (q) PCR and droplet digital polymerase chain reaction (ddPCR)-based approaches, it was shown that HPV-positive OPSCC patients exhibited detectable circulating tumor human papillomavirus DNA (ctHPV DNA) at diagnosis in cellular preparations, in swabs from the oropharynx, sinonasal, or in saliva [29–32].

Blood-based molecular diagnostics were also used not only as a diagnostic tool for early diagnosis but also for monitoring of treatment and early recurrence detection in HNSCC patients. Such liquid biopsy-based techniques are effective in the detection of somatic mutations in cell-free DNA, released from cancer cells, or in methylation status characterization [27, 28]. Different reports proved that all the abovementioned novel methods for HPV detection exhibit high specificity, sensitivity, and reproducibility, acceptable for future clinical use. Nevertheless, the cost, especially for the molecular methods, remains high [33, 34]. Additionally, more data especially in combined detection platforms are needed in order for these applications to become part of guidelines for HPV detection, in particular HNSCC cases at different anatomical sites in relation to the type of available sampling [33–36]. A next-generation sequencing (NGS)-based HPV liquid biopsy test called CaptHPV uses probes designed for more than 200 HPV genotypes and variants followed by NGS library preparation and sequencing proposed by Sastre-Garau et al. [37] This test provided high sensitivity and specificity across various HPV-associated cancers (including a small number of HPV-positive OPSCC cases). NGS-based liquid biopsies have the ability to overcome some of the limitations of ddPCR, such as the number of genotypes that can be detected. NGS-based ctHPV DNA detection,

however, still presents the disadvantage of higher cost, more complex informatics, and sample volume.

Further work is needed to optimize ctHPV DNA as a routine diagnostic tool, either used alone or in combination with standard-of-care cytology or tissue-based tests, for the diagnosis and monitoring of patients with HPV-positive OPSCC.

8.3 Diagnostic Workflow Recommendations

There is a lack of HPV diagnostic tests that have obtained regulatory approval. The current approach involves utilizing p16 IHC as a surrogate marker with high sensitivity for detecting transcriptionally active HPV in OPSCC tissue samples and cell block preparations. However, challenges arise when dealing with cystic lesions, small primary tumors, and lymph node metastasis with low cellularity in a FNA material, and there are no established guidelines for interpreting p16 immunoexpression in such cases.

The testing of the E6 oncoprotein has been clinically utilized for HPV detection in HNSCC cases, particularly in tissue samples. DNA PCR techniques demonstrate reproducibility with high sensitivity and specificity. RT-PCR for HPV mRNA E6/E7 offers high sensitivity and specificity but necessitates the use of fresh or frozen specimens. HPV DNA ISH allows for the direct visualization of the virus within tumor cells in tissue samples and cell block preparations, exhibiting high sensitivity and specificity.

The detection of HPV circulating tumor DNA (ctDNA) in noninvasive samples, such as swabs or plasma, using ultrasensitive ddPCR, has generated increasing clinical interest in HNSCC, although limited data are available. E6 serology could be considered for monitoring HPV-positive OPSCC patients, particularly for early detection of residual disease or recurrence.

Table 8.1 Different methods used for HPV status detection in HNSCC for screening/early detection, diagnosis, and disease monitoring

Screening/early detection	HPV ctDNA
Diagnosis/prognosis	p16 IHC DNA PCR RT PCR HPV DNA ISH
Surveillance/disease monitoring	HPV ctDNA (ddPCR) E6 serology

Table 8.1 summarizes the diverse methods utilized for HPV status detection in HNSCC, spanning screening, early detection, diagnosis, and disease monitoring, providing an overview of current diagnostic approaches in clinical practice.

References

1. Kombe Kombe AJ, et al. Epidemiology and burden of human papillomavirus and related diseases, molecular pathogenesis, and vaccine evaluation. Front Public Heal. 2021;8:552028.
2. Williams J, Kostiuk M, Biron VL. Molecular detection methods in HPV-related cancers. Front Oncol. 2022;12
3. de Martel C, Plummer M, Vignat J, Franceschi S. Worldwide burden of cancer attributable to HPV by site, country and HPV type. Int J Cancer. 2017;141:664–70.
4. Dayyani F, et al. Meta-analysis of the impact of human papillomavirus (HPV) on cancer risk and overall survival in head and neck squamous cell carcinomas (HNSCC). Head Neck Oncol. 2010;2:15.
5. Rahman QB, Iocca O, Kufta K, Shanti RM. Global burden of head and neck cancer. Oral Maxillofac Surg Clin North Am. 2020;32:367–75.
6. Serrano B, Brotons M, Bosch FX, Bruni L. Epidemiology and burden of HPV-related disease. Best Pract Res Clin Obstet Gynaecol. 2018;47:14–26.
7. Castellsagué X, et al. HPV involvement in head and neck cancers: comprehensive assessment of biomarkers in 3680 patients. JNCI J Natl Cancer Inst. 2016;108
8. Lam EWH, et al. Prevalence, clinicopathological characteristics, and outcome of human papillomavirus-associated oropharyngeal cancer in southern Chinese patients. Cancer Epidemiol Biomarkers Prev. 2016;25:165–73.
9. Shaikh MH, et al. Prevalence and types of high-risk human papillomaviruses in head and neck cancers from Bangladesh. BMC Cancer. 2017;17:1–11.
10. Lim MY, Dahlstrom KR, Sturgis EM, Li G. Human papillomavirus integration pattern and demographic, clinical, and survival characteristics of patients with oropharyngeal squamous cell carcinoma. Head Neck. 2016;38:1139–44.
11. Fakhry C, et al. Distinct biomarker and behavioral profiles of human papillomavirus-related oropharynx cancer patients by age. Oral Oncol. 2020;101:104522.
12. Del Mistro A, et al. Age-independent increasing prevalence of human papillomavirus-driven oropharyngeal carcinomas in north-East Italy. Sci Reports 2020 101. 2020;10:1–10.
13. Rettig EM, et al. Oropharyngeal cancer is no longer a disease of younger patients and the prognostic advantage of human papillomavirus is attenuated among older patients: analysis of the National Cancer Database. Oral Oncol. 2018;83:147–53.
14. Lassen P, et al. Prognostic impact of HPV-associated p16-expression and smoking status on outcomes following radiotherapy for oropharyngeal cancer: the MARCH-HPV project. Radiother Oncol. 2018;126:107–15.
15. Ang KK, et al. Human papillomavirus and survival of patients with oropharyngeal cancer. N Engl J Med. 2010;363:24–35.
16. Li H, et al. Association of Human Papillomavirus Status at head and neck carcinoma subsites with overall survival. JAMA Otolaryngol Head Neck Surg. 2018;144:519–25.
17. Brierley J.D., Gospodarowicz M.K. & Wittekind C. TNM classification of malignant tumours, 8th. Union Int. Cancer Control 1–272 (2017).
18. Amin, M. B. et al. American joint committee on cancer (AJCC). AJCC cancer staging manual. AJCC cancer staging manual (2017).
19. Lewis JS, et al. Human papillomavirus testing in head and neck carcinomas: guideline from the College of American Pathologists. Arch Pathol Lab Med. 2018;142:559–97.
20. Furniss CS, et al. Human papillomavirus 16 and head and neck squamous cell carcinoma. Int J Cancer. 2007;120:2386–92.
21. Fakhry C, Gillison ML. Clinical implications of human papillomavirus in head and neck cancers. J Clin Oncol. 2006;24:2606.
22. Fakhry C, et al. Human papillomavirus testing in head and neck carcinomas: ASCO clinical practice guideline endorsement of the college of American pathologists guideline. J Clin Oncol. 2018;36:3152–61.
23. Begum S, Gillison ML, Nicol TL, Westra WH. Detection of human Papillomavirus-16 in fine-needle aspirates to determine tumor origin in patients with metastatic squamous cell carcinoma of the head and neck. Clin Cancer Res. 2007;13:1186–91.
24. Boscolo-Rizzo P, Schroeder L, Romeo S, Pawlita M. The prevalence of human papillomavirus in squamous cell carcinoma of unknown primary site metastatic to neck lymph nodes: a systematic review. Clin Exp Metastasis. 2015;32:835–45.

25. Bussu F, et al. HPV and EBV infections in neck metastases from occult primary squamous cell carcinoma: another virus-related neoplastic disease in the head and neck region. Ann Surg Oncol. 2015;22(Suppl 3):979–84.
26. Jordan RC, et al. Validation of methods for oropharyngeal cancer HPV statusdetermination in United States cooperative group trials. Am J Surg Pathol. 2012;36:945.
27. Hindson CM, et al. Absolute quantification by droplet digital PCR versus analog real-time PCR. Nat Methods 2013 1010. 2013;10:1003–5.
28. Hindson BJ, et al. High-throughput droplet digital PCR system for absolute quantitation of DNA copy number. Anal Chem. 2011;83:8604–10.
29. Walline MH, et al. High-risk human papillomavirus detection in oropharyngeal, nasopharyngeal, and oral cavity cancers: comparison of multiple methods. JAMA Otolaryngol Head Neck Surg. 2013;139:1320–7.
30. Robinson M, Schache A, Sloan P, Thavaraj S. HPV specific testing: a requirement for oropharyngeal squamous cell carcinoma patients. Head Neck Pathol. 2012;6:83.
31. Chernesky M, et al. HPV E6 oncoproteins and nucleic acids in neck lymph node fine needle aspirates and oral samples from patients with oropharyngeal squamous cell carcinoma. Papillomavirus Res (Amsterdam, Netherlands). 2018;6:1–5.
32. Menegaldo A, et al. Detection of HPV16/18 E6 Oncoproteins in head and neck squamous cell carcinoma using a protein Immunochromatographic assay. Laryngoscope. 2021;131:1042–8.
33. Chera BS, et al. Rapid clearance profile of plasma circulating tumor HPV type 16 DNA during Chemoradiotherapy correlates with disease control in HPV-associated oropharyngeal cancer. Clin Cancer Res. 2019;25:4682.
34. Chera BS, et al. Plasma circulating tumor HPV DNA for the surveillance of cancer recurrence in HPV-associated oropharyngeal cancer. J Clin Oncol. 2020;38:1050–8.
35. Augustin JG, et al. HPV detection in head and neck squamous cell carcinomas: what is the issue? Front Oncol. 2020;10
36. Prigge ES, Arbyn M, von Knebel Doeberitz M, Reuschenbach M. Diagnostic accuracy of p16INK4a immunohistochemistry in oropharyngeal squamous cell carcinomas: a systematic review and meta-analysis. Int J Cancer. 2017;140:1186–98.
37. Sastre-Garau X, et al. A NGS-based blood test for the diagnosis of invasive HPV-associated carcinomas with extensive viral genomic characterization. Clin Cancer Res. 2021;27:5307–16.

Adam Kowalewski Pathologist at the Prof. F. Łukaszczyk Oncology Center and Assistant Professor at the University of Science and Technology in Bydgoszcz. He is currently pursuing a European Masters in Molecular Pathology at the University Côte d'Azur. His research and inventions primarily focus on advancing minimally invasive diagnostics, understanding cancer evolution, and exploring alternative treatment approaches.

Theocharis Stamatios Professor of Pathology at National and Kapodistrian University of Athens, Greece. His research interests include, among others, biomarkers in pathology and cytopathology, molecular pathology and toxicology.

Lineage and Molecular Marker Integration in Diagnosis and Differential Diagnosis of Neck Tumors

Adel K. El-Naggar

9.1 Introduction

The neck region is composed of several organ tissue types and lymph node groups, and the host of diverse primary and metastatic neoplasms (Fig. 9.1). The diagnosis and differential diagnosis of tumors in this region, therefore, mandate an integrated clinical, radiological, and pathological approach. The vast majority of neck masses and neoplasms are readily visible and accessible to noninvasive sampling either by fine needle aspiration (FNA) or core tissue biopsies and in general, light-optic evaluation of cytological smears and biopsies provides diagnostic information on

Fig. 9.1 Lymph node distribution in the neck region

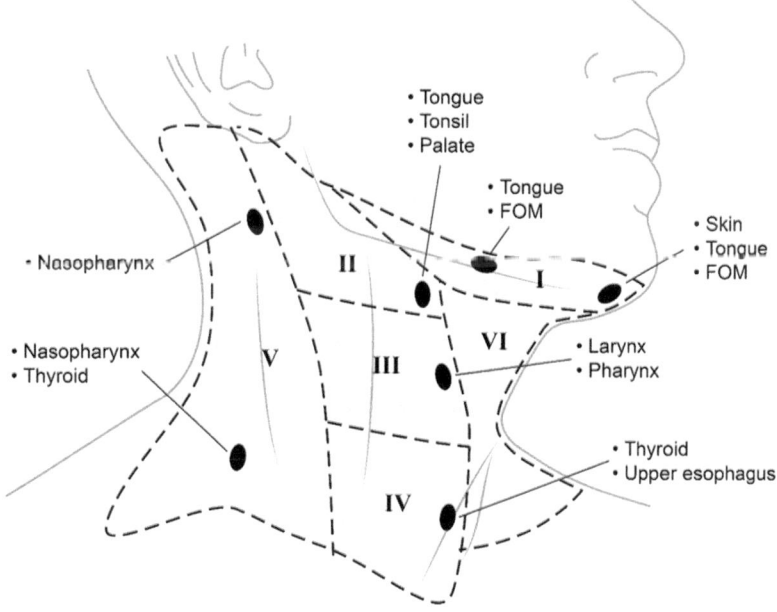

A. K. El-Naggar (✉)
UT M.D. Anderson Cancer Center,
Houston, TX, USA
e-mail: anaggar@mdanderson.org

the majority of cases. Incremental and expanding new techniques and genetic platforms have led to plethora of potential diagnostic, biological, and therapeutic markers, mandating knowledge and familiarities of the validity of their utilization and potential pitfalls of these methods' diagnostic and clinical practices. Accordingly, the optic assessment complemented with lineage markers should remain the basic diagnostic principal with the optional use of certain molecular testing as deemed to be complementary [1–7].

9.2   Anatomic Sites and Organs of the Neck Region

The neck regions are anatomically defined superiorly by the hyoid bone, laterally by the carotid artery, and inferiorly by the sternal notch and the brachiocephalic artery (Fig. 9.1 and Table 9.1).

This region encompass multiple organs including larynx, hypopharynx, trachea, esophagus, thyroid, parathyroid, cervical thymus, submandibular salivary gland, heterotopic salivary tissues, and multiple lymph node compartments (Fig. 9.2). Of the later, the prelaryngeal (Delphian) and tracheal and the paratracheal nodes are the most commonly affected nodes.

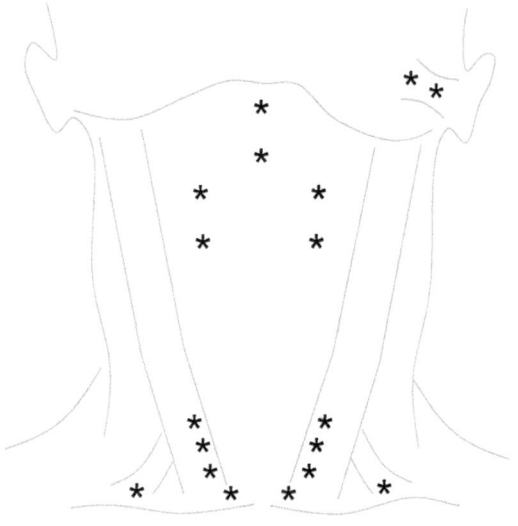

Fig. 9.2 Sites of salivary heterotopic remnants in the neck

Table 9.1 Neck nodes sites and potential metastatic sources

Level	Anatomic site	Possible origin
I	Submental/ submandibular	Oral cavity, lip, anterior tongue, oropharynx
II	Digastric and upper jugular nodes	Larynx, nasopharynx, base of tongue, parotid
III	Middle jugular component	Oral cavity, larynx, hypopharynx, thyroid, oropharynx
IV	Inferior jugular nodes	Larynx, hypopharynx, esophagus, thyroid
V	Supraclavicular	Larynx, hypopharynx, thyroid, lung and other distant sources

9.3 Diagnostic Materials and Phenotypic Assessment

The neck region is an accessible region to noninvasive sampling, processing, and storage of core biopsies and fine needle aspiration (FNA) materials for diagnostic and biomarker testing [8–10]. Generally, accurate diagnosis can readily be made on optic assessment, of the vast majority of thyroid, salivary, and mucosal-based malignancies.

Core biopsies are particularly valuable in initial presurgical assessment and subsequent utilization of tissue for follow-up and response to therapy. Combined cytomorphological evaluation and biological markers especially those adapted to immunohistochemistry (IHC) are central to accurate diagnosis and providing complementary biological information for clinical management. Lineage and transcription factor (TF) markers are supplemental to assist in diagnosis and differential diagnosis [11, 12].

9.3.1 Definition of Biomarkers

The National Cancer Institute (USA) has broadly defined biomarker as "a biological molecule formed in blood, other body fluids, or tissues that is a sign of normal or abnormal process" (https://www.cancer.gov/publications/dictionaries/cancer-terms/). Alterations in DNA, RNA, and protein products are potential markers for cancer diagnosis and classification, behavior, and response to therapy. Markers are generally categorized into lineage and biological in nature [13, 14].

A. *Lineage-based Diagnostic Markers*

  Ancillary diagnostic markers are primarily lineage associated to determine tumor derivation and typically include antibodies to epithelial (keratin, EMA), mesenchymal (SMA, disseminate), melanocytic, neural, and lympho-reticular markers. These are typically standardized, adapted to immunohistochemistry, and routinely utilized by accredited pathology laboratories [15, 16].

B. *Biological and Therapeutic-Associated Markers*

  Recent advances in cancer genomic and proteomic investigations have provided wealth information on alterations associated with development and progression of human malignancies and allowed investigators to link certain alterations to tumor development, progression, and biological behavior of solid tumors. Identifying critical events associated with development and progression of cancer subtypes is fundamental to translational diagnostic and therapeutic surrogate markers of these tumors. Multiple variations and technical modifications are available, and these can selectively be used to serve specific objective and conditions. The specificity and prevalence of molecular alterations, however, must be considered in the utilization for diagnosis and classification of neck tumors [17–19].

  Considering the plethora of publications documenting certain fusion genes and molecular alterations in solid tumors and especially in the head and neck region, the clinical application of a given marker without rigorously designed, and executed prospective, clinical trial should be considered tentative. Nonetheless, the empirical use of complementary markers to optic evaluation can be supportive, and the availability of genomic transcriptomic and proteomic provides wealth of information for targeted studies to identify functional protein to be adapted in a multiplex immunohistochemistry [20–22].

9.4 Molecular Techniques

Technical and genomic advances have led to the development of wide varieties of instrumentation and methods for protein, RNA, and DNA analyses of human tumors. These efforts, however, have provided new targets and novel biological pathways to numerous human neoplastic conditions. A brief overview of major technical advances in the field of genetic, molecular, and proteomic methods is presented.

9.4.1 Sample Sources and Nature

The neck is an excellent site to access and to harvest diagnostic materials. The main shortcomings, however, are the limited materials for an expanding need for ancillary testing requiring great care for optimum processing and utilizations [23, 24].

(a) *Cytological Smears and Cell Blocks*
    Scraping of smear preparation is suitable for limited RNA and is also ideal for in situ hybridization. Cell blocks can also be a source for targeted molecular testing by RT-PCR-based target markers [25].
(b) *Formalin-Fixed Paraffin-Embedded Tissues*
    Core tissue biopsies and excised lesioned tissues fixed for 6 to 20 hours in 10% buffered formalin are typically available for limited RNA, protein, and DNA testing. For better RNA stabilization and preservation, RNA, later kits can be used. Flash-frozen samples in liquid nitrogen and transfer to -20 °C are ideal for source for DNA, RNA, and proteins [26].
(c) *Nucleic Acid Extraction*
    The solid-phase approach is the preferred method for its reproducibility and yield from a small and limited sample and is based on the adsorption of DNA/RNA to silica in the presence of alcohol or guanidine thiocyanate salt. Nucleic acid extracted from cell trypsate

after protein digestion is precipitated using alcohol and added to a silica-impregnated filter. Cell debris is excluded. Filters are washed, and DNA/RNA is eluted with distilled water. Sample suitability and representation depends on percentage of tumor cells [27].

(i) *Nucleic Acid-based Techniques*
    Amplification methods are the most readily used in clinical laboratories for scant materials. Customized microarray-based platforms using DNA and RNA are being used in clinical oncology settings while advanced genome-wide sequencing techniques are currently limited for clinical application. The following are the most common methods in the clinical use (Table 9.2).

(a) *Polymerase Chain Reaction (PCR)*
    PCR is the most popular method of amplifying nucleic acids especially for limited clinical specimens. The methods simply entail amplification of targeted DNA template by a pair of primers complementary to the sense and antisense strands of the target in a thermocycler, and detailed steps of the procedures are standardized. The PCR yield is referred to as amplicons and is typically used for electrophoresis in situ and DNA sequencing. There are also multiple variations of PCR types including nested PCR, where the initial amplicon is subjected to a second round of amplification for highly

Table 9.2 Molecular methods for DNA, RNA, and protein alterations

Source	Alteration	Cytogenetics	FISH	DNA/RNA	Genomic array	Target seq.	Proteomics	IHC
DNA	Mutation	Yes	Yes	Yes	Yes	Yes	No	No
	Amplification	Yes	Yes	Yes	Yes	Yes	No	No
	Deletion	Yes	Yes	Yes	Yes	Yes	No	No
	Fusion genes	Yes	Yes	Yes	No	Yes	No	No
	Methylation	No	No	Yes	Yes	No	No	No
RNA	mRNA	No	No	Yes	No	Yes	No	No
	Gene fusion	No	Yes	Yes	No	Yes	No	No
	miRNA	No	No	No	No	Yes	No	no
	Transcription	No	No	No	No	Yes	No	No
Protein	Level	No	No	No	No	No	Yes	No
	Alterations	No	No	No	No	No	Yes	Yes

FISH fluorescence in situ hybridization, *IHC* immunohistochemistry, *RNA* ribonucleic acid, *seq.* sequencing

accurate qualitative assays, multiplex PCR, using two different DNA templates. It has to be realized by practicing pathologists, however, that molecular results can be affected by PCR errors and such possibility should be considered. Reagent contamination and sample contamination are not uncommon and should be eliminated. These include carry-over during the multistep PCR procedure and sample processing [28, 29].

(b) *Reverse-Transcriptase PCR*

In this technique, RNA is reverse-transcribed into complementary DNA (cDNA) using reverse-transcriptase enzyme. cDNA product is further used as a template to detect mRNA, gene fusion, and foreign targets. This technique is typically used in diagnostic kits of limited gene panels in oncology practice and detection of fusion genes transcripts [30, 31].

(c) *Real-Time PCR (RT PCR)*

This technique allows operators to monitor PCR quantification in real-time san electrophoresis of RNA and DNA targets. It requires fluorescent chromogen or labeled probes to bind to DNA and the fluorescence intensity, which reflects the amplicon content calculated with a standard control. The technique detects genetic alteration (mutation, detection, gene fusions, and SNPS) and is currently in use in most laboratories [32–34].

(d) *Fluorescence In Situ Hybridization (FISH)*

It is a well-established technique applicable to tissue and cytological materials of certain lymphoproliferative and solid tumors by most pathology laboratories.

This test is typically useful for scant specimen for genomic amplification and translocation detection in cytological smears and unstained sections of paraffin-embedded tissues. Detailed procedural preparations of specimens and optimal technical steps of this technique are well established and standardized. Appropriate positive and negative controls, however, are critical especially in diagnostic settings along with a standard operation procedure that details criteria of

positive and negative results for selected targets [35–37].

1. *Chromogenic ISH (CISH)*

In this method, conventional FISH except fluorescent probe labeling is substituted using peroxidase or alkaline phosphatase to convert chromogen to a visible colored product. It entails tagging target (DNA or RNA) with antibody to digoxigenin by another antibody labeled with an enzyme (peroxidase or alkaline phosphatase).

The technique is generally preferred in a clinical setting for light microscopic assessment, automation, and light quality of cytological preparations. Currently, CISH is preferred for better cellular definition, evaluation by light microscopy, subject to automation, and dual color advantages [38–40]. Recently, dual-color CISH assay for chromosome 17 and HER-2 gene was approved by the FDA for breast cancer.

2. *Comparative Genomic and Array Hybridization*

Both techniques provide broad screening of the molecular alterations by comparing extracted normal and matching tumor DNA samples hybridized to metaphase chromosome preparations. The array variant is more refined and provides detailed genetic information but insensitive to minor genetic alteration sand variations. They are also unsuitable for clinical purposes unless adapted to specific targets [41–43].

(ii) *Comprehensive Genomic and Proteomic Platforms*

Recently, high throughput genomic and proteomic platforms have been used in human malignancies and led to the availability a plethora of data resources for exploration (Table 9.3). These include the following:

A. *DNA/RNA Microarray*

Both DNA and RNA platforms are applied to survey broad DNA sequence and RNA expression transcripts with great accuracy.

Table 9.3 Biomarker screening strategy

Source	Alterations	Method
DNA	Sanger sequencing Mutations Translocations	HT Targeted
RNA	Genes fusion Transcription factor Micro-RNA	HT Targeted
Protein	Antibodies Peptides	HT Antibody-based

HT high throughput

The technique is based on imprinting short DNA sequences onto a solid phase that used hybridization to cDNA or cRNA. There are different platforms for printing microarray with the most commonly used printing probe on solid surface (Affymetrix) or microscopic beads (Illumina). Limited and custom-designed assays have been developed and being used in clinical oncology to triage patients for treatment or clinical trial [44–52].

B. *Sequencing Techniques*
  1. *Targeted DNA Sequencing (Sanger Method)*
     The basic principal of this method, which is developed by Sanger et al 43, is the inclusion of 2′, 3′ dinucleotide triphosphates (DD NTPs) as DNA chain terminator. This chain-terminator process requires a single stranded DNA template, a primer, DNA polymerase enzyme, control NTPs, and DD NTPs that terminate elongation.
     Different DD NTPs (ATP, GTP, CTP, and TTP) is labeled differently. The product of the sequencing process and capillary electrophoresis, a pattern of different fragments with variable fluorescent dye, can be subjected to analysis by sequencing instruments [53, 54].
  2. *Pyro-Sequencing*
     Is a direct sequencing technique based on the detection of inorganic phosphate (PPI) released during DNA synthesis and DNA polymerase nucleotide incorporation. PPI released is converted to ATP using ATP enzyme (sulfurylase) to induce

lactase enzyme to oxidize its substrate and produce visible light that is proportional to the number of incorporated nucleotides, and the resulted template can be measured. Although rapid and less costly than Sanger, it is limited by the short reads length [55, 56].
  3. *Next Generation Sequencing*
     This platform utilizes massive parallel sequencing of DNA and RNA that can simultaneously sequence >100,000 DNA/RNA fragments. Several platforms by different manufactures, and are mainly used for broad genomic analysis and are currently not suitable for clinical applications [57–63].

C. *Protein-based Platforms*
   Proteins are the end products of genomic and transcriptomic alterations and modification and are critical to biomarkers applications in pathology. Proteomics directly identifies candidate proteins that can be adjusted to be assayed by immunohistochemistry. The vast majority of lineage and biological markers available in pathology practice are protein-based adjusted to be assessed by different techniques available in pathology laboratories. Recently, large-scale protein analysis of these techniques has been conducted, leading to the discovery of a vast amount of information on protein structures and functions in major human malignancies.

   These techniques range in scale and sophistication and include electrophoresis, liquid chromatography, spectroscopy, mass spectrometry, and antibody-based microarray.

   Although impractical for routine laboratories, knowledge of these techniques and their findings are crucial to pathologists. Information on novel protein and their variants are critical to expanding IHC biomarker discovery and applications [64–67].

   Recent technical advances in sample preparation, liquid-phase separation, mass spectrometry, and bioinformatics of fresh and archived tissues allowed for detailed and expensive proteomic interrogation and linked the findings to genomic origin. Although these data broadly provide detailed information on largest protein domains, alternative splicing, and post-transcriptional modification, the broad variation of these events remain to complicate analysis and hinder standardization. Rational efforts to provide detailed characterization functional proteins in different cancer types are under way and will ultimately lead to the utilization of this method in diagnosis, stratification, and therapy.

1. *Mass Spectrometry*

   Mass spectrometry enables detection of structural, chemical modification, and degradation of proteins, and post-translational modification. Notably, a customized reversed-phase protein assay (RPPA) has been developed and used to identifying total and phosphorylases proteins in solid tumors. Although limited in scope, it can be customized to target relevant protein in different tumor types [65, 68–79].

2. *Immunohistochemistry (IHC)*

   IHC is currently the foreseeable future and is the principle technique for protein product assessment on paraffin sections and fixed cellular preparation for lineage and biomarkers in clinical pathology. The major advantage of the technique over emerging molecular testing methods and platforms is the simultaneous integration of optic morphological localization of biomarker expression of targeted tissues [80–83].

9.5 Genomic Pathways of Diagnostic and Clinical Utility

A. *Transcription Factors*

Transcription factors (TFs) are important protein products that regulate gene expression by binding to regulatory elements of DNA. Different isoforms of transcription factors are common as a result of alternative splicing, and under physiological conditions, a proper balance of different isoforms is needed to maintain specific transcriptional factor. Alteration in transcriptional factor by alternative splices generally leads to uncontrolled proliferation, defective differentiation, and cell death programs. It is increasingly used to complement established immunohistochemistry in pathology practice. There are more than 2000 different types of TFs, and different sets of these factors are expressed in each cell types to directly activate or repress specific programs. These are different categories of transcription factors that affect different processes [84–89].

The following are the most studies and characterized transcription factors with potential clinical implications:

(a) *Signal Transducer and Activator of Transcription (STATS)*

   This TF mediates transcriptions of a variety of cytokines, growth hormones, and factors in normal and neoplastic states. It is ubiquitously expressed and activates different genes in a cell and an organ context manner. STAT3 has two main isoforms; the most common is STAT3β, which plays regulatory and transcriptional pathways, and STAT3α, which plays a role in endometrial and ovarian carcinomas, glioma, and acute myeloid leukemia [90–92].

(b) *Transcription factor-7 like-2 (TCF7L2)*

   It is also known as T cell-specific transcription factor 4 (TCF4). This TF is a member of the high mobility group (HMG) box-containing transcription machinery. Its binding to nuclear β-Catenin leads to activation of cell growth, proliferation, apoptosis, and inflammation. Notably, JCF7L2 is reported to be downregulated in colon cancer [93–95].

(c) *Wilm's Tumor Factor (WT1)*

   WT1 is a key transcriptional factor in cell cycle, proliferation, differentiation, and cell death programs. It is expressed in urogenital organs of developing embryos and in adult kidneys, CNS, and hematopoietic cells. Alteration of the WT1 is common in Wilm's tumor and breast and may be useful in certain diagnostic challenges [96–98].

(d) *Melanocyte-Inducing Transcription Factor (MITF)*

MITF plays a central role in cell differentiation, proliferation, and cell death programs and comprises of multiple isoforms of different findings, as a result of alternative promoters. Two different isoforms, as a result of splice variants, are of differential prognostic significance in melanoma. Splice variants at exon6 give rise to (+) and (-) isoforms. The MITF(-) is highly in melanoma and cutaneous metastasis biology and diagnosis [99–101].

(e) *Nuclear Factor of Activated T Cells (NFAT2/NAFTC1)*

This transcriptional factor plays a role in immune response and regulation of genes linked to cell proliferation, cell death, and has been linked to melanoma tumorigenesis, colorectal and pancreatic cancer progression and metastasis, and Burkitt's lymphoma [102–106].

(f) *Kruppel-like Factor 6 (KLF6)*

KLF6 is highly expressed in different organs especially placenta, thymus, prostate, intestine, and spleen. It plays a role in cell growth, differentiation hematopoiesis, fibrosis, and liver cell regeneration. Alteration of this KLF6 has been reported in prostate, head and neck, ovarian, and lung cancers [107–111].

(g) *TTF-1*

This transcription factor is highly sensitive and a specific marker for thyroid and pulmonary lineage. TTF-1 is a transcription factor expressed in thyroid follicular cells, pneumocytes, and thyroid c-cells. In the lung, TTF1 is expressed in type II pneumocytes and nonciliated bronchial epithelial cells, and in the thyroid gland, it is expressed in follicular cell-derived differentiated carcinoma and typically negative in most poorly differentiated and anaplastic thyroid carcinomas and poorly differentiated nonsmall cell lung carcinoma [112–115]. TTF1 is commonly used in routine pathology practice for differential diagnosis and unknown primary investigations.

(h) *PAX Family Transcription Factors*

The PAX family of genes is considered to function as oncogenes and as lineage-associated markers for certain embryonic tissues in a distinct spatial and an organ context manner. The most clinically relevant members are the following:

These transcription factors are increasingly being applied in diagnosis and differential diagnosis in routine pathology settings.

(i) *PAX2 and PAX8: (Wilm's tumor and thyroid follicular cancer)*

PAX-2 is expressed in the epithelial components of Wilm's tumor and in renal cell carcinoma. PAX-8 is also expressed in Wilm's tumor and papillary thyroid carcinoma [116].

(ii) *PAX5: Brain and Lymphomas*

The PAX5 is highly expressed in astrocytoma and a small percentage of non-Hodgkin's lymphoma and especially medulloblastoma of children. A small percentage of non-Hodgkin lymphomas manifest translation t(9;14)(p13;q32), PAX5/IGH. Fusion of an EM enhancer close to the PAX5 gene leads to its overexpression [117–121].

(iii) *PAX3 and PAX7*

Both transcription factors are expressed in Rhabdomyosarcoma. The alveolar subtype of this entity is characterized by translocation between chromosomes 2 and 13, t(2;13) (q35;q14), resulting in fusion between PAX3 and the

FKHR transcription factor and a second translocation between chromosomes 1 and 13, t(1;13) (p36;q14), resulting in fusion between PAX7 and the FKHR gene on Ewing's small-celled tumors.

PAX3 has also been reported to be expressed in peripheral neuroectodermal tumors [122, 123].

(i) *SOX Family Transcription Factor*

The sex-determining (SR4) DNA region on chromosome Y is the location for the Sox genes. All Sox genes share the high mobility region and binds to corresponding DNA sequences. The SOX family comprises of at least 20 members; of these, only nine are currently characterized. In general, the majority of the SOX factors are biological mediations and linked to cellular differentiation and proliferations, and their diagnostic utilization is limited and rarely used in routine pathology. The SOX genes are also critical to the development and functions of the nervous systems, skeletal muscle, eye development pigment formation, and immune systems [124, 125]. Only those commonly available members of SOX family with potential diagnostic utility are to be discussed.

(a) *SOX4*

It is uniquely overexpressed in differentiated thyroid carcinoma and can be useful in selected and challenging instances [126].

(b) *SOX8*

SOX8 transcription factor has been used as a marker of tumor progression in triple negative breast cancer and hepatocellular carcinoma [127, 128].

(c) *SOX9*

Nuclear SOX9 is characteristically expressed in gastric carcinoma and has been reported to be consistently present in both primary and metastatic lesions. Sox 9 also in Sertoli cells and cartilage formation may be helpful in differentiating testicular germ cells and cartilaginous tumors [129, 130].

(d) *SOX10*

SOX10 transcription factor is encoded by the SOX gene located on the long arm and encodes a protein of 33 a.a. It plays an important role in stem cell, lineage, and differentiation of neural crest cells, melanocyte, thyroid, and adrenal medullar cells. It has also been linked to myoepithelial cell development and is being utilized in pathology practices in salivary, breast, neural, and soft tissue tumors as an ancillary marker [131–133].

(e) *SOX11*

SOX11 gene is mapped to chromosome 2p25-3 and is involved in neural commitment and phenotype. SOX11 is also expressed in keratinocytes and other epithelial-derived mucosa. It may be used on ancillary markers in certain types of lymphomas (mantel cell), pancreas, and differential diagnosis of metastatic ovarian and breast [134].

(f) *SOX17*

SOX-17 is preferentially expressed in the gastro-intestinal tract especially in the upper sites (esophagus, stomach, and small intestines) and can be selectively used in the differential diagnosis of unknown primaries [135].

B. *Fusion Genes and Chromosomal Translocations*

Structural chromosomal alterations resulting from in gene fusion are considered a driver event in certain solid tumors especially sarcoma. Fusion genes and their products as a result of chromosomal translocations have been considered a significant factor affecting transcription and protein function of tumors. The association of certain chromosomal translocations and gene fusion with certain tumor types has been considered a potential diagnostic marker. However, the specific and lineage restriction of these events to a given tumor type has yet to be realized. At present, therefore, the diagnostic role of these events exclusive of the phenotypic diagnosis should be guarded. They may, however, in certain instances support the histological diagnosis, but negative finding should not overrule diagnosis biologically and therapeutically. These events may in the future be of a significant clinical and therapeutic potential [136–138].

9.6 Primary and Metastatic Tumors

I. Metastasis to Neck Nodes
  1. *Cystic Squamous Carcinoma*
     Metastatic cystic squamous carcinoma of known primary is commonly encountered and involves different compartments dependent on the site of the primary. Metastasis may not uncommonly precede the identification of a primary especially of the oropharyngeal sites.
     Potential sites of origin include base of tongue, tonsil, and oropharynx and nasopharynx are typically the source. A simple positive p16 immunostaining can suggest oropharyngeal origin. This may be followed by in situ viral testing for HPV and EBV, which is needed [139–141].
  2. *Carcinoma of Unknown Origin*
     The definition of carcinoma of unknown primary (CUP), however, entails a histologically confirmed metastatic carcinoma in a patient with no known primary identifiable origin after clinical and radiological examination. Lineage and biological markers of neck metastasis are complex and should be integrated based on knowledge of the technical, scoring, and differential expression of tumors of different organs. The utilization of ancillary tests, therefore, should be tailored and prioritized based on whether the target lesion is native or alien to this region. Broadly, for pathologists and cytologists',

biomarkers are categorized as diagnostic, prognostic, predictive, and surrogate [142–144].

The primary source of diagnostic material is fine needle aspiration (FNA) and core tissue biopsy complemented with the selective use of ancillary testing including lineage, transcription factors, and molecular expression and alterations for head and neck. Customized panel of markers can be used for supraclavicular node metastasis including genomic platform tailored for tumors of different origins to complement optic assessment. In the majority of specialized medical centers, tumors of unknown origins are triaged to special clinics. A standard initial procedure is fine needle aspiration and core tissue biopsy. The location of the affected node(s) in the neck may provide initial guidance to possible primary especially at supraclavicular locations (Table 9.1 and Fig. 9.1) [9, 145]

  3. *Infraclavicular Metastasis Sources*
     The majority of these instances are from the lung, breast, and gastrointestinal tract primaries, but other sources are not uncommon. Therefore, the application and integration of markers of both lineage and biological nature should be based on the tailored to the most relevant differential diagnosis based on the optic evaluation of the primary tumor type. Negative findings of biomarkers and genetic alterations are not uncommon and should not be the sole reason to exclude a given phenotypic diagnosis and the possibility of a second malignancy. Future and current specific applications of certain molecular and biomarkers, however, will increasingly be critical in the follow-up of tumors progression, treatment selection, and toxicity and response especially using FNA and core biopsies. Not infrequently, incidents of metastatic carcinoma commonly to supraclavicular lymph nodes with no known history or clinical detectable primary are encountered [146–150].

II. *Primary Organ-based Tumors of the Neck*

1. *Salivary Gland Tumors*

Salivary gland tumors originating from submandibular and parotid glands can present as upper neck masses, and FNA is the initial source of diagnostic materials. They may also, rarely, arise in heterotopic salivary remnant in the neck (Fig. 9.2).

Salivary gland tumors are generally cellularly and structurally heterogeneous circumscription, and the invasion of host stroma is currently the main differentiating factor in benign and malignant diagnosis. This is especially the case in myoepithelial-dominate pleomorphic adenoma, basal cell tumors, myoepithelial tumors, and carcinoma arising in pleomorphic adenoma. Similarly, differentiation between reactive and neoplastic oncocytic nodule may not infrequently pose diagnostic challenges.

Molecular and biomarkers of common tumors in the posterior parotid and submandibular glands are illustrated in Fig. 9.3.

(a) *Pleomorphic Adenoma*

Currently, none of the genetic, molecular, and phenotypic markers are specific or diagnostic of this entity. Nonetheless, the PLAG1 gene on chromosome 3p21 has been considered a frequent and specific [151, 152] gene alteration. The diagnostic and differential diagnostic utility of this alteration is minimal.

(b) *Warthin's and Oncocytric Lesion*

Cytological diagnosis of Warthin's is straight unless a rare development of mucoepidermoid carcinoma is suspected. Simple mucicarmine stain is needed for continuing MEC [153].

(c) *Myoepithelial Tumors*

Pure myoepithelial tumors are rare and may display wide range of cytological variations. The majority is likely originated from pleomorphic adenoma. The difference between benign and malignant categories is based on the invasive nature of the lesion. In addition to morphology p63 and smooth muscle action, calponin and keratin are useful markers in identification and classification.

Currently, no known biomarkers and genetic alterations have been linked to these tumors to be considered a diagnostic marker [154–156].

(d) *Mucoepidermoid Carcinoma*

It is the most common malignant epithelial neoplasm and the entity with defined low, intermediate, and high grades. Low-grade tumors are largely cystic with small foci of cellular clusters. Intermediate grade is generally cellular with small cystic regions and composed epidermal-like clusters with mucinous features. High-grade MEC is mainly occasional small cystic and scattered mucin-forming cells. Simple mucin stain to detect intracellular mucin is the main ancillary tests. Fusion genes as a result of chromosomal translocation t(11:19)(q21; p13) leading to CRTC1/MAML2 gene fusion have been iden-

Fig. 9.3 Salivary glands

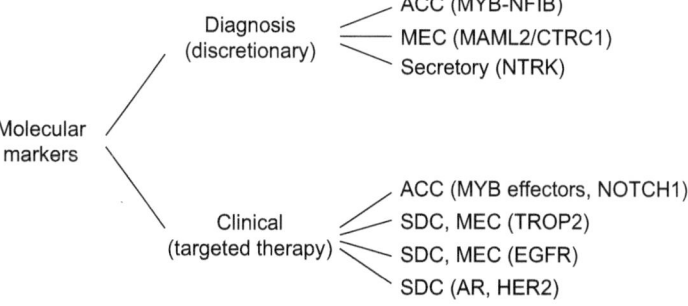

Molecular markers

Diagnosis (discretionary)
- ACC (MYB-NFIB)
- MEC (MAML2/CTRC1)
- Secretory (NTRK)

Clinical (targeted therapy)
- ACC (MYB effectors, NOTCH1)
- SDC, MEC (TROP2)
- SDC, MEC (EGFR)
- SDC (AR, HER2)

tified in more than 50% of this entity. Generally, but fusion testing is not needed. In certain circumstances especially poorly differentiated carcinoma with visible mucin, fusion detection may be helpful in confirming MEC arising in Warthin's tumor but negative cannot exclude this diagnosis. Currently, no known targeted molecular therapy for patients with fusion positive MEC and the fusion has also been detected in other solid tumors [157–159].

(e) *Adenocarcinoma/Salivary Duct Carcinoma*

These entities closely resemble mammary ductal carcinoma and express androgen receptor, HER-2, and EGFR expression. Both forms also either arise de novo or in longstanding pleomorphic adenoma. The malignant component either de novo or in the setting of pleomorphic adenoma is identical in their biomarker expression and genomic composition. FNA of the latter may not target the carcinoma component. Also in contrast to breast, IHC is only used in assessing HER-2 expression, and high expression is similar to that of breast. In general, diagnosis is mainly based on cytohistological evaluation and could be assisted with AR and HER-2 if positive. Lack of high HER-2 and negative AR findings are not uncommon, and it does not exclude the diagnosis of adenocarcinoma. No known genetic alteration or fusion genes are consistently identified in this entity [160–162].

(f) *Adenoid Cystic Carcinoma*

Adenoid cystic carcinoma is the second most common primary malignancy of minor and major salivary glands and is uniquely formed of dual epithelial and myoepithelial cells. Loss of myoepithelial cells is coincident with the development of the solid form. Cytologically, it may be difficult to firmly establish the diagnosis, and the exclusion of salivary and nonsalivary basal cell tumors could be a challenge.

The differential diagnosis may also include pleomorphic adenoma, epimyoepithelial carcinoma, and polymorphous adenocarcinoma. Firm diagnosis, however, may not be essential for surgically excisable cases. ACC is characterized by chromosomal translocations including t(6;9) and t(8;9), leading to fusion transcripts of MYB-NFIB and MYBL1-NFIB. Irrespective of these fusions, MYB expression is commonly expressed. At least 30–40% ACC lack these fusions with no documented evidence of difference in behavior or response. Currently, known pre- or postexcision targeted small molecule therapy are available. NOTCH1 mutation, however, has been identified recently and is currently being tested in small subset of patients [31, 163–167].

(g) *Acinic Cell Carcinoma*

Acinic cell carcinoma is a relatively uncommon, salivary malignancy that may rarely present as metastasis. Not uncommonly, in comparison to other salivary malignancies, high-grade undifferentiated carcinoma transformation emerges and is commonly associated with poor prognosis. The diagnosis can be difficult on FNA and limited biopsy materials, but histopathological diagnosis is generally straightforward. Genomic and molecular analyses of these tumors provide little specific and/or diagnostic certainty. New potential marker of pathological and clinical assessment of acinic cell carcinoma, the NR4A3, has recently been identified in a genomic study of those tumors as a result of variable chromosomal translocation. Adaptation of the orphan nuclear receptor to archival tissue will serve as a novel marker in practice [168–172].

(h) *Secretory Carcinoma*

Previously, a variant of acidic cell carcinoma secretory carcinoma, identical to their mammary counterpart, has been extracted from this malignancy. The Translocation involving chromosomes 12q13 and 15q15 resulting in the fusion gene transcript ETV6-NTRK3 is nonrestricted to secretory carcinoma of either salivary or mammary carcinoma. It is critical to know that approximately half of these tumor types is fusion negative. For diagnostic purposes, fusion detection may confirm the diagnosis but negative results do not confirm the diagnosis. The significance of this alteration, however, rests on the stratification of patients with progressive disease to NTRK small molecule therapy [173–175].

(i) *Basal cell salivary neoplasms*

Basal cell salivary tumors are classified histopathologically into adenoma and adenocarcinoma based on the postsurgical assessment of invasive nature. Both forms share identical cytomorphological and structural features. Accordingly, early diagnosis by noninvasive mass is unattainable. Moreover, their presurgical differential diagnosis from adenoid cystic carcinoma poses significant challenges. Basal cell tumors histologically, biologically, and genetically low-grade malignancy with few genetic alterations of minimum diagnosis impact. A small subset of these tumors, however, carries mutation of the CYLD gene. The diagnostic significant of this alteration is unknown [176–181].

2. *Primary Mesenchymal Neoplasms of the Neck*

(a) *Synovial Sarcoma*

Synovial sarcoma in the neck region accounts for approximately 10% of all soft tissue subtypes. It is generally presented in young patients typically in oropharynx and hypopharynx. They also detected near joints in the upper neck. Diagnosis is fairly formed straight and typically by-phasic computed tomography (CT), and core biopsy provides sufficient information for diagnosis along with lineage-associated markers including keratin and EMA. Detection of the t(X; 18) (p11.2; q11.2) translocation resulting in SYT-SSX1 or SYT-SSX2 fusion transcripts confirms the diagnosis, but negative results are not exclusionary [182, 183].

(b) *Chordoma*

Chordomas are not uncommon especially at the spheno-occipita and base of skull regions. The diagnosis can be readily made on excisional or core tissue biopsy with the aid of keratin, GMA, and occasionally S100. Differential diagnosis from chondrosarcoma, recurrent pleomorphic adeno, and metastatic mucinous carcinoma should be considered. No consistent or specific chromosomal or genetic alterations to aid diagnosis is currently known [184–186].

3. *Carotid Body Neoplasms and Paraganglioma*

These tumors are infrequent but may lead to differential diagnostic difficulties with carcinoid tumor, neuroendocrine carcinoma, medullary thyroid carcinoma, and forms of thyroid neoplasms. They are typically negative for cytokeratin stains and neuroendocrine markers. Negative calcitonin and TTF-1 exclude medullary carcinoma [187–189].

4. *Thyroid Neoplasms*

Thyroid tumors are the most common primary neck neoplasms, and in principal, all presurgical diagnosis is based on (FNA) analysis. The diagnosis of the papillary and medullary carcinomas subtypes can be ascertained by FNA with and without ancillary testing. Assessing FNA findings of follicular neoplasms is limited by the inability to evaluate capsular and confirming capsular invasion and vascular permeation. The diagnosis of medullary thyroid carcinoma, in contrast, is typically aided by immunohistochemistry for calcitonin and other neuroendocrine markers [190, 191].

Presurgical diagnosis based on molecular analysis remains a subject of intensive studies. These efforts, however, have to take in consideration the protracted follow- up of patients to evaluate patients with and without alterations. Presurgical classification of follicular thyroid masses is a subject of intense investigations. Diagnosis of malignancy remains largely based on the postsurgical finding of capsular and vascular invasions.

The most common molecular alteration in this category is RAS gene mutations and PAX8/PPARγ of gene rearrangement (75%). It is also not uncommon for these alterations to be detected in noncarcinoma follicular lesion. Whether these lesions are premalignant or incidental is unknown. The diagnostic value of this alteration, along with BRAF protein, however, remains uncertain (Fig. 9.4 and Table 9.4) [192]

(a) *Papillary Thyroid Carcinoma*

In this form, alteration of the BRAF and RAS genes and rearrangements of the RET and PTC genes have been characterized. Although these alterations are not mutually exclusive, they are linked to MAPK pathway activation. The frequency of the BRAF mutualization ranges between 35% and 75% and largely involves the 1799 nucleotides resulting in transversion change of thymine to adenine

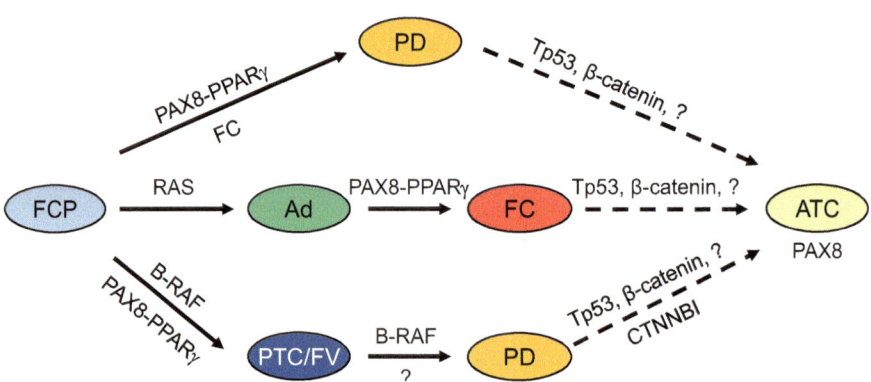

Fig. 9.4 Diagram of thyroid tumorigenesis and current molecular uncut and associated with their evolution. FCP follicular cell precursor, Ad adenoma, PTC papillary thyroid carcinoma, FV follicular variant, FC follicular carcinoma, PD poorly differentiated, ATC anaplastic thyroid carcinoma

Table 9.4 Incidence of gene mutations in thyroid tumors

Alterations	Braf (%)	RAS-F (%)	PTEN (%)	CTNNB1 (%)	TP53 (%)	ALK IDH1 (%)
PTC	45	0	1–2	0	0	0
F-PTC	15	30–45	0	0	0	0
FTA	0	20–25	0	0	0	0
FTC	0	30–45	15–20	0	0	0
ATC	25	20–30	20–30	60	60	10

at codon 600 (V600E). Other less frequent changes can occur as well, although with much less frequency, and the prognostic significance of this alteration remains uncertain. The second molecular alteration in PTC is chromosomal inversion involving the 3′ segment of the PTC1 or PTC3 genes on chromosome 10. This alteration comprises approximately 15 to 20% of PTC especially those linked to radiation exposure in children and young adults. Alterations in the RAS gene family have been reported in PTC and also in FTC and some adenomas. The association of alterations of these glues to activation of the MAPK and PI3K/AKT pathways underscores a role in tumorigenesis [193–199].

(b) *Follicular Thyroid Neoplasms*

Follicular-forming neoplasms represent a spectrum of well-encapsulated and invasive forms. The potential malignant progression of the encapsulated type to the invasive form is certain, and a clinical follow-up is required. The integration of molecular alterations in the cytological and histopathological interpretation may be helpful, although consistent and frequent genetic alteration of these tumors is infrequent. The most common alteration is mutations of the RAS genes. Both follicular adenomas and carcinomas carry RAS gene mutations in approximately 40 to 60% of the cases. The second common alterations of follicular thyroid neoplasm is rearrangements of the PAX8-PPARγ as a consequence to a translocation between t(2:3)(q13; p25) that lead to overexpression of the PPARγ protein that can be evaluated by routine IHC [197, 200–205].

(c) *Poorly Differentiated and Anaplastic Thyroid Carcinoma*

Poorly differentiated thyroid carcinoma is difficult to diagnose presurgically, and medullary thyroid carcinoma, paraganglioma, and metastasis to thyroid should be excluded [206]. Thyroglobulin and PAX18 are markers that can be utilized.

Anaplastic carcinoma, however, are highly diverse and may manifest sarcomatoid carcinoma with and without squamous features, giant cell, and spectrum of cellular anaplasia. They can be clinically predicted by rapid and aggressive local growth. Not uncommonly, they may arise in PTC, but they have reported in follicular and medullary subtypes. The differential diagnosis, especially, if significant rapid growth is lacking, is spindle cell melanoma, sarcomatoid squamous carcinoma of dermal, and for head–neck sites and sarcoma. Except for perhaps melanoma, lineage and biological markers should be cautiously utilized [207–209]. No specific genetic and/or molecular alterations have been reported in these tumors. However, mutations of P53, β-catenin, RAS, and P13K genes have been reported with widely variable frequency in both forms [197, 210–216].

(d) *Medullary Carcinoma*

The majority of medullary carcinoma are sporadic and characterized by mutation of the RET gene in approximately 20 to 70% of adult patients. The majority of identified mutations affect codon q18. RET mutation in familial is germ line. In MEN2A, the mutation is limited to codon 634 of the gene in contrast to familial cases. This mutation can be targeted by small molecule inhibitor of RET kinase [217, 218].

(e) *Neoplasms of Undetermined Malignancy*

Approximately 30% of thyroid nodules are classified as undetermined of follicular neoplasm per the Bethesda System for reporting thyroid cytopathology (TBSRTC). Although considerable improvements have been achieved using consensus criteria in assessing intermediate category of thyroid follicular nodular, definitive clinical management of these lesions remains uncertain due to the variability of platforms used, lack of information on the fate of nonresected patients and prospective clinical trials of surgically resected lesions. The applications of these platforms can be considered empirical and the incorporation of genetic information in definitive diagnosis must await.

Recently, molecular analysis of these lesions has been the subject of intense investigation with a tendency to advocate surgery for lesion with genetic alterations. A major issue is the long-term follow-up of patients with histologically benign lesions with molecular alterations. The use of molecular testing to guide clinical decision of thyroid nodules especially in intermediate cytological categories remains unclear. This is due to the lack of defined guidelines for management decisions based on molecular findings irrespective of cytological categorization. Therefore, the inclusion of molecular testing in clinical management of thyroid nodules of undetermined cytology must await a prospective multi-institutional prospective trial where all patients undergo surgery and independent, blinded, cytopathological conformities. Integration of phenotypic assessment and tissue-based markers is critical to diagnosis, especially in cases of unknown primary [219–221].

(f) *Paraganglioma*

Primary paraganglioma of the thyroid is rare but should be considered in the differential diagnosis of sporadic medullary carcinoma. A comparative genomic analysis of few examples of thyroid paraganglioma and medullary thyroid carcinoma reported a negative calcitonin and positive NDUFA4L2 (NADH dehydrogenase 1 alpha subcomplex, 4-like 2) and COXIV2 (Cytochrome c oxidase subunit IV isoform 2) to be limited to paraganglioma [222–226]

(g) *Metastasis*

Metastasis to thyroid is not uncommon and should be considered in early assessment especially in patients with history of renal cell carcinoma and melanoma. In addition, consideration for differentiating between medullary thyroid carcinoma and primary thyroid paraganglioma should be kept as a possibility in rare instances. A panel of histochemical markers dependent on the optic features could be used [226–228].

5. *Parathyroid Neoplasms*

Reactive, benign lesions and malignant parathyroid carcinoma are primarily a surgical disease. Presurgical fine needle aspiration and core biopsy are rarely required or practiced in presurgical evaluation. These procedures can be used for recurrent and widely invasive parathyroid carcinoma. Occasional instances of locally invasive nodular thyroid hyperplasia and parathyroid carcinoma are encountered and lead to differential diagnostic difficulties [229–232].

References

1. Hayes DF, Bast RC, Desch CE, Fritsche H Jr, Kemeny NE, Jessup JM, et al. Tumor marker utility grading system: a framework to evaluate clinical utility of tumor markers. J Natl Cancer Inst. 1996;88(20):1456–66.

2. Ioannidis JP, Panagiotou OA. Comparison of effect sizes associated with biomarkers reported in highly cited individual articles and in subsequent meta-analyses. JAMA. 2011;305(21):2200–10.
3. Morris JS, Luthra R, Liu Y, Duose DY, Lee W, Reddy NG, et al. Development and validation of a gene signature classifier for consensus molecular subtyping of colorectal carcinoma in a CLIA-certified setting. Clin Cancer Res. 2021;27(1):120–30.
4. Vo TT, Vivot A, Porcher R. Impact of biomarker-based design strategies on the risk of false-positive findings in targeted therapy evaluation. Clin Cancer Res. 2018;24(24):6257–64.
5. Lih CJ, Harrington RD, Sims DJ, Harper KN, Bouk CH, Datta V, et al. Analytical validation of the next-generation sequencing assay for a nationwide signal-finding clinical trial: molecular analysis for therapy choice clinical trial. J Mol Diagn. 2017;19(2):313–27.
6. Fumagalli D, Desmedt C, Ignatiadis M, Loi S, Piccart M, Sotiriou C. Gene profiling assay and application: the predictive role in primary therapy. J Natl Cancer Inst Monogr. 2011;2011(43):124–7.
7. Chen A, Flaherty K, O'Dwyer PJ, Giantonio B, Marinucci DM, Lee JW, et al. Tumor genomic profiling practices and perceptions: a survey of physicians participating in the NCI- MATCH Trial. JCO Precis Oncol. 2020:4.
8. Giusti L, Iacconi P, Ciregia F, Giannaccini G, Donatini GL, Basolo F, et al. Fine-needle aspiration of thyroid nodules: proteomic analysis to identify cancer biomarkers. J Proteome Res. 2008;7(9):4079–88.
9. Eisele DW, Sherman ME, Koch WM, Richtsmeier WJ, Wu AY, Erozan YS. Utility of immediate on-site cytopathological procurement and evaluation in fine needle aspiration biopsy of head and neck masses. Laryngoscope. 1992;102(12 Pt 1):1328–30.
10. Sgariglia R, Nacchio M, Migliatico I, Vigliar E, Malapelle U, Pisapia P, et al. Moving towards a local testing solution for undetermined thyroid fine-needle aspirates: validation of a novel custom DNA-based NGS panel. J Clin Pathol. 2022;75(7):465–71.
11. Berger MF, Mardis ER. The emerging clinical relevance of genomics in cancer medicine. Nat Rev Clin Oncol. 2018;15(6):353–65.
12. Mansfield AS, Park BH, Mullane MP. Identification, prioritization, and treatment of mutations identified by next-generation sequencing. Am Soc Clin Oncol Educ Book. 2018;38:873–80.
13. Henry NL, Hayes DF. Cancer biomarkers. Mol Oncol. 2012;6(2):140–6.
14. Mishkin GE, Kohn EC. Biomarker development: bedside to bench. Clin Cancer Res. 2022;28(13):2722–4.
15. Jo VY, Demicco EG. Update from the 5th edition of the World Health Organization classification of head and neck tumors: soft tissue tumors. Head Neck Pathol. 2022;16(1):87–100.
16. Meyer MT, Watermann C, Dreyer T, Ergün S, Karnati S. 2021 update on diagnostic markers and translocation in salivary gland tumors. Int J Mol Sci. 2021;22(13):6771.
17. Kamps R, Brandão RD, van den Bosch BJ, Paulussen AD, Xanthoulea S, Blok MJ, Romano A. Next-generation sequencing in oncology: genetic diagnosis, risk prediction and cancer classification. Int J Mol Sci. 2017;18(2):308.
18. Lohmann K, Klein C. Next generation sequencing and the future of genetic diagnosis. Neurotherapeutics. 2014;11:699–707.
19. George S, Bertagnolli MM. Linking genotype to phenotype: bench to bedside. Clin Cancer Res. 2022;28(13):2725–7.
20. Cui M, Cheng C, Zhang L. High-throughput proteomics: a methodological mini-review. Lab Invest. 2022;102(11):1170–81.
21. Füzéry AK, Levin J, Chan MM, Chan DW. Translation of proteomic biomarkers into FDA approved cancer diagnostics: issues and challenges. Clin Proteomics. 2013;10(1):1–14.
22. Mani DR, Krug K, Zhang B, Satpathy S, Clauser KR, Ding L, et al. Cancer proteogenomics: current impact and future prospects. Nat Rev Cancer. 2022;22(5):298–313.
23. Haverstick DM, Groszback AR. Specimen collection and processing. In: Bruns DE, editor. Fundamentals of molecular diagnostics. St. Louis: Elsevier Health Sciences; 2007. p. 25–37.
24. Zehnbauer BA. Clinical testing of patient's specimens. In: Pfeifer JD, editor. Molecular genetic testing in surgical pathology. Philadelphia: Lippincott Williams & Wilkins; 2006. p. 171–85.
25. Shafigh E, Siadaty S. Comparison of smear cytology and cell blocks in detection of respiratory cancer. Ann Saudi Med. 2005;25(6):514.
26. Mansour A, Chatila R, Bejjani N, Dagher C, Faour WH. A novel xylene free deparaffinization method for the extraction of proteins from human derived formalin-fixed paraffin embedded (FFPE) archival tissue blocks. MethodsX. 2014;1:90–5.
27. Smith Zagone MJ, Pulliam JF, Farkas DH. Molecular pathology methods. In: Leonard DG, Bagg A, Caliendo AM, Deerlin VM, Kaul KL, editors. Molecular pathology in clinical practice. New York: Springer; 2007. p. 15–40.
28. Kramer MF, Coen DM. Enzymatic amplification of DNA by PCR: standard procedures and optimization. Curr Prot Mol Biol. 2001;56(1):15.1.1–4.
29. Wickham CL, Boyce M, Joyner MV, Sarsfield P, Wilkins BS, Jones DB, Ellard S. Amplification of PCR products in excess of 600 base pairs using DNA extracted from decalcified, paraffin wax embedded bone marrow trephine biopsies. Mol Pathol. 2000;53(1):19–23.
30. Cave H, Acquaviva C, Bieche I, Brault D, de Fraipont F, Fina F, et al. RT-PCR in clinical diagnosis. Ann Biol Clin (Paris). 2003;61(6):635–44.

31. Mitani Y, Li J, Rao PH, Zhao YJ, Bell D, Lippman SM, et al. Comprehensive analysis of the MYB-NFIB gene fusion in salivary adenoid cystic carcinoma: incidence, variability, and clinicopathologic significance. Clin Cancer Res. 2010;16(19):4722–31.

32. Bustin SA, Benes V, Nolan T, Pfaffl MW. Quantitative real-time RT-PCR—a perspective. J Mol Endocrinol. 2005;34(3):597–601.

33. Gabert J, Beillard E, Van der Velden V, Bi W, Grimwade D, Pallisgaard N, et al. Standardization and quality control studies of 'real-time'quantitative reverse transcriptase polymerase chain reaction of fusion gene transcripts for residual disease detection in leukemia–a Europe Against Cancer program. Leukemia. 2003;17(12):2318–57.

34. Mocellin S, Rossi CR, Pilati P, Nitti D, Marincola FM. Quantitative real-time PCR: a powerful ally in cancer research. Trends Mol Med. 2003;9(5):189–95.

35. Perry A. Fluorescence *in situ* hybridization. In: Pfeifer JD, editor. Molecular genetic testing in surgical pathology. Philadelphia: Lippincott Williams & Wilkins; 2006. p. 72–85.

36. Cappuzzo F, Finocchiaro G, Rossi E, Janne PA, Carnaghi C, Calandri C, et al. EGFR FISH assay predicts for response to cetuximab in chemotherapy refractory colorectal cancer patients. Ann Oncol. 2008;19(4):717–23.

37. Moroni M, Veronese S, Benvenuti S, Marrapese G, Sartore-Bianchi A, Di Nicolantonio F, et al. Gene copy number for epidermal growth factor receptor (EGFR) and clinical response to antiEGFR treatment in colorectal cancer: a cohort study. Lancet Oncol. 2005;6(5):279–86.

38. Lambros MB, Natrajan R, Reis-Filho JS. Chromogenic and fluorescent in situ hybridization in breast cancer. Hum Pathol. 2007;38(8):1105–22.

39. Mollerup J, Henriksen U, Müller S, Schønau A. Dual color chromogenic in situ hybridization for determination of HER2 status in breast cancer: a large comparative study to current state of the art fluorescence in situ hybridization. BMC Clin Pathol. 2012;12(1):1–7.

40. Bartlett JM, Campbell FM, Ibrahim M, O'Grady A, Kay E, Faulkes C, et al. A UK NEQAS ISH multicenter ring study using the Ventana HER2 dual-color ISH assay. Am J Clin Pathol. 2011;135(1):157–62.

41. Kallioniemi A, Kallioniemi OP, Sudar D, Rutovitz D, Gray JW, Waldman F, Pinkel D. Comparative genomic hybridization for molecular cytogenetic analysis of solid tumors. Science. 1992;258(5083):818–21.

42. Shinawi M, Cheung SW. The array CGH and its clinical applications. Drug Discov Today. 2008;13(17–18):760–70.

43. Rao PH, Roberts D, Zhao YJ, Bell D, Harris CP, Weber RS, El-Naggar AK. Deletion of 1p32-p36 is the most frequent genetic change and poor prognostic marker in adenoid cystic carcinoma of the salivary glands. Clin Cancer Res. 2008;14(16):5181–7.

44. Brown PO, Botstein D. Exploring the new world of the genome with DNA microarrays. Nat Genet. 1999;21(1 Suppl):33–7.

45. Bilitewski U. DNA microarrays: an introduction to the technology. Methods Mol Biol. 2009;509:1–14.

46. Bumgarner R. Overview of DNA microarrays: types, applications, and their future. Curr Protoc Mol Biol. 2013; Chapter 22:Unit 22 1.

47. Lenoir T, Giannella E. The emergence and diffusion of DNA microarray technology. J Biomed Discov Collab. 2006;1:11.

48. Fan JB, Gunderson KL, Bibikova M, Yeakley JM, Chen J, Garcia EW, et al. [3] illumina universal bead arrays. Meth Enzymol. 2006;410:57–73.

49. Auer H, Newsom DL, Kornacker K. Expression profiling using Affymetrix GeneChip microarrays. Methods Mol Biol. 2009;509:35–46.

50. Alexander EK, Kennedy GC, Baloch ZW, Cibas ES, Chudova D, Diggans J, et al. Preoperative diagnosis of benign thyroid nodules with indeterminate cytology. N Engl J Med. 2012;367(8):705–15.

51. Wallden B, Storhoff J, Nielsen T, Dowidar N, Schaper C, Ferree S, et al. Development and verification of the PAM50-based Prosigna breast cancer gene signature assay. BMC Med Genomics. 2015;8:54.

52. Slodkowska EA, Ross JS. MammaPrint 70-gene signature: another milestone in personalized medical care for breast cancer patients. Expert Rev Mol Diagn. 2009;9(5):417–22.

53. Smith LM, Sanders JZ, Kaiser RJ, Hughes P, Dodd C, Connell CR, et al. Fluorescence detection in automated DNA sequence analysis. Nature. 1986;321(6071):674–9.

54. Smith LM, Fung S, Hunkapiller MW, Hunkapiller TJ, Hood LE. The synthesis of oligonucleotides containing an aliphatic amino group at the 5′ terminus: synthesis of fluorescent DNA primers for use in DNA sequence analysis. Nucleic Acids Res. 1985;13(7):2399–412.

55. Nyren P, Pettersson B, Uhlen M. Solid phase DNA minisequencing by an enzymatic luminometric inorganic pyrophosphate detection assay. Anal Biochem. 1993;208(1):171–5.

56. Ronaghi M, Uhlen M, Nyren P. A sequencing method based on real-time pyrophosphate. Science. 1998;281(5375):363–5.

57. Wang Z, Gerstein M, Snyder M. RNA-Seq: a revolutionary tool for transcriptomics. Nat Rev Genet. 2009;10(1):57–63.

58. Anderson MW, Schrijver I. Next generation DNA sequencing and the future of genomic medicine. Genes (Basel). 2010;1(1):38–69.

59. Tucker T, Marra M, Friedman JM. Massively parallel sequencing: the next big thing in genetic medicine. Am J Hum Genet. 2009;85(2):142–54.

60. Kukurba KR, Montgomery SB. RNA sequencing and analysis. Cold Spring Harb Protoc. 2015;2015(11):951–69.

61. Garcia EP, Minkovsky A, Jia Y, Ducar MD, Shivdasani P, Gong X, et al. Validation of OncoPanel: a targeted next-generation sequencing assay for the detection of somatic variants in cancer. Arch Pathol Lab Med. 2017;141(6):751–8.

62. Marchetti A, Del Grammastro M, Filice G, Felicioni L, Rossi G, Graziano P, et al. Complex mutations & subpopulations of deletions at exon 19 of EGFR in NSCLC revealed by next generation sequencing: potential clinical implications. PLoS One. 2012;7(7):e42164.

63. Best MG, Sol N, Kooi I, Tannous J, Westerman BA, Rustenburg F, et al. RNA-seq of tumor-educated platelets enables blood-based pan-cancer, multiclass, and molecular pathway cancer diagnostics. Cancer Cell. 2015;28(5):666–76.

64. Bischoff R, Permentier H, Guryev V, Horvatovich P. Genomic variability and protein species—improving sequence coverage for proteogenomics. J Proteomics. 2016;134:25–36.

65. Baker H, Patel V, Molinolo AA, Shillitoe EJ, Ensley JF, Yoo GH, et al. Proteome-wide analysis of head and neck squamous cell carcinomas using laser-capture microdissection and tandem mass spectrometry. Oral Oncol. 2005;41(2):183–99.

66. Liu AY, Zhang H, Sorensen CM, Diamond DL. Analysis of prostate cancer by proteomics using tissue specimens. J Urol. 2005;173(1):73–8.

67. Seccia V, Navari E, Donadio E, Boldrini C, Ciregia F, Ronci M, et al. Proteomic investigation of malignant major salivary gland tumors. Head Neck Pathol. 2020;14(2):362–73.

68. Mehta S, Zhang J. Liquid–liquid phase separation drives cellular function and dysfunction in cancer. Nat Rev Cancer. 2022;22(4):239–52.

69. Tong X, Tang R, Xu J, Wang W, Zhao Y, Yu X, Shi S. Liquid–liquid phase separation in tumor biology. Signal Trans Targeted Ther. 2022;7(1):221.

70. Shi SR, Liu C, Dalglcy DM, Lee C, Taylor CR. Protein extraction from formalin-fixed, paraffin-embedded tissue sections: quality evaluation by mass spectrometry. J Histochem Cytochem. 2006;54(6):739–43.

71. Murph M, Tanaka T, Pang J, Felix E, Liu S, Trost R, et al. Liquid chromatography mass spectrometry for quantifying plasma lysophospholipids: potential biomarkers for cancer diagnosis. Meth Enzymol. 2007;433:1–25.

72. Giltnane JM, Rimm DL. Technology insight: identification of biomarkers with tissue microarray technology. Nat Clin Pract Oncol. 2004;1(2):104–11.

73. Haab BB. Antibody arrays in cancer research. Mol Cell Proteomics. 2005;4(4):377–83.

74. Kallioniemi O-P, Wagner U, Kononen J, Sauter G. Tissue microarray technology for high-throughput molecular profiling of cancer. Hum Mol Genet. 2001;10(7):657–62.

75. Menschaert G, Fenyö D. Proteogenomics from a bioinformatics angle: a growing field. Mass Spectrometry Rev. 2017;36(5):584–99.

76. Low TY, Mohtar MA, Ang MY, Jamal R. Connecting proteomics to next-generation sequencing: proteogenomics and its current applications in biology. Proteomics. 2019;19(10):1800235.

77. Gustafsson OJ, Arentz G, Hoffmann P. Proteomic developments in the analysis of formalin-fixed tissue. Biochim Biophys Acta. 2015;1854(6):559–80.

78. Addis MF, Tanca A, Pagnozzi D, Crobu S, Fanciulli G, Cossu-Rocca P, Uzzau S. Generation of high-quality protein extracts from formalin-fixed, paraffin-embedded tissues. Proteomics. 2009;9(15):3815–23.

79. Vitorino R, Choudhury M, Guedes S, Ferreira R, Thongboonkerd V, Sharma L, et al. Peptidomics and proteogenomics: background, challenges and future needs. Exp Rev Proteomics. 2021;18(8):643–59.

80. Varma M, Jasani B. Diagnostic utility of immunohistochemistry in morphologically difficult prostate cancer: review of current literature. Histopathology. 2005;47(1):1–16.

81. Zhu S, Schuerch C, Hunt J. Review and updates of immunohistochemistry in selected salivary gland and head and neck tumors. Arch Pathol Lab Med. 2015;139(1):55–66.

82. Marur S, D'Souza G, Westra WH, Forastiere AA. HPV-associated head and neck cancer: a virus-related cancer epidemic. Lancet Oncol. 2010;11(8):781–9.

83. Bailey S, Wallwork B. Differentiating between benign and malignant thyroid nodules: 'An evidence-based approach in general practice'. Aust J Gen Pract. 2018;47(11):770–4.

84. Escobar-Hoyos L, Knorr K, Abdel-Wahab O. Aberrant RNA splicing in cancer. Annu Rev Cancer Biol. 2019;3(1):167–85.

85. Park E, Pan Z, Zhang Z, Lin L, Xing Y. The expanding landscape of alternative splicing variation in human populations. Am J Hum Genet. 2018;102(1):11–26.

86. Belluti S, Rigillo G, Imbriano C. Transcription factors in cancer: when alternative splicing determines opposite cell fates. Cells. 2020;9(3):760.

87. Cusanovich DA, Pavlovic B, Pritchard JK, Gilad Y. The functional consequences of variation in transcription factor binding. PLoS Genet. 2014;10(3):e1004226.

88. Lambert SA, Jolma A, Campitelli LF, Das PK, Yin Y, Albu M, et al. The human transcription factors. Cell. 2018;172(4):650–65.

89. Nebert DW. Transcription factors and cancer: an overview. Toxicology. 2002;181–182:131–41.

90. Maritano D, Sugrue ML, Tininini S, Dewilde S, Strobl B, Fu X, et al. The STAT3 isoforms alpha and beta have unique and specific functions. Nat Immunol. 2004;5(4):401–9.

91. Tang JZ, Kong XJ, Banerjee A, Muniraj N, Pandey V, Steiner M, et al. STAT3alpha is oncogenic for endometrial carcinoma cells and mediates the oncogenic effects of autocrine human growth hormone. Endocrinology. 2010;151(9):4133–45.

92. Schaefer LK, Ren Z, Fuller GN, Schaefer TS. Constitutive activation of Stat3alpha in brain

tumors: localization to tumor endothelial cells and activation by the endothelial tyrosine kinase receptor (VEGFR-2). Oncogene. 2002;21(13):2058–65.

93. Wenzel J, Rose K, Haghighi EB, Lamprecht C, Rauen G, Freihen V, et al. Loss of the nuclear Wnt pathway effector TCF7L2 promotes migration and invasion of human colorectal cancer cells. Oncogene. 2020;39(19):3893–909.

94. Jin T, Liu L. Minireview: the Wnt signaling pathway effector TCF7L2 and type 2 diabetes mellitus. Mol Endocrinol. 2008;22(11):2383–92.

95. Jin T. Current understanding on role of the Wnt signaling pathway effector TCF7L2 in glucose homeostasis. Endocrine Rev. 2016;37(3):254–77.

96. Call KM, Glaser T, Ito CY, Buckler AJ, Pelletier J, Haber DA, et al. Isolation and characterization of a zinc finger polypeptide gene at the human chromosome 11 Wilms' tumor locus. Cell. 1990;60(3):509–20.

97. Silberstein GB, Van Horn K, Strickland P, Roberts CT Jr, Daniel CW. Altered expression of the WT1 wilms tumor suppressor gene in human breast cancer. Proc Natl Acad Sci U S A. 1997;94(15):8132–7.

98. Yang L, Han Y, Saurez Saiz F, Minden M. A tumor suppressor and oncogene: the WT1 story. Leukemia. 2007;21(5):868–76.

99. Levy C, Khaled M, Fisher DE. MITF: master regulator of melanocyte development and melanoma oncogene. Trends Mol Med. 2006;12(9):406–14.

100. Yajima I, Kumasaka MY, Thang ND, Goto Y, Takeda K, Iida M, et al. Molecular network associated with MITF in skin melanoma development and progression. J Skin Cancer 2011;2011.

101. Bismuth K, Maric D, Arnheiter H. MITF and cell proliferation: the role of alternative splice forms. Pigment Cell Res. 2005;18(5):349–59.

102. Rao A, Luo C, Hogan PG. Transcription factors of the NFAT family: regulation and function. Annual Rev Immunol. 1997;15(1):707–47.

103. Mancini M, Toker A. NFAT proteins: emerging roles in cancer progression. Nat Rev Cancer. 2009;9(11):810–20.

104. Tripathi MK, Deane NG, Zhu J, An H, Mima S, Wang X, et al. Nuclear factor of activated T-cell activity is associated with metastatic capacity in colon cancer. Cancer Res. 2014;74(23):6947–57.

105. Flockhart RJ, Armstrong JL, Reynolds NJ, Lovat PE. NFAT signalling is a novel target of oncogenic BRAF in metastatic melanoma. Br J Cancer. 2009;101(8):1448–55.

106. Qin JJ, Nag S, Wang W, Zhou J, Zhang WD, Wang H, Zhang R. NFAT as cancer target: mission possible? Biochim Biophys Acta. 2014;1846(2):297–311.

107. Narla G, Heath KE, Reeves HL, Li D, Giono LE, Kimmelman AC, et al. KLF6, a candidate tumor suppressor gene mutated in prostate cancer. Science. 2001;294(5551):2563–6.

108. Teixeira MS, Camacho-Vanegas O, Fernandez Y, Narla G, DiFeo A, Lee B, et al. KLF6 allelic loss is associated with tumor recurrence and markedly decreased survival in head and neck squamous cell carcinoma. Int J Cancer. 2007;121(9):1976–83.

109. DiFeo A, Narla G, Hirshfeld J, Camacho-Vanegas O, Narla J, Rose SL, et al. Roles of KLF6 and KLF6-SV1 in ovarian cancer progression and intraperitoneal dissemination. Clin Cancer Res. 2006;12(12):3730–9.

110. DiFeo A, Feld L, Rodriguez F, Wang C, Beer DG, Martignetti JA, Narla G. A functional role for KLF6-SV1 in lung adenocarcinoma prognosis and chemotherapy response. Cancer Research. 2008;68(4):965–70.

111. DiFeo A, Martignetti JA, Narla G. The role of KLF6 and its splice variants in cancer therapy. Drug Resistance Updates. 2009;12(1–2):1–7.

112. Lau SK, Luthringer DJ, Eisen RN. Thyroid transcription factor-1: a review. Appl Immunohistochem Mol Morphol. 2002;10(2):97–102.

113. Bingle CD. Thyroid transcription factor-1. Int J Biochem Cell Biol. 1997;29(12):1471–3.

114. Bejarano PA, Nikiforov YE, Swenson ES, Biddinger PW. Thyroid transcription factor-1, thyroglobulin, cytokeratin 7, and cytokeratin 20 in thyroid neoplasms. Appl Immunohistochem Mol Morphol. 2000;8(3):189–94.

115. Miettinen M, Franssila KO. Variable expression of keratins and nearly uniform lack of thyroid transcription factor 1 in thyroid anaplastic carcinoma. Hum Pathol. 2000;31(9):1139–45.

116. Eccles MR, Yun K, Reeve AE, Fidler AE. Comparative in situ hybridization analysis of PAX2, PAX8, and WT1 gene transcription in human fetal kidney and Wilms' tumors. Am J Pathol. 1995;146(1):40–5.

117. Bharti B, Shukla S, Tripathi R, Mishra S, Kumar M, Pandey M, Mishra R. Level of PAX5 in differential diagnosis of non-Hodgkin's lymphoma. Indian J Med Res. 2016;143(Supplement):S23–31.

118. Stuart ET, Kioussi C, Aguzzi A, Gruss P. PAX5 expression correlates with increasing malignancy in human astrocytomas. Clin Cancer Res. 1995;1(2):207–14.

119. Kozmik Z, Sure U, Ruedi D, Busslinger M, Aguzzi A. Deregulated expression of PAX5 in medulloblastoma. Proc Natl Acad Sci U S A. 1995;92(12):5709–13.

120. Iida S, Rao PH, Nallasivam P, Hibshoosh H, Butler M, Louie DC, et al. The t(9;14)(p13;q32) chromosomal translocation associated with lymphoplasmacytoid lymphoma involves the PAX-5 gene. Blood. 1996;88(11):4110–7.

121. Busslinger M, Klix N, Pfeffer P, Graninger PG, Kozmik Z. Deregulation of PAX-5 by translocation of the Emu enhancer of the IgH locus adjacent to two alternative PAX-5 promoters in a diffuse large-cell lymphoma. Proc Natl Acad Sci U S A. 1996;93(12):6129–34.

122. Kelly KM, Womer RB, Sorensen PH, Xiong QB, Barr FG. Common and variant gene fusions predict distinct clinical phenotypes in rhabdomyosarcoma. J Clin Oncol. 1997;15(5):1831–6.

123. Davis RJ, Barr FG. Fusion genes resulting from alternative chromosomal translocations are over-expressed by gene-specific mechanisms in alveolar rhabdomyosarcoma. Proc Natl Acad Sci U S A. 1997;94(15):8047–51.

124. Grimm D, Bauer J, Wise P, Kruger M, Simonsen U, Wehland M, et al. The role of SOX family members in solid tumours and metastasis. Semin Cancer Biol. 2020;67(Pt 1):122–53.

125. Castillo SD, Sanchez-Cespedes M. The SOX family of genes in cancer development: biological relevance and opportunities for therapy. Exp Opin Ther Targets. 2012;16(9):903–19.

126. Kuo C-Y, Hsu Y-C, Liu C-L, Li Y-S, Chang S-C, Cheng S-P. SOX4 is a pivotal regulator of tumorigenesis in differentiated thyroid cancer. Mol Cell Endocrinol. 2023;578:112062.

127. Tang H, Chen B, Liu P, Xie X, He R, Zhang L, et al. SOX8 acts as a prognostic factor and mediator to regulate the progression of triple-negative breast cancer. Carcinogenesis. 2019;40(10):1278–87.

128. Zhang S, Zhu C, Zhu L, Liu H, Liu S, Zhao N, et al. Oncogenicity of the transcription factor SOX8 in hepatocellular carcinoma. Med Oncol. 2014;31(4):918.

129. Lefebvre V, Li P, de Crombrugghe B. A new long form of Sox5 (L-Sox5), Sox6 and Sox9 are coexpressed in chondrogenesis and cooperatively activate the type II collagen gene. EMBO J. 1998;17(19):5718–33.

130. Fan Y, Li Y, Yao X, Jin J, Scott A, Liu B, et al. Epithelial SOX9 drives progression and metastases of gastric adenocarcinoma by promoting immunosuppressive tumour microenvironment. Gut. 2023;72(4):624–37.

131. Ohtomo R, Mori T, Shibata S, Tsuta K, Maeshima AM, Akazawa C, et al. SOX10 is a novel marker of acinus and intercalated duct differentiation in salivary gland tumors: a clue to the histogenesis for tumor diagnosis. Mod Pathol. 2013;26(8):1041–50.

132. Ivanov SV, Panaccione A, Nonaka D, Prasad ML, Boyd KL, Brown B, et al. Diagnostic SOX10 gene signatures in salivary adenoid cystic and breast basal-like carcinomas. Br J Cancer. 2013;109(2):444–51.

133. Miettinen M, McCue PA, Sarlomo-Rikala M, Biernat W, Czapiewski P, Kopczynski J, et al. Sox10—a marker for not only schwannian and melanocytic neoplasms but also myoepithelial cell tumors of soft tissue: a systematic analysis of 5134 tumors. Am J Surg Pathol. 2015;39(6):826–35.

134. Psilopatis I, Schaefer JI, Arsenakis D, Bolovis D, Levidou G. SOX11 and epithelial- mesenchymal transition in metastatic serous ovarian cancer. Biomedicines. 2023;11(9):2540.

135. Kuo IY, Wu CC, Chang JM, Huang YL, Lin CH, Yan JJ, et al. Low SOX17 expression is a prognostic factor and drives transcriptional dysregulation and esophageal cancer progression. Int J Cancer. 2014;135(3):563–73.

136. Edwards PA. Fusion genes and chromosome translocations in the common epithelial cancers. J Pathol. 2010;220(2):244–54.

137. Mertens F, Johansson B, Fioretos T, Mitelman F. The emerging complexity of gene fusions in cancer. Nat Rev Cancer. 2015;15(6):371–81.

138. Perry JA, Seong BKA, Stegmaier K. Biology and therapy of dominant fusion oncoproteins involving transcription factor and chromatin regulators in sarcomas. Annual Rev Cancer Biol. 2019;3:299–321.

139. Micheau C, Klijanienko J, Luboinski B, Richard J. So-called branchiogenic carcinoma is actually cystic metastases in the neck from a tonsillar primary. Laryngoscope. 1990;100(8):878–83.

140. Regauer S, Mannweiler S, Anderhuber W, Gotschuli A, Berghold A, Schachenreiter J, et al. Cystic lymph node metastases of squamous cell carcinoma of Waldeyer's ring origin. Br J Cancer. 1999;79(9–10):1437–42.

141. Thompson LD, Heffner DK. The clinical importance of cystic squamous cell carcinomas in the neck: a study of 136 cases. Cancer. 1998;82(5):944–56.

142. Haskell CM, Cochran AJ, Barsky SH, Steckel RJ. Metastasis of unknown origin. Curr Probl Cancer. 1988;12(1):5–58.

143. Califano J, Westra WH, Koch W, Meininger G, Reed A, Yip L, et al. Unknown primary head and neck squamous cell carcinoma: molecular identification of the site of origin. J Natl Cancer Inst. 1999;91(7):599–604.

144. Issing WJ, Taleban B, Tauber S. Diagnosis and management of carcinoma of unknown primary in the head and neck. Eur Arch Otorhinolaryngol. 2003;260(8):436–43.

145. Keller LM, Galloway TJ, Holdbrook T, Ruth K, Yang D, Dubyk C, et al. p16 status, pathologic and clinical characteristics, biomolecular signature, and long-term outcomes in head and neck squamous cell carcinomas of unknown primary. Head Neck. 2014;36(12):1677–84.

146. Batsakis JG, Bautina E. Metastases to major salivary glands. Ann Otol Rhinol Laryngol. 1990;99(6 Pt 1):501–3.

147. Tracy JC, Mildenhall NR, Wein RO, O'Leary MA. Breast cancer metastases to the head and neck: case series and literature review. Ear Nose Throat J. 2017;96(3):E21–E4.

148. Howlett DC, Skelton E, Moody AB. Establishing an accurate diagnosis of a parotid lump: evaluation of the current biopsy methods—fine needle aspiration cytology, ultrasound-guided core biopsy, and intraoperative frozen section. Br J Oral Maxillofac Surg. 2015;53(7):580–3.

149. Burke C, Thomas R, Inglis C, Baldwin A, Ramesar K, Grace R, Howlett DC. Ultrasound- guided core biopsy in the diagnosis of lymphoma of the head and neck. A 9 year experience. Br J Radiol. 2011;84(1004):727–32.

150. Zuur CL, van Velthuysen ML, Schornagel JH, Hilgers FJ, Balm AJ. Diagnosis and treatment of isolated neck metastases of adenocarcinomas. Eur J Surg Oncol. 2002;28(2):147–52.

151. Sahlin P, Mark J, Stenman G. Submicroscopic deletions of 3p sequences in pleomorphic adenomas with t(3;8)(p21;q12). Genes Chromosomes Cancer. 1994;10(4):256–61.

152. Kas K, Voz ML, Roijer E, Astrom AK, Meyen E, Stenman G, Van de Ven WJ. Promoter swapping between the genes for a novel zinc finger protein and beta-catenin in pleiomorphic adenomas with t(3;8)(p21;q12) translocations. Nat Genet. 1997;15(2):170–4.

153. Goonewardene SA, Nasuti JF. Value of mucin detection in distinguishing mucoepidermoid carcinoma from Warthin's tumor on fine needle aspiration. Acta Cytol. 2002;46(4):704–8.

154. El-Naggar A, Batsakis J, Luna M, Goepfert H, Tortoledo M. DNA content and proliferative activity of myoepitheliomas. J Laryngology Otology. 1989;103(12):1192–7.

155. Batsakis JG, el-Naggar AK. Myoepithelium in salivary and mammary neoplasms is host- friendly. Adv Anat Pathol. 1999;6(4):218–26.

156. Hasegawa M, Hagiwara S, Sato T, Jijiwa M, Murakumo Y, Maeda M, et al. CD109, a new marker for myoepithelial cells of mammary, salivary, and lacrimal glands and prostate basal cells. Pathol Int. 2007;57(5):245–50.

157. Tonon G, Modi S, Wu L, Kubo A, Coxon AB, Komiya T, et al. t(11;19)(q21;p13) translocation in mucoepidermoid carcinoma creates a novel fusion product that disrupts a Notch signaling pathway. Nat Genet. 2003;33(2):208–13.

158. Saade RE, Bell D, Garcia J, Roberts D, Weber R. Role of CRTC1/MAML2 translocation in the prognosis and clinical outcomes of mucoepidermoid carcinoma. JAMA Otolaryngol Head Neck Surg. 2016;142(3):234–40.

159. Bell D, Luna MA, Weber RS, Kaye FJ, El-Naggar AK. CRTC1/MAML2 fusion transcript in Warthin's tumor and mucoepidermoid carcinoma: evidence for a common genetic association. Genes Chromosomes Cancer. 2008;47(4):309–14.

160. Mitani Y, Rao PH, Maity SN, Lee YC, Ferrarotto R, Post JC, et al. Alterations associated with androgen receptor gene activation in salivary duct carcinoma of both sexes: potential therapeutic ramifications. Clin Cancer Res. 2014;20(24):6570–81.

161. Williams MD, Roberts D, Blumenschein GR Jr, Temam S, Kies MS, Rosenthal DI, et al. Differential expression of hormonal and growth factor receptors in salivary duct carcinomas: biologic significance and potential role in therapeutic stratification of patients. Am J Surg Pathol. 2007;31(11): 1645–52.

162. Williams MD, Roberts DB, Kies MS, Mao L, Weber RS, El-Naggar AK. Genetic and expression analysis of HER-2 and EGFR genes in salivary duct carci-

noma: empirical and therapeutic significance. Clin Cancer Res. 2010;16(8):2266–74.

163. Persson M, Andren Y, Mark J, Horlings HM, Persson F, Stenman G. Recurrent fusion of MYB and NFIB transcription factor genes in carcinomas of the breast and head and neck. Proc Natl Acad Sci U S A. 2009;106(44):18740–4.

164. Mitani Y, Liu B, Rao PH, Borra VJ, Zafereo M, Weber RS, et al. Novel MYBL1 gene rearrangements with recurrent MYBL1-NFIB fusions in salivary adenoid cystic carcinomas lacking t(6;9) translocations. Clin Cancer Res. 2016;22(3):725–33.

165. Brayer KJ, Frerich CA, Kang H, Ness SA. Recurrent fusions in MYB and MYBL1 define a common, transcription factor-driven oncogenic pathway in salivary gland adenoid cystic carcinoma. Cancer Discov. 2016;6(2):176–87.

166. Ferrarotto R, Mitani Y, Diao L, Guijarro I, Wang J, Zweidler-McKay P, et al. Activating NOTCH1 mutations define a distinct subgroup of patients with adenoid cystic carcinoma who have poor prognosis, propensity to bone and liver metastasis, and potential responsiveness to notch1 inhibitors. J Clin Oncol. 2017;35(3):352–60.

167. Ho AS, Ochoa A, Jayakumaran G, Zehir A, Valero Mayor C, Tepe J, et al. Genetic hallmarks of recurrent/metastatic adenoid cystic carcinoma. J Clin Invest. 2019;129(10):4276–89.

168. Batsakis JG, Regezi JA, Luna MA, el-Naggar A. Histogenesis of salivary gland neoplasms: a postulate with prognostic implications. J Laryngol Otol. 1989;103(10):939–44.

169. Skalova A, Sima R, Vanecek T, Muller S, Korabecna M, Nemcova J, et al. Acinic cell carcinoma with high-grade transformation: a report of 9 cases with immunohistochemical study and analysis of TP53 and HER-2/neu genes. Am J Surg Pathol. 2009;33(8):1137–45.

170. Haller F, Bieg M, Will R, Korner C, Weichenhan D, Bott A, et al. Enhancer hijacking activates oncogenic transcription factor NR4A3 in acinic cell carcinomas of the salivary glands. Nat Commun. 2019;10(1):368.

171. Lee DY, Brayer KJ, Mitani Y, Burns EA, Rao PH, Bell D, et al. Oncogenic orphan nuclear receptor NR4A3 interacts and cooperates with MYB in acinic cell carcinoma. Cancers (Basel). 2020;12(9):2433.

172. Wong KS, Marino-Enriquez A, Hornick JL, Jo VY. NR4A3 immunohistochemistry reliably discriminates acinic cell carcinoma from mimics. Head Neck Pathol. 2021;15(2):425–32.

173. Skalova A, Vanecek T, Sima R, Laco J, Weinreb I, Perez-Ordonez B, et al. Mammary analogue secretory carcinoma of salivary glands, containing the ETV6-NTRK3 fusion gene: a hitherto undescribed salivary gland tumor entity. Am J Surg Pathol. 2010;34(5):599–608.

174. Balanza R, Arrangoiz R, Cordera F, Munoz M, Luque-de-Leon E, Moreno E, et al. Mammary analog secretory carcinoma of the parotid gland: a case

report and literature review. Int J Surg Case Rep. 2015;16:187–91.

175. Guilmette J, Dias-Santagata D, Nose V, Lennerz JK, Sadow PM. Novel gene fusions in secretory carcinoma of the salivary glands: enlarging the ETV6 family. Hum Pathol. 2019;83:50–8.

176. Batsakis JG, Luna MA, el-Naggar AK. Basaloid monomorphic adenomas. Ann Otol Rhinol Laryngol. 1991;100(8):687–90.

177. Batsakis JG, Luna MA. Basaloid salivary carcinoma. Ann Otol Rhinol Laryngol. 1991;100(9 Pt 1):785–7.

178. Jo VY, Sholl LM, Krane JF. Distinctive patterns of CTNNB1 (beta-Catenin) alterations in salivary gland basal cell adenoma and basal cell adenocarcinoma. Am J Surg Pathol. 2016;40(8):1143–50.

179. Wilson TC, Ma D, Tilak A, Tesdahl B, Robinson RA. Next-generation sequencing in salivary gland basal cell adenocarcinoma and basal cell adenoma. Head Neck Pathol. 2016;10(4):494–500.

180. Rito M, Mitani Y, Bell D, Mariano FV, Almalki ST, Pytynia KB, et al. Frequent and differential mutations of the CYLD gene in basal cell salivary neoplasms: linkage to tumor development and progression. Mod Pathol. 2018;31(7):1064–72.

181. Choi HR, Batsakis JG, Callender DL, Prieto VG, Luna MA, El-Naggar AK. Molecular analysis of chromosome 16q regions in dermal analogue tumors of salivary glands: a genetic link to dermal cylindroma? Am J Surg Pathol. 2002;26(6):778–83.

182. Bertolini F, Bianchi B, Pizzigallo A, Tullio A, Sesenna E. Synovial cell sarcoma of the neck. Case report and review of the literature. Acta Otorhinolaryngol Ital. 2003;23(5):391–5.

183. Coindre JM, Pelmus M, Hostein I, Lussan C, Bui BN, Guillou L. Should molecular testing be required for diagnosing synovial sarcoma? A prospective study of 204 cases. Cancer. 2003;98(12):2700–7.

184. Coffin CM, Swanson PE, Wick MR, Dehner LP. An immunohistochemical comparison of chordoma with renal cell carcinoma, colorectal adenocarcinoma, and myxopapillary ependymoma: a potential diagnostic dilemma in the diminutive biopsy. Mod Pathol. 1993;6(5):531–8.

185. Yamaguchi T, Suzuki S, Ishiiwa H, Shimizu K, Ueda Y. Benign notochordal cell tumors: a comparative histological study of benign notochordal cell tumors, classic chordomas, and notochordal vestiges of fetal intervertebral discs. Am J Surg Pathol. 2004;28(6):756–61.

186. Tallini G, Dorfman H, Brys P, Dal Cin P, De Wever I, Fletcher CD, et al. Correlation between clinicopathological features and karyotype in 100 cartilaginous and chordoid tumours. A report from the Chromosomes and Morphology (CHAMP) Collaborative Study Group. J Pathol. 2002;196(2):194–203.

187. Wieneke JA, Smith A. Paraganglioma: carotid body tumor. Head Neck Pathol. 2009;3:303–6.

188. Luna-Ortiz K, Rascon-Ortiz M, Villavicencio-Valencia V, Granados-Garcia M, Herrera-

GA. Carotid body tumors: review of a 20-year experience. Oral oncology. 2005;41(1):56–61.

189. Lee SM, Policarpio-Nicolas MLC. Thyroid paraganglioma. Arch Pathol Lab Med. 2015;139(8):1062–7.

190. Castro MR, Gharib H. Thyroid nodules and cancer. When to wait and watch, when to refer. Postgrad Med. 2000;107(1):113–6, 9–20, 23–4.

191. Sclabas GM, Staerkel GA, Shapiro SE, Fornage BD, Sherman SI, Vassillopoulou-Sellin R, et al. Fine-needle aspiration of the thyroid and correlation with histopathology in a contemporary series of 240 patients. Am J Surg. 2003;186(6):702–9; discussion 9–10.

192. Xing M. Molecular pathogenesis and mechanisms of thyroid cancer. Nat Rev Cancer. 2013;13(3):184–99.

193. Santarpia L, Myers JN, Sherman SI, Trimarchi F, Clayman GL, El-Naggar AK. Genetic alterations in the RAS/RAF/mitogen-activated protein kinase and phosphatidylinositol 3- kinase/Akt signaling pathways in the follicular variant of papillary thyroid carcinoma. Cancer. 2010;116(12): 2974–83.

194. Santarpia L, Sherman SI, Marabotti A, Clayman GL, El-Naggar AK. Detection and molecular characterization of a novel BRAF activated domain mutation in follicular variant of papillary thyroid carcinoma. Hum Pathol. 2009;40(6):827–33.

195. Cohen Y, Xing M, Mambo E, Guo Z, Wu G, Trink B, et al. BRAF mutation in papillary thyroid carcinoma. J Natl Cancer Inst. 2003;95(8):625–7.

196. Xing M, Westra WH, Tufano RP, Cohen Y, Rosenbaum E, Rhoden KJ, et al. BRAF mutation predicts a poorer clinical prognosis for papillary thyroid cancer. J Clin Endocrinol Metab. 2005;90(12):6373–9.

197. Nikiforova MN, Nikiforov YE. Molecular genetics of thyroid cancer: implications for diagnosis, treatment and prognosis. Expert Rev Mol Diagn. 2008;8(1):83–95.

198. Kimura ET, Nikiforova MN, Zhu Z, Knauf JA, Nikiforov YE, Fagin JA. High prevalence of BRAF mutations in thyroid cancer: genetic evidence for constitutive activation of the RET/PTC-RAS-BRAF signaling pathway in papillary thyroid carcinoma. Cancer Res. 2003;63(7):1454–7.

199. Soares P, Trovisco V, Rocha AS, Lima J, Castro P, Preto A, et al. BRAF mutations and RET/PTC rearrangements are alternative events in the etiopathogenesis of PTC. Oncogene. 2003;22(29): 4578–80.

200. Sobrinho-Simoes M, Eloy C, Magalhaes J, Lobo C, Amaro T. Follicular thyroid carcinoma. Mod Pathol. 2011;24:S10–S8.

201. Haugen BR, Sawka AM, Alexander EK, Bible KC, Cetin AM, Doherty GM, et al. American Thyroid Association guidelines on the management of thyroid nodules and differentiated thyroid cancer task force review and recommendation on the proposed renaming of encapsulated follicular variant papillary thyroid carcinoma without invasion to noninva-

sive follicular thyroid neoplasm with papillary-like nuclear features. Thyroid. 2017;27(4):481–3.

202. Esapa CT, Johnson SJ, Kendall-Taylor P, Lennard TW, Harris PE. Prevalence of Ras mutations in thyroid neoplasia. Clin Endocrinol (Oxf). 1999;50(4):529–35.

203. Motoi N, Sakamoto A, Yamochi T, Horiuchi H, Motoi T, Machinami R. Role of ras mutation in the progression of thyroid carcinoma of follicular epithelial origin. Pathol Res Pract. 2000;196(1):1–7.

204. Nikiforova MN, Lynch RA, Biddinger PW, Alexander EK, Dorn GW 2nd, Tallini G, et al. RAS point mutations and PAX8-PPAR gamma rearrangement in thyroid tumors: evidence for distinct molecular pathways in thyroid follicular carcinoma. J Clin Endocrinol Metab. 2003;88(5):2318–26.

205. Marques AR, Espadinha C, Catarino AL, Moniz S, Pereira T, Sobrinho LG, Leite V. Expression of PAX8-PPAR gamma 1 rearrangements in both follicular thyroid carcinomas and adenomas. J Clin Endocrinol Metab. 2002;87(8):3947–52.

206. Volante M, Collini P, Nikiforov YE, Sakamoto A, Kakudo K, Katoh R, et al. Poorly differentiated thyroid carcinoma: the Turin proposal for the use of uniform diagnostic criteria and an algorithmic diagnostic approach. Am J Surg Pathol. 2007;31(8):1256–64.

207. Besic N, Hocevar M, Zgajnar J, Pogacnik A, Grazio-Frkovic S, Auersperg M. Prognostic factors in anaplastic carcinoma of the thyroid-a multivariate survival analysis of 188 patients. Langenbecks Arch Surg. 2005;390(3):203–8.

208. Brignardello E, Gallo M, Baldi I, Palestini N, Piovesan A, Grossi E, et al. Anaplastic thyroid carcinoma: clinical outcome of 30 consecutive patients referred to a single institution in the past 5 years. Eur J Endocrinol. 2007;156(4):425–30.

209. Elliott DD, Sherman SI, Busaidy NL, Williams MD, Santarpia L, Clayman GL, El- Naggar AK. Growth factor receptors expression in anaplastic thyroid carcinoma: potential markers for therapeutic stratification. Hum Pathol. 2008;39(1):15–20.

210. Smallridge RC, Marlow LA, Copland JA. Anaplastic thyroid cancer: molecular pathogenesis and emerging therapies. Endocr Relat Cancer. 2009;16(1):17–44.

211. Nikiforov YE. Genetic alterations involved in the transition from well-differentiated to poorly differentiated and anaplastic thyroid carcinomas. Endocr Pathol. 2004;15(4):319–27.

212. Boltze C, Roessner A, Landt O, Szibor R, Peters B, Schneider-Stock R. Homozygous proline at codon 72 of p53 as a potential risk factor favoring the development of undifferentiated thyroid carcinoma. Int J Oncol. 2002;21(5):1151–4.

213. Garcia-Rostan G, Zhao H, Camp RL, Pollan M, Herrero A, Pardo J, et al. ras mutations are associated with aggressive tumor phenotypes and poor prognosis in thyroid cancer. J Clin Oncol. 2003;21(17):3226–35.

214. Quiros RM, Ding HG, Gattuso P, Prinz RA, Xu X. Evidence that one subset of anaplastic thyroid carcinomas are derived from papillary carcinomas due to BRAF and p53 mutations. Cancer. 2005;103(11):2261–8.

215. Rao AS, Kremenevskaja N, von Wasielewski R, Jakubcakova V, Kant S, Resch J, Brabant G. Wnt/beta-catenin signaling mediates antineoplastic effects of imatinib mesylate (gleevec) in anaplastic thyroid cancer. J Clin Endocrinol Metab. 2006;91(1):159–68.

216. Garcia-Rostan G, Costa AM, Pereira-Castro I, Salvatore G, Hernandez R, Hermsem MJ, et al. Mutation of the PIK3CA gene in anaplastic thyroid cancer. Cancer Res. 2005;65(22):10199–207.

217. Kouvaraki MA, Shapiro SE, Perrier ND, Cote GJ, Gagel RF, Hoff AO, et al. RET proto- oncogene: a review and update of genotype–phenotype correlations in hereditary medullary thyroid cancer and associated endocrine tumors. Thyroid. 2005;15(6):531–44.

218. Drosten M, Pützer BM. Mechanisms of disease: cancer targeting and the impact of oncogenic RET for medullary thyroid carcinoma therapy. Nat Clin Pract Oncol. 2006;3(10):564–74.

219. Ali S. Cibas eS The Bethesda system for reporting thyroid cytopathology. New York: Springer; 2010.

220. Bellevicine C, Ciarrocchi A, Friedlaender A, Malapelle U, de Biase D. Editorial: molecular characterization of thyroid lesions in the era of "Next-Generation" techniques. Front Endocrinol (Lausanne). 2022;13:955185.

221. Patel J, Klopper J, Cottrill EE. Molecular diagnostics in the evaluation of thyroid nodules: current use and prospective opportunities. Front Endocrinol (Lausanne). 2023;14:1101410.

222. LaGuette J, Matias-Guiu X, Rosai J. Thyroid paraganglioma: a clinicopathologic and immunohistochemical study of three cases. Am J Surg Pathol. 1997;21(7):748–53.

223. Ferri E, Manconi R, Armato E, Ianniello F. Primary paraganglioma of thyroid gland: a clinicopathologic and immunohistochemical study with review of the literature. Acta Otorhinolaryngol Ital. 2009;29(2):97–102.

224. Gonzalez Poggioli N, Lopez Amado M, Pimentel MT. Paraganglioma of the thyroid gland: a rare entity. Endocr Pathol. 2009;20(1):62–5.

225. Grajower MM. Malignant paraganglioma of thyroid. Endocr Pract. 2006;12(6):696–7.

226. Castelblanco E, Gallel P, Ros S, Gatius S, Valls J, De-Cubas AA, et al. Thyroid paraganglioma. Report of 3 cases and description of an immunohistochemical profile useful in the differential diagnosis with medullary thyroid carcinoma, based on

complementary DNA array results. Hum Pathol. 2012;43(7):1103–12.

227. Papi G, Fadda G, Corsello SM, Corrado S, Rossi ED, Radighieri E, et al. Metastases to the thyroid gland: prevalence, clinicopathological aspects and prognosis: a 10-year experience. Clin Endocrinol (Oxf). 2007;66(4):565–71.

228. Chung AY, Tran TB, Brumund KT, Weisman RA, Bouvet M. Metastases to the thyroid: a review of the literature from the last decade. Thyroid. 2012;22(3):258–68.

229. Morrison C, Farrar W, Kneile J, Williams N, Liu-Stratton Y, Bakaletz A, et al. Molecular classification of parathyroid neoplasia by gene expression profiling. Am J Pathol. 2004;165(2):565–76.

230. Juhlin CC, Villablanca A, Sandelin K, Haglund F, Nordenstrom J, Forsberg L, et al. Parafibromin immunoreactivity: its use as an additional diagnostic marker for parathyroid tumor classification. Endocr Relat Cancer. 2007;14(2):501–12.

231. Cetani F, Ambrogini E, Faviana P, Vitti P, Berti P, Pinchera A, Marcocci C. Spontaneous short-term remission of primary hyperparathyroidism from infarction of a parathyroid adenoma. J Endocrinol Invest. 2004;27(7):687–90.

232. Cetani F, Ambrogini E, Viacava P, Pardi E, Fanelli G, Naccarato AG, et al. Should parafibromin staining replace HRTP2 gene analysis as an additional tool for histologic diagnosis of parathyroid carcinoma? Eur J Endocrinol. 2007;156(5):547–54.

Adel K. El-Naggar is the Professor of pathology and Director of the Head and Neck Pathology Section and the Subspecialty Head and Neck Fellowship Training Program at MD Anderson Cancer Center, Houston, TX, USA. He has authored and co-authored more than 600 peer-reviewed publications. He is the lead editor of the WHO tumor classification of the head and neck area.

Lester J. Layfield

10.1 Introduction

The head and neck is a complex area with a combination of anatomic sites, tissue types, and a variety of lesions each presenting significant challenges for their pathological diagnosis. The proper neck contains structures predominately represented by lymph nodes and also includes benign cysts and primary neoplasms [1]. Salivary gland tissue is found not only within the major salivary glands but also within widely distributed minor salivary glands. Salivary gland neoplasms present a wide range of morphological appearances associated with significant differences in therapeutic approach for benign neoplasms, low-grade malignancies, and high-grade malignancies. Preoperative distinction of benign from malignant neoplasms is necessary for appropriate therapy. The thyroid gland demonstrates clinically and radiographically a wide variety of nodules variably representing hyperplastic processes (nodular goiter), adenomas, and a variety of malignancies [2]. Preoperative evaluation is necessary to direct the extent of surgery performed if any is necessary. While generally uncommon, lesions within the base of the skull present diagnostic challenges due to their deep-seated loca-

L. J. Layfield (✉)
Department of Pathology and Anatomical Sciences,
Columbia, MO, USA

tion and difficulty in adequate sampling for morphological diagnosis. Finally, many head and neck lesions present as mucosal abnormalities occurring over a wide area and extending from the subglottic region to the nasopharynx, nasal sinuses, and oral cavity. With a few exceptions, these mucosal lesions are best investigated by direct grasp excisional or incisional biopsy.

Techniques for investigation of abnormalities of the head and neck include fine-needle aspiration (FNA) [3–14], core needle biopsy, and frozen section study of tissues obtained at the time of open biopsy. Frozen section is generally performed to determine the extent of the subsequent resection [15]. This review discusses the biopsy techniques available for each anatomical site and compares the characteristics of each technique including its diagnostic accuracy, potential hazards, and limitations to other techniques currently and historically used for investigation of lesions occurring in the head and neck.

10.2 Biopsy of Lesions of the Neck

Abnormalities of the cervical region often requiring tissue analysis for diagnosis include lymphadenopathy of infectious, reactive, or neoplastic etiology, developmental and acquired cystic lesions, and a small number of primary neoplasms. Primary neoplasms of the neck include carotid body tumors, lipomas, synovial sarcomas, and nerve sheath tumors. Carotid body tumors may undergo FNA but generally are excised following characterization of their vascular nature and precise location by imagining studies.

sensitivity of 100% and a specificity of 98.6% [19]. Because open biopsy of cervical lymph nodes is associated with a relatively high cost and some patient morbidity, alternate techniques have been utilized including core needle biopsy and FNA cytology.

10.3 Biopsy Techniques for Cervical Lymphadenopathy

Cervical lymphadenopathy has a variety of etiologies including reactive lymphadenopathy of unknown etiology, infectious agents including tuberculosis, Kikuchi's disease, lymphoma, and metastases [16]. Biopsy of cervical lymph nodes is not without hazard. Excisional biopsy of lymph nodes must be carefully planned with appropriate positioning of the incision. Recently, intraoperative sentinel lymph node biopsy has gained popularity for the evaluation of potential nodal metastases not only for melanoma but also for squamous cell carcinomas arising in the head and neck region [17, 18]. Frozen section evaluation of sentinel lymph nodes shows good diagnostic accuracy but the false-negative rate has been reported to be as high as 7.9% [17, 18]. Similar accuracy has been found for frozen section evaluation of nonsentinel lymph nodes with suspected metastatic disease, where the frozen section accuracy has been reported to be 98.9% with a

10.4 Core Needle Biopsy for Suspected Metastatic Disease

Core needle biopsy of cervical lymphadenopathy has been de-empathized in relationship to FNA because of concerns over patient discomfort and potential local complications including bleeding and needle tract tumor cell implantation. Despite these concerns, core needle biopsy of cervical lymph nodes has been performed at a number of institutions. Reported studies have demonstrated good diagnostic accuracy at times exceeding that achievable with FNA [3, 4]. In comparison to FNA, core needle biopsy has demonstrated a considerably lower nondefinitive diagnosis rate (5% for core needle biopsy and as high as 52% for FNA) [20, 21]. Diagnostic accuracy of core biopsy as judged by agreement with final histopathological diagnosis has varied from 86.9% to 100% [20–25]. Table 10.1 lists the reported diagnostic accuracies for core needle biopsy of cervical lymphadenopathy due to metastatic squamous cell carcinoma.

Table 10.1 Accuracy of core needle biopsy for diagnosis of cervical lymphadenopathy as reported in the literature

Author	# Cases	Sensitivity	Specificity	Accuracy[a]
Kim [16]	155	100%	100%	94%
Saha [20]	48	NR[+]	NR[+]	97%
Han [22]	6695	99.7%	100%	99.5%
Lo [23]	260	84.5%	100%	86.9%
Oh [24]	79	91.6%	100%	98.6%

NR[+] not reported

[a]Accuracy for separation of benign from malignant

10.5 Core Needle Biopsy for Infectious Disease

Not all cases of cervical lymphadenopathy are due to metastatic disease, and a number of infectious etiologies have been successfully investigated by core needle biopsy including tuberculous lymphadenitis [26] and toxoplasmosis [27]. In a series of 55 patients undergoing both core needle biopsy and subsequent excision of the involved cervical node, core needle biopsy was shown to have very high diagnostic accuracy [26]. Similarly, ultrasound-guided core needle biopsy has been shown to have superior accuracy to FNA for the diagnosis of Kikuchi's disease [28]. In that study, FNA was found to have a sensitivity of 44.7%, while core needle biopsy had a diagnostic sensitivity of 95.6% when compared with excisional biopsy [28]. Other non-neoplastic entities amenable to core needle biopsy include sarcoid.

10.6 Core Biopsy for Diagnosis of Lymphoproliferative Diseases

The utility of core needle biopsy for the diagnosis of lymphomas remains in question. In a study of 56 patients with both core biopsies and excisional biopsies of lymph nodes, core needle biopsy gave a correct diagnosis of lymphoma in only 66% of cases [29]. The technique was inconclusive in 14% of cases and incorrectly identified the type of lymphoma present in 18%. In 2% of cases, core needle biopsy resulted in a false-negative diagnosis, but no false-positive diagnoses of lymphoma were recorded [29]. In the majority of reported studies, core needle biopsy has good accuracy for the diagnosis of lymphoma, but assigning a specific subtype of lymphoma is less accurate [30–36]. Hence, the issue regarding the utility of core biopsy for the diagnosis of lymphoma is whether or not core needle biopsy can result in sufficiently specific diagnoses of lymphoma to allow type-specific therapy without excisional biopsy of the lymph node. Results in published studies have been variable concerning whether or not core needle biopsy is sufficiently accurate to be the only biopsy necessary for appropriate therapy. In studies by Allin, et al. [30] and Pedersen, et al. [31], core needle biopsy resulted in sufficiently specific diagnoses to serve as the only biopsy method necessary. However, in a study by Kwon, core needle biopsy yielded sufficiently specific diagnoses in only 69.2% of the patient [32]. In the meta-analysis reported by Warshavsky, et al. [33], actionable lymphoma diagnoses secondary to core needle biopsy were obtained in 30% to 96.3% of cases [33]. Warshavsky, et al. [33] concluded that core needle biopsy of enlarged lymph nodes suspected to be lymphoma was a generally accurate technique and they concluded that the choice of the initial diagnostic method should depend upon clinical and institutional considerations. Burke, et al. [34] had similar findings with 60 of 83 core needle biopsies (72.2%), making a diagnosis of lymphoma sufficiently specific for therapy. In an additional 7 patients (8.4%), core needle biopsy was only suggestive of lymphoma but clinical management preceded on the basis of the diagnosis without surgical excision. In Burke's study, 81% of core needle biopsies provided sufficient information to allow definitive treatment [34].

Core needle biopsy appears to be a sufficiently accurate method for the investigation of lymphadenopathies due to primary lymphoproliferative disorders and infectious etiologies [26–28, 30–36]. In a series of 147 patients, histopathological diagnoses were obtained in 137 (93.2%) [36]. This series included examples of tuberculous lymphadenitis, Kikuchi's disease, nonspecific lymphadenitis, and lymphoma. Core needle biopsy is not without its hazards, like local hemorrhage, needle tract implantations, delayed wound healing, and even carotid artery rupture in post radiation patients being reported [22, 37]. Needle tract implantations have been reported following core needle biopsy and may occur in the immediate post biopsy or delayed periods [37]. The true incidence of core needle biopsy tract tumor implantations is difficult to estimate, but Shah and Ethunandan [37] estimated that such implantations occur following approximately 0.0011% of core needle biopsies. The incidence following FNA appears to be considerably less at an estimated incidence of 0.00012% [37]. Overall, core needle biopsy appears to be a generally safe and effective biopsy technique for the investigation of lymphadenopathy due to nonspecific causes, infectious etiologies, lymphomas, and metastatic malignancies. Core needle biopsy may represent an important "fall back" technique for the investigation of lymphadenopathy when multiple FNAs have been nondiagnostic.

10.7   Fine-Needle Aspiration and the Diagnosis of Lymphoma

For decades, FNA has been used for the diagnosis of lymphoma often in association with ancillary testing for clonality [38–53]. These early studies demonstrating the efficacy of FNA for the diagnosis of lymphoma were performed when lymphoma classification was less complex and diagnostic requirements for the initiation of therapy were simpler. In many cases, the demonstration of large-cell morphology and B-cell monoclonality was sufficient for treatment. Immunocytochemical analysis was shown to be valuable in the separation of reactive processes from lymphomas [52]. In a study of 158 FNA lymph node specimens, Carter, et al. [53] reported that 118 of 158 (75%) lymph nodes were definitively diagnosed as lymphoma. This series contained two false-positive diagnoses and four false-negative diagnoses. Subclassification of the cytological specimens was attempted in 60 needle aspirates and was identical to the histological subclassification in 51 (85%) [53]. Despite these encouraging findings, Hehn, et al. [54] published a comprehensive study questioning the clinical utility of FNA as a technique for the diagnosis of lymphoma [54]. They reviewed 115 FNA procedures and found that only 27 of the 93 FNA attempts at initial diagnosis (29%) supplied a specific and complete histological diagnosis following an accepted classification system. Moreover, only 9 of 22 (41%) FNAs performed for recurrent disease gave a classification for the lymphoma in an accepted system. Of greater concern, in the 67 FNAs with paired excisional biopsies, only 8 of 67 (12%) had cytological diagnoses, which correlated with subsequent excisional biopsy diagnosis. These authors concluded that FNA for lymphoma diagnosis was not helpful, not cost effective, and often resulted in misguiding subsequent therapy [54]. This publication resulted in a reassessment of the utility of FNA for the diagnosis of lymphoma. In the associated editorial, Austen, et al. [55] listed a number of methodological concerns regarding the manuscript by Hehn, et al. [54] Nonetheless, the manuscript by Hehn, et al. [54] and the subsequent editorial resulted in a number of studies reevaluating the accuracy and utility of FNA for the diagnosis of lymphoma. Caraway discussed issues impacting the successful utilization of FNA for the diagnosis of lymphoma and ongoing developments in technique and ancillary testing positively impacting the accuracy and ability to subtype lymphomas [56]. Ancillary testing such as flow cytometry and molecular diagnostics will undoubtedly improve FNA's ability for accurate diagnosis and subclassification of lymphomas.

Studies following that of Hehn, et al. [54] have addressed some of the issues raised in that publication (Table 10.2). Two large meta-analyses have more clearly defined the diagnostic accuracy in the recognition of lymphoma but have not successfully addressed the issues concerning subtyping and clinical utility [57–58]. Wong, et al. [57] demonstrated a pooled sensitivity and specificity of FNA for diagnosing lymphoma of 93% and 97%, respectively. They also pointed out that there was significant heterogeneity among studies reporting sensitivity and specificity for lymphoma in their meta-analysis. The study did not address accuracy of subtyping of lymphoma or its clinical utility in selecting modern specific therapy. A systemic review and meta-analysis by Labarca, et al. [58] documented poorer sensitivity but somewhat higher specificity. In that study, sensitivity for the diagnosis of lymphoma was only 66.2% while specificity was 99.3%. Unsurprisingly, the sensitivity for the diagnosis of recurrent lymphoma was higher at 78% and specificity remained excellent at 99.5%

Table 10.2 Sensitivity and specificity for diagnosis of lymphoma and diagnostic accuracy for clinically useful assignment of lymphoma subtype

Author	Sensitivity for lymphoma	Specificity for lymphoma	Accuracy for useful assignment of lymphoma subtype
Sigaard [29]	98%	100%	84%
Allin [30]	NG*	NG*	94.5%
Pedersen [31]	96.7%	100%	82.8%
Burke [34]	NG*	NG*	81% (adequate for treatment)
Kwon [32]	NG*	NG*	69.2%
Warshavsky [33]	NG*	NG*	80.1% to 97.1% (depending on subtype)

NG not given in text

in their view of 14 studies. Labarca, et al. [58] analyzed the impact of rapid on-site evaluation and needle size (21-g vs 22-g). These authors did not find any differences in diagnostic accuracy with or without the use of ROSE. Needle size did not appear to have an impact on diagnostic accuracy for initial diagnosis of lymphoma but sensitivity increased with larger needle size for patients with suspected recurrent lymphoma. The study by Labarca, et al. [58] found that the accuracy of FNA was sufficient to utilize it as a first-line modality, and its accuracy was similar to mediastinoscopy for lymphoma. In individual studies included in the meta-analysis, immunophenotyping and genetic analysis did improve overall sensitivity.

In a large single institution's study, Jelloul, et al. [59] found good accuracy in the recognition of lymphoma, but subtyping was achievable in only 40% of cases studied by FNA. In that study, a definitive diagnosis of lymphoma relied on ancillary testing. They concluded that the use of FNA and core needle biopsy with ancillary testing was effective in providing a definitive diagnosis of lymphoma. Improved sensitivity and specificity for cytological diagnosis of lymphoma were also documented by Das [60]. Other recent studies have confirmed the high sensitivity (95.5%) and specificity (98.7%) for FNA diagnosis of lymphoma in cervical lymph nodes [61].

Despite the findings of good to excellent diagnostic sensitivity and specificity for the cytological diagnosis of lymphoma [59–61], issues remain concerning the technique's ability to accurate subtype lymphomas. Without accurate subtyping, the applicability of FNA to the diagnosis of lymphoma and its ability to aid oncologists in the selection of appropriate modern therapy remains questionable. Moreover, the cytological diagnosis of lymphoma may be especially limited in certain types of non-Hodgkin's lymphomas including marginal zone lymphoma and other hypocellular variants [62, 63]. Further studies using flow cytometry and molecular analysis will be necessary to fully establish FNA's utility for the diagnosis and subtyping of lymphomas without subsequent node excision.

While FNA appears to be a highly accurate technique for the identification of nodal disease including primary lymphoproliferative processes and metastatic disease, a significant number of FNAs will not yield a specific diagnosis, and a number of terms have been used to characterize not-fully diagnostic samples. In general, FNAs with nondefinitive diagnoses and nondiagnostic FNAs are repeated or result in node excision. Recently, a proposal has been made in which a classification system of five categories is used to aid in the stratification of these not-fully diagnostic aspirates [64]. The categories are similar to those proposed by the Papanicolaou Society of Cytopathology for Cytologic Categorization of Pancreaticobiliary and Respiratory Cytology. The true clinical impact of the "Sydney System" is not yet known but many surgeons may simply prefer to excise the lymph node in question regardless of the "Sydney" categorization.

10.8 Management and Biopsy Techniques for Cystic Masses of the Neck

The discovery of a cystic mass within the neck raises an important differential diagnosis, the nature of which is largely dependent on the patient age. Separation of benign cysts from cystic malignancies is therapeutically important and will determine subsequent patient management. In individuals below the age of 40 years, the majority of cystic masses will be benign embryological remnants, whereas in patients over 40 years of age, a high percentage will represent cystic metastases. Cimberg, et al. [65] reported that 22% of patients admitted for workup of assumed branchial cysts had metastatic carcinoma of thyroid, salivary gland, or squamous etiology. In their experience, FNA was unhelpful in two-thirds of cases [65]. Andrews, et al. reported a similar experience [66]. They reported three cases clinically thought to be branchial cysts but on tissue examination were found to be cystic lymph node metastases of squamous cell carcinomas. All three cancers arose from tonsilar primaries. Studies have shown that up to 80% of cysts thought to be branchial cleft cysts in patients over 40 years of age were in fact metastatic squamous cell carcinomas. Thus, patients over 40 years of age presenting with a lateral cystic neck mass require a high degree of suspicion for malignancy. Pan-endoscopy should be performed along with ipsilateral tonsillectomy and blind biopsies of Waldeyer's ring [66]. Cimberg, et al. [65] recommended approaching neck cysts in an adult as if they were malignant. Cimberg, et al. [65] recommended a preoperative through head and neck examination to identify potential primary carcinomas. If none are found, it should be followed by FNA of the mass. A negative report should be considered inconclusive. When a definitive diagnosis of carcinoma cannot be made, the cystic lesions should be resected and gross examination should be performed in the operating room with frozen section of any suspicious areas.

Biopsy techniques available for the analysis of cystic masses of the lateral neck include FNA, core needle biopsy, and frozen section evaluation. Tavet, et al. [67] retrospectively reviewed 135 patients presenting with lateral cystic neck masses. They found that FNA had lower sensitivity than core needle biopsy or frozen section with sensitivity being 59%, 83%, and 93%, respectively. In their study, frozen section had a significantly better negative predictive value when compared to either FNA or core needle biopsy. The positive predictive value was similar for all three biopsy techniques. In the opinion of Tavet, et al. [67], FNAs should be used initially on lateral cystic neck masses as the method has sufficient sensitivity (59%) to justify its initial usage. When FNAs are inconclusive, core needle biopsy or frozen sections should be performed. Begebie, et al. [68] had a similar experience finding that the sensitivity of FNA was 75%, while that of frozen section was 100%. They concluded that adult patients may undergo FNA to establish the diagnosis of malignancy but a benign FNA should be considered as inconclusive. Cytological evaluation of material obtained by FNA from a cystic neck mass is difficult with a significant risk for under and over diagnosis. Burgess, et al. [69] found that increased nuclear/cytoplasmic ratio, irregularity of nuclear outline, and nuclear hyperchromasia were all key features for the diagnosis of metastatic squamous cell carcinoma. Branchial cleft cysts showed benign squamous cells with only mild nuclear atypia. Additionally, the background of necrotic debris with relatively few neutrophils favored the diagnosis of malignancy over branchial cleft cysts. Nordemar, et al. [70] proffered the use of image cytometry DNA analysis of FNA material to aid in the separation of branchial cleft cysts from cystic metastases of squamous cell carcinoma. This method adds considerable expense and is currently not widely available.

The workup of cysts within the lateral neck is diagnostically challenging. The workup differs considerably between pediatric patients and adults over the age of 40 years. In pediatric patients, branchial cleft cysts are considerably more common than cystic metastases, while in patients over 40 years of age, cystic metastases far outnumber branchial cleft cysts. Both the cytopathologists and clinicians need to bear this in mind when formulating workup and therapy of these lesions.

10.9 Biopsy Techniques for Deep-Seated Lesions of the Nasopharynx and Base of the Skull

A number of important but relatively uncommon tumors occur within deep structures of the base of the skull, nasopharynx, parapharyngeal, and retropharyngeal spaces. These neoplasms include but are not limited to meningioma, olfactory neuroblastoma, paranasal sinus carcinoma, schwannoma, chondrosarcoma, chordoma, and carcinomas of the paranasal sinuses. Accurate diagnosis of these lesions is important since their clinical behavior varies considerably. Surgical approach for diagnosis of these neoplasms is difficult and may be associated with significant patient morbidity. This makes surgical biopsy challenging and less desirable than more minimally invasive techniques such as core needle biopsy and FNA. While frozen section evaluation of intraoperative specimens is possible and has good accuracy, such an approach is not optimal due to the highly invasive nature of the surgery.

FNA and core needle biopsy represent minimally invasive alternatives, and a number of approaches and guidance techniques have been developed for accurate biopsy of deep-seated lesions of the parapharyngeal, retropharyngeal, and the base of skull lesions [71–77]. Magnetic resonance imaging (MRI) appears to give superior definition to lesions arising in these areas but requires the use of special low ferromagnetic needles. Computerized axial tomography (CT) appears to be the most commonly utilized guidance technique, but intraoral ultrasound guidance has been used for some deep-seated lesions of the head and neck [77]. The most common approaches are the following: (1) transfacial with the tract passing lateral to the maxilla and lateral to the pterygoid plate; (2) lateral through the mandibular notch between the coronoid process

and mandibular condyle; and (3) retromandibular through the parotid gland [72]. These approaches and biopsy techniques have been found to be highly accurate (87% to 95%) for the separation of benign from malignant neoplasms by core needle or FNA biopsy [72–76]. The definitive selection of the superior biopsy technique (FNA vs core needle biopsy) is not possible based on the relatively scant literature published. Intraoral ultrasound-guided biopsy techniques have been suggested for some deep-seated masses of the head and neck, but insufficient data have been published to fully evaluate the advantages of this approach.

10.10 Primary Neoplasms of the Neck Including Paraspinal Lesions

A limited number of primary neoplasms are found within the neck and include lymphangioma, carotid body paraganglioma, lipoma, schwannoma, neurofibroma, synovial sarcoma, rhabdomyosarcoma, malignant peripheral nerve sheath tumor, and liposarcoma. Many of these will present as palpable masses and can be easily biopsied by either FNA or core needle biopsy. Since many represent mesenchymal lesions, the relative accuracies of FNA and core needle biopsy are the same as those at other body sites, and the comparable accuracies of FNA and core needle biopsies have been investigated [78, 79]. Investigation of carotid body paragangliomas by minimally invasive techniques presents some special circumstances. Early experience of FNA with carotid paragangliomas suggested a risk of myocardial infarction but the risk of that presently appears minimal. Carotid body tumors are by their nature, relatively deep-seated lesions often recognized initially by symptomatology and imaging studies. Appropriate imaging studies will define the precise location, high vascularity, and probable diagnosis of the carotid body tumor. This may result in making biopsy unnecessary and excision with possible intraoperative frozen section the initial diagnostic and therapeutic option. Despite this, FNA has been utilized for the diagnosis of carotid body paragangliomas and shown to be a safe technique but of variable diagnostic accuracy [80, 81]. From the available literature, core biopsies do not appear to be a biopsy technique utilized for the investigation of carotid body tumors.

10.11 Biopsy Techniques for the Salivary Gland Lesions

The tissue diagnosis of salivary gland nodules and masses can be approached by three techniques: operative excision with frozen section evaluation to determine the extent of surgery including the potential need for a neck dissection, core needle biopsy, and FNA. Traditionally, salivary gland nodules were investigated by surgical excision of the nodule often associated with intraoperative frozen section. The technique is invasive and not without hazards including potential damage to the facial nerve. Despite nearly five decades of experience with frozen section evaluation of salivary gland lesions, controversy remains as to its diagnostic accuracy, utility, and integration with FNA cytology. The introduction of the Milan System with its indeterminant categories of atypia of unknown significance, salivary gland neoplasm of uncertain malignant potential and suspicious for malignancy, has resulted in reevaluation of the utility and appropriate usage of frozen section evaluation [82, 83]. Accuracy rates reported for frozen section in the literature have varied widely with sensitivities of as low as 61% to as high as 98.5% [84–91]. Specificity has varied from 96% to 100% [84–91].

Overall diagnostic accuracy of frozen section for the separation of benign neoplasms from malignancies has been above 90% in the majority of studies but the exact diagnosis of the type of malignancy present has been as low as 51% [84, 86, 90]. Table 10.3 documents the published accuracy rates for frozen section evaluation of salivary gland nodules. In the majority of published studies, frozen section has been more accurate in separating benign neoplasms from malignancies than FNA cytology, but occasional studies have documented a higher accuracy rate for FNA [92, 93]. Frozen section evaluation also has higher accuracy for the specific identification of salivary gland malignancies [86].

Despite frozen section's high diagnostic accuracy for the separation of benign from malignant salivary gland neoplasms [94], less invasive techniques were sought to determine if a salivary gland nodule was benign or malignant. Core needle biopsy represents such a minimally invasive technique and offers a potential advantage of material appropriate for histopathological evaluation. In recent years, considerable debate has occurred as to whether FNA or core needle biopsy should be the preferred initial biopsy technique for the investigation of salivary gland tumors. While imaging studies are helpful in the assessment of salivary gland nodules, they are not substitutes for either FNA or core needle biopsy [95]. FNA clearly has some advantages over core needle biopsy in that it can be quickly performed and interpreted on site, is associated with little pain, does not require local anesthesia, and has an extremely low incidence of needle tract tumor cell implantation or other complications. On the other hand, core needle biopsy has

Table 10.3 Accuracy of frozen section for evaluation of salivary gland tumors

Author	# Cases	Sensitivity	Specificity
Heller [84]	310	69%	96%
Mantsopoulos [85]	669	91%	100%
Dindzans [86]	110	94%	97%
Wheelis [87]	256	89.6%	98.1%
Carralho [89]	153	61.5%	98%
Olsen [91]	1339	98.5%	99%

a higher diagnostic accuracy in some studies and is more likely to be able to specifically categorize the type of malignancy present. However, the technique has some drawbacks in that it generally requires at least overnight processing, requires localized anesthesia, has a higher incidence of needle tract implantations, and risk injuries to such structures as the facial nerve branches as well as an increased likelihood for local hemorrhage [95]. In a meta-analysis of five relevant studies, Witt and Schmidt [96] documented summary estimates of sensitivity for a diagnosis of 96% and summary estimates for a specificity of 100%. Accuracy varied little between studies, and few complications were documented with only a 1.6% risk of hematoma per procedure [96]. In comparison to the relative uniformity of results for core needle biopsy, FNA has greater variability in diagnostic accuracy between centers reporting results [97]. Reported diagnostic accuracy for core needle biopsy is very high [98], and in some studies, core needle biopsy has been shown to be significantly more accurate in identifying malignancies (99% vs 87%) and was superior to FNA in providing a specific diagnosis (93% vs 74%) [99]. In a recent systemic review and meta-analysis, Cho, et al. [100] demonstrated a significantly higher summarized sensitivity for core needle biopsy over FNA (92% vs 65%) and a higher specificity for core needle biopsy than FNA (100% vs 97%). A more recent study by Bugracengiz, et al. [101] confirmed the higher sensitivity of core needle biopsy over FNA (100% vs 40%), but specificity was identical for the two techniques. The accuracy rates, sensitivities, and specificities in these comparison studies yield lower accuracy rates for FNA than those reported in individual studies of the accuracy of FNA and in a larger meta-analysis [102]. In the meta-analysis by Schmidt, et al. [102], the accuracy rate for separation of benign from malignant by FNA was 96%, and the summary estimates for sensitivity and specificity were 80% and 97%, respectively. These differences in reported accuracy, sensitivity, and specificity for FNA may indicate that many of the comparison studies summarize data from institutions lacking high levels of expertise in obtaining and interpreting fine-needle aspirates. Additional comparison studies and meta-analyses in this area will be necessary to more definitively document the relationship between accuracies of core needle biopsy and FNA. The choice of initial diagnostic technique (FNA vs core needle biopsy) may depend on regional preferences and the availability of a team of cytopathologists, radiologists, and otolaryngologists adept at the technique of FNA.

10.12   Fine-Needle Aspiration in the Diagnosis of Salivary Gland Lesions

Early reports of the experience with FNA indicated good sensitivity and excellent specificity [103]. This led to the wide acceptance of the technique for the investigation of salivary gland nodules both in Europe and in the United States. Acceptance of the technique was aided by the fact that it could be performed in clinics with almost immediate evaluation and results reporting. In a systemic review and meta-analysis by Schmidt, et al. [102], the high diagnostic accuracy, sensitivity, and specificity were confirmed, but heterogeneity of results was seen between institutions [102]. Some reports documented significantly lower degrees of sensitivity (59%) and diagnostic accuracy (93.8%) [104]. Low sensitivities (81% to 85%) have also been reported in other studies [104–105]. In summary, FNA has excellent specificity for the diagnosis of malignancy but less sensitivity. The Milan System for Reporting Salivary Gland Cytopathology was developed to improve the diagnostic accuracy and maintain a high level of sensitivity and specificity for the diagnostic categories of neoplasms, benign and malignant [106, 107]. This system reports risks of malignancy for each category with the benign category having a malignancy risk of less than 5% and the malignant category having a malignancy risk of approximately 90%. These malignancy risks are in line with the meta-analysis findings reported by Schmidt, et al. [102].

10.13 Summary of Diagnostic Techniques for the Investigation of Salivary Gland Nodules

The optimal method for obtaining the diagnosis in salivary gland nodules has not been definitively established but the available literature appears to suggest the initial use of FNA when individuals competent and well trained in the technique are available as part of the patient care team. Such individuals are not always readily available as indicated by the study of Schmidt, et al. [102] When significant expertise in the technique and interpretation of fine-needle aspirates is lacking, core needle biopsy may be the preferable technique as it has generally higher diagnostic sensitivity and a greater ability to subtype the malignancy present. The workup of a salivary gland nodule is a multidisciplinary undertaking requiring input from clinicians, radiologists, and pathologists. In 2020, the French Society of Otorhinolaryngology-Head and Neck surgery (SFORL) issued guidelines for the preliminary treatment of pleomorphic adenomas [108]. The recommendations for the workup of salivary gland pleomorphic adenomas are applicable to the workup of all suspected primary neoplasms of the salivary gland. The society recommended that MRIs should be performed of the parotid gland and head and neck lymph node levels. This should be followed by FNA particularly in tumors difficult to be characterized by MRI. Frozen section biopsy should be performed to confirm the diagnosis and adapt the surgical procedure in case of intraoperative findings of malignancy. Additionally, the performance of frozen section can aid in distinction of high- and low-grade malignancies allowing the performance of a neck lymph node dissection when necessary. The routine inclusion of imaging modalities and frozen section in the preoperative and intraoperative workup of a salivary gland nodule significantly impacts the clinical value of some of the categories of the Milan system. The management recommendations for the categories salivary gland neoplasm of uncertain malignant potential (SUMP), suspicious for malignancy, and malignant all include recommendations for surgery. The category neoplasm: benign may use clinical follow-up in a minority of cases. The type and extent of surgery may differ for the categories neoplasm: benign, salivary gland neoplasm of uncertain malignant potential; suspicious for malignancy, and malignant. The Milan System contains different recommendations for the use of imaging studies and intraoperative frozen section. These differences are largely negated by the current recommendations of SFORL, where imaging studies and intraoperative frozen section are invariably performed. The extent of future use of intraoperative frozen section is difficult to predict, but currently, the majority of otolaryngologists, head and neck surgeons, do perform preoperative imaging studies following the recommendations of SFORL. When imaging studies are not congruent with FNA findings, either core needle biopsy or intraoperative frozen section should be performed to better identify the type of neoplasm present and select the appropriate operative procedure including the potential for neck dissection.

10.14 Biopsy Techniques for Nodules of the Thyroid Gland

Thyroid nodules are relatively common in the adult population with the majority representing hyperplastic nodules often resulting clinically in multinodular goiter. The majority of thyroid nodules are benign, but diagnostic workup is required to separate the frequent benign nodules from the relatively uncommon malignancies. Traditionally, this was achieved by the use of ultrasound evaluation and radio-nucleotide uptake studies. When the findings of these two studies suggested a malignancy, operative intervention occurred with lobectomy and intraoperative frozen section. At most body sites, frozen section is a highly accurate technique but not without occasional false-negative and false-positive diagnoses [109, 110]. The evaluation of follicular lesions of the thyroid by frozen section has questionable accuracy [111, 112]. However, before the implementation of FNA as an alternative technique, lobectomy of clinically and imaging suspicious nodules was the only technique for tissue diagnosis. Thus, standard management of suspicious thyroid nodules was lobectomy with intraoperative frozen section. Further operative intervention was predicated on the diagnosis of malignancy by frozen section evaluation. While frozen section was highly accurate for the recognition of papillary and medullary carcinoma, its diagnostic accuracy and sensitivity for follicular lesions of the thyroid was considerably less [113–115]. In general, the diagnosis of follicular lesions of the thyroid requires complete evaluation of the capsule surrounding the follicular nodule. This requires multiple sections of the nodule each carefully evaluated for the presence or absence of capsular invasion and/or vascular invasion. This process is time consuming and requires multiple sections. Such evaluation is not possible during intraoperative evaluation due to time constraints and processing issues.

Since the widespread use and availability of FNA, the paradigm concerning intraoperative frozen section evaluation has shifted [116, 117].

With the realization that frozen section evaluation of follicular lesions of the thyroid was unlikely to separate benign from malignant lesions, the use of frozen sections became restricted to a relatively small number of diagnostic scenarios. Some authors have recommended its use for the category, suspicious for papillary thyroid carcinoma [118], but even in this area, caution is advised by most experts. The majority of experts have expressed the opinion that intraoperative frozen section has little to contribute to decision-making in patients diagnosed with thyroid cancer by preoperative FNA or to the diagnosis of lesions classified as follicular or Hurthle cell neoplasm by FNA [115–119].

10.15 Core Biopsy in the Diagnosis of Thyroid Nodules

Core biopsy represents an alternative to FNA for the minimally invasive diagnosis of thyroid nodules. Initially, it was used as a direct competitor to FNA and has been preferred by some authors over FNA [120]. These authors favor the first-line use of core needle biopsy because of apparent improved accuracy for the diagnosis of thyroid nodules, the reduction of inconclusive or false-negative results, and diminishing the number of unnecessary operative procedures [120]. The second approach utilizing core needle biopsy uses the technique as a follow-up methodology for thyroid nodules with initially indeterminant fine-needle aspirates including nondiagnostic specimens, follicular neoplasms, and nodules judged as suspicious for malignancy [121–125].

Issues for consideration when evaluating the utility of core biopsy include [1] relative costs of core needle biopsy and FNA; [2] patient discomfort; [3] safety; [4] speed of diagnosis; and [5] core biopsy-associated limitations of histological analysis of specimens for diagnosis of follicular neoplasms. Trimeoli and Cresenzi [121] evaluated the available literature on each of these issues [121]. At many institutions, core needle biopsy is slightly more expensive than FNA for the investigation of a thyroid nodule. Additionally, in the clinic setting, rapid on-site evaluation may be available for FNA while core needle biopsy is associated with approximately one working day delay in availability of results. Relatively, little information exists to the frequency of significant complications associated with core needle biopsy and FNA, but in a retrospective study of 350 consecutive patients, Chen, et al. [126] did not detect any significant immediate or delayed procedure-related complications for either biopsy techniques [126]. Two studies evaluated the patients' reporting of pain between the two techniques, and neither study found a significant difference between the patients' tolerability of the technique or their differential perception of pain [127, 128]. Jaw, et al. [37] in a meta-analysis found that the frequency of needle tract implantations following core biopsy was significantly higher than following FNA (0.0011% vs 0.000125).

An important aspect of core needle biopsy is that the technique produces a histological specimen with very limited sampling or no sampling of the follicular neoplasm's capsule or a specimen large enough to exclude lymphovascular invasion. This limits its diagnostic utility for the evaluation of purely follicular lesions. Additionally, core needle biopsy-derived histological specimens generally have poorer cytological detail than properly prepared cytological specimens. The relative advantages and disadvantages of core needle biopsy have been summarized by Yoon, et al. [129]

The utilization of core needle biopsy as the initial diagnostic technique for the workup of a thyroid nodule has been well studied and reported on in a large number of studies. These are well summarized in three systematic reviews and meta-analyses [130–132]. Two of the three studies [130, 131] show no significant difference for diagnostic accuracy between the core needle biopsy and FNA. The study by Wolinski, et al. [132] demonstrated that core needle biopsy yielded a higher proportion of diagnostic results than conventional FNA. This study also suggested that core needle biopsy may reduce the number of unnecessary thyroidectomies, and core needle biopsy was associated with significantly fewer nondiagnostic results [132]. The findings of these three studies have been largely substantiated by later publications [133]. Some later studies favored the primary use of FNA because it was more easily performed, better accepted by patients, and had a lower cost benefit ratio [133].

Because core needle biopsy is not significantly superior to FNA in the diagnosis of thyroid nodules and is associated with some disadvantages, FNA remains the procedure of choice for the initial investigation of thyroid nodules. However, core needle biopsy may provide some advantages when initial FNA is either nondiagnostic or indeterminant [122–125]. A meta-analysis reviewing four eligible studies containing 1028 patients demonstrated that core needle biopsy was associated with significantly lower rates of nondiagnostic results (3.65%) compared to repeat FNA (6.4%). Core needle biopsy also demonstrated significantly higher summary estimates of sensitivity (89.8%) than did repeat FNA (60.6%) [133]. Summary specificities did not differ between the two techniques. These and other studies indicate that the combination of FNA and core needle biopsy is a safe and clinically useful technique [135], and patients with a prior non-diagnostic or inconclusive FNA should undergo core needle biopsy. This is especially true when there are two prior nondiagnostic FNAs [135].

10.16 Fine-Needle Aspiration for the Diagnosis of Thyroid Nodules

Currently, FNA is the predominant technique for the investigation of thyroid nodules. This is due to the technique's ease of performance, generally high acceptance by patients, relatively low cost, and adequate diagnostic accuracy. Reported sensitivities of FNA have averaged 0.68 with average specificities of 0.92 [130]. The technique is most accurate for the recognition of papillary thyroid carcinoma and is less able to evaluate the benign or malignant nature of purely follicular pattern lesions. The inability of FNA to specifically diagnose follicular carcinomas has led to the development of the Bethesda System for Reporting Thyroid Cytopathology (BSRTC) [136]. This system uses a number of intermediate or indeterminant categories to insure the high diagnostic sensitivity and specificity of the categories: benign and malignant. The six categories used by the Bethesda System for Reporting Thyroid Cytology (BSRTC) are nondiagnostic, benign, atypia of undetermined significance or follicular lesion of undetermined significance, follicular neoplasm or suspicious for follicular neoplasms, suspicious for malignancy, and malignant. Each category is associated with an estimated risk of malignancy (%) as well as management and follow-up recommendations. The benign category is associated with a malignancy risk of approximately 0 to 3%, while the malignant category has an estimated malignancy risk running from 97% to 99% [136]. The categories atypia of undetermined significance/follicular lesion of undetermined significance, follicular neoplasm or suspicious for follicular neoplasm, and suspicious for malignancy are associated with progressive risks for malignancy running from 10% to 30% to 50% to 75%. This stepwise increase in risk of malignancy is helpful for planning of the follow-up.

Currently, FNA is the most commonly utilized of the three techniques available. While the categories benign and malignant have high sensitivities and specificities, [130–132] a number of specimens will be assigned to one of the indeterminant categories including nondiagnostic, atypia of indeterminant significance/follicular lesion of indeterminant significance, follicular neoplasm or suspicious for follicular neoplasm, and suspicious for malignancy. These categories require further workup on the part of the endocrinologists treating the patient. In many cases, the recommendation has been to repeat the fine-needle aspirate or send the material to a recognized expert. While this may reclassify the specimen, a significant number will remain in one of the indeterminant categories. The follow-up of these specimens is repeat FNA, potentially repeated twice. If the second repeat fine-needle aspirate does not yield a more definitive diagnosis, some authors recommend the use of core needle biopsy to better characterize the specimen [134]. This approach is based on the higher diagnostic sensitivity of core needle biopsy and the ability of core needle biopsy to better classify the type of malignancy present [99–101]. Repeat FNA of thyroid nodules should be performed under ultrasound guidance to ensure the most accurate needle placement possible.

10.17   Biopsy of Parathyroid Lesions

The identification and biopsy of parathyroid lesions is a complex undertaking with scans and operative intervention. In general, enlarged parathyroid glands are studied intraoperatively by frozen section and venous levels of parathyroid hormone. This approach appears to be the most expeditious in that it is both diagnostic and often therapeutic at the time of operation.

A few reports of FNA of parathyroid tumors have been made in the literature, and the technique appears to be extremely helpful in differentiating parathyroid tumors from thyroid nodules [137]. Additionally, measurement of parathormone levels in needle aspirates derived from cervical masses can be helpful in differential diagnosis [138].

At present, core needle biopsy appears to have little place in the workup of parathyroid nodules.

References

1. Bhasker N. Review of head and neck masses in the Indian population based on prevalence and etiology with emphasis on primary diagnostic modalities. Cureus. 2021;13(7):e16249.
2. Laco J, Daum O, Zambo I, Ondic O, Svajdien M. Intra operative diagnosis of the head and neck lesions, thyroid and parathyroid gland, bone and soft tissue, and genitourinary tract. Cesk Patol. 2018;54(2):72–80.
3. Soumya WA, Ooi EH, Lockwood C. Accuracy of core needle biopsy compared to fine-needle biopsy for the diagnosis of neoplasm in patients with suspected head and neck cancers: a systematic review protocol of diagnostic test accuracy. JBI Evid Synth. 2020;18(7):1602–8.
4. Kraft M, Laeng H, Schmuziger N, Arnoux A, Gurtler N. Comparison of ultrasound-guided core-needle biopsy and FNA in the assessment of head and neck lesions. Head Neck. 2008;30(11):1457–63.
5. Bayrak BY, Ozkara SK. FNA of non-thyroidal head and neck masses: correlation of the cyto-histopathological diagnoses, causes of inconsistency and traps. Ann Diagn Pathol. 2019;39:15–20.
6. Peters BR, Schnadig VJ, Quinn FB Jr, Hokanson JA, Zaharopoulos P, McCracken MM, et al. Interobserver variability in the interpretation of FNA biopsy of head and neck masses. Arch Otolaryngol Head and Neck Surg. 1989;115(12):1438–42.
7. Merkle EM, Lewin JS, Ashoff AJ, Stepnick DW, Duerk JL, Lanzieri CF, Strauss LM. Percutaneous magnetic resonance image-guided biopsy and spiration in the head and neck. Laryngoscope. 2000;110(3 part 1):382–5.
8. Amoedo MK, Tying CJ, Vieira Pinto Barbosa PN, Bezerra de Melo RA, Arrada Almeida MF, Chojniak R, Vierira Bitencourt AG. Computed tomography-guided percutaneous biopsy of head and neck

masses: techniques, outcomes, and complications. Radiol Bras. 2021;54(5):295–302.

9. Russ JE, Scanlon EF, Christ MA. Aspiration cytology of head and neck masses. Am J Surg. 1978;136(3):342–7.

10. Young JE, Archibald SD, Shier KJ. Needle aspiration cytology biopsy in head and neck masses. Am J Surg. 1981;142(4):484–9.

11. Slack RW, Croft CB, Crome LP. FNA cytology in the management of head and neck masses. Clinotolaryngol Allied Sci. 1985;10(2):93–6.

12. Layfield LJ. FNA in the diagnosis of head and neck lesions: a review and discussion of problems in differential diagnosis. Diagn Cytopathol. 2007;32(12):798–805.

13. Gertner R, Podoshin L, Fradis M. Accuracy of FNA biopsy in neck masses. Laryngoscope. 1984;94(10):1370–1.

14. Horrath L, Kraft M. Evaluation of ultrasound and FNA in the assessment of head and neck lesions. Eur Arch Otorhinolaryngol. 2019;276(10):2903–11.

15. Wenig BM. Intraoperative consultation (IOC) in mucosal lesions of the upper aerodigestive tract. Head Neck Pathol. 2008;2(2):131–44.

16. Kim BM, Kim EK, Kim MJ, Yang WI, Park CS, Park SI. Sonographically guided core needle biopsy of cervical lymphadenopathy in patients without known malignancy. J Ultrasound Med. 2007;26(5):585–91.

17. Terada A, Hasegawa Y, Yatabe Y, Hana N, Ozawa T, Hirakawa H, et al. Follow-up after intraoperative sentinel node biopsy of N0 Neck oral cancer patients. Eur Arch Otorhinolaryngol. 2011;268(3):429–35.

18. Liu J, Wang Z-I, Liu L, Xue L-Y, Liu K, Huang H, Xu Z-G. Application value of sentinel node biopsy in early-stage oral tongue cancer with clinically negative neck. Zhonshua Zhong Liu Zu Zhi. 2013;35(6):459–62.

19. Neduvanchery S, Gochhait D, Srinivas BH, Harichandrakumar KT, Subramanian P, Shukkur N, et al. Comparison of intraoperative imprints cytology with frozen section for lymph node metastasis in patients with head and neck squamous cell carcinoma. Diagn Cytopathol. 2021;49(2):252–7.

20. Saha S, Woodhouse NR, Gok G, Ramesan K, Moody A, Howlett DC. Ultrasound guided core biopsy, FNA cytology and surgical excision biopsy in the diagnosis of metastatic squamous cell carcinoma in the head and neck: an eleven-year experience. Eur J Radiol. 2011;80(3):792–5.

21. Howlett DC, Harpet B, Quante M, et al. Diagnostic adequacy and accuracy of FNA cytology in neck lump assessment: results from a regional cancer network over a one-year period. Journal Laryngology and Otology. 2007;121:571–9.

22. Han F, Xu M, Xie T, Wang JW, Lin QG, Guo ZX, et al. Efficacy of ultrasound-guided core needle biopsy in cervical lymphadenopathy: a retrospective study of 6,695 cases. Eur Radiol. 2018;28(5):1809–17.

23. Lo T, Wang CP, Chen CH, Yang TL, Lou PJ, Lo JY, et al. Diagnostic performance of core needle biopsy for nodal recurrences in patients with head and neck squamous cell carcinoma. Sci Rep. 2022;12(1):2048.

24. Oh KH, Woo JS, Cho JG, Baek SK, Jung KY, Kwon SY. Efficacy of ultrasound-guided core needle gun biopsy in diagnosing cervical lymphadenopathy. Eur Ann Otorhinolaryngol Head Neck Dis. 2016;133(6):401–4.

25. Ryu KH, Lee JH, Jung SW, Kim HJ, Lee JY, Chung SR, et al. US-guided core-needle biopsy versus US-guided fine-needle aspiration of suspicious cervical lymph nodes for staging workup of non-head and neck malignancies: a propensity score matching study. J Surg Oncol. 2017;116(7):870–6.

26. Altuwairgi O, Baharron S, Alkabab Y, Alsufi E, Almowegei M, L-Jahdali HA. Ultrasound-guided core biopsy in the diagnostic work-up of tuberculous lymphadenitis in Saudi Arabia, refining the diagnostic approach. Case series and review of literature. J Infect Public Health. 2014;7(5):371–6.

27. Cho W, Kim MK, Sim JS. Ultrasound-guided core needle biopsy of cervical lymph nodes in the diagnosis of toxoplasmosis. J Clin Ultrasound. 2017;45(4):192–6.

28. Park SG, Koo HR, Jang K, Myung JK, Song CM, Ji YB, et al. Efficacy of ultrasound-guided needle biopsy in the diagnosis of Kikuchi-Fujimoto disease. Laryngoscope. 2021;131(5):E1519–23.

29. Sigaard RK, Weenervuldt K, Munksgaard L, Rahbek Gjerdrum LM, Homoe P. Core needle biopsy is an inferior tool for diagnosing cervical lymphoma compared to lymph node excision. Acta Oncol. 2021;60(7):904–10.

30. Allin D, David S, Jacob A, Mir N, Gibbins GA. Use of cre biopsy in diagnosing cervical lymphadenopathy: a viable alternative to surgical excisional biopsy of lymph node? Ann R Coll Surg Engl. 2017;99(3):242–4.

31. Pedersen OM, Aarstad HJ, Lokeland T, Bostad L. Diagnostic yield of biopsies of cervical lymph nodes using a large (14-guage) core biopsy needle. A PMIS. 2013;121(12):1119–30.

32. Kwon M, Yim C, Baek HJ, Lee JS, Seo JH, Kim JP, et al. Ultrasound guided core needle biopsy of cervical lymph nodes for diagnosing head and neck lymphoma compared with open surgical biopsy: exploration for factors that shape diagnostic yield. Am J. Otolaryngol. 2018;39(6):679–84.

33. Warshavsky A, Rosen R, Perry C, Muhanna N, Ungar OJ, Carmel-Neiderman NN, et al. Core needle biopsy for diagnosing lymphoma in cervical lymphadenopathy: meta-analysis. Head Neck. 2020;42(10):3051–60.

34. Burke C, Thomas R, Inglis C, Baldwin A, Ramesar K, Grace R, et al. Ultrasound-guided core biopsy in the diagnosis of lymphoma of the head and neck. A Song9-year experience. Br J Radiol. 2011;84:727–32.

35. Ryu YJ, Cha W, Jeong WJ, Choi SI, Ahn SH. Diagnostic role of core needle biopsy in cervical lymphadenopathy. Head Neck. 2015;37(2):229–31.

36. Song JT, Cheong HJ, Kee SY, Lee J, Sohn JW, Kim MJ, et al. Disease spectrum of cervical lymphadenitis: analysis based on ultrasound-guided core-needle gun biopsy. J Infect. 2007;55(4):310–6.

37. Shah KSV, Ethunandau M. Tumor seeding after FNA and core biopsy of the head and neck -a systematic review. Br J. Oral Maxillofac Surg. 2016;54(3):260–5.

38. Hsu C, Leung BS, Lau SK, Sham JS, Choy D, Engzell U. Efficacy of FNA and sampling of lymph nodes in 1,484 Chinese patients. Diagn Cytopathol. 1990;6(3):154–9.

39. Mondal A, Mukherjee D, Chatterjee DN, Saha AM, Mukherjee AL. FNA biopsy cytology in diagnosis of cervical lymphadenopathies. J Indian Med Assoc. 1989;87(12):281–3.

40. Steel BL, Schwartz MR, Ramzy I. Fine needle aspiration biopsy in the diagnosis of lymphadenopathy in 1,103 patients. Role, limitations and analysis of diagnostic pitfalls. Acta Cytol. 1995;39(1):76–81.

41. Baatenberg RJ, Rongen RJ, Verwoerd CD, vanOverhagen H, Lameris JS, Knegt P. Ultrasound-guided FNA biopsy of neck nodes. Arch Otolaryugol Head Neck Surg. 1991;17(4):402–4.

42. Vanden Brekel MW, Castelijus JA, Stel HV, Luth WJ, Valk J, vander Waal I, Snow GB. Occultmerastatic neck disease: detection with US and US-guided FNA cytology. Radiology. 1991;180(2):457–61.

43. Du W, Fang Q, Dai L, Fan J. FNA biopsy versus frozen section examination in assessing cervical lymph node metastasis in primary clinically positive neck papillary thyroid carcinoma. Diagn Cytopathol. 2022;50(5):217–22.

44. Rammeh S, Romdhane E, Sassi A, Belhajkucem L, Blei A, Ksentini M, et al. Accuracy of FNA cytology of head and neck masses. Diagn Cytopathol. 2019;47(5):394–9.

45. Sandhya KN, Girija KL, Venugopal M, Thomas V, Ramachandran S, Asish R. Cervical lymph node evaluation in oral squamous cell carcinoma using ultrasound guided FNA cytology-a descriptive diagnostic evaluation study in a tertiary care center. Contemp Clin Dent. 2020;11(3):256–60.

46. Horvath A, Prekopp P, Polony G, Szekely E, Tamas L, Danos K. Accuracy of the preoperative diagnostic workup in patients with head and neck cancers undergoing neck dissection in terms of nodal metastases. Eur Arch Otorhinolaryngol. 2021;278(6):2041–6.

47. Sejwal P, Jaigwal M, Pandey S. Utility of fine needle aspiration cytology as a low cost tool to diagnose cervical lymphadenopathy. Iran J Pathol. 2018;13(3):340–7.

48. Kotowski U, Brkic FF, Koperek O, Nemec SF, Pensanidis C, Altorjai G, er al. Accuracy of FNA cytology in suspicious neck nodes after radiotherapy: retrospective analysis of 100 patients. Clin Otolaryngol. 2019;44(3):384–8.

49. Orell SR, Skinner JM. The tying of non-Hodgkins lymphomas using fine needle aspiration cytology. Pathology. 1982;14(4):389–94.

50. Russell J, Orell SR, Skinner JM, Seshadri R. Fine needle aspiration cytology in the management of lymphoma. Aust NZ J Med. 1983;13(4):365–8.

51. Levitt S, Cheng L, DuPuis MH, Layfield LJ. Fine needle aspiration diagnosis of malignant lymphoma with confirmation by immunoperoxidase staining. Acta Cytol. 1985;29(5):895–902.

52. Tani EM, Christensson B, Ponit A, Skoog L. Immunocytochemical analysis and cytomorphologic diagnosis on fine needle aspirates of lymphoproliferative disease. Acta Cytol. 1988;32(2):209–15.

53. Carter TR, Feidman PS, Innes D Jr, Frierson HF Jr, Frigy AF. The role of fine needle aspiration cytology in the diagnosis of lymphoma. Acta Cytol. 1988;32(6):848–53.

54. Hehn ST, Grogan TM, Miller TP. Utility of FNA as a diagnostic technique in lymphoma. J Clinoncol. 2004;22(15):3046–52.

55. Austin RM, Bridsong GG, Sidawy MK, Kamisnsky SB, Benstein BD, Chibas EB. Fine needle aspiration is a feasible and accurate technique in the diagnosis of lymphoma. J Clin Oncol. 2004;23(35):9029.

56. Caraway NP. Evolving role of FNA biopsy in diagnosing lymphoma: past, present, and future. Cancer Cytopathol. 2015;123(7):389–93.

57. Wang H, Shankar Hariharan V, Sarma S. Diagnostic accuracy of FNA cytology for lymphoma: a systematic review and meta-analysis. Diag Cytopathol. 2021;49(9):975–86.

58. Labarca G, Sierra-Ruiz M, Kheir F, Folch E, Majid A, Mehta H, et al. Diagnostic accuracy of endobronchial ultrasound transbronchial needle aspiration in lymphoma. A systematic review and meta-analysis. Ann Am Thorac Soc. 2019;16(11):1432–9.

59. Jelloul FZ, Navarro M, Navale P, Hagan T, Cocker RS, Das K, et al. Diagnosis of lymphoma using FNA biopsy and core-needle biopsy: a single-institution experience. Acta Cytol. 2019;63:198–205.

60. Das DK. Contribution of immunocytochemistry to the diagnosis of usual and unusual lymphoma cases. J Cytol. 2018;35(3):163–9.

61. Houcine Y, Romdhane F, Blei A, Ksentini M, Aloui R, Lahiani R, et al. Evaluation of fine0needle aspiration cytology in the diagnosis of cervical lymph node lymphomas. J Craniomaxillofac Surg. 2018;46(7):1117–20.

62. Senturk A, Babaoglu E, Kilic H, Dogan HT, Hasanoglu HC, et al. Endobronchial ultrasound-guided transbronchial needle aspiration in the diagnosis of lymphoma. Asian Pac J Cancer Prev. 2014;15:4169–73.

63. Dhooria S, Mehta RM, Madan K, Biswanath G, Sehgal IS, Chhajed PN, et al. A multicenter study on the utility of EBUS-TBNA and EUS-B-FNA in the diagnosis of mediastinal lymphoma. J Bronchology Interv Pulmonol. 2019;26:199–209.

64. Al-Abbadi M, Barroca H, Bode-Lesniewska B, Calaminici M, Caraway NP, Chhieng DF, et al. A proposal for the performance, classification, and reporting of lymph node FNA cytopathology: the Sydney System. Acta Cytol. 2020;64(4):306–22.

65. Cinberg JZ, Silver CE, Molnar JJ, Vogl SE. Cervical cysts: cancer until proven otherwise? Laryngoscope. 1982;92(1):27–30.

66. Andrews PJ, Giddings CEB, Su AP. Management of lateral cystic swellings of the neck, in the over 40's age group. J Laryngol Otol. 2003;117(4):318–20.

67. Tabet P, Saydy N, Letouorneau-Guillon L, Gologan O, Bissada E, Ayad T, et al. Cystic masses of the lateral neck: diagnostic value comparison between FNA core-needle biopsy, and frozen section. Head and Neck. 2019;41(8):2696–703.

68. Begbie F, Visvanathan V, Clark LJ. Fine needle aspiration cytology versus frozen section in branchial cleft cysts. J Laryngol Otol. 2015;129(2):174–8.

69. Burgess KL, Hartwick RWJ, Bedard YC. Metastatic squamous cell carcinoma presenting as a neck cyst: differential diagnosis from inflamed branchial cleft cyst in fine-needle aspirates. Acta Cytol. 1993;17(4):494–8.

70. Nordemar S, Tani E, Hogmo A, Jangard M, AuenG M-WW. Image cytometry DNA-analysis of fine needle aspiration cytology to aid cytomorphology in the distinction of branchial cleft cyst from cystic metastasis of squamous cell carcinoma: a prospective study. Laryngoscope. 2004;114(11):1997–2000.

71. Wenokur R, Andrews JC, Abemayor E, Bailet J, Layfield L, Canalis RF, et al. Magnetic resonance imaging-guided FNA for the diagnosis of skull base lesions. Skull Base Surg. 1992;2(3):167–70.

72. Caldemeyer KS, Pritz MB. CT-guided percutaneous FNA biopsy of posterior skull base lesions. Skull Base Surg. 1999;9(2):161–5.

73. Spearman M, Curtin H, Duscnbery D, Janecka LP, Reyna EL. Computed tomography-directed FNA of skull base parapharyngeal and infratemporal fossa masses. Skull Base Surg. 1995;5(4):199–205.

74. Connor SEJ, Chaudhary N. CT-guided percutaneous core biopsy of deep face and skull-base lesions. Clin Radiol. 2008;63(9):986–94.

75. Zhu JH, Yang R, Guo YX, Wang J, Liu XJ, Guo CB. Navigation-guided core needle biopsy for skull base and parapharyngeal lesions: a five-year experience. Int J Oral Maxillofac Surg. 2021;50(1):7–13.

76. Matsaki T, Miura K, Tada Y, Masubuchi T, Fashimi C, Kanno C, et al. Classification of tumors by imaging diagnosis and preoperative FNA cytology in 120 patients with tumors in the parapharyngeal space. Head Neck. 2019;41(5):1277–81.

77. Wong KT, Tsang RKY, Tse GMK, Yuen EHY, Ahuja AT. Biopsy of deep-seated head and neck lesions under intraoral ultrasound guidance. AJNR. 2006;27(8):1654–7.

78. Layfield LJ, Schmidt RL, Sangle N, Crim JR. Diagnostic accuracy and clinical utility of biopsy in musculoskeletal lesions: comparison of fine-needle aspiration, core and open biopsy techniques. Diagn Cytopathol. 1014;42(6):476–86.

79. Leonetti JP, Donzelli JJ, Littooy FN, Farrell BP. Perioperative strategies in the management of carotid body tumors. Otolaryngol Head Neck Surg. 1997;117(1):111–5.

80. Fleming MV, Oertel YC, Rodriguez ER, Fidler WJ. FNA of six carotid body paragangliomas. Diagn Cytopathol. 1993;9(5):510–5.

81. Kapila K, Tewari MC, Verma. Paragangliomas – a diagnostic dilemma on fine-needle aspirates. Indian J. Cancer. 1993;30(4):152–7.

82. Choy KC, Bandele MM, Fu EW, Li H, Gan JYJ. Risk stratification of parotid neoplasms based on intraoperative frozen section and preoperative FNA cytology. Eur Arch Otorhinolaryngol. 2022;279(4):2117–31.

83. Pastorello RG, Rodriguez EF, McCormick BA, Calsavara VF, Chen LC, Zarka MA. Is there a role for frozen section evaluation of parotid masses after preoperative cytology or biopsy diagnosis? Head Neck Pathol. 2021;15(3):859–65.

84. Heller KS, Attie JN, Dubner S. Accuracy of frozen section in the evaluation of salivary tumors. Am J Surg. 1993;166:424–7.

85. Mantsopoulos K, Bessas Z, Sievert M, Muller SK, Koch M, Agaimy A, et al. Frozen section of parotid gland tumours: the head and neck pathologist as a key member of the surgical team. J Clin Med. 2022;11(5):1249.

86. Dindzans LJ, Van Nostrand AW. The accuracy of frozen section diagnosis of parotid lesions. J Otolaryngol. 1984;13(6):382–6.

87. Wheelis RF, Yarington JRCT. Tumors of the salivary glands. Comparison of frozen section diagnosis with final pathologic diagnosis. Arch Otolaryngol. 1984;110(2):76–7.

88. Rigual NR, Milley P, Lore' JM, Kaufman S. Accuracy of frozen-section diagnosis in salivary gland neoplasms. Head Neck Surg. 1986;8(6):442–6.

89. Carralho MB, Soares JM, Rapoport A, Sebrinho JA, Fava AS, Kanda JL, et al. Perioperative frozen section examination in parotid gland tumors. Sao Paulo Med J. 1999;117(6):233–7.

90. Mianroodi AAA, Sigston EA, Vallance NA. Frozen section for parotid surgery: should it become routine? ANZ J Surg. 2006;76(8):736–9.

91. Olsen KD, Moore EJ, Lewis JE. Frozen section pathology for decision making in parotid surgery. JAMA Otolaryngol Head Neck Surg. 2013;139(12):1275–8.

92. Seethals RR, LiVolsi VA, Baloch ZW. Relative accuracy of FNA and frozen section in the diagnosis of lesions of the parotid gland. Head Neck. 2005;27(3):217–23.

93. Cohen MB, Ljung BM, Boles R. Salivary gland tumors. FNA vs frozen section diagnosis. Archotolaryngol Head Neck Surg. 1986;112(8):867–9.

94. Miller RH, Calcaterra TC, Paglia DE. Accuracy of frozen section diagnosis of parotid lesions. Ann Otol Rhinol Laryngol. 1979;88(4):573–6.

95. Zbaren P, Trantafyllou A, Devaney KO, Vanderpoorter V, Hellquist H, Rinaldo A, et al. Preoperative diagnostic of parotid gland neoplasms: FNA cytology or core needle biopsy? Eur Arch Otorhinolaryngol. 2018;275(11):2609–13.

96. Witt BL, Schmidt RL. Ultrasound-guided core needle biopsy of salivary gland lesions: a systematic review and meta-analysis laryngoscope. 2014;124(3):695–700.

97. Haldar S, Sinnott JD, Tekeli KM, Turner SS, Howlett DC. Biopsy of parotid masses: review of current techniques. World J Radiol. 2016;8(5):501–5.

98. Del Cura JL, Coronado G, Zabula R, Korta I, Lopez I. Accuracy and effectiveness of ultrasound-guided core-needle biopsy in the diagnosis of focal lesions in the salivary glands. EurRadiol. 2018;28(7):2934–41.

99. Novoa E, Gurtler N, Arnoux A, Kraft M. Diagnostic value of core needle biopsy and FNA in salivary gland lesions. Head Neck. 2016;38 Suppl 1:E 346-52.

100. Cho J, Kim J, Lee JS, Chee CG, Kim Y, Choi SII. Comparison of core needle biopsy and FNA in diagnosis of malignant salivary gland neoplasm: systematic review and meta-analysis. Head Neck. 2020;42(10):3041–50.

101. Bugra Cengiz A, Tansuker HD, Gul R, Emre F, Demirbas T, Oktay MF. Comparison of preoperative diagnostic accuracy of FNA and core biopsy in parotid gland neoplasms. Eur Arch Otorhinolaryngol. 2021;278(10):4067–74.

102. Schmidt RL, Hall BH, Wilson AR, Layfield LJ. A systematic review and meta-analysis of the diagnostic accuracy of FNA cytology for parotid gland lesions. Am J Clin Pathol. 2011;136(1):45–59.

103. Mavec P, Eneroth CM, Franzen S, S, Moberger G, Zajicek J. Aspiration biopsy of salivary gland tumours: I. Correlationof cytologic reports from 652 aspiration biopsies with clinical and histologic findings. Acta Oto-Laryngologic. 1964;58:471–84.

104. Yildiz S, Seneldir L, Karaca CT, Toros SZ. FNA cytology of salivary gland tumors before the Milan System: ten years of experience at a tertiary care center in Turkey. Medeni Med J. 2021;36(3):233–40.

105. Inancli HM, Kanmuz MA, Ural A, Dilek GB. FNA biopsy: in the diagnosis of salivary gland neoplasms compared with hisopathology. Indian J Otolaryngol Head and Neck Surg. 2013;65(Suppl 1):121–5.

106. Baloch Z, Field AS, Katabi N, Wenig BM. The Milan system for reporting salivary gland cytopathology. In: Faquin WC, Rossi ED, editors. The Milan system for reporting salivary gland cytopathology. 1st ed. Cham: Springer; 2018. p. 1–9.

107. Layfield LJ, Tan P, Glasgow BJ. FNA of salivary gland lesions. Comparison with frozen sections and histologic findings. Arch Pathol Lab Med. 1987;111(4):346–53.

108. Vergez S, Fakhry N, Cartier C, Kennel T, Courtade M, Uro-Coste E, et al. Guidelines of the French Society of Otorhinolaryngology -Head and Neck Surgery (SFORL), part I: primary treatment of pleomorphic adenoma. Eur Ann Otohinoloryngol Head Neck Dis. 2021;138(4):269–74.

109. Nakazawa H, Rosen P, Lane N, Lattes R. Frozen section experience in 3000 cases. Accuracy, limitations, and value in residency training. Am J Clin Pathol. 1968;49:41–51.

110. Bredahl E, Simonsen J. Routine performance of intro-operative frozen microscopy with particular reference to diagnostic accuracy. Acta Pathol Microbiol Scand Suppl. 1970;212:104.

111. Paphavasit A, Thompson GB, Hay ID, et al. Follicular and Harthle cell thyroid neoplasms. Is frozen-section evaluation worthwhile? Arch Surg. 1997;132:674–8.

112. Montone KT, LiVolsi V. Frozen section analysis of thyroidectomy specimens: experience over a 12-year period. Pathol Case Rev. 1998.

113. DeMay RM. Frozen section of thyroid? Just say no. Am J Clin Pathol. 1998;110:423–4.

114. LiVolsi BZW. Use and abuse of frozen section in the diagnosis of follicular thyroid lesions. Endocr Pathol. 2005;16(4):285–93.

115. Sanabria A, Zafereo M, Thompson LDR, Hernandez-Prera JC, Kowalski LP, Nixon IJ, er al. Frozen section in thyroid gland follicular neoplasms: it's high time to abandon it! Surg Oncol. 2021;36:76–81.

116. Kopald KH, Layfield LJ, Mohrmann R, Foshag LJ, Giuliano AE. Clarifying the role of FNA cytologic evaluation and frozen section examination in the operative management of thyroid cancer. Arch Surg. 1989;124(10):1201–4.

117. Tallini G, Gallo C. FNA and intraoperative consultation in thyroid pathology: when and how? Int J Surg Pathol. 2011;19(2):141–4.

118. Ye Q, Woo JS, Zhao Q, Wang P, Huang P, Chen L, et al. FNA versus frozen section in the evaluation of malignant thyroid nodules in patients with the diagnosis of suspicious for malignancy or malignancy by FNA. Arch Pathol Lab Med. 2017;141(5):684–9.

119. Boyd LA, Earnhardt RC, DunnJT FHF, Hank JB. Preoperative evaluation and predictive value of FNA and frozen section of thyroid nodules. J Am Coll Surg. 1998;187(5):494–502.

120. Kim HC, Kim YJ, Hau HY, Yi JM, Baek JH, Park SY, et al. First-line use of core needle biopsy for high-yield preliminary diagnosis of thyroid nodules. AJNR Am J Neuroradiol. 2017;382(2):357–63.

121. Trimboli P, Crescenzi A. Thyroid core needle biopsy: taking stock of the situation. Endocrine. 2015;48(3):779–85.

122. Choi WJ, Back JH. Role of core biopsy for patients with indeterminate FNA cytology. Endocrine. 2014;45(1):1–2.

123. Qui XY, Dong XY, Huang ZL, Hu QH, Chen SX, Fan XM. Role of core-needle biopsy in thyroid nod-

ules with initially non-diagnostic cytologic results. Radiology. 2014;270(2):629–30.

124. Hakala T, Kholova I, Sand J, Saaristo P, Kellokampu-Lehtinen P. A core needle biopsy provides more malignancy-specific results than FNA biopsy in thyroid nodules suspicious for malignancy. J Clin Pathol. 2013;66(12):1046–50.

125. Hahn SY, Shin JH, Han BK, Ko EY, Ko ES. Ultrasonography-guided core needle biopsy for the thyroid nodule: does the procedure hold any benefit for the diagnosis when FNA cytology analysis shows inclusive results? Br J Radiol. 2013;86(1025):20130007.

126. Chen BT, Jain AB, Dagis A, Chu P, Vora L, Maghami E. Comparison of efficiency and safety of ultrasound-guided core needle biopsy vs FNA for evaluating thyroid nodules. Endocr Pract. 2015;21(2):128–35.

127. Carpi A, Rossi G, Nicolini A, Iervasi G, Russo M, Mechanick J. Does large needle aspiration biopsy add pain to the thyroid nodule evaluation? PLoS One. 2013;8(3):e58016.

128. Stangierski A, Wolinski K, Martin K, Leitgeber O, Ruchala M. Core needle biopsy of thyroid nodules-evaluation of diagnostic utility and pain experience. Neruo Endocrinol Lett. 2013;34(8):798–801.

129. Yoon JH, Kim EK, Kwak JY, Moon HJ. Effectiveness and limitations of core needle biopsy in the diagnosis of thyroid nodules: review of current literature. J Pathol Transl Med. 2015;49(3):230–5.

130. Li L, Chen BD, Shu HF, Wu S, Wei D, Zhang JQ, et al. Comparison of pre-operation diagnosis of thyroid cancer with fine needle aspiration and core-needle biopsy: a meta-analysis. Asian Pac J Cancer Prev. 2014;15(17):7187–93.

131. Cao H, Kuo RH, Hsieh MC. Comparison of core-needle biopsy and FNA in screening for thyroid malignancy 6 systematic review and meta-analysis. Curr Med Res Opin. 2016;32(7):1291–301.

132. Wolinski K, Stangierski A, Ruchala M. Comparison of diagnostic yield of core-needle and FNA biop-sies of thyroid lesions: systematic review and meta-analysis. Eur Radiol. 2017;27(1):431–6.

133. Pisani T, Bononi M, Nagar C, Angelini M, Bezzi M, Vecchione A. Fine needle and core biopsy techniques in the diagnosis of nodular thyroid pathologies. Anti cancer Res. 2000;20(C):3843–7.

134. Suh CH, Baek JH, Kim KW, Sung TY, Kim TY, Song DE. The role of core-needle biopsy for thyroid nodules with initially non-diagnostic FNA results: a systematic review and meta-analysis. Endocr Pract. 2016;22(6):679–88.

135. Samir AE, Vij A, Seale MK, Desai G, Halpern E, Faquin WC. Ultrasound-guided percutaneous thyroid nodule core biopsy: clinical utility in patient with prior nondiagnostic fine-needle aspirate. Thyroid. 2012;22(5):461–7.

136. Baloch ZW, Cooper DS, Gharib H, Alexander EK. Overview of diagnostic terminology and reporting. In: Ali SZ, Cibas ES, editors. The Bethesda system for reporting thyroid cytopathology. 2nd ed. Cham: Springer; 2018. p. 1–6.

137. Solbiati L, Montali G, Croce F, Bellotti E, Giangrande A, Ravetto C. Parathyroid tumors detected by FNA biopsy under ultrasonic guidance. Radiology. 1983;148(3):793–7.

138. Sacks BA, Pallotta JA, Cole A, Hanwitz J. Diagnosis of parathyroid adenomas: efficacy of measuring parathormone levels in needle aspirates of cervical masses. AJR Am J Roentgenol. 1994;163(5):1223–6.

Lester J. Layfield is a Professor of pathology at the Department of Pathology and Laboratory Medicine, Columbia, MO, USA. He has published over 450 peer-reviewed manuscripts, the majority of which are related to cytopathology. He has presented at numerous national and international meetings, including the ECC, USCAP, and the ASC. His areas of interest include cytopathology of bone and soft tissue lesions, head and neck lesions, and pancreaticobiliary cytology.

Differential Cytological Diagnosis of Salivary Tumors

11

Jerzy Klijanienko and Philippe Vielh

11.1 Introduction

Since there is no specific radiological or clinical diagnostic criteria for an accurate diagnosis, preoperative fine-needle aspiration (FNA) became a classical diagnostic technique in salivary gland tumors.

FNA is a rapid, repetitive, and noninvasive technique. However, FNA may be assisted by the rapid on situ evaluation (ROSE) using Diff-Quik stain, which will allow fast (1 minute) initial diagnosis. ROSE permits an appreciation of quality of cellular material and eventually indicates further cytoponcture passes. If the ROSE diagnosis is not clear, additional passes to obtain cellular material for immunocytochemistry using liquid-based cytology or cell-block for or for molecular analyses may be indicated. Similarly, samples for flow cytometry may be realized in case of possibility of malignant lymphoma. Finally, paraffin inclusion or core-needle biopsy may be indicated for theranostic purposes in some instances (usually metastatic disease).

Palpable lesions may be sampled using palpation-guided technique, whereas nonpalpable lesions may be sampled using ultrasound-guided technique. It is recommended that cytoponctures are performed in a room with a microscope and with a water access, which is necessary for ROSE staining.

In case of suspicious diagnosis of malignancy, frozen-section procedure may be programmed and an operative strategy may be definitely established before surgery. Radical surgery versus salivary gland preservation may be therefore defined. Similarly, when the results are malignant, lymph node clearance may also be programmed.

Finally, ROSE allows the patient and the surgeon to plan their occupations. Negative results, which are common in salivary glands, also have an important psychological impact on the patient.

11.2 FNA in Salivary Gland Tumors: Statistics of Excellence

Salivary gland tumors are rarc, and their therapeutic management should be centralized in a specialized oncology centers. Depending of experience, performances of preoperative FNA may vary from center to center (Table 11.1). Early series before 1995 [1–5] are usually not sufficiently informative since diagnostic nomenclature and comprehension have substantially changed. Until recent times, certain carcinomatous entities (like mucoepidermoid carcinoma or

J. Klijanienko (✉)
Institute Curie, Pathology, Paris, France
e-mail: jerzy.klijanienko@curie.fr

P. Vielh
Medipath & American Hospital of Paris,
Neuilly/Seine, France

© The Author(s), under exclusive license to Springer Nature Switzerland AG 2024
J. Klijanienko et al. (eds.), *Diagnostic Procedures in Patients with Neck Masses*,
https://doi.org/10.1007/978-3-031-67675-8_11

Table 11.1 FNA performance in salivary gland tumors. Selected series including few historical reports [1–3]

References	Year	Number of cases	Accuracy %	Sensitivity %	Specificity %
[1]	1967	690	64	95	89
[2]	1973	216	86	99	95
[3]	1989	119	87.7	80.9	94.3
[4]	1990	79	80	84	98.4
[5]	1993	582	93	99	97
[6]	1995	325	85	99	94
[21]	1997	153		97.4	96.9
[22]	1998	816	97	98	98
[20]	2000	1253	94	97	95
[23]	2010	382	83	99	93
[24]	2014	182	94	100	99

acinic cell carcinoma) were classified as "tumor" because indolent carcinological evolution was observed in low-grade forms. Adenomas were also initially classified as monomorphic adenomas and pleomorphic adenomas. Moreover, certain entities were not yet recognized: salivary duct carcinoma, hyalinizing clear cell carcinoma, or sialoblastoma. Because of rarity of salivary tumors, it was difficult to collect representative series, and the time of education was long, taking few decades in the literature. In 1995, Orell et al. [6] have revisited publications of salivary gland tumors and established referential points. Up to 2000, Klijanienko and Vielh reported a series of publications referring to particular entities of salivary gland tumors [7–19]. Identified morphological parameters in specific lesions were described and analyzed in a monograph, which was published in 2000 [20].

Collective comparison of large and more recently (after 1995) published series shows that FNA is a highly accurate procedure in salivary gland tumors, with an accuracy of higher than 85%, a sensitivity of higher than 97%, and a specificity of higher than 93%.

FNA performances may vary in particular entities. High-grade malignancies are composed from atypical cells, which can be easily recognized on smears. Low-grade malignancies may present diagnostic challenge since moderate or weak cytonuclear atypia may simulate benign tumors.

Table 11.2 shows FNA performances in benign salivary lesions in our hands. Comparing

the three most frequent salivary adenomas which were published previously [7, 8, 17], benign, suspicious/false positive, and unsatisfactory diagnostic categories are 93.1%, 3.2%, and 3.7%, respectively. In the group of other pseudotumoral benign conditions (lymphoepithelial lesion, cysts, Küttner tumor), benign, suspicious/false positive, and unsatisfactory diagnostic categories are 87%, 4.2%, and 8.8%, respectively. Combining adenomas and benign pseudotumors, benign, suspicious/false positive, and unsatisfactory diagnostic categories are 92.5%, 3.3%, and 4.2%, respectively.

Analyzing particular benign lesions, we found that pleomorphic adenoma, basal cell adenoma, and Warthin tumor are relatively easy to diagnose by FNA, whereas Küttner tumor (atrophic chronic sialadenitis) is more difficult and may be misdiagnosed as low-grade mucoepidermoid carcinoma, especially in submandibular localizations.

Table 11.3 show FNA performances in malignancies. FNA performances are more heterogeneous in malignancies. Comparing the results from our published series [9–19, 25], malignant, suspicious, false-negative, and unsatisfactory rate are 80.5%, 4.6%, 11.9%, and 3%, respectively.

Analyzing particular malignant entities, we found that all high-grade carcinomas like adenoid cystic carcinoma, salivary duct carcinoma, and primary squamous cell carcinomas are relatively easy to diagnose, whereas low-grade carcinomas like acinic cell carcinoma, low-grade mucoepidermoid carcinoma, and carcinoma ex pleomorphic adenomas are more difficult with a high rate

Table 11.2 Diagnostic FNA accuracy: Benign lesions from our published series [7, 8, 17]. Selected entities

Type	Number of cases	Benign %	Suspicious/False Positive %	Unsatisfactory %
Pleomorphic adenoma	1747	94	3	3
Basal cell adenoma	42	83.3	16.7	0
Warthin tumor	265	92.1	2.3	5.7
Subtotal adenomas	**2189**	**93.1**	**3.2**	**3.7**
Benign lymphoepithelial lesion	49	96	2	2
Cysts	48	85.4	6.3	8.3
Küttner tumor	89	78.7	5.6	15.7
Subtotal pseudotumors	**216**	**87**	**4.2**	**8.8**
Total benign	**2405**	**92.5**	**3.3**	**4.2**

Table 11.3 Diagnostic FNA accuracy: Selected malignant entities. Based mainly on our previously published series [9–19, 25]

Type	Number of cases	Malignant %	Suspicious %	False Negative %	Unsatisfactory %
Adenoid Cystic Carcinoma	247	83	3.2	12.2	1.6
Acinic Cell carcinoma	158	74.4	3.8	19	2.5
Mucoepidermoid carcinoma	169	58.6	8.9	23	9.5
Salivary Duct Carcinoma	54	92.6	1.8	5.6	0
Carcinoma ex Pleomorphic Adenoma	68	54.4	8.8	35.3	1.5
Primary Squamous Cell Carcinoma	73	91.8	1.4	4.1	2.7
TOTAL MALIGNANT	1355	80.5	4.6	11.9	3

of false-negative diagnoses. Acinic cell carcinoma may be misdiagnosed with sialadenosis, low-grade mucoepidermoid carcinoma with Warthin tumor or salivary cyst, and carcinoma ex pleomorphic adenoma with pleomorphic adenoma, especially when a carcinomatous component is intraadenoma and of low-grade malignancy.

11.3   Differential FNA Components in Salivary Tumors

As previously published [20], both benign and malignant salivary tumors may be classified according to the predominant cell type (Table 11.4). Smears from salivary tumors are usually cell-rich and stroma-rich. Recognizing the nature of the stroma and secretions is as important as recognizing these cellular elements in this pathology. It is therefore essential to use a stain that allows morphological analysis of the stromal tissue. The exclusive use of Papanicolaou may limit the morphological spectrum and therefore diminish the quality observation. It seems logical to use May Grunwald Giemsa (MGG) or Diff Quik and eventually Papanicolaou stains in parallel in order to be able to recognize correctly the nature of the connective tissue (Fig. 11.1).

Epithelial cells (acinic cells, ductal cells, myoepithelial cells, mucus-secreting cells, squamous cells, oncocytic cells, naked nuclei) and connective cells (lymphocytes, chondrocytes, osteoblasts, fibroblasts) constitute the cellular material.

Chondromyxoid, hyaline globules, tubular formations, nonspecific connective debris, osteoid, mucus, crystals, inflammatory infiltrations, and necrosis constitute the stroma and the secretion material (Fig. 11.2).

Acinic cells, which are well differentiated, are large. Nuclei are small, with fine chromatin and minute nucleoli. In MGG, cytoplasm is grayish, micro-, or macrovacuolated. Moderately or poorly differentiated acinic cells are less specific

Table 11.4 Salivary gland tumoral entities depending of cellular predominance of the smears

Predominant cytology pattern	Salivary tumor entity
Myoepithelial cells	Pleomorphic adenoma
	Adenoid cystic carcinoma
	Polymorphous carcinoma
	Epithelial-myoepithelial carcinoma
	Clear cell carcinoma
	Basal cell adenocarcinoma
Basal cells	Basal cell adenoma
	Canalicular adenoma
	Basal cell adenocarcinoma
	Adenoid cytic carcinoma
	Metastases
Oncocytic cells	Oncocytoma
	Warthin tumor
	Salivary duct carcinoma
	Oncocytic carcinoma
Squamous cells	Primary or secondary squamous cell carcinoma
	High-grade mucoepidermoid carcinoma
	Warthin tumor with squamous metaplasia
	Basal cell adenoma with squamous metaplasia
Poorly-differentiated malignant cells	Large cell undifferentiated carcinoma
	Squamous cell carcinoma
	Primary or metastatic neuroendocrine carcinoma
Chondromyxoid stroma	Pleomorphic adenoma
Mucus	Mucoepidermoid carcinoma
	Warthin tumor
	Pleomorphic adenoma
	Metastases
	Salivary cysts
	Küttner tumor
Necrosis	High-grade malignancies
	Squamous cell carcinoma
	Warthin tumor
	Inflammatory processes
	Metastases
Lymphocytes	Enlarged lymph node
	Malignant lymphoma
	Benign lymphoepithelial lesion
	Warthin tumor
	Acinic cell carcinoma
	Mucoepidermoid carcinoma
Cystic component	Salivary cyst
	Warthin tumor
	Acinic cell carcinoma
	Mucoepidermoid carcinoma
	Pleomorphic adenoma
	Primary or metastatic squamous cell carcinoma

Table 11.4 (continued)

Predominant cytology pattern	Salivary tumor entity
Naked nuclei	Acinic cell carcinoma
	Basal cell adenocarcinoma
	Sialadenosis
Paucicellular smear	Küttner tumor
	Fibrous tumors
	Lipomas
	Hemangiomas
	Sialadenosis
	Warthin tumor
	Salivary cyst
	Missed target

and adopt noncharacteristic epithelial morphology. They are isolated or clustered (Figs. 11.3 and 11.4).

Ductal cells are small-sized and frequently basaloid. Nuclei are regular with delicate chromatin. In MGG, cytoplasm are dark and grayish. Cells are usually clustered and associated to naked nuclei. Papanicolaou stain highlights their presence. They are usually clustered (Figs. 11.5, 11.6, and 11.7).

Myoepithelial cells may present in pleomorphism. Myoepithelial cells are plasmacytoid with eccentric nuclei. Nuclei are roundish or irregular with granular chromatin. In MGG, cytoplasm are blue and homogeneous. Some cytoplasmic vacuolization or clarification may be seen. Occasionally, myoepithelial cells are spindle or round. They are usually dispersed (Figs. 11.8, 11.9, 11.10, 11.11, and 11.12).

Mucus-secreting cells may be goblet or vacuolated cells with various-sized nuclei. Clear, vegetal cells may be observed in mucoepidermoid carcinoma. They are usually in small clusters (Fig. 11.13).

Squamous cells are pleomorphic. Well-differentiated, keratinizing cells are spindle, polygonal or roundish in shape. Nuclei are small and dark. Cytoplasm shows keratinization. Poorly differentiated cells are large, atypical, and necrotic. Frequently squamous cells are associated with necrosis. They are isolated or clustered. Benign-looking squamous cells are seen in squamous metaplasia (Figs. 11.14, 11.15, and 11.16).

Oncocytic cells may show pleomorphism. In some tumors, oncocytic cells are moderately large with small nuclei with delicate chromatin in

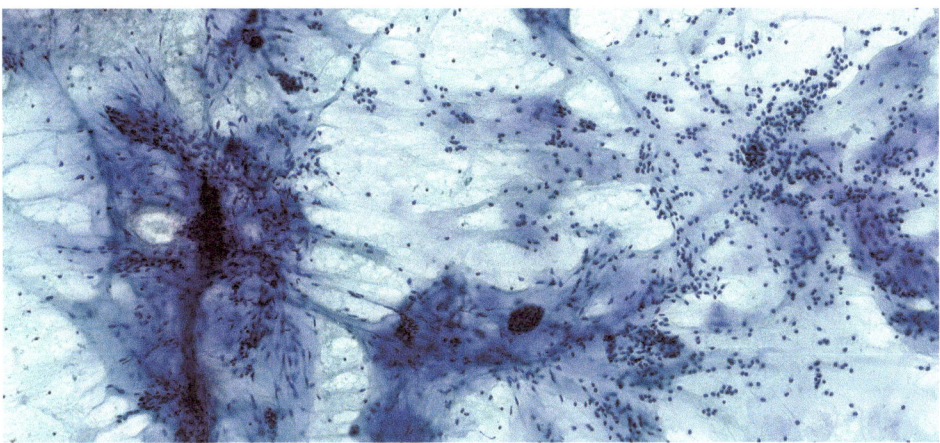

Fig. 11.1 Pleomorphic adenoma. Tinctorial specificities are less evident using Papanicolaou stain

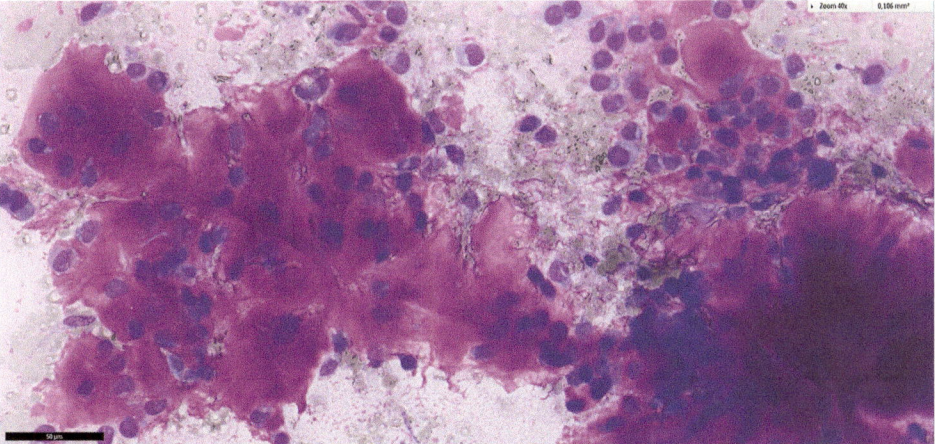

Fig. 11.2 Pleomorphic adenoma. Chondromyxoid stroma and plasmacytoid myoepithelial cells

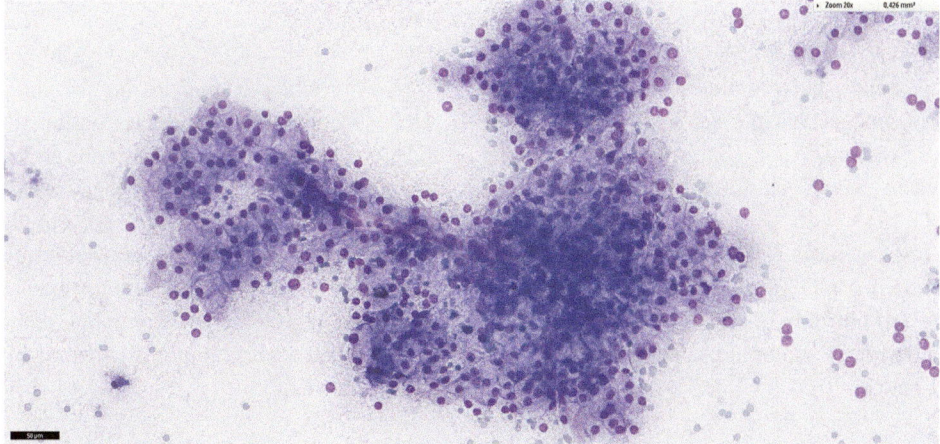

Fig 11.3 Well-differentiated acinic cell carcinoma. Acinic cells and naked nuclei

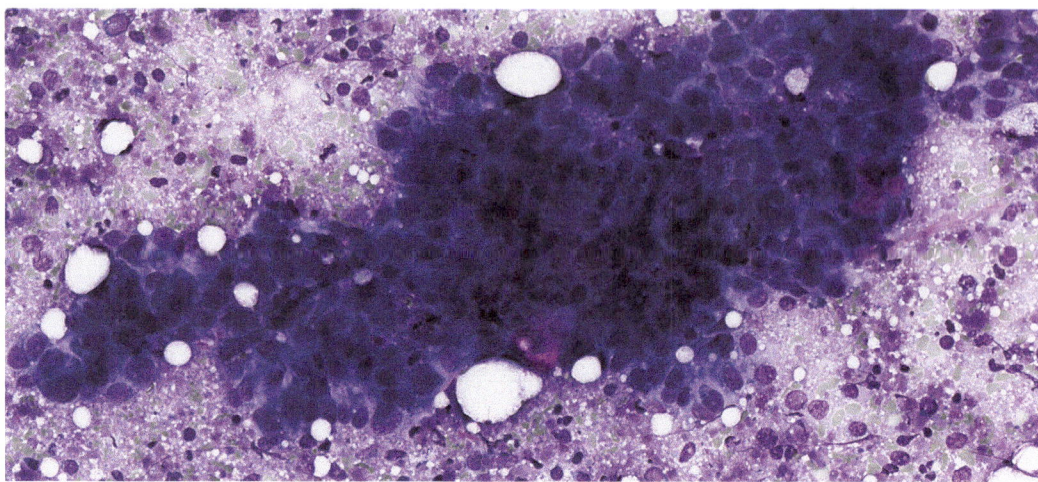

Fig 11.4 Poorly differentiated acinic cell carcinoma. Necrosis and atypia

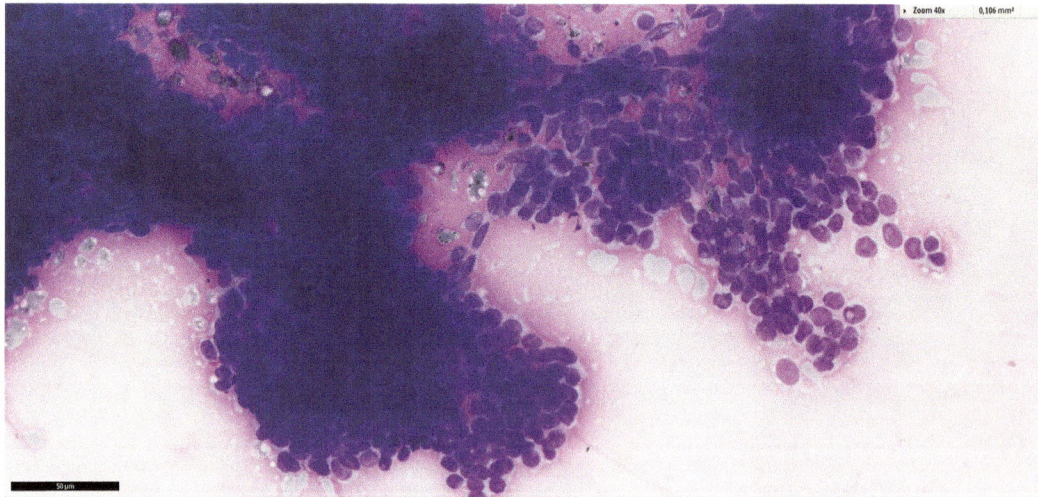

Fig 11.5 Basal cell adenoma. Ductal basaloid cells

single, small, but prominent nucleoli. In other tumors, oncocytic cells are large and polymorphous: roundish, polygonal, or spindle-shaped. They are usually clustered (Figs. 11.17, 11.18, and 11.19).

Chondromyxoid is characteristic pink–magenta in MGG. Chondromyxoid is irregular in shape and fibrillary in high power. Its presence is specific for pleomorphic adenoma (Figs. 11.1, 11.2, and 11.20).

Hyaline globules and tubular formations are composed of connective debris within roundish and elongated deposits. Usually cells are attached around or in the internal part (negative and positive). Hyaline globules are present in epimyoepithelial tumors like pleomorphic adenoma, adenoid cystic carcinoma, polymorphous adenocarcinoma, epithelial-myoepithelial carcinoma, and basal cell adenocarcinoma (Figs. 11.6, 11.20, 11.21, and 11.22).

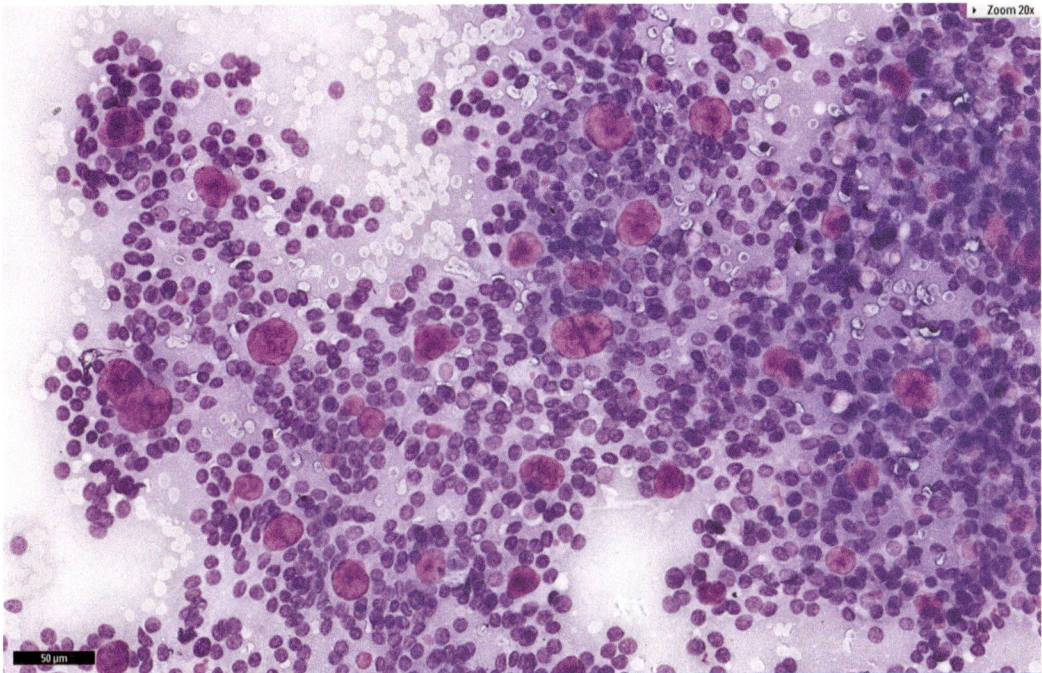

Fig 11.6 Basal cell adenocarcinoma. Ductal basaloid cells and hyaline globules

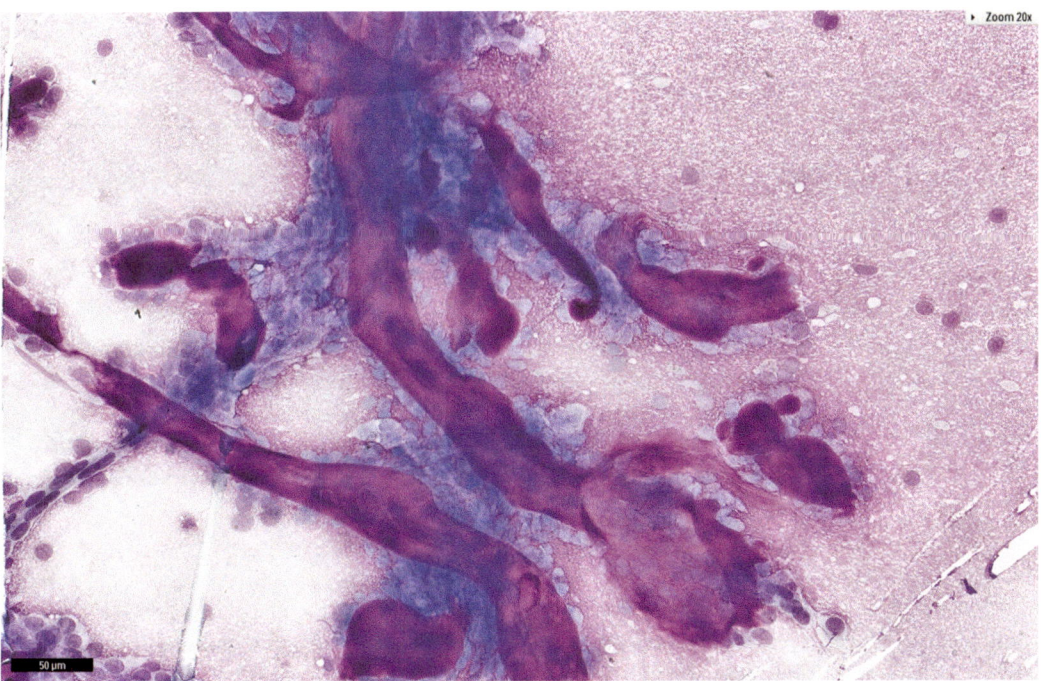

Fig 11.7 Adenoid cystic carcinoma. Tubular structures and basaloid cells

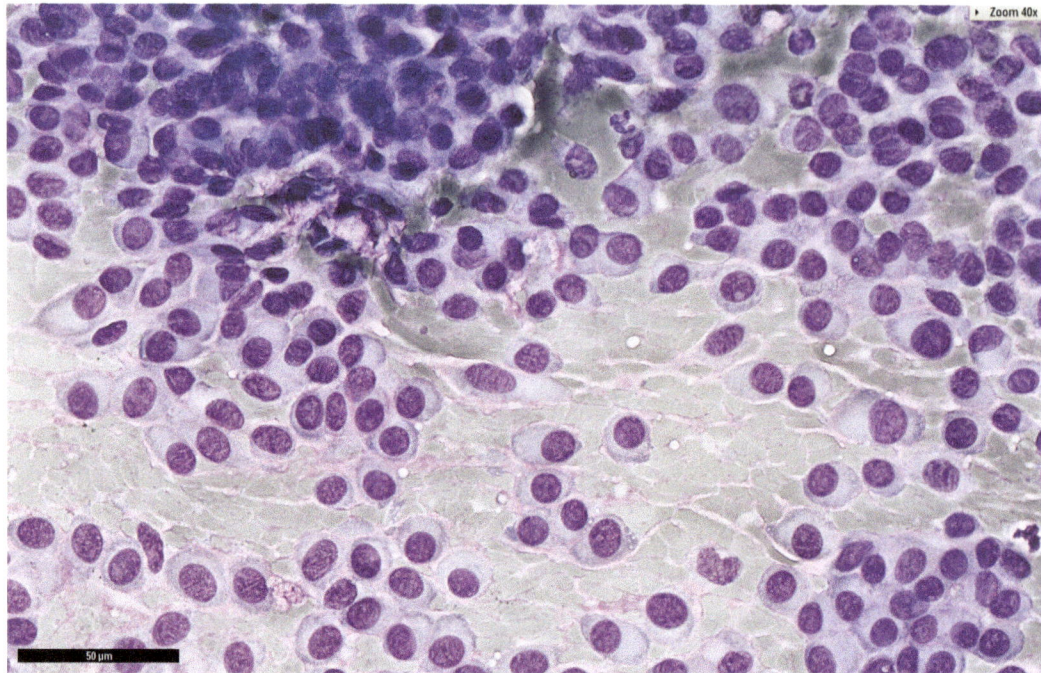

Fig 11.8 Myoepithelioma. Plasmacytoid myoepithelial cells

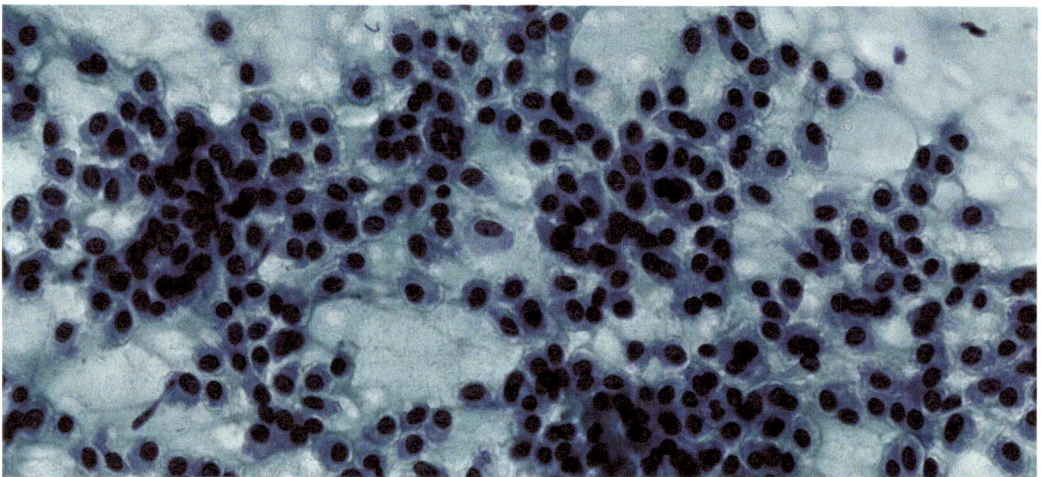

Fig 11.9 Myoepithelioma. Plasmacytoid myoepithelial cells without chondromyxoid

Nonspecific connective debris present as ill-limited fragments of connective tissue. They stain pinkish in MGG. Naked nuclei may be associated with connective tissue. They are usually present in basal cell adenomas (Fig. 11.23).

Osteoid is rare in salivary tumors. Usually, it is seen as yellowish or intensively red ill-delimited deposits in MGG. It is seen in rare pleomorphic adenomas or bone-forming sarcomas (Fig. 11.24).

Mucus may stain differently in MGG. Usually, it is metachromatic going from translucent to dark blue. Papanicolaou stain allows better to appreciate its content and analysis of "sub-

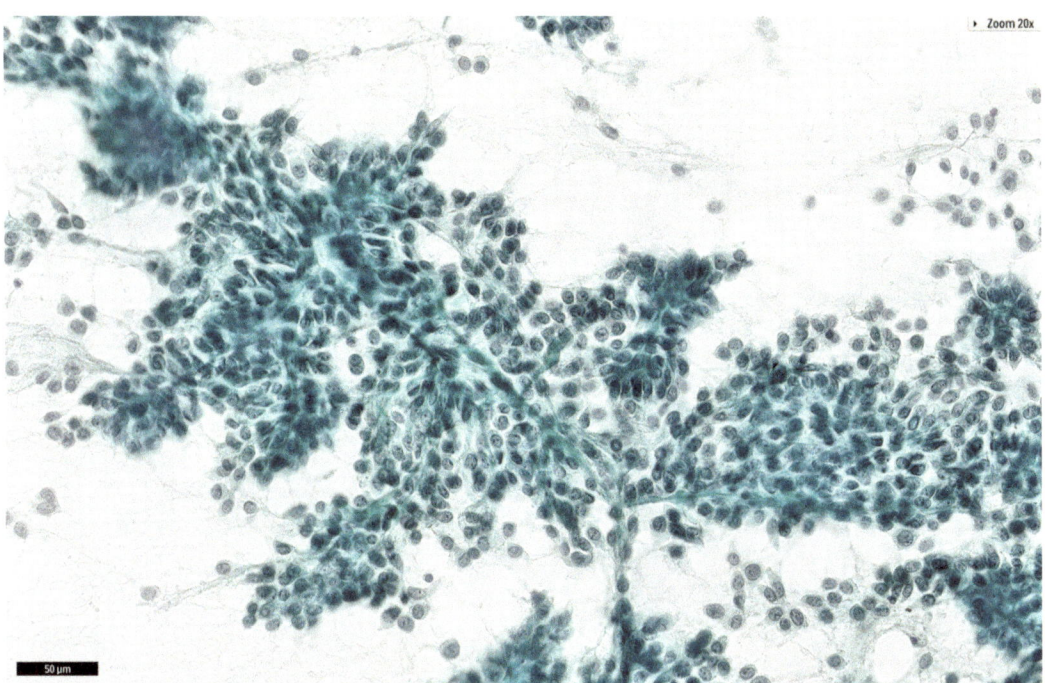

Fig 11.10   Myoepithelioma. Spindle-shaped myoepithelial cells

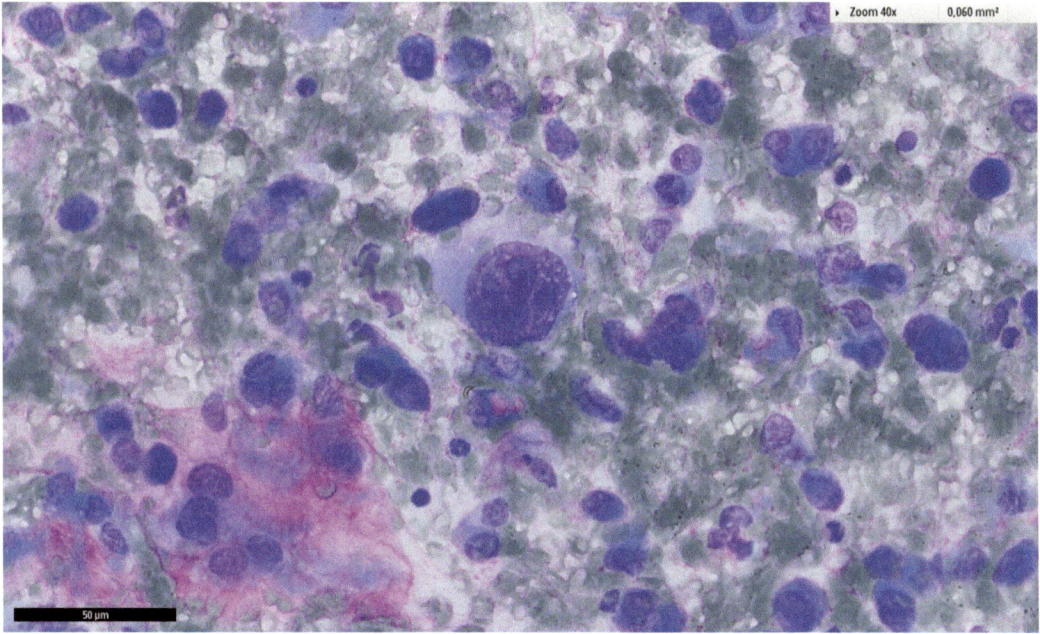

Fig 11.11   Pleomorphic adenoma. Atypical myoepithelial cells which are not indicative of malignant transformation

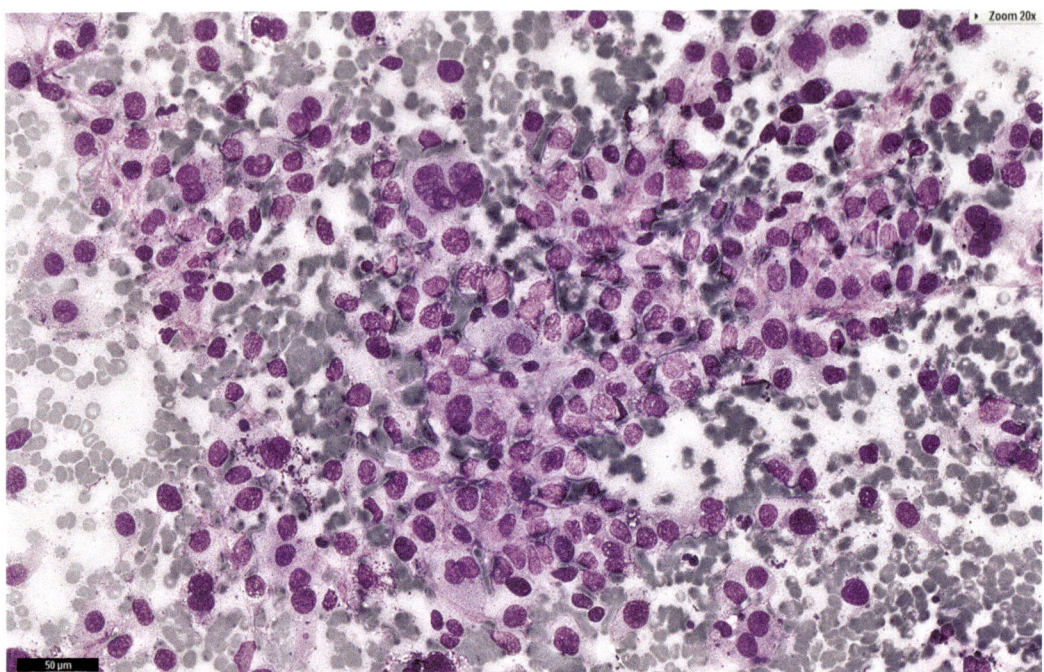

Fig 11.12 Myoepithelial carcinoma. Malignant myoepithelial cells

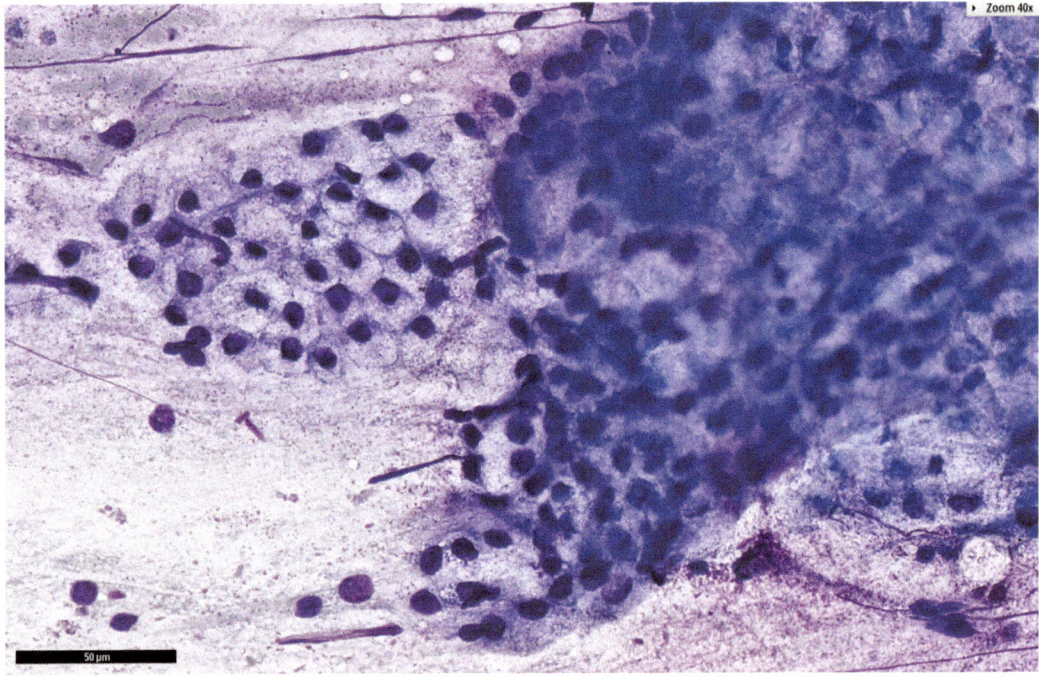

Fig 11.13 Mucoepidermoid carcinoma. Mucus secreting cells of vegetal morphology

Fig 11.14 Primary
squamous cell
carcinoma. Squamous
keratinizing cells

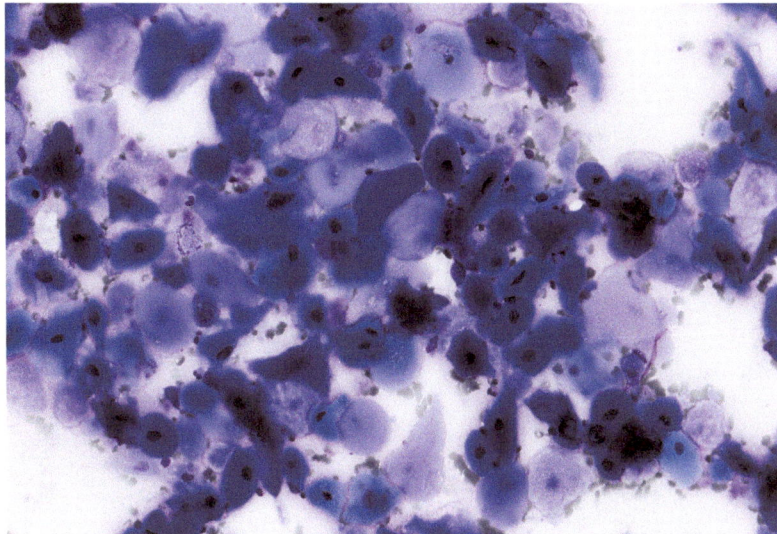

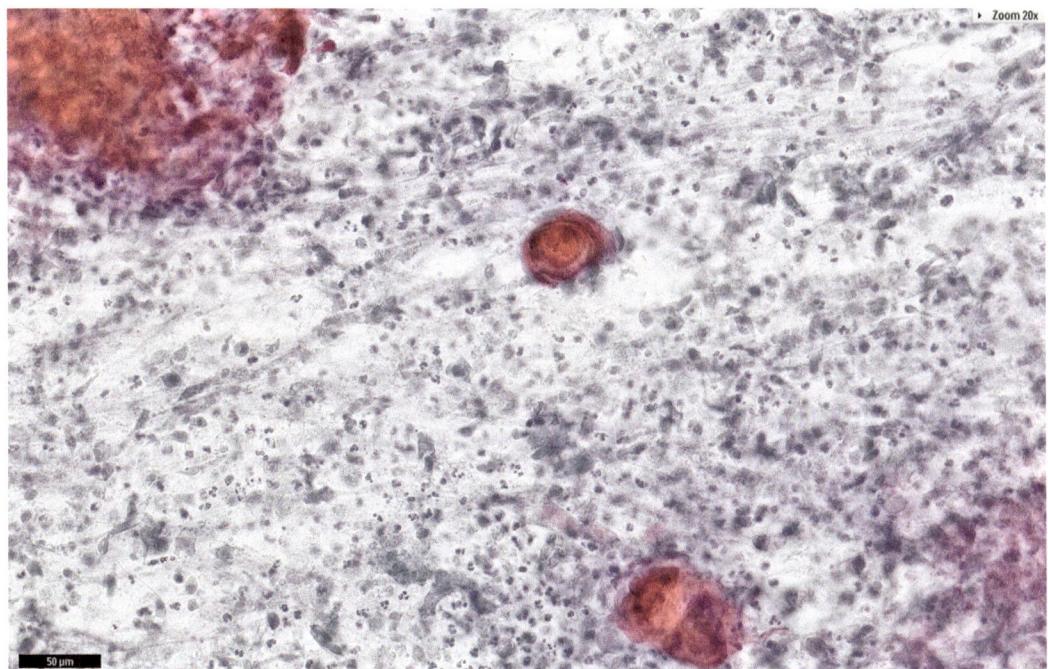

Fig 11.15 Mucoepidermoid carcinoma. Squamous cells and necrotic background

merged" cells. Mucus is present in large part of mucoepidermoid carcinoma, but similar substance is also observed in Warthin tumors, sialolithiasis, salivary cysts, and Küttner tumors (Figs. 11.25, 11.26, and 11.27).

Crystals are usually elements in favor of benignity. They are polymorphous and frequently translucent. They are present in some pleomorphic adenomas, salivary cysts, and inflammatory chronic processes (Fig. 11.28).

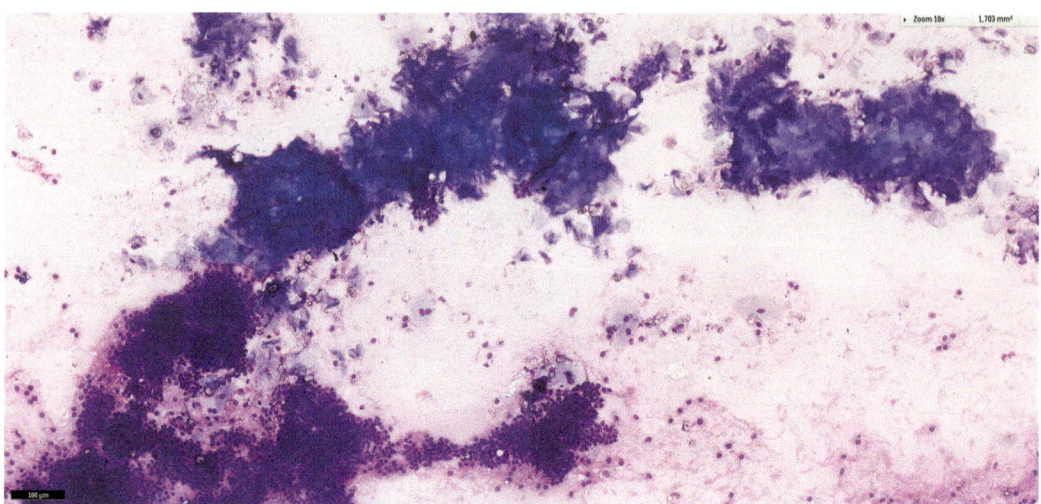

Fig 11.16 Pleomorphic adenoma. Metaplastic squamous cells

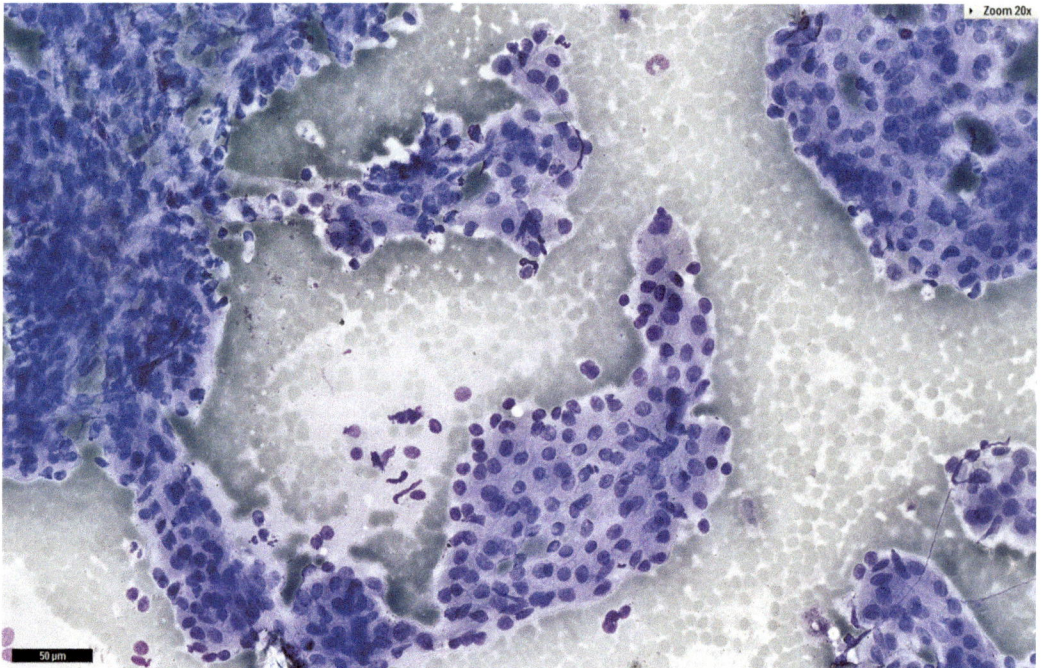

Fig 11.17 Oncocytoma. Oncocytic cells

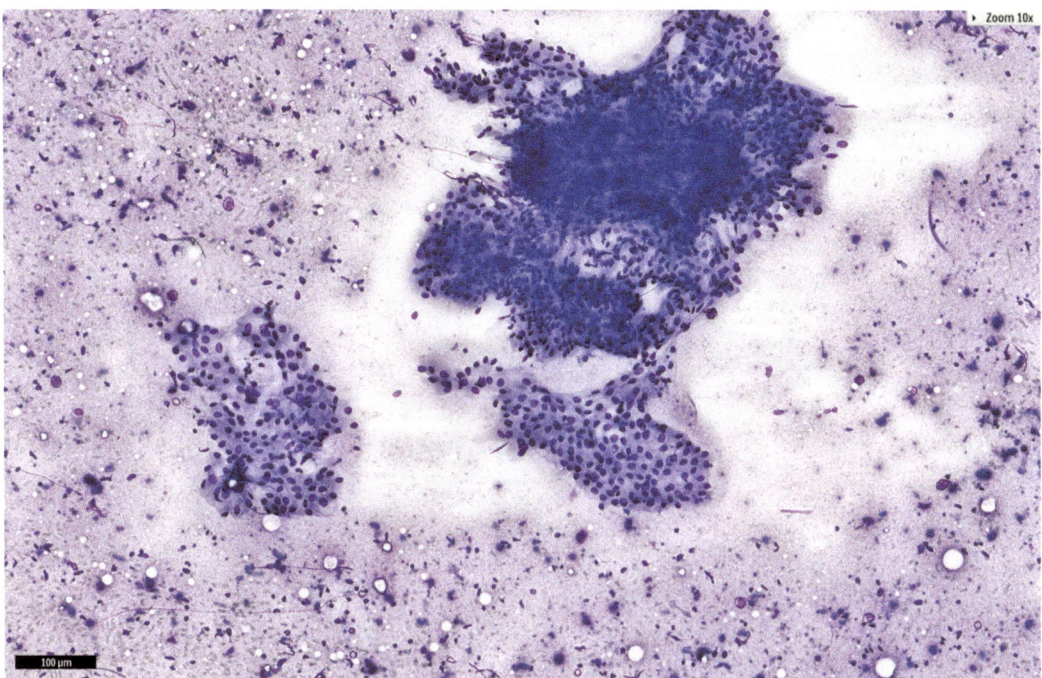

Fig 11.18 Warthin tumor. Clusters of oncocytic cells. Necrotic and lymphocytic background

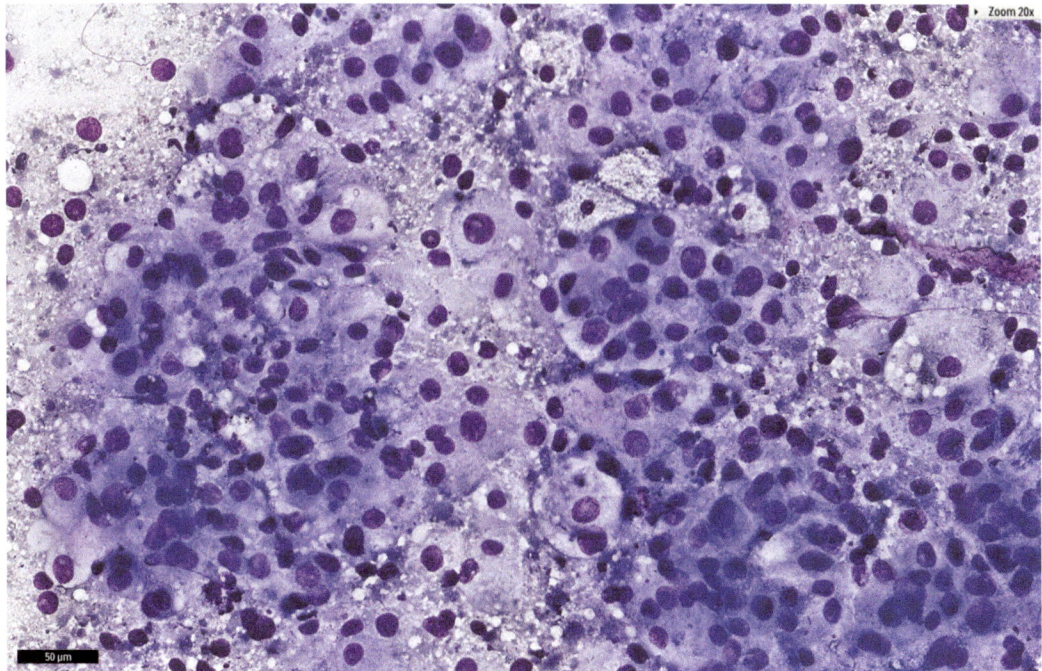

Fig 11.19 Oncocytic carcinoma. Malignant oncocytic cells

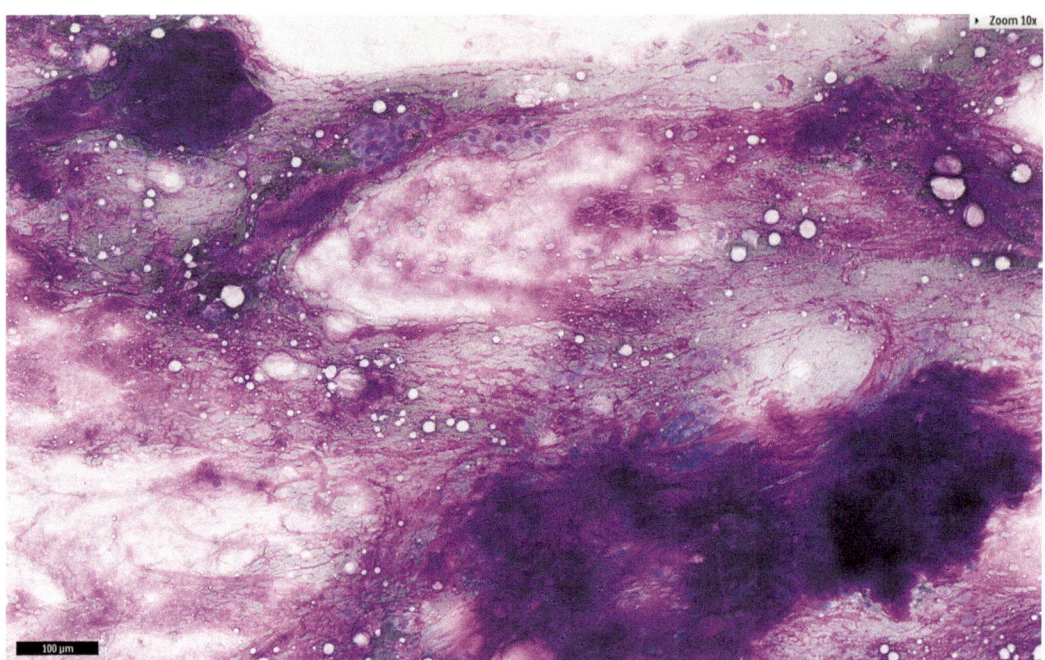

Fig 11.20 Pleomorphic adenoma with predominant chondromyxoid which stains intensively magenta

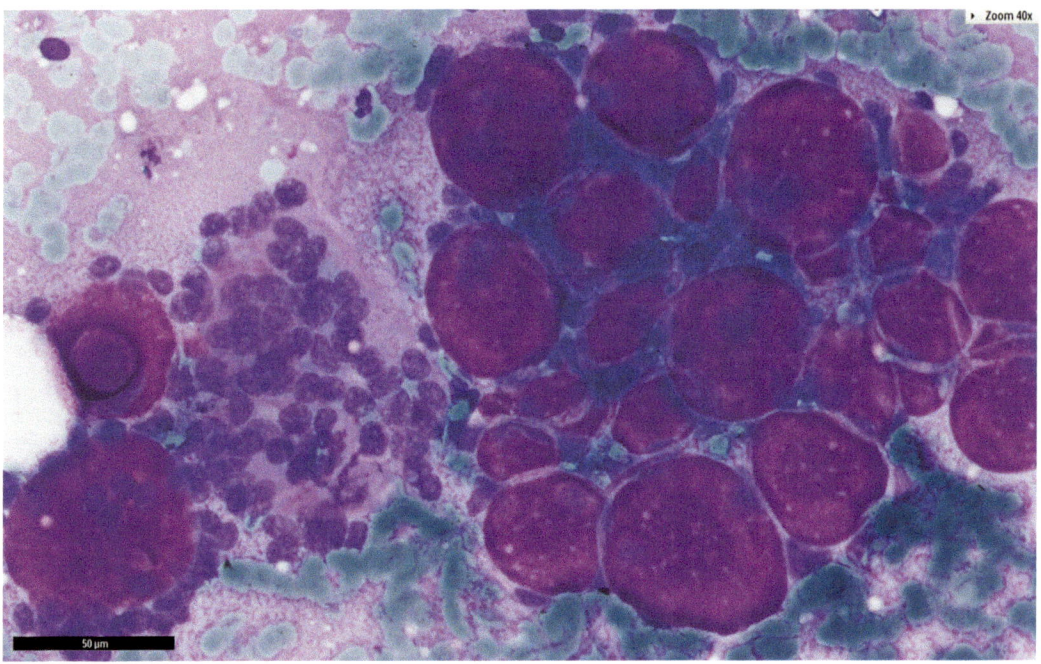

Fig 11.21 Adenoid cystic carcinoma. Hyaline globules

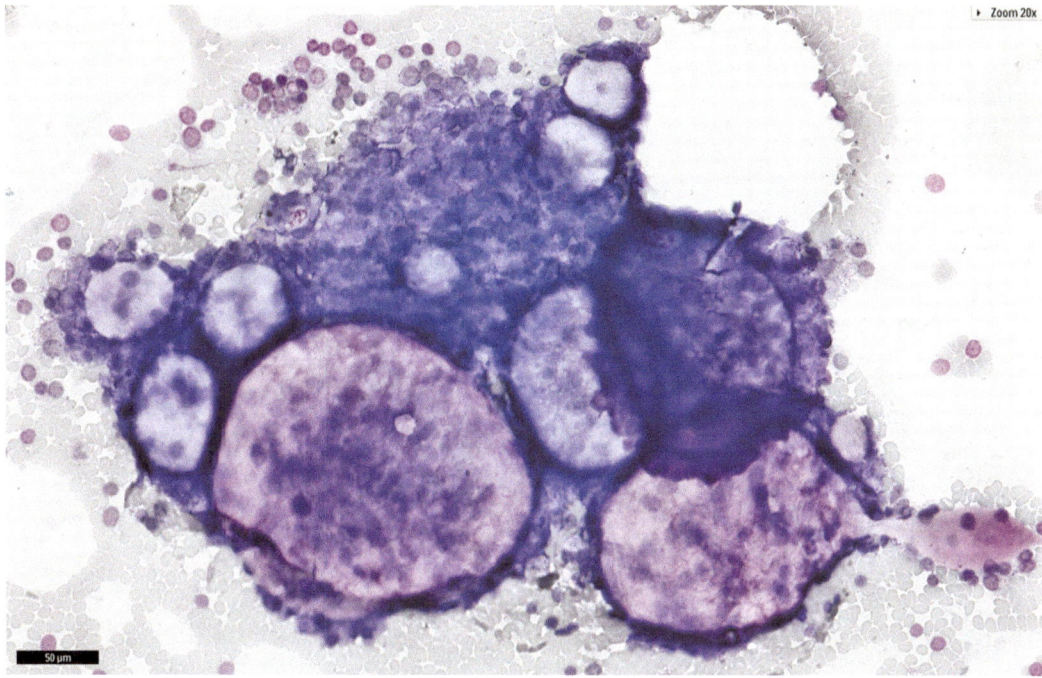

Fig 11.22 Epithelial-myoepithelial carcinoma. Hyaline globules

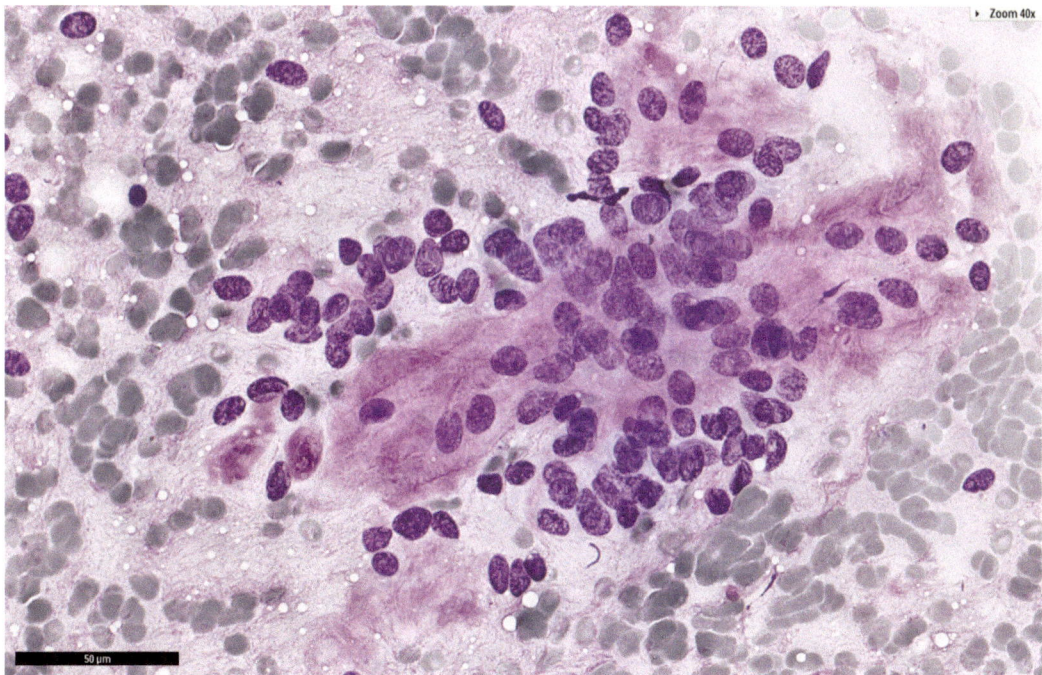

Fig 11.23 Basal cell adenoma. Nonspecific connective fragments and naked nuclei

Fig 11.24 Parotid
radio-induced
osteosarcoma. Atypical
malignant osteoblasts
and osteoid

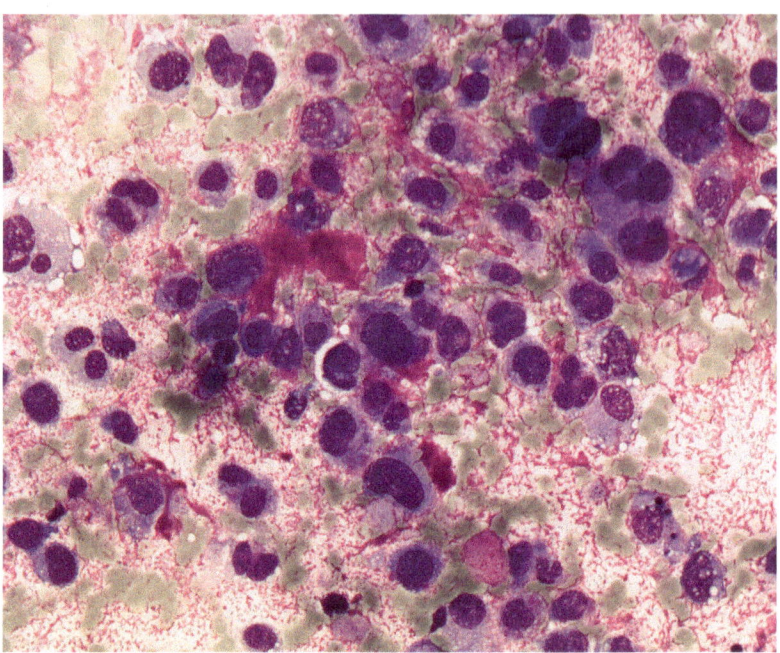

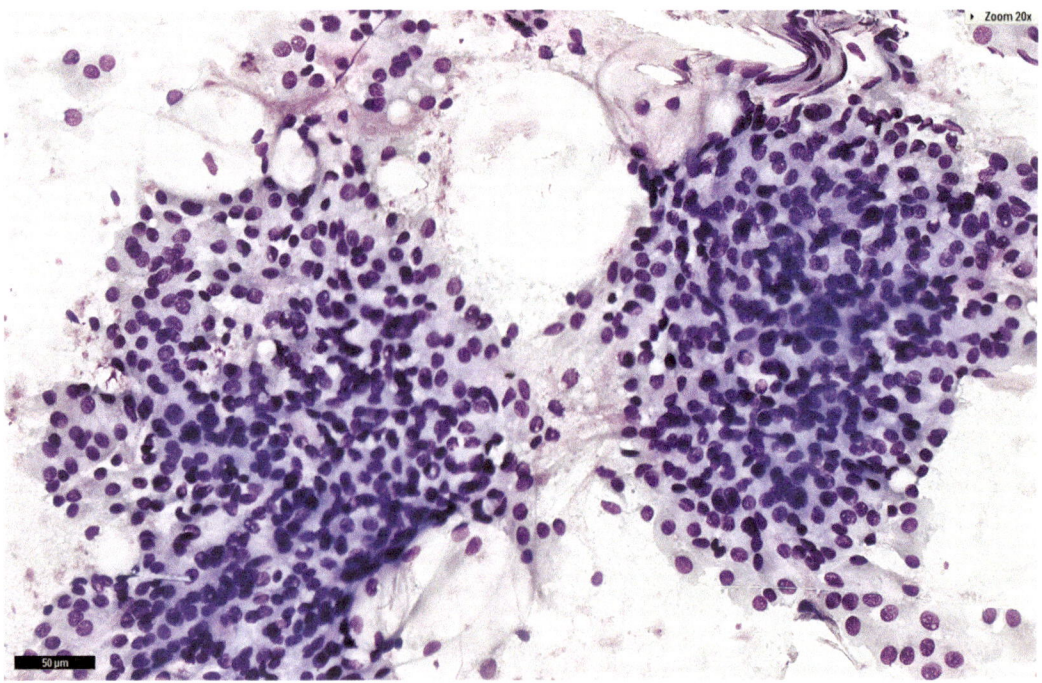

Fig 11.25 Mucoepidermoid carcinoma. Intermediate cells and mucoid background

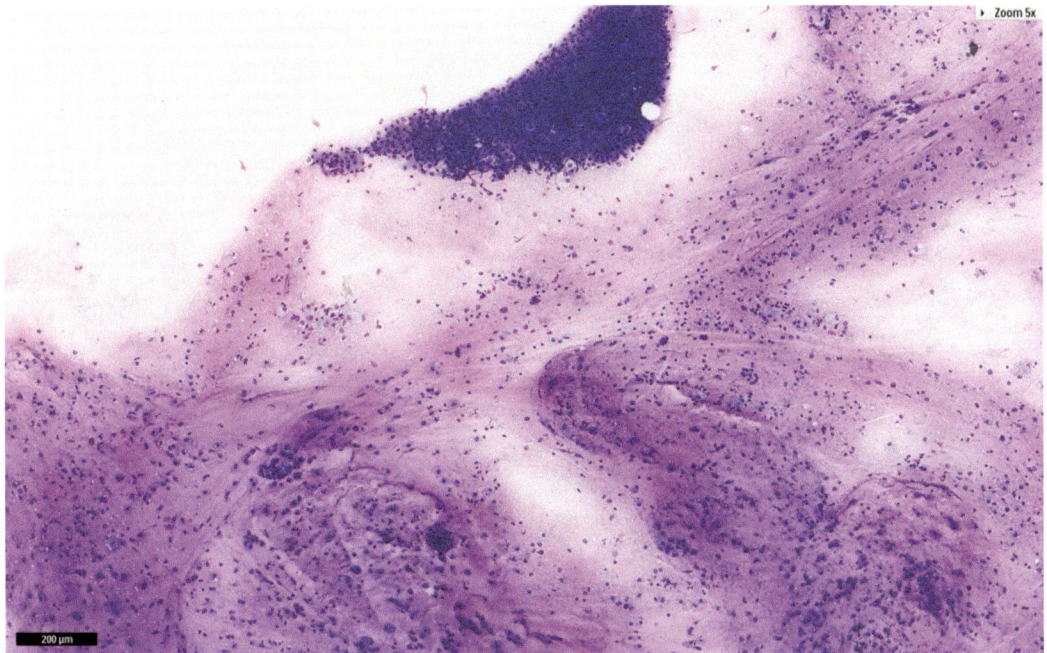

Fig 11.26   Warthin tumor. Mucus

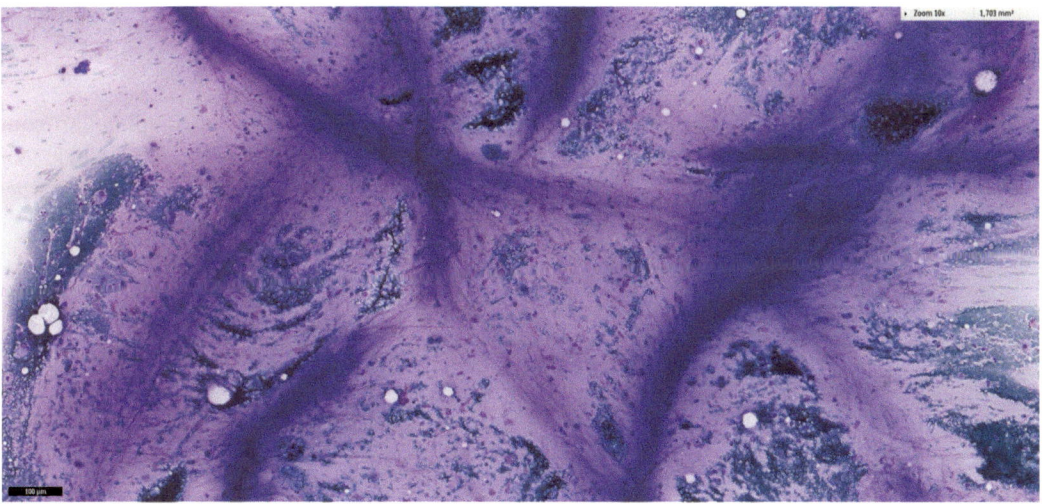

Fig 11.27   Küttner tumor. Mucus and inflammatory cells

Fig 11.28 Salivary
cyst. Crystals

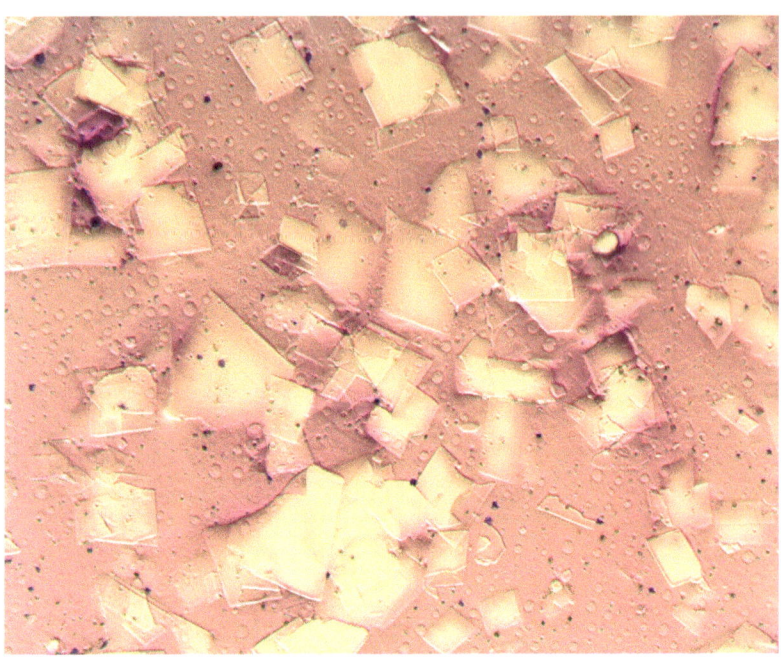

11.4 Diagnostic Criteria and Differential FNA Diagnosis in Salivary Tumors

The combination of different cellular and stromal/secretion elements allows accurate cytological typing.

11.4.1 Cell-Rich and Stroma-Rich Tumors

Myoepithelial cells and chondromyxoid secretion suggest pleomorphic adenoma (Figs. 11.1, 11.2, and 11.20).

Oncocytic cells, lymphocytes, necrosis, and mast cells within oncocytic clusters suggest Warthin tumor (Fig. 11.18 and 11.26).

Basaloid dark cells without necrosis nor atypia, nonspecific connective debris, and naked nuclei suggest basal cell adenoma, and in lip localization, it suggests canalicular adenoma (Figs. 11.5 and 11.23).

Basaloid dark cells, hyaline globules, tubular structures, and naked nuclei suggest adenoid cystic carcinoma, epithelial-myoepithelial carcinoma, and basal cell adenocarcinoma. In pleomorphic, adenocarcinoma nuclei are elongated and clarified (Figs. 11.6, 11.7, 11.12, 11.21, 11.22, 11.29, and 11.30).

Intermediate epithelial cells, epithelial "squamoid" cells, mucus-secreting cells, lymphocytic background, and mucus suggest mucoepidermoid carcinoma (Figs. 11.13, 11.15, and 11.25).

11.4.2 Cell-Rich and Stroma-Poor Tumors

Acinic cells (isolated and clustered) and naked nuclei suggest well-differentiated acinic cell carcinoma (Fig. 11.3).

Epithelial cells or roundish, plasmacytoid or polygonal cells with variable cytonuclear atypia, oncocytic metaplasia, and possibility of necrotic background suggest salivary duct carcinoma (Fig. 11.31).

Poorly differentiated malignant cells and necrotic background suggest large-cell undifferentiated carcinoma (Fig. 11.32).

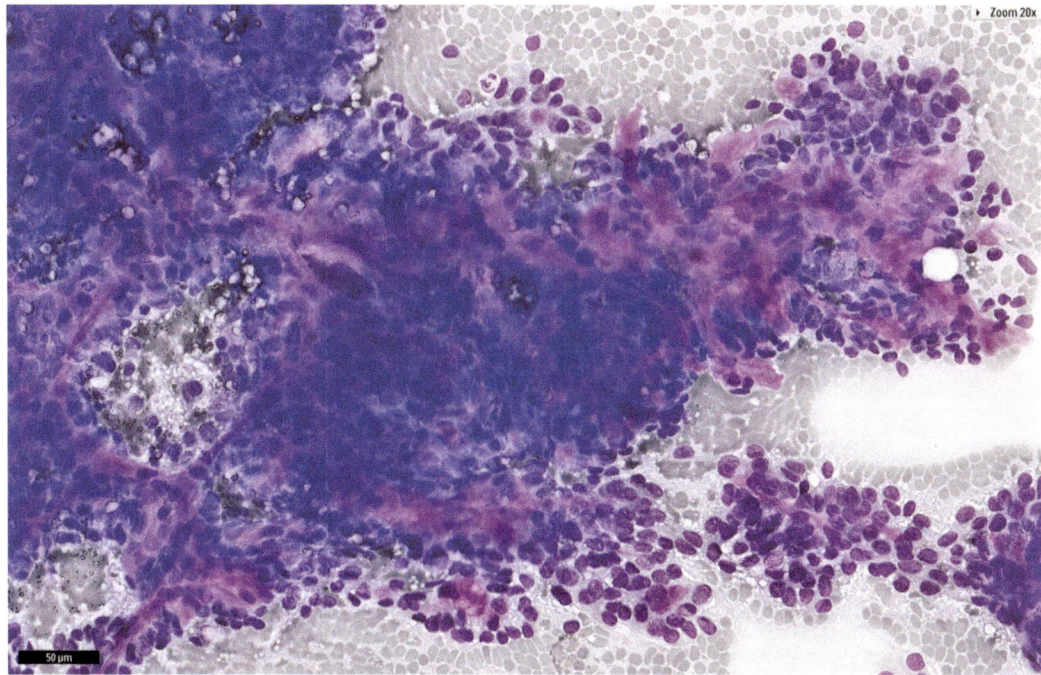

Fig 11.29 Epithelial-myoepithelial carcinoma. Tubular connective structures

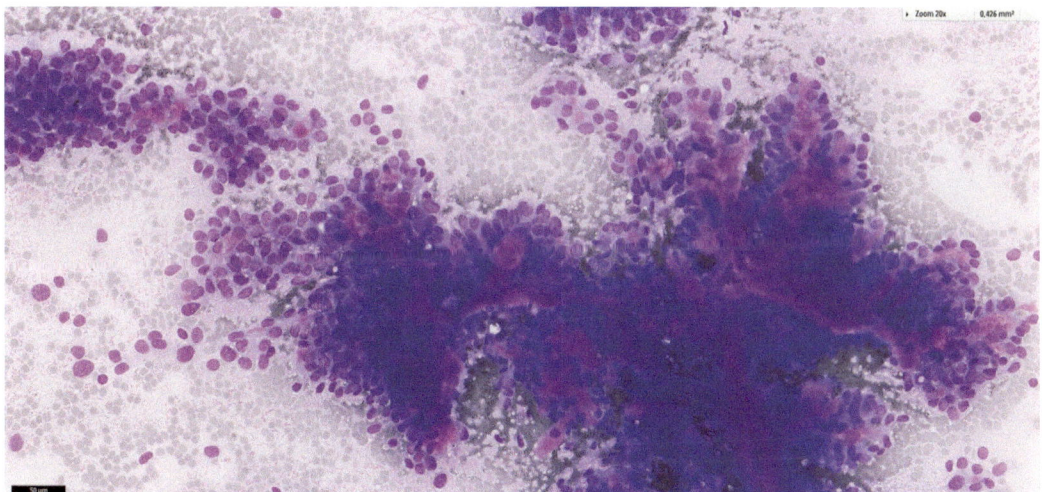

Fig 11.30 Polymorphous adenocarcinoma. Tubular structures and hyaline globules

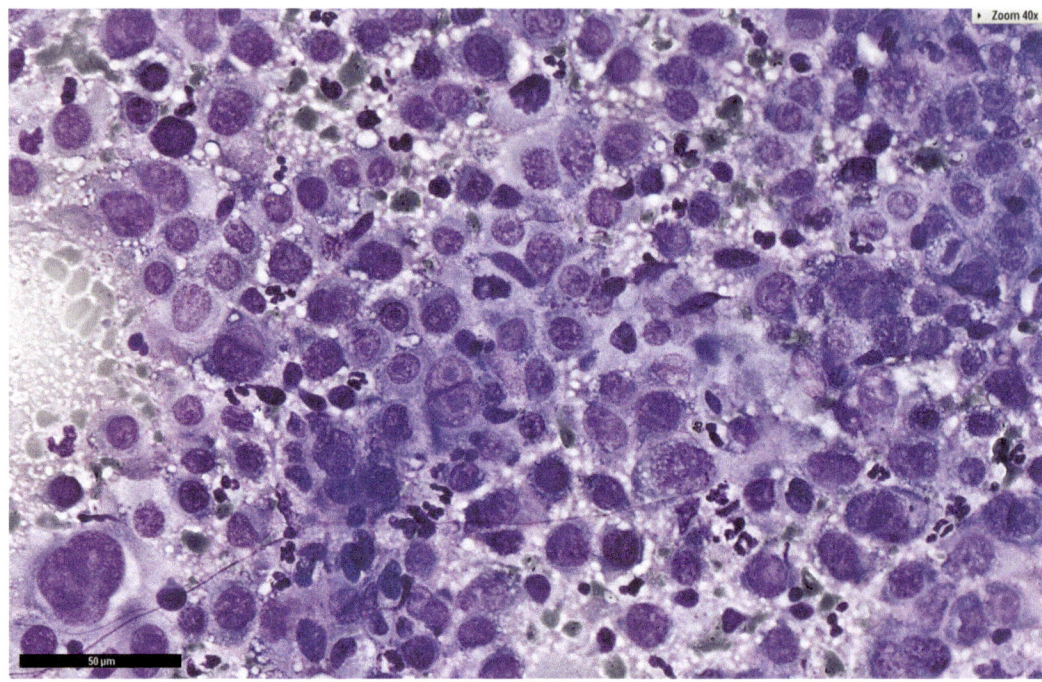

Fig 11.31 Salivary duct carcinoma. Malignant epithelial cells and necrotic background

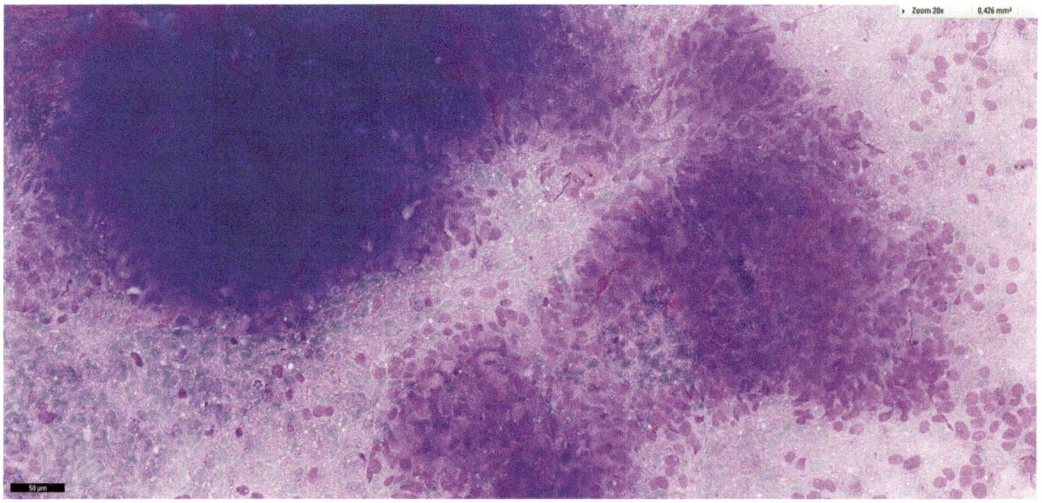

Fig 11.32 Large cell undifferentiated carcinoma. Nonspecific malignant cells and necrotic background

Spindle-shaped or plasmacytoid cells suggest cellular pleomorphic adenoma or myoepithelioma (Figs. 11.8, 11.9, and 11.10).

Small, sometimes large but delicate epithelial cells with nuclear molding, palisading, and smearing artifacts suggest primary or metastatic neuroendocrine carcinoma (Figs. 11.33 and 11.34).

Squamous cells with atypia and necrosis suggest primary or metastatic squamous cell carcinoma or high-grade mucoepidermoid carcinoma (Figs. 11.14 and 11.15).

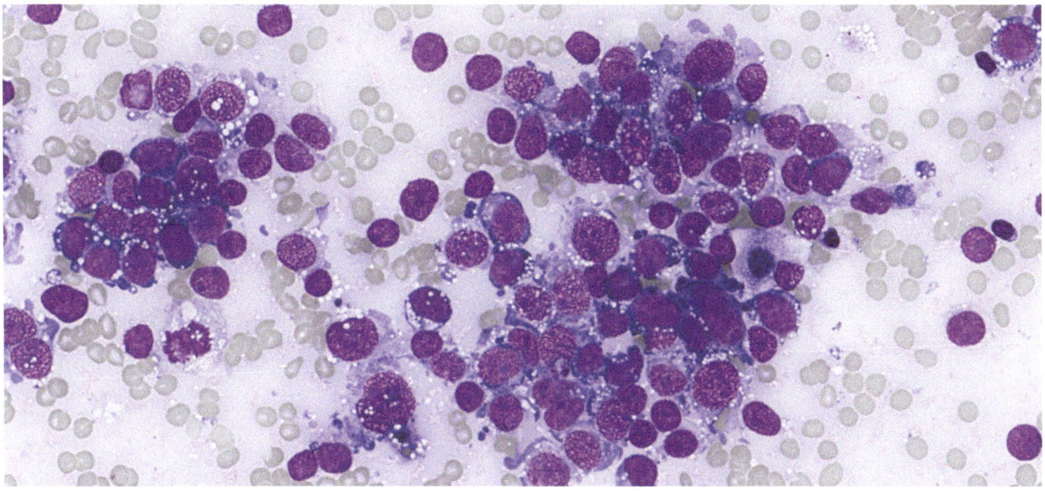

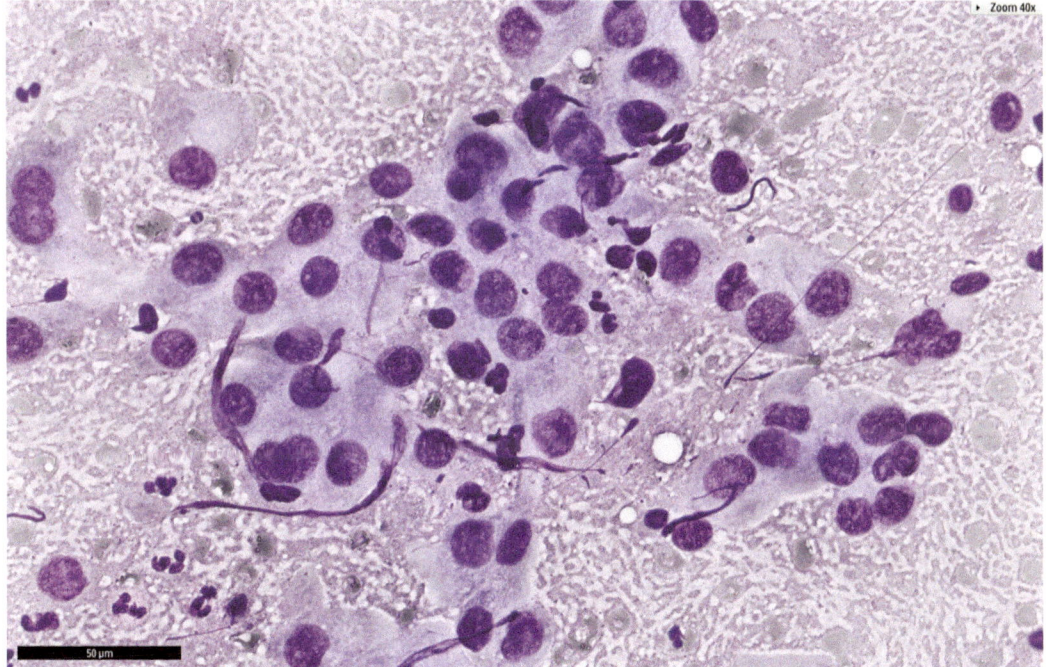

Fig 11.33 Parotid metastasis from INI1 deficient sinus carcinoma

Fig 11.34 Salivary duct carcinoma. Oncocytic-like cells

Polymorphous and oncocytic-like cells occasionally with nuclear inclusion and binucleation suggest oncocytic or myoepithelial carcinoma and also metastatic melanoma (Figs. 11.35 and 11.36).

Clarified nuclei are usually seen in polymorphous adenocarcinoma (Fig. 11.37).

Polymorphous lymphocytes suggest enlarged lymph node. Cellular monotony, lympho-glandular bodies, cytonuclear atypia, and necrosis suggest malignant lymphoma (Fig. 11.36).

Unusual cellular component may suggest metastatic tumor.

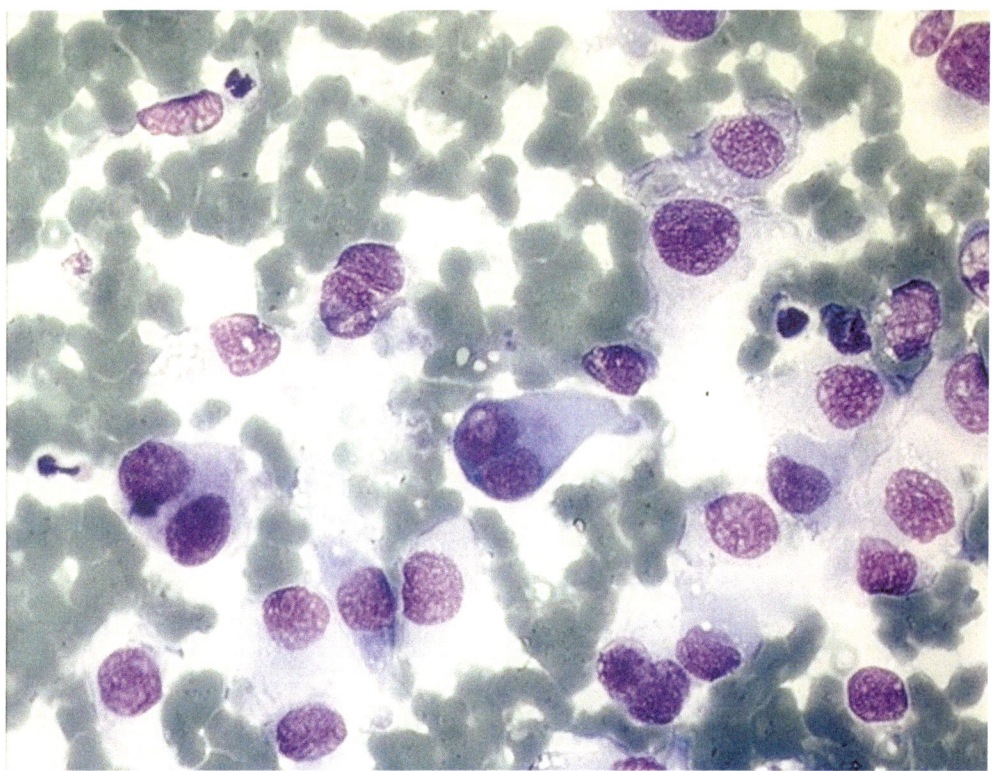

Fig 11.35 Metastatic malignant melanoma to the parotid gland. Cells with large cytoplasm and binucleated cells

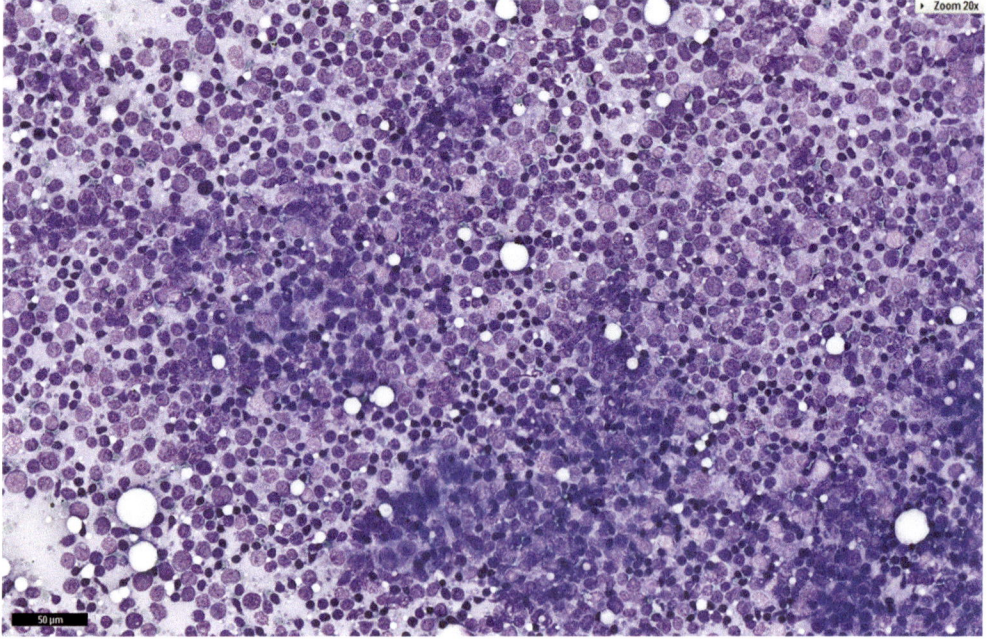

Fig 11.36 Malignant lymphoma in parotid lymph node

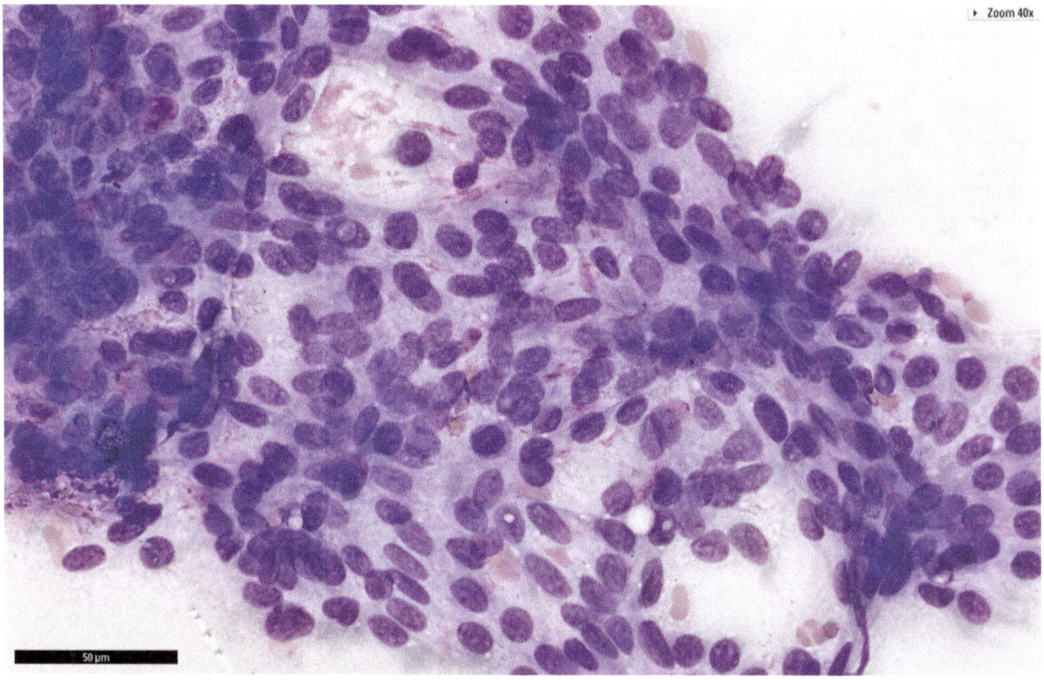

Fig 11.37 Polymorphous adenocarcinoma. Clarified nuclei

11.4.3 Cell-Poor and Stroma/Secretion-Rich Tumors

Clear or mucoid fluid with or without crystals suggest salivary cyst of various etiologies (Fig. 11.28).

Metachromatic mucus containing scant cells of "macrophagic" morphology suggests low-grade mucoepidemoid carcinoma, salivary cyst, or Warthin tumor. Nonrecognition of this substance is the source of false-negative diagnoses in mucoepidermoid carcinoma (Figs. 11.26 and 11.27).

Abundant chondromyxoid with occasional plasmocytoid cells suggests pleomorphic adenoma and chondromyxoid subtype (Figs. 11.2 and 11.20).

Abundant "chondroid" with rare, clarified cells of big size and occasional cytonuclear atypia suggests chordoma (Fig. 11.38).

11.4.4 Cell-Poor and Stroma/Secretion-Poor Tumors

Scant dark, "atypical" epithelial cells, connective fragments, inflammatory cells, and mucus suggest Küttner tumor. This can be a source of false-positive diagnoses (Fig. 11.27).

Rare, nonspecific connective fragments with occasional spindle cells are suggestive of fibromatosis.

Lipomateous material suggests lipoma.

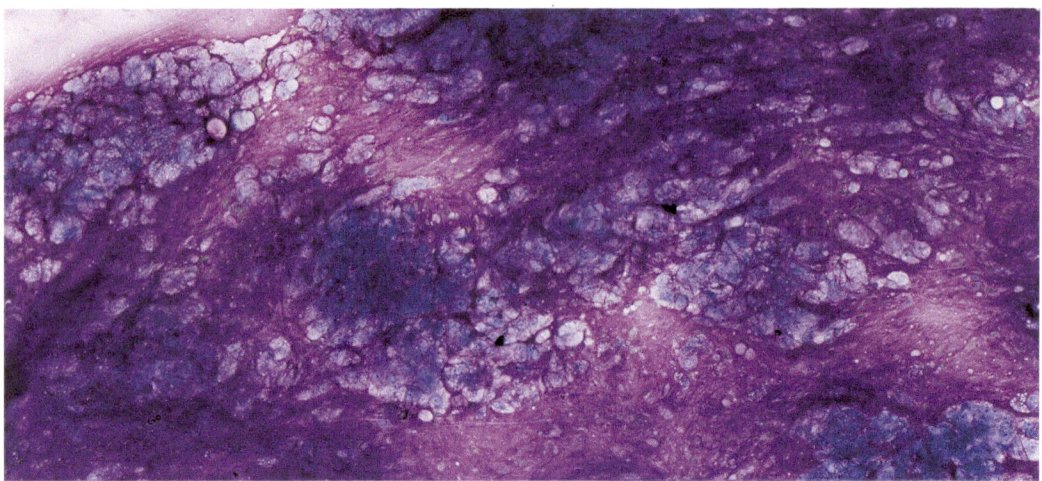

Fig 11.38 Chordoma. Pinkish background and physaliferous cells mimicking pleomorphic adenoma

11.5   Further Applications

Recently, Milan system for reporting salivary gland cytopathology was proposed in adult and pediatric tumors [26, 27]. This was shown to be of great clinical–pathological utility.

References

1. Mavec P, Eneroth CM, Franzen S, Moberger G, Zajicek J. Aspiration biopsy of salivary gland tumours. I. Correlation of cytologic reports from 652 aspiration biopsies with clinical and histologic findings. Acta Otolaryngol. 1964;58:471–84. https://doi.org/10.3109/00016486409121406.
2. Persson PS, Zettergren L. Cytologic diagnosis of salivary gland tumors by aspiration biopsy. Acta Cytol. 1973;17(4):351–4.
3. Jayaram N, Ashim D, Rajwanshi A, Radhika S, Banerjee CK. The value of fine-needle aspiration biopsy in the cytodiagnosis of salivary gland lesions. Diagn Cytopathol. 1989;5(4):349–54. https://doi.org/10.1002/dc.2840050402.
4. Young JA, Smallman LA, Thompson H, Proops DW, Johnson AP. Fine needle aspiration cytology of salivary gland lesions. Cytopathology. 1990;1(1):25–33. https://doi.org/10.1111/j.1365-2303.1990.tb00323.x.
5. MacLeod CB, Frable WJ. Fine-needle aspiration biopsy of the salivary gland: problem cases. Diagn Cytopathol. 1993;9(2):216–24. https://doi.org/10.1002/dc.2840090222; discussion 224–5. PMID: 8390349
6. Orell SR. Diagnostic difficulties in the interpretation of fine needle aspirates of salivary gland lesions: the problem revisited. Cytopathology.

1995;6(5):285–300. https://doi.org/10.1111/j.1365-2303.1995.tb00574.x.
7. Klijanienko J, Vielh P. Fine-needle sampling of salivary gland lesions. I. Cytology and histology correlation of 412 cases of pleomorphic adenoma. Diagn Cytopathol. 1996;14(3):195–200. https://doi.org/10.1002/(SICI)1097-0339(199604)14:3<195::AID-DC1>3.0.CO;2-H.
8. Klijanienko J, Vielh P. Fine-needle sampling of salivary gland lesions. II. Cytology and histology correlation of 71 cases of Warthin's tumor (adenolymphoma). Diagn Cytopathol. 1997;16(3):221–5. https://doi.org/10.1002/(sici)1097-0339(199703)16:3<221::aid-dc5>3.0.co;2-i.
9. Klijanienko J, Vielh P. Fine-needle sampling of salivary gland lesions. III. Cytologic and histologic correlation of 75 cases of adenoid cystic carcinoma: review and experience at the Institut Curie with emphasis on cytologic pitfalls. Diagn Cytopathol. 1997;17(1):36–41. https://doi.org/10.1002/(sici)1097-0339(199707)17:1<36::aid-dc7>3.0.co;2-n.
10. Klijanienko J, Vielh P. Fine-needle sampling of salivary gland lesions. IV. Review of 50 cases of mucoepidermoid carcinoma with histologic correlation. Diagn Cytopathol. 1997;17(2):92–8. https://doi.org/10.1002/(sici)1097-0339(199708)17:2<92::aid-dc3>3.0.co;2-q.
11. Klijanienko J, Vielh P. Fine-needle sample of salivary gland lesions. V: Cytology of 22 cases of acinic cell carcinoma with histologic correlation. Diagn Cytopathol. 1997;17(5):347–52. https://doi.org/10.1002/(sici)1097-0339(199711)17:5<347::aid-dc7>3.0.co;2-7.
12. Klijanienko J, Vielh P. Salivary carcinomas with papillae: cytology and histology analysis of polymorphous low-grade adenocarcinoma and papillary cystadenocarcinoma. Diagn Cytopathol.

1998;19(4):244–9. https://doi.org/10.1002/(sici)1097-0339(199810)19:4<244::aid-dc3>3.0.co;2-a.

13. Klijanienko J, El-Naggar AK, Servois V, Rodriguez J, Validire P, Vielh P. Mucoepidermoid carcinoma ex pleomorphic adenoma: nonspecific preoperative cytologic findings in six cases. Cancer. 1998;84(4):231–4.

14. Klijanienko J, Vielh P. Cytologic characteristics and histomorphologic correlations of 21 salivary duct carcinomas. Diagn Cytopathol. 1998 Nov;19(5):333–7. https://doi.org/10.1002/(sici)1097-0339(199811)19:5<333::aid-dc4>3.0.co;2-p.

15. Klijanienko J, Vielh P. Fine-needle sampling of salivary gland lesions. VI. Cytological review of 44 cases of primary salivary squamous-cell carcinoma with histological correlation. Diagn Cytopathol. 1998;18(3):174–8. https://doi.org/10.1002/(sici)1097-0339(199803)18:3<174::aid-dc2>3.0.co;2-e.

16. Klijanienko J, El-Naggar AK, Vielh P. Fine-needle sampling findings in 26 carcinoma ex pleomorphic adenomas: diagnostic pitfalls and clinical considerations. Diagn Cytopathol. 1999;21(3):163–6. https://doi.org/10.1002/(sici)1097-0339(199909)21:3<163::aid-dc3>3.0.co;2-2.

17. Klijanienko J, el-Naggar AK, Vielh P. Comparative cytologic and histologic study of fifteen salivary basal-cell tumors: differential diagnostic considerations. Diagn Cytopathol. 1999;21(1):30–4. https://doi.org/10.1002/(sici)1097-0339(199907)21:1<30::aid-dc9>3.0.co;2-9.

18. Lussier C, Klijanienko J, Vielh P. Fine-needle aspiration of metastatic nonlymphomatous tumors to the major salivary glands: a clinicopathologic study of 40 cases cytologically diagnosed and histologically correlated. Cancer. 2000;90(6):350–6.

19. Klijanienko J, Lagacé R, Servois V, Lussier C, El-Naggar AK, Vielh P. Fine-needle sampling of primary neuroendocrine carcinomas of salivary glands: cytohistological correlations and clinical analysis. Diagn Cytopathol. 2001;24(3):163–6. https://doi.org/10.1002/1097-0339(200103)24:3<163::aid-dc1034>3.0.co;2-i.

20. Klijanienko J, Vielh P. Salivary gland tumours. In: Orell SR, editor. Monographs in clinical cytology, vol. 15. Basel: Karger; 2000.

21. Cristallini EG, Ascani S, Farabi R, Liberati F, Macciò T, Peciarolo A, Bolis GB. Fine needle aspiration biopsy of salivary gland, 1985–1995. Acta Cytol. 1997;41(5):1421–5. https://doi.org/10.1159/000332853.

22. Boccato P, Altavilla G, Blandamura S. Fine needle aspiration biopsy of salivary gland lesions. A reappraisal of pitfalls and problems. Acta Cytol. 1998;42(4):888–98. https://doi.org/10.1159/000331964. PMID: 9684573.

23. Christensen RK, Bjørndal K, Godballe C, Krogdahl A. Value of fine-needle aspiration biopsy of salivary gland lesions. Head Neck. 2010;32(1):104–8. https://doi.org/10.1002/hed.21151.

24. Pastore A, Borin M, Malagutti N, Di Laora A, Beccati D, Delazer AL, Bianchini C, Stomeo F, Ciorba A, Pelucchi S. Preoperative assessment of salivary gland neoplasms with fine needle aspiration cytology and echography: a retrospective analysis of 357 cases. Int J Immunopathol Pharmacol. 2013;26(4):965–71. https://doi.org/10.1177/039463201302600416.

25. Klijanienko J, El-Naggar AK, Servois V, Rodriguez J, Desjardins L, Schlienger P, Validire P, Vielh P. Histologically similar, synchronous or metachronous, lacrimal salivary-type and parotid gland tumors: a series of 11 cases. Head Neck. 1999;21(6):512–6. https://doi.org/10.1002/(sici)1097-0347(199909)21:6<512::aid-hed3>3.0.co;2-u.

26. Rossi ED, Faquin WC, Baloch Z, Barkan GA, Foschini MP, Pusztaszeri M, Vielh P, Kurtycz DFI. The Milan System for Reporting Salivary Gland Cytopathology: analysis and suggestions of initial survey. Cancer Cytopathol. 2017;125(10):757–66. https://doi.org/10.1002/cncy.21898. Epub 2017 Jul 14

27. Maleki Z, Saoud C, Viswanathan K, Kilic I, Tommola E, Griffin DT, Heider A, Petrone G, Jo VY, Centeno BA, Saieg M, Mikou P, Fadda G, Ali SZ, Kholová I, Wojcik EM, Barkan GA, Eisele DW, Bellevicine C, Vigliar E, Wiles AB, Al-Ibraheemi A, Allison DB, Dixon GR, Chandra A, Walsh JM, Baloch ZW, Faquin WC, Krane JF, Rossi ED, Pantanowitz L, Troncone G, Callegari FM, Klijanienko J. Application of the Milan System for Reporting Salivary Gland Cytopathology in pediatric patients: an international, multi-institutional study. Cancer Cytopathol. 2022;130(5):370–80. https://doi.org/10.1002/cncy.22556.

Jerzy Klijanienko Professor of pathology at Institut Curie, Paris, France. President of 43rd European Congress of Cytology 2021 in Wroclaw, Poland and past president of European Federation of Cytology Societies 2019–2021. Vice-president of French Society of Clinical Cytology. Author of around 200 publications, 4 books, 30 chapters, and around 200 abstracts. Author/co-author/editor of two "WHO blue books" concerning cytology in soft tissue tumors and breast tumors. Co-author of *The Milan System for Reporting Salivary Gland Cytopathology*.

Philippe Vielh is a Professor of pathology at Medipath and American Hospital of Paris, France. He is the Former President of the French Society of Cytology (SFCC), President of the 31st European Congress of Cytology in 2005 (Paris, France), and Secretary General of the European Federation of Cytology Societies (EFCS) for 7 years (2005–2012). He chaired the 18th International Congress of Cytology in Paris (2013) and served as President of the International Academy of Cytology (IAC) for 3 years (2013–2016). He has been the Chair of the European Society of Pathology (ESP) Cytopathology Working Group since 2018.

The Milan System for Classifying Salivary Gland Cytopathology

Esther Diana Rossi and William C. Faquin

Fine needle aspiration (FNA) is widely accepted as an accurate diagnostic test with important first-line implications for the management of salivary gland lesions [1–9]. Its popularity resides in the fact that it is rapid and easy to perform, minimally invasive, safe, and inexpensive. Salivary gland FNA is most effective when performed using ultrasound guidance, and it shows a range of sensitivities and specificities from 92.3% to 97% depending upon on a wide variety of factors [1–9]. False-negative (FN) and false-positive (FP) diagnoses are uncommon although in some cases, inadequate/non-diagnostic FNAs due to sampling issues can cause limitations. One reason for the success of salivary gland FNA is that it performs remarkably well in diagnosing the most common salivary gland tumors, pleomorphic adenoma (PA) and Warthin tumor (WT) due to their characteristic cytomorphologic features [10]. In most cases, FNA can also differentiate between low-grade and high-grade carcinomas as reported by Johnson et al. [11]. While salivary gland FNA can reliably distinguish neoplastic from non-neoplastic lesions, the greatest limitation might be its ability to distinguish between less common benign tumors and low-grade carcinomas (e.g., basal cell adenoma versus basal cell adenocarcinoma), although ancillary testing can be useful in many cases [10–13].

12.1 Salivary Gland FNA and the Need for Uniform Reporting

The recent 2022 World Health Organization (WHO) classification system of tumors of the salivary glands recognizes 36 benign and malignant epithelial tumors along with several emerging entities [10]. Salivary gland tumors represent one of the highest morphologic, phenotypic, and genotypic diversities encountered in any single-organ system. It is also among the most difficult areas for cytology and surgical pathology [12–16]. The reason is mostly due to similarities in microscopic features between different benign and low-grade salivary gland tumors and the inability of FNA or core biopsy to assess for invasion. The heterogeneous nature of salivary gland tumors combined with non-neoplastic lesions has led to the frequent use of morphological descriptions of the FNA specimen rather than a defined diagnosis with clear-cut implications for clinical management [17–20]. This approach has the

E. D. Rossi (✉)
Division of Anatomic Pathology and Histology, Agostino Gemelli School of Medicine, Università Cattolica del Sacro Cuore, Rome, Italy
e-mail: esther.rossi@policlinicogemelli.it

W. C. Faquin
Department of Pathology, Massachusetts General Hospital and Harvard Medical School, Boston, MA, USA
e-mail: WFAQUIN@mgh.harvard.edu

J. Klijanienko et al. (eds.), *Diagnostic Procedures in Patients with Neck Masses*,
https://doi.org/10.1007/978-3-031-67675-8_12

consequence of being inconsistent in the format and terminology used for reporting the results between different institutions and pathologists. All these factors contributed to the development of a uniform reporting system for salivary gland cytology. The result was the publication of the Milan System for Reporting Salivary Gland Cytopathology in February 2018 [12–18].

12.2 The Milan System for Reporting Salivary Gland Cytopathology, an Overview

The Milan System for Reporting Salivary Gland Cytopathology (MSRSGC) was modeled after other cytology reporting systems used for different organs and tissues, including the Bethesda System for Reporting Thyroid Cytopathology [19–25]. The MSRSGC is the result of a joint effort by an international task force of cytopathologists, surgical pathologists, and head and neck surgeons who first met in 2015 in Milan, Italy, during the European Congress of Cytology. The MSRSGC was endorsed by the American Society of Cytopathology and the International Academy of Cytology, and its main goal was to standardize the reporting of salivary gland cytology, and promote better communication between clinicians and institutions, and ultimately improve patient care [12–18]. The general format is based on six diagnostic categories covering non-neoplastic, benign, and malignant lesions of the salivary glands. Similar to other cytology reporting systems, the MSRSGC includes a ROM and specific management algorithm for each diagnostic category that may be used to guide decision-making and patient counseling [12–18]. The system is an evidence-based system so that the ROM for each category was based on a rigorous review of all the published literature since 1980.

In the MSRSGC, each diagnostic category is associated with definitions, morphologic criteria, diagnostic category explanations, and sample reports for each. Since its implementation, the MSRSGC has obtained international acceptance among cytologists and clinicians, and has been adopted by many institutions around the globe.

Furthermore, it has been endorsed by the 2021 ASCO guidelines for the management of patients with salivary gland cancer, and by the 2022 WHO Classification of Head and Neck tumors [10, 24]. The publication of the MSRSGC in 2018 was followed by the publication of more than 100 papers from various countries including reviews and meta-analyses, which have confirmed the value and role of the MSRSGC as a practical and useful reporting system [12–18, 26–35]. The large amount of data from published studies using the MSRSGC served as a basis for the Second Edition of the MSRSGC The latter includes more highly refined ROMs for each diagnostic category, a new chapter on imaging studies for salivary glands, updates on the application of ancillary studies to salivary gland FNA, as well as updated nomenclature and entities in keeping with the latest 2022 WHO classification. The global enthusiasm for the MSRSGC is also reflected in recent translations of the atlas into Japanese and Chinese which were published in 2019 and 2022, respectively.

12.2.1 Summary of the Diagnostic Categories in the Updated Milan System

The MSRSGC maintains six diagnostic categories that are summarized below and in

I. *Non-diagnostic*

The "Non-diagnostic" (ND) category is defined by insufficient quantitative and/or qualitative cellular material to make a cytologic diagnosis.

Features include:

- Insufficient cells
- Artifacts such as air-drying, obscuring blood, poor preservation, and staining
- Normal salivary gland elements in the setting of a clinically or radiologically defined mass
- Nonmucinous cyst fluid without epithelial cells (can be designated "ND, cyst fluid only")

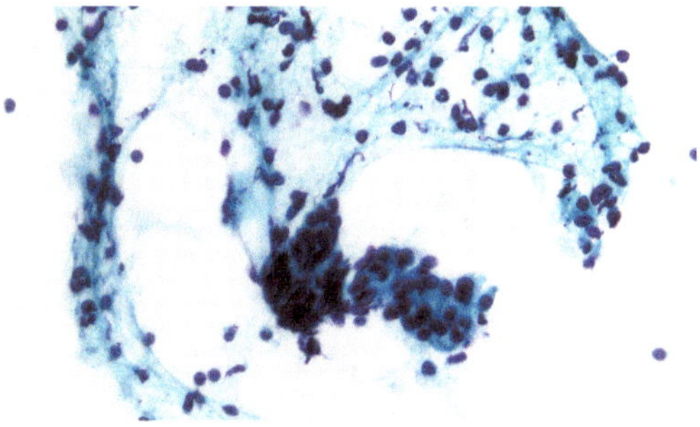

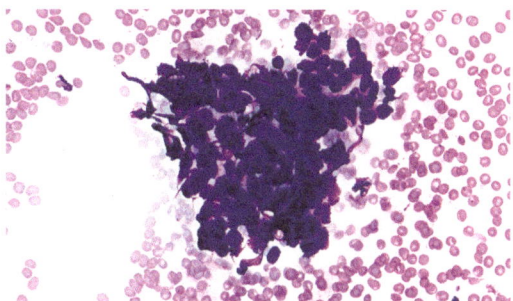

Fig. 12.1 FNA of chronic sialadenitis classified as "Non-neoplastic" (Papanicoloau stain)

Fig. 12.2 FNA showing a hypocellular aspirate with atypical features which are indefinite for a neoplasm. This case is classified as "AUS" (Diff-Quik stain)

The MSRSGC recommends that the rate of ND salivary gland FNAs should be < 10% and not greater than 20%.

II. *Non-neoplastic*

The "Non-neoplastic" (NN) category is characterized by samples that lack evidence of a neoplastic process (Fig. 12.1). Several entities included in this category are acute sialadenitis, chronic sialadenitis (including IgG4-related disease), granulomatous sialadenitis, sialolithiasis, and benign lymphoepithelial lesion/lymphoepithelial sialadenitis (LESA). Correlation with clinical and radiological findings is crucial to ensure that the FNA is representative of the salivary gland lesion and to minimize false-negative results. Lymph node aspirates from enlarged intra- and peri-parotid lymph nodes are frequently included in the ND category, and correlation with flow cytometry is recommended.

III. *Atypia of Undetermined Significance (AUS)*

The major indication for performing FNA on the salivary gland lesions is to identify whether a lesion is a non-neoplastic or neoplastic process, as this has implications for clinical management. The introduction of the "AUS" category was intended for those cases that are indefinite for a neoplasm due to a variety of reasons (Fig. 12.2).

Features include:

- Atypia indefinite for a neoplasm.
- Squamous, oncocytic, or other metaplastic changes indefinite for a neoplasm.

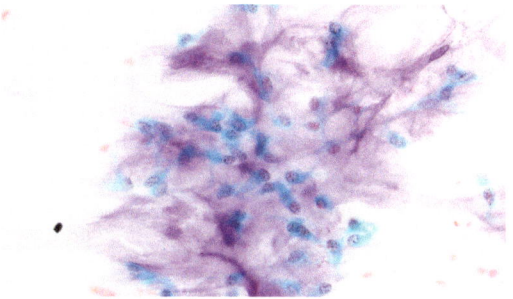

Fig. 12.3 This aspirate demonstrates classic features of pleomorphic adenoma and is classified as "Neoplasm-Benign" (Papanicoloau stain)

- Low cellularity specimens that are suggestive, but not definitive, of a neoplasm.
- Artifacts limiting the distinction between a non-neoplastic and neoplastic process.
- Mucinous cystic lesions with absent or very scant epithelial cells.
- Atypical lymphocytes in which a lymphoproliferative disorder cannot be excluded.

IVA. *Neoplasm: Benign*

In the MSRSGC, the use of the "Neoplasm: Benign" category is reserved for classic benign neoplasms diagnosed based on established cytologic criteria (Fig. 12.3). A majority of tumors in this category will be PA and WT, which, in most cases, can be accurately diagnosed by FNA. Other entities included in this category are lipoma, schwannoma, lymphangioma, and hemangioma.

IVB. *Neoplasm: Salivary Gland Neoplasm of Uncertain Malignant Potential (SUMP)*

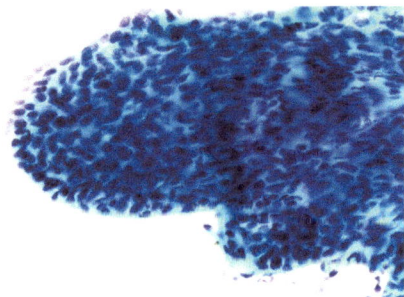

Fig. 12.4 FNA of a basaloid neoplasm indefinite for malignancy, classified as "Neoplasm: SUMP" (Papanicoloau stain)

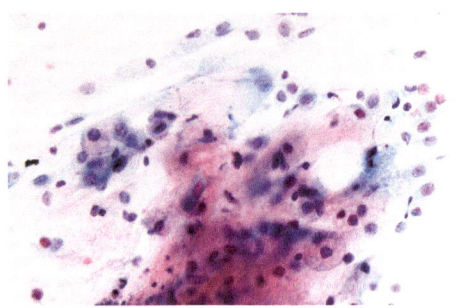

Fig. 12.5 This aspirate shows background mucin and cytologic features highly susicious for low-grade mucoepidermoid carcinoma, and is classified as "Suspicious for Malignancy" (Papanicoau stain)

A second subset of salivary gland neoplasms is classified in the "Neoplasm: SUMP" category. This category is reserved for FNA specimens that have cytologic features diagnostic of a neoplasm, but a specific entity cannot be defined and, most importantly, a malignant neoplasm cannot be excluded (Fig. 12.4). A majority of lesions in the SUMP subcategory will be cellular benign neoplasms, neoplasms with atypical features, and low-grade carcinomas. In terms of formulating a differential diagnosis, entities in the SUMP category can be further subclassified as "cellular basaloid neoplasm," "cellular oncocytic/oncocytoid neoplasm," and "cellular neoplasm with clear cell features."

V. *Suspicious for Malignancy*

The "Suspicious for Malignancy" (SUS) category includes cases with a severe degree of atypia and which are highly suggestive of malignancy (Fig. 12.5). The purpose of separating this category from the "Malignant" category is to ensure that the positive predictive value of the "Malignant" category remains high, approaching 100%.

Features include:

- Markedly atypical cells with artifacts precluding a definitive diagnosis of malignancy (e.g., obscuring blood or inflammation, poor cellular preservation) or poor smear preparation which limits cytomorphological assessment.

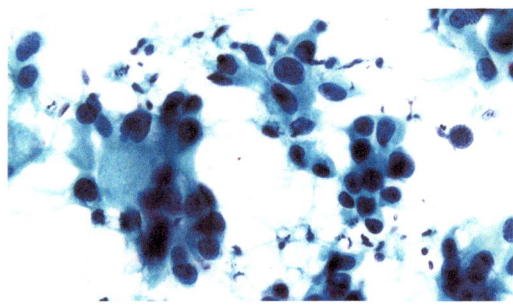

Fig. 12.6 FNA of a high-grade carcinoma consistent with salivary duct carcinoma; classified as "Malignant" (Papanicoloau stain)

- Rare markedly atypical cells in a sparsely cellular sample.
- Atypical lymphocytes suspicious for lymphoma, but lacking sufficient material for ancillary studies.

VI. *Malignant*

The "Malignant" category is used for specimens that have cytomorphological features, either alone or in combination with ancillary studies (see below), that are diagnostic of malignancy (Fig. 12.6). When possible, a specific classification of the tumor type should be made. In addition, the tumor should be graded as low-grade versus high-grade when feasible. This diagnostic category also includes secondary (metastatic) tumors and lymphoid malignancies.

12.3 Risk of Malignancy and the Milan System

Each diagnostic category of the MSRSGC is associated with an implied ROM (Table 12.1) based on the published literature. In this way, each diagnostic category can provide more meaningful information for the treating clinician and the patient.

12.3.1 Report Format in the Milan System

The purpose of the MSRSGC is not to change any of the well-known diagnostic cytomorphologic criteria for salivary gland lesions or the way that salivary gland lesions are evaluated. Instead, the MSRSGC provides a practical, uniform format for reporting the FNA interpretation with the ultimate result of better communication and improved patient care.

In the MSRSGC, the cytology report should start with an adequacy statement, followed by the diagnostic category, and a brief description of the cytologic features including a specific classification of the lesion when possible. If the latter is not possible, a concise comment on the reason for the categorization of the lesion is recommended. The MSRSGC Atlas, now in its second edition, is designed to be user-friendly and incorporates many examples of reports with explanatory notes.

12.3.2 Role of Ancillary Studies

Both the first and the second editions of the salivary Atlas emphasize the role of ancillary techniques in making a definite diagnosis [35–40]. Ancillary studies including IHC for salivary gland FNA are needed only in a minority of cases since most cases (e.g., PA and WT) can be accurately diagnosed by cytomorphology alone. The use of ancillary techniques should be considered when they can change the clinical management or clinical risk within the MSRSGC. While approximately half of ACC, AciCC, SC, and MEC are diagnosed as malignant by cytomorphology alone (46%), many of these cases are diagnosed as SUMP (43%) or SUS (11%) (PMID: 31104944). For several of them, the evaluation of their specific genetic alterations and/or immunoprofiles can be extremely useful for a diagnosis as malignant.

In these last decades, numerous papers have demonstrated that the majority of SGT is characterized by specific genetic alterations that can be used for diagnostic purposes. The most common molecular alterations were included in the latest WHO definitions of several SGTs including MEC, ACC, SC, polymorphous adenocarcinoma, and hyalinizing clear cell carcinoma. The 2021 ASCO Guidelines recommend that pathologists perform ancillary testing (IHC or molecular studies) on FNAs and CNBs to support diagnosis and ROM [24]. Hence, several new immunomarkers have been developed and can be very useful to

Table 12.1 Comparison of Milan system I and II edition-Risk of malignancy

	ROM (I ed-2018)	ROM (II ed-2023)	Management
Non-diagnostic	25%	15%	Clinical and/o radiologica correlation. Repeat FNA
Non-neoplastic	10%	11%	Follow-up
Atypia of undetermined significance-AUS	20%	30%	Repeat FNA and/or surgery
Neoplastic Benign	< 5%	< 3%	Conservative surgery
Neoplasms of Unceratin malignant potential-SUMP	35%	35%	Conservative surgery
Suspicious for malignancy	60%	83	Surgery
Malignant	>90%	98%	Surgery

refine the differential diagnostic list or to favor a specific entity when cytomorphology alone is not sufficient. A new approach was the adoption of antibodies to identify protein surrogates of specific genetic alterations that are overexpressed in a subset of SGTs, including MYB (*MYB-NFIB* fusion in AdCC), PLAG-1 (*PLAG-1* rearrangement in PA and carcinomas-ex-PA), and more recently pan-TRK and NR4A3 expression for SC and AciCC, respectively. Additionally, some centers have developed their own comprehensive customizable NGS SGT-specific panels to detect specific gene alterations, including mutations, fusions, and RNA gene expression alterations, in order to facilitate the diagnosis and classification of SGT.

12.4 Clinical Implications

A detailed discussion of clinical management is beyond the scope of this chapter; however, combined with the clinical history, physical exam, and imaging studies (including ultrasound (US), contrast-enhanced computed tomography (CT), or magnetic resonance imaging (MRI) with contrast), FNA plays an essential role in helping to define the correct management of salivary gland lesions. This would include observation for non-neoplastic lesions, limited resection for benign tumors and low-grade carcinomas, or more radical surgical resection, and possible adjuvant therapy for selected cases of high-grade malignancy.

In summary, the role of FNA in the preoperative assessment of salivary gland lesions has been emphasized by an abundance of published literature, and its use has been endorsed in the ASCO guidelines for the management of salivary gland cancer. The purpose of the first and second editions of the MSRSGC is to provide a universally accepted and consistent reporting structure for salivary gland FNA. The primary goals of the MSRSGC are to improve cytopathologist–clinician communication and provide assistance with clinical decision-making.

References

1. Faquin WC, Powers CN. Salivary gland cytopathology, Essentials in cytopathology series, vol. 5. New York: Springer; 2008.
2. Jain R, Gupta R, Kudesia M, et al. Fine needle aspiration cytology in diagnosis of salivary gland lesions: a study with histologic comparison. Cyto J. 2013;10:5.
3. Colella G, Cannavale R, Flamminio F, et al. Fine-needle aspiration cytology of salivary gland lesions: a systematic review. J Oral Maxillofac Surg. 2010;68:2146–53.
4. Schmidt RL, Hunt JP, Hall BJ, et al. A systematic review and meta-analysis of the diagnostic accuracy of frozen section for parotid gland lesions. Am J Clin Pathol. 2011;136:729–38.
5. Faquin WC, Rossi ED, editors. The Milan System for Reporting Salivary Gland Cytopathology. Cham: Springer; 2018.
6. Pusztaszeri M, Rossi ED, Baloch ZW, et al. Salivary gland fine needle aspiration and introduction of the Milan Reporting System. Adv Anat Pathol. 2019;26:84–92.
7. Hughes JH, Volk EE, Wilbur DC. Cytopathology Resource Committee, College of American Pathologists. Pitfalls in salivary gland fine-needle aspiration cytology: lessons from the College of American Pathologists Interlaboratory Comparison Program in Nongynecologic Cytology. Arch Pathol Lab Med. 2005;129:26–31.
8. Tyagi R, Dey P. Diagnostic problems of salivary gland tumors. Diagn Cytopathol. 2015;43:495–509.
9. El-Naggar AK, Chan J, Takata T, Grandis J, Blootweg P. WHO classification of tumours. Pathology and genetics of head and neck tumours. 4th ed. Lyon: IARC Press; 2022.
10. Wei S, Layfield L, LiVolsi VA, et al. Reporting of fine needle aspiration (FNA) specimens of salivary gland lesions: a comprehensive review. Diagn Cytopathol. 2017;45:820–7.
11. Johnson DN, Onenerk M, Krane J, et al. Cytologic grading of primary malignant salivary gland tumors: a blinded review by an international panel. Cancer Cytopathol. 2020;128(6):392–402.
12. Rossi ED, Faquin WC, Baloch Z, et al. The Milan System for Reporting Salivary Gland Cytopathology: analysis and suggestions of initial survey. Cancer. 2017;125:757–66.
13. Layfield LJ, Baloch ZW, Hirschowitz SL, et al. Impact on clinical follow-up of the Milan System for salivary gland cytology: a comparison with a traditional diagnostic classification. Cytopathology. 2018;29:335–42.
14. Rossi ED, Baloch Z, Pusztaszeri M, et al. The Milan System for Reporting Salivary Gland Cytopathology (MSRSGC): an ASC-IAC-sponsored system for reporting salivary gland fine-needle aspiration. J Am Soc Cytopathol. 2018;7:111–8.

15. Pusztaszeri M, Baloch Z, Vielh P, et al. Application of the Milan system for reporting risk stratification in salivary gland cytopathology. Cancer Cytopathol. 2018;126:69–70.

16. Rossi ED, Faquin WC, Baloch Z, et al. The Milan System for Reporting Salivary Gland Cytopathology: analysis and suggestions of initial survey. Cancer Cytopathol. 2017;125:757–66.

17. Barbarite E, Puram SV, Derakhshan A, et al. A call for universal acceptance of the Milan System for Reporting Salivary Gland Cytopathology. Laryngoscope. 2020;130:80–5.

18. Rossi ED, Faquin WC. The Milan System for Reporting Salivary Gland Cytopathology (MSRSGC): an international effort toward improved patient care-when the roots might be inspired by Leonardo da Vinci. Cancer Cytopathol. 2018;126:756–66.

19. Rossi ED, Wong LQ, Bizzarro T, Petrone G, Mule A, Fadda G, Baloch ZM. The impact of FNAC in the management of salivary gland lesions: institutional experiences leading to a risk based classification scheme. Cancer Cytopathol. 2016;124:388–96.

20. Griffith CC, Pai RK, Schneider F, Duvvuri U, Ferris RL, Johnson JT, Seethala RR. Salivary gland tumor fine needle aspiration cytology. A proposal for a risk stratification classification. Am J Clin Pathol. 2015;143:839–53.

21. Sundling KE, Kurtycz DFI. Standardized terminology systems in cytopathology. Diagn Cytopathol. 2019;47:53–63.

22. Grapsa D, Politi E. Standardized categorical reporting of cytopathology results. Diagn. Cytopathol. 2013;41:917–21.

23. Crothers BA, Tench WD, Schwartz MR, et al. Guidelines for the reporting of nongynecologic cytopathology specimens. Arch Pathol Lab Med. 2009;133:1743–56.

24. Geiger JI, Ismaila N, Beadle B, et al. Management of salivary gland malignancy: ASCO Guidelines. J Clin Oncol. 2021;39(17):1909–41.

25. Ali SZ, Cibas ED, editors. The Bethesda system for reporting thyroid cytopathology: definitions, criteria and explanatory notes. New York: Springer; 2017.

26. Behaeghe M, Vander Poorten V, Hermans R, et al. The Milan System for Reporting Salivary Gland Cytopathology: single center experience with cell blocks. Diagn Cytopathol. 2020; https://doi.org/10.1002/dc.24515.

27. Iskandar ME, Bonomo G, Avadhani V, et al. Evidence for overestimation of the prevalence of malignancy in indeterminate thyroid nodules classified as Bethesda category III. Surgery. 2015;157:510–7.

28. Maleki Z, Miller JA, Arab SE, et al. "Suspicious" salivary gland FNA: risk of malignancy and interinstitutional variability. Cancer. 2018;126:94–100.

29. Viswanathan K, Sung S, Scognamiglio T, et al. The role of the Milan System for Reporting Salivary Gland Cytopathology: a 5-year institutional experience. Cancer Cytopathol. 2018;126:541–51.

30. Wang H, Malik A, Maleki Z, et al. "Atypical" salivary gland fine needle aspiration: risk of malignancy and interinstitutional variability. Diagn Cytopathol. 2017;45:1088–94.

31. Rohilla M, Singh P, Rajwanshi A, et al. Three-year cytohistological correlation of salivary gland FNA cytology at a tertiary center with the application of the Milan system for risk stratification. Cancer Cytopathol. 2017;125:767e775.

32. Thiryayi SA, Low YX, Shelton D, et al. A retrospective 3-year study of salivary gland FNAC with categorisation using the Milan reporting system. Cytopathology. 2018;29:343–8.

33. Liu H, Ljungren C, Lin F, et al. Analysis of histologic follow-up and risk of malignancy for salivary gland neoplasm of uncertain malignant potential proposed by the Milan System for Reporting Salivary Gland Cytopathology. Cancer Cytopathol. 2018;126:490–7.

34. Rossi ED, Faquin WC. The Milan System for Reporting Salivary Gland Cytopathology: the clinical impact so far. Considerations from theory to practice. Cytopathology. 2020;31:181–4.

35. Jalaly JB, Farahani SJ. Baloch, ZW. The Milan System for Reporting Salivary Gland Cytopathology: a comprehensive review of the literature: Diag Cytopathol; 2020. p. 1–10.

36. Maleki Z, Baloch Z, Lu R, et al. Application of the Milan System for Reporting Submandibular Gland Cytopathology: an international, multi-institutional study. Cancer Cytopathol. 2019;127:306–15.

37. Lubin D, Buonocore D, Wei XJ, et al. The Milan System at Memorial Sloan Kettering: utility of the categorization system for in-house salivary gland fine-needle aspiration cytology at a comprehensive cancer center. Diagn Cytopathol. 2020;48:183–90.

38. Kurtycz DFI, Rossi ED, Baloch Z, et al. Milan Interobserver Reproducibility Study (MIRST): Milan System 2018. J Am Soc Cytopathol. 2020;9:116–25.

39. Jo V, Krane J. Ancillary testing in salivary gland cytology: a practical guide. Cancer Cytopathol. 2018;126(Suppl 8):627–42.

40. Wong KS, Marino-Enriquez A, Hornick JL, Jo VY. NR4A3 immunohistochemistry reliably discriminates acinic cell carcinoma from mimics. Head Neck Pathol. 2021;15(2):425–32.

Esther Diana Rossi, Professor of pathology at Catholic University of Rome, Italy. Responsible of the task force for salivary gland lesions of the American Society of Cytopathology (ASC), co-editor of the new classification system for salivary gland Cytopathology Author and Member of the second edition of *The Bethesda System for Thyroid Cytopathology.*

William C. Faquin is the Professor of pathology at Harvard Medical School, Boston, MA, USA. He has authored over 400 peer-reviewed publications. He is the Editor-in-Chief for *Cancer Cytopathology*, which is one of the three journals of the American Cancer Society. He is a co-author of *The Bethesda System for Reporting Thyroid Cytopathology*, co-chair of the College of American Pathologists' Evidence-Based Guidelines Committee for the testing of head and neck squamous cell carcinomas for high-risk HPV, and co-chair of *The Milan System for Reporting Salivary Gland Cytopathology*, sponsored by the ASC and IAC.

FNAB of Lymph Nodes in the Head and Neck region

13

Andrew S. Field, Sharron Liang, and William Sewell

13.1 Introduction

Lymph node fine needle aspiration biopsies (FNAB) in the head and neck (H&N) region are one of the most common sites for FNAB apart from the thyroid and salivary gland. There is a long tradition of performing FNAB of palpable lymph nodes in this region, but over the past 20 years ultrasound has become the most common modality used to direct the FNAB. The use of FNAB of H&N lymph nodes to diagnose infections such as mycobacterial infections and to diagnose metastatic carcinoma and melanoma is well established and accepted as a minimally invasive, accurate and cost-effective diagnostic procedure, similarly for confirming recurrent lymphomas. However, the use of FNAB to make the primary diagnosis of many lymphomas supported by ultrasound, immunocytochemistry (ICC), flow cytometry, fluorescent in situ hybridization (FISH) and cytogenetic findings is regarded by some as routine and by others as contentious.

A. S. Field (✉)
School of Clinical Medicine, University of New South Wales Sydney, Sydney, NSW, Australia

Medical School, University of Notre Dame, Sydney, NSW, Australia

Department of Anatomical Pathology, St Vincent's Hospital, Sydney, NSW, Australia

International Academy of Cytology, Freiburg im Breisgau, Germany

IAC WHO IARC Cytopathology Joint Standing Editorial Board, Lyon, France

WHO Classification of Tumours Standing Editorial Board, Lyon, France
e-mail: Andrew.Field@svha.org.au

S. Liang
Anatomical Pathology Department, St Vincent's Hospital, Sydney, NSW, Australia
e-mail: Sharron.liang@svha.org.au

W. Sewell
School of Clinical Medicine, University of New South Wales Sydney, Sydney, NSW, Australia

Garvan Institute of Medical Research, Darlinghurst, NSW, Australia
e-mail: w.sewell@garvan.or.gau

13.2 Pre-FNAB Assessment of History, Laboratory Data and Lesion Site

The commonest cause of lymphadenopathy in the H&N region apart from nonspecific infection is metastatic carcinoma. It is essential to have a good clinical history, especially of any previous malignancy in the region or at any other site, and to correlate any imaging, full blood count or other pathology tests including serology results before performing the FNAB.

The site of the lymph node often assists in the pre-FNAB assessment by suggesting a differential diagnosis, although nonspecific infections, viral infections and bacterial infections of the oro-

© The Author(s), under exclusive license to Springer Nature Switzerland AG 2024
J. Klijanienko et al. (eds.), *Diagnostic Procedures in Patients with Neck Masses*,
https://doi.org/10.1007/978-3-031-67675-8_13

pharynx or larynx or systemic infections are the commonest causes of H&N lymphadenopathy. The type of infection may vary depending on the patient's country; for example, a patient with an enlarged cervical lymph node in countries having endemic mycobacterial infection will have this as among the most likely causes, while in a high-income country (HIC), this may not be considered initially except in the immune compromised. However, clinical information and the site of the lymph node contribute to the pathologist's development of a differential diagnosis.

B-cell and T-cell lymphomas (non-Hodgkin lymphomas) affect any of the H&N lymph nodes and may be bilateral. Classic Hodgkin lymphoma can present unilaterally and may involve the supraclavicular and cervical lymph nodes more commonly. Occipital lymph nodes may be associated with metastases from carcinomas of the scalp and skin of the H&N region, and in a younger patient, they may suggest toxoplasmosis. Post- and pre-auricular lymph nodes similarly can be involved by metastases from the scalp, face, parotid glands and lesions of the ear canal and ear. Upper cervical lymph nodes and mid-cervical lymph nodes may be involved by metastases from lip and skin primaries, oropharyngeal primaries such as nasopharyngeal and squamous cell carcinomas including HPV-related carcinomas, and salivary gland carcinomas. Assessment of mid-cervical lymph nodes should always consider the possibility of a laryngeal pouch or thyroglossal duct cyst when the site is more towards the midline, and a branchial cleft cyst if the lesion is more lateral. Lower cervical lymph nodes may have metastases from the H&N region and also from lung and the abdomen. Supraclavicular lymph nodes can have metastases from the H&N, as well as from the lung, breast and abdomen.

13.3 Lymph Node Fine Needle Aspiration Biopsy Procedure

Fundamental to all FNAB cytopathology is that it is crucial to perform the FNAB with good technique and to make good quality direct smears,

and this applies to FNAB of H&N lymph nodes.

At the time of the procedure, rapid on-site evaluation (ROSE) is very valuable to not only guide the proceduralist to attain adequate material but also to triage the lymph node material in the best possible way for ancillary testing and the most cost-effective selection of tests. For example, an FNAB of a lymph node yielding metastatic carcinoma does not need flow cytometry, and a case providing lymphoid material in most situations needs flow cytometry and possibly a cell block.

When the FNAB is performed under ultrasound direction, there is a tendency to only use one line of approach and to aim for any particular cortical thickening or other lesion seen on the ultrasound. Often local anaesthetic is placed in one position in the skin and each puncture is made through this same position. This decreases the ability of the FNAB to sample the node widely. Under ultrasound direction, the needle is placed into and through the lesion in the lymph node, ultrasound images are taken to demonstrate 'that the needle is in the lesion', and then the needle is passed and withdrawn backwards and forwards within the node or lesion or in some cases minimally moved with aspiration applied. The risks are that the needle will remain too long in the tissue including the lymph node and that fibrin clotting will occur resulting in a fibrin cast of the needle lumen being deposited as a coiled 'snake' on the slides, or that the over-emphasis of 'aspiration' will produce mainly blood from the lymph node's ample vasculature.

Ideally, a better technique is to keep the needle in the tissue and lymph node for a minimum 'dwell time'. If ultrasound is used, then the operator must be aware of the absolute requirement for the speed of the procedure to prevent clotting in the needle and the minimization of bleeding within the lesion. The needle can be introduced attached to a syringe ideally within a holder to allow the other hand to help fix the lymph node so that it ideally does not move during the procedure and should be passed rapidly to and fro within the node and then withdrawn rapidly to expel the material onto slides. Alternatively, the 23- or 25-gauge needle alone can be held between the thumb and first fingertips and used without a syringe and without aspiration. This method allows an excellent sensitive feel of the needle as it passes through the skin and lymph node capsule into the node. The needle is rapidly passed in and out of the lesion or in varying directions to sample the lymph node, making sure changes in the direction of the needle are made when the needle is almost withdrawn from the node, and then the needle is withdrawn. If there is concern regarding the nature of the lesion being possibly cystic, a syringe with the plunger removed can be attached to the needle and the needle is held in the same way. Each cytopathologist and proceduralist will have their favourite technique, and it may vary with the lymph node and expected findings. For example, a needle *attached to* a syringe in a holder may be used for a presumed metastatic lesion and the needle by itself for expected lymphomas.

Ideally, FNAB of lymph nodes should be performed by a cytopathologist who has experienced the 'short loop' of performing and immediately assessing the outcome of their skill or lack of skill in performing the FNAB and benefitted greatly from this to produce a skilled proceduralist, or an interventional radiologist who has been well trained in the procedure, and taken feedback at ROSE and final reporting of their cases to improve their skills. This is the most crucial component of the lymph node FNAB. If the proceduralist cannot provide material from the FNAB, the procedure has failed.

The second most crucial step is the rapid making of good-quality smears from the material deposited on the slides. This is a grossly underrated skill and often left to a poorly trained assistant or trainee, but it is a skill that must be developed to make FNAB of lymph nodes possible. Rapid assessment of the amount and type of material deposited on the slide should be followed, if possible, by specimen splitting onto at least two, if not three or more slides. Material smeared on the first slide should immediately go into alcohol fixation without even a quick look by the proceduralist, and material smeared on a second slide should be rapidly air-dried using a hair dryer on low heat or a warming plate. The air-

dried slide can be stained with the Giemsa stain, and the alcohol-fixed slide with the Papanicolaou, or in some laboratories, with H&E stain. If smears are not performed well, the FNAB procedure is at risk of being a waste of time. Poor performance of the FNAB itself and the making of smears are the greatest causes of poor results in the FNAB of lymph nodes of the head and neck.

Ideally, smears should be prepared by alcohol fixation for Pap stains and air-drying for Giemsa smears. Some cytopathologists prefer the Pap stain for its nuclear and nucleolar detail, and it is very effective for staining keratin, the assistance it provides in assessing small-cell lymphomas and the ability to look into three-dimensional tissue fragments. Others prefer the Giemsa stain which allows for the assessment of lymphoid material, which can be reactive or lymphomatous, and other haematological lesions, and also effectively stains stromal components and background components such as mucin. Ideally, it is recommended that both stains should be used. Direct smears can also be used for acid-fast mycobacterial, fungal and other special stains.

Ancillary testing is dependent on ROSE. If ROSE is not utilized, then a protocol should be developed so that a number of specimens are taken at the time of the FNAB, and then decisions are made once the stained slides have been viewed in the laboratory by the cytopathologists, as to which tests will be used. For example, FNAB of an immune-compromised patient with a swollen lymph node in the cervical region of the neck would require alcohol and air-dried slides, extra air-dried slides for auramine or acid-fast stains for mycobacteria and fungi, material directly squirted into a sterile container for mycobacterial cultures and PCR, and needle rinsings or a separate pass in buffered saline or Hanks' transport medium for flow cytometry and/or cell block. On the other hand, if the FNAB is of a cervical lymph node in a patient with a history of carcinoma of the H&N region, then in addition to the direct smears, needle rinsings in buffered saline or Hanks' medium or a separate pass can be placed in a container for preparation of a cell block for immunocytochemistry (ICC) and potentially next generation sequencing (NGS).

Fluorescent in situ hybridization (FISH) may also be needed in some cases, such as potential salivary gland carcinomas. Direct smears can be used for NGS and FISH if cell block material is not available.

Flow cytometry is a powerful tool to distinguish between reactive and lymphomatous samples, and is of particular usefulness in small-cell lymphomas, including mantle cell lymphoma, small lymphocytic lymphoma/chronic lymphocytic leukaemia, lymphoplasmacytic lymphoma, marginal zone lymphoma and lymphoblastic lymphoma (Table 13.3). Lymph node FNAB samples can be easily dispersed into single-cell suspensions suitable for flow cytometry analysis. Lymph nodes contain CD3 positive T-cells admixed with CD19 and CD20 positive B-cells, which in reactive samples are largely negative for CD5 and CD10. Assessment of light chain restriction by flow cytometry is an effective way to distinguish between reactive and lymphoma cases. In reactive cases, the B-cell kappa: lambda light chain ratio is normally between 1:1 and 3:1, whereas in lymphoma, the monoclonal B-cells are restricted to the expression of either kappa or lambda. Lymphoma cases often contain admixed non-neoplastic B-cells, but lymphoma B-cells can be identified by the use of flow cytometry software to select populations and display their light chain properties. For example, B-cells that are positive for CD5 or CD10, or that are unusually dim or bright for CD19 or CD20, can be selected by software to display their light chain properties. If a monoclonal B-cell population is present, it will usually be revealed by this approach, even in the presence of large numbers of polyclonal B-cells.

Liquid-based cytopathology (LBC) for lymph node FNAB is used by some pathologists. It decreases problems with the requirement for good direct smearing techniques, reduces air-drying artefacts of alcohol-fixed smears and reduces the skill required of the proceduralist in these facets of effective FNAB of lymph nodes. However, well-made direct smears provide pattern recognition information that is a vital part of the assessment of FNAB of lymph nodes, and this is lost in LBC to a great degree, as are many of the characteristic findings in Pap smears. Further, there are no Giemsa smears to assess and the cost for LBC is greater. LBC samples can be processed for NGS.

13.4 Standardized Reporting of Head and Lymph Nodes

The Sydney system for lymph node FNAB reporting, an IAC initiative that brought more than 30 cytopathologists with an interest in lymph node FNAB together, has recently been published and recommends categorization of all lymph node FNAB as one of five categories described by a specific terminology. Numbers are not used in FNAB cytopathology reporting because they detract from the information provided to the clinician and cause poor communication errors.

- *Insufficient/Inadequate/Nondiagnostic:* This category is defined as cases with insufficient material due to low or absent cellularity, poor quality smearing or staining, and obscuring material such as ultrasound gel, heavy blood contamination or perhaps necrosis. The term 'nondiagnostic' is used by some cytopathologists for cases where there is good lymphoid material that appears benign but there is high clinical suspicion or imaging features of a suspicious nodal lesion. Other cytopathologists prefer to issue a 'Benign' categorization, describe the material present and attach a caveat 'that the material may not be representative of the lesion seen on imaging'. A reporting cytopathologist or group of cytopathologists within a department should select an approach and one term, and stick to it consistently.
- *Benign:* This category is defined as cases with unequivocal benign features, and includes infectious and inflammatory lesions and reac-

tive lymph nodes, for example, mycobacterial granulomatous lymphadenitis.

- *Atypical:* This category is defined as cases with mainly benign features but some features are present that raise the possibility of a neoplastic process, and includes cases of 'atypical lymphoid cells of uncertain significance', for example, lymph nodes with features most suggestive of a follicular hyperplasia but where some features raise the possibility of a low-grade follicular lymphoma. This category maintains the high negative predictive value of a 'Benign' category.
- *Suspicious of malignancy*: This category is defined as cases where there may be limited material or discrepant benign and malignant features. This category maintains the high positive predictive value of a 'Malignant' diagnosis.
- *Malignant:* This category is defined as cases with unequivocal malignant features, such as metastasis to a lymph node or a high-grade lymphoma.

The 'Atypical' and 'Suspicious of malignancy' categories should be kept to a minimum in numbers and their rates within practice should be monitored, recognizing that their rates may differ between different practices and in different countries, such as comparing an oncology hospital in a high-income country (HIC) and a general hospital practice in a low to middle-income country (LMIC).

Recently, as part of the joint project between the IAC, WHO and IARC, a WHO reporting system for lymph node cytopathology has been developed by an international Expert Editorial Board. Importantly, a consensus has been reached on definitions of the categories and the key diagnostic cytopathological criteria of each lesion within the 'Benign' and 'Malignant' categories, and sections on specimen preparation and appropriate ancillary testing have been included. Each category is tied to a risk of malignancy, which with a brand-new reporting system will be based on a review of the literature available, and a recommendation for further diagnostic management. The Sydney system and WHO system are similar in their categories, and the latter will include any changes in the forthcoming fifth edition of the WHO Classification of Haematopoietic Tumours. Both systems recognize the importance of special stains, such as an acid-fast stain for mycobacteria demonstrating mycobacteria in a granulomatous FNAB, ICC that may confirm the type of metastatic carcinoma found in a malignant FNAB (Tables 13.1 and 13.2) and flow cytometry that may confirm and subtype the lymphoma found on FNAB (Table 13.3). These ancillary tests are an essential part of all FNAB of lymph nodes and may change the final category or make more specific the cytopathology diagnosis, but they may vary in their availability in LMIC. The WHO System emphasizes the cytopathology diagnostic features and the differential diagnosis based on these features so that it can be used globally in all conditions.

Table 13.1 Immunocytochemistry lineage marker for metastases to lymph nodes

	Pancytokeratin, EMA, CEA	Melanocytic markers: HMB45, MART1	Lymphoid markers: CD45, CD20 (B- cells), CD3 (T cells)	SALL4	Vimentin	Neuroendocrine markers, synaptophysin, chromogranin, INSM1
Carcinoma	+	−	−	−	−	−
Melanoma	−	+	−	−	−	−
Lymphoma	−	−	+	−	−	−
Sarcoma	−	−	−	−	+	−
Germ cell tumour	+	−	−	+	−	−
Neuroendocrine tumours	+	−	−	−	−	+

Table 13.2 Immunocytochemistry site-specific marker for metastases to lymph nodes

	CK7	CK20	TTF-1	CDX2	SATB2	GATA3	PAX8	GCDFP1	ER	Thyroglobulin	S100P	NKX3.1	Other
Oesophagus	+	−	−	−/+	−	−	−	−	−	−	−	−	
Stomach	+	+	−	−/+	−	−	−	−	−	−	−	−	
Lung	+	−	+	−	−	−	−	−	−	−	−	−	Napsin A +
Colorectal	−	+	−	+	+	−	−	−	−	−	−	−	
Breast	+	−	−	−	−	+	−	+	−/+	−	−	−	
Pancreas	+	+	−	−	−	−	−	−	−	−	+	−	SMAD4 loss
Liver	−	−	−	−	−	−	−	−	−	−	−	−	HepPar1 +; Glypectin 3 +
Genitourinary bladder	+	+	−	−	−	+	−	−	−	−	−	−	Uroplakin +
Prostate	−	−	−	−	−	−	−	−	−	−	−	+	PSA +, PMSA +
Female gynecological tract	+	−	−	−	−	−	+	−	−/+	−	−	−	WT1 + for sercus carcinoma
Kidney	−/+	−	−	−	−	−	+	−	−	−	−	−	PAX2 +
Thyroid (follicular or papillary)	+	−	+	−	−	−	+	−	−	+	−	−	
Medullary thyroid	+	−	+	−	−	−	−	−	−	−	−	−	Calcitonin +, Neuroendocrine markers +

Table 13.3 Phenotype of commoner B-cell lymphoma

Lymphoma type	CD5	CD10	CD19	CD20	CD23	CD200
CLL/SLL	+	−	+	+*	+	+
DLBCL	±	±	+	+	±	±
FL	−	+	+	+	±	±
LPL	−/±	−	+	+/±	−/±	−
MCL	+	−	+	+	−/±	−/±
Nodal MZL	−/±	−	+	+	−	+

Abbreviations: *CLL/SLL* chronic lymphocytic lymphoma/small lymphocytic leukaemia, *DLBCL* diffuse large B-cell lymphoma, *FL* follicular lymphoma, *LPL* lymphoplasmacytic lymphoma, *MCL* mantle cell lymphoma, *Nodal MZL* nodal marginal zone lymphoma
Symbols: +, typically positive; −, typically negative; ±, variable expression; −/±, usually negative, may be positive; +/±, usually positive, may be negative; *, dim expression

The aim of all FNAB cytopathology is to provide as accurate a diagnosis as possible, beginning with the cytopathology report, and then provide well-triaged material for ancillary tests, finishing with an integrated report that includes any further testing. The components of this report have been recommended by the Sydney and WHO Systems, but how they are included in the final report will be determined by local formatting, IT systems and local usage. These components include the following:

- Clinical and imaging information
- The exact site of the lymph node biopsy
- Diagnostic summary that includes the site of the FNAB, the category of the report and as specific a diagnosis as possible, or if not, a differential diagnosis
- Microscopy report that may be brief in cases with a specific diagnosis and more descriptive in cases requiring a differential diagnosis
- Ancillary testing

13.5   Lymph Node Fine Needle Aspiration Biopsy Assessment of Direct Smears

The assessment of FNAB direct smears requires two basic steps: assessment of the *smear pattern* on the slide and then *assessment of tissue fragments and dispersed cells and the background*. If there are epithelial tissue fragments in a lymph node FNAB, which may or may not have residual lymphoid material or other features such as necrosis, then the initial diagnosis of *metastatic carcinoma* is suggested and can be confirmed by high-power assessment confirming the epithelial cells and their type as far as possible.

If there are no tissue fragments and the material consists of *dispersed single cells,* then a high-power assessment of the cell type is required. If the material is lymphoid then the prominent lymphoid cell types have to be established. Some carcinomas such as lobular carcinoma of the breast (Figs. 13.1 and 13.2) and signet ring carcinoma of the stomach and other tumours such as metastatic melanoma can produce dispersed single cells, but often there will be residual lymphocytes and the two cell types can be recognized. Assessment of the cell type will demonstrate the metastatic cells.

If there are tissue fragments representing granulomas consisting of epithelioid histiocytes with or without multinucleated giant cells, then assessment of the background for necrosis, the type of granulomas and the accompanying lymphocytes, neutrophils or eosinophils can further define the diagnosis. Specific causes of *granulomatous lymphadenitis* (Figs. 13.3, 13.4, 13.5 and 13.6), such as fungi, mycobacteria and pigment of various types can be looked for on the standard and special stains. Rarely, Hodgkin lymphoma and some metastatic carcinomas, in particular squamous cell carcinomas and metastatic seminomas, may be associated with a granulomatous component.

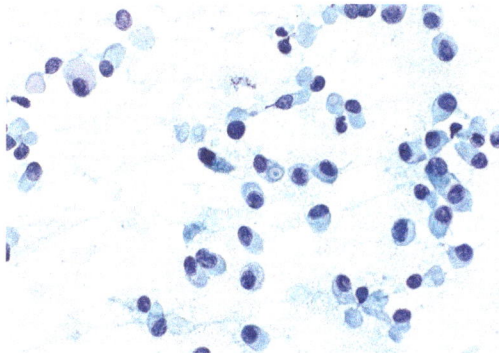

Fig. 13.1 Metastatic lobular carcinoma with discohesive dispersed single cells with mildly enlarged mildly pleomorphic nuclei lacking prominent nucleoli. Centrally, a cell shows an intracytoplasmic vacuole containing a mucin droplet ('targetoid body') in the eccentric cytoplasm. Pap ×60

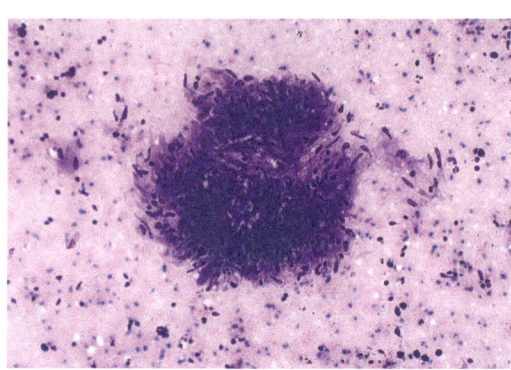

Fig. 13.4 Loosely cohesive non-necrotising epithelioid granuloma, with epithelioid histiocytes with elongated 'footprint in the sand' nuclei. Embedded lymphocytes within the granuloma are noted. The patient had a history of sarcoidosis. Giemsa ×20

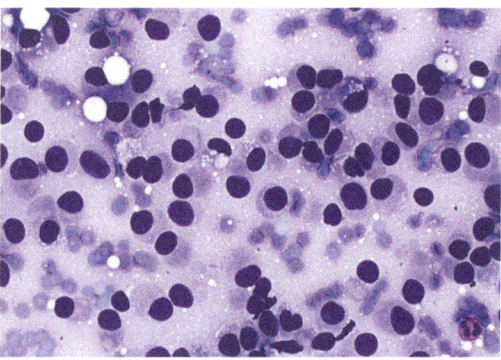

Fig. 13.2 Metastatic lobular carcinoma with discohesive dispersed single cells. Giemsa ×60

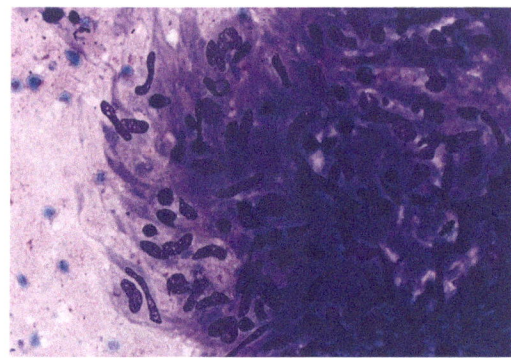

Fig. 13.5 Loosely cohesive epithelioid granuloma with elongated nuclei of epithelioid histiocytes. Giemsa ×60

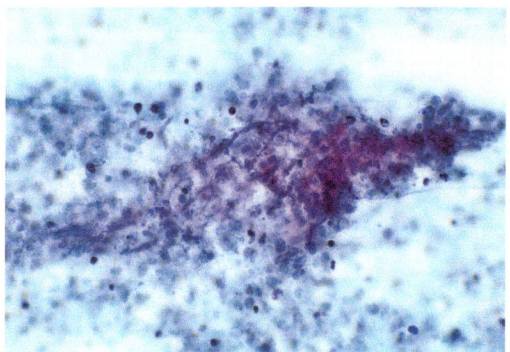

Fig. 13.3 Caseating necrosis in a patient with a history of multidrug-resistant mycobacterial infection. Pap ×60

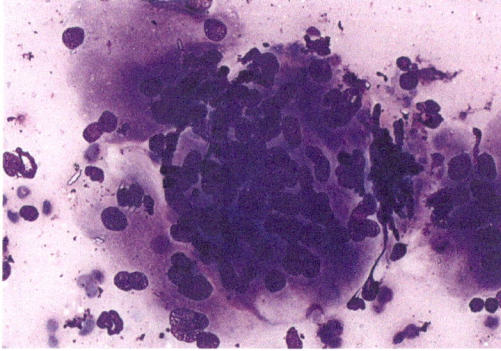

Fig. 13.6 Loosely cohesive epithelioid non-necrotising granuloma with multinucleated giant cells and elongated nuclei of epithelioid histiocytes. The patient had a history of sarcoidosis. Giemsa ×60

Suppurative lymphadenitis, suppurative granulomatous lesions and lymphoid reactive and neoplastic processes produce dispersed cells. Large numbers of neutrophils in various stages of degeneration with a variable number of histiocytes and lymphocytes are present in a background of fibrin and debris. Aggregates of neutrophils, fibrin and histiocytes are present. Occasionally suppurative infections will include tissue fragments of acutely inflamed epithelium or fragments of granulation tissue in a background of neutrophils, macrophages, degenerate cells and fibrinous debris. Careful assessment of the epithelium in the tissue fragments looking for a low N:C ratio, uniformity of nuclear shape, chromatin and nucleoli is required, although there may be a uniform increase in cell and nuclear size and some anisonucleosis. Occasional metastatic carcinomas can be associated with a suppurative or suppurative granulomatous response. Kimura's disease has a high cellularity with a polymorphous population made up of markedly increased eosinophils with admixed lymphocytes, plasma cells and histiocytes. Free eosinophilic necrosis with free eosinophil granules may be seen suggestive of the eosinophilic abscesses seen in Kimura's disease.

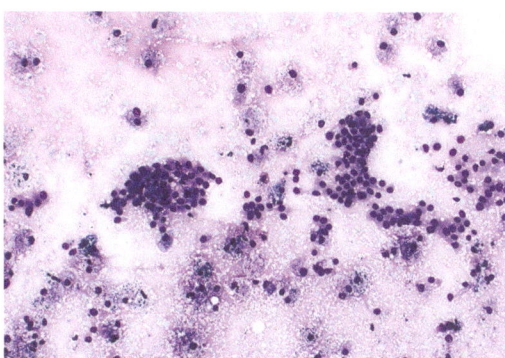

Fig. 13.7 Metastatic papillary thyroid carcinoma with tissue fragments and a prominent cystic background with hemosiderophages. Giemsa ×20

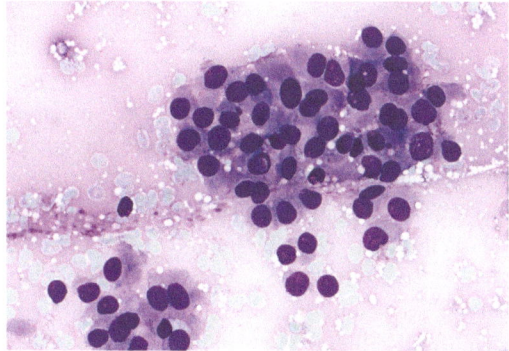

Fig. 13.8 Metastatic papillary thyroid carcinoma with tissue fragments with classic nuclear features including crowding, grooves, nuclear membrane irregularities, fine chromatin and nuclear pseudoinclusions. Giemsa ×60

13.6 Metastases to Lymph Nodes in the Head & Neck Region

The most common metastatic carcinoma in the H&N region is squamous cell carcinoma (SCC), and nasopharyngeal carcinoma (NPC) must be considered in this differential diagnosis along with Merkel cell carcinoma, basal cell carcinoma and metastatic melanoma. Salivary gland and thyroid carcinomas should also be considered especially in the cervical region, and these will have very similar features to their primaries, although papillary carcinoma of the thyroid (Figs. 13.7 and 13.8) often produces cystic degenerative lesions in lymph nodes on imaging and FNAB. Almost any other carcinoma can metastasize to H&N lymph nodes, including lung and breast cancers to lower cervical and supraclavicular nodes, but with far lower frequency. In the situation where the metastasis does not have the features of metastasis from one of these common H&N primary sites, then a review of the clinical history and imaging, a review by a more experienced cytopathologist and judicious application of ICC and in some cases, NGS is required (Tables 13.1 and 13.2).

Keratinizing well-differentiated squamous cell carcinoma shows scattered sheets and small tissue fragments that may include keratin pearls in a background of abundant anucleate squamous cells and keratinous debris (Fig. 13.9). There are pyknotic nuclei in keratinized cells with polygonal, spindle or tadpole dense sky blue (Giemsa stain) or orange (Pap stain) cytoplasm, and often only occasional tissue fragments of cells with central round to pleomorphic nuclei with coarse

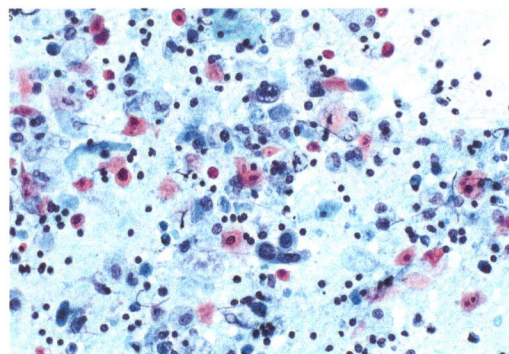

Fig. 13.9 Metastatic keratinizing squamous cell carcinoma with atypical cytoplasmic shapes including spindle and tadpole cells, containing enlarged, pleomorphic nuclei with granular chromatin and prominent nucleoli in some cells. Pap ×40

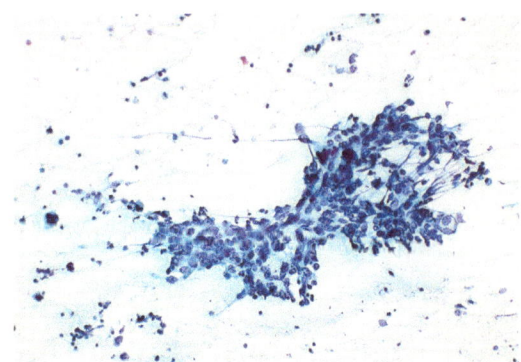

Fig. 13.10 Poorly differentiated squamous cell carcinoma with large cohesive tissue fragments containing malignant cells and apoptotic debris. The nuclei are centrally located and the cytoplasm is dense suggesting squamous differentiation. Excision showed a metastatic p16-positive squamous cell carcinoma. Pap ×20

chromatin and often single nucleoli and well defined cytoplasmic borders. The diagnosis should only be made on the basis of the nuclear features of these well-preserved cells to avoid false positive diagnoses of branchial cleft cyst epithelium and other squamous cysts in FNAB of lymph nodes in or near salivary glands. There may be a granulomatous and occasionally suppurative reaction in the background.

Poorly differentiated squamous cell carcinoma presents as more cellular smears with sheets and tissue fragments of large cells with often well-defined pale to denser cytoplasm, central round to pleomorphic nuclei and prominent nucleoli with perinucleolar clearing in some cells (Figs. 13.10 and 13.11). There is usually focal poorly developed keratinization and necrotic material in the background and some dispersal of single cells. ICC markers for SCC including p40 and CK5/6 are positive. CK7 and melanoma markers are negative. The distinction of a lung or other SCC metastasis from an H&N SCC is not possible. There is probably an argument for doing a p16 in these cases (Table 13.2).

Nasopharyngeal carcinoma (NPC) presents as cellular smears with tissue fragments of cells often associated with a background of lymphocytes and plasma cells. The usually large cells show moderately well-defined cytoplasm although some syncytial sheets may be present. The N:C ratio is usually moderate to high; the

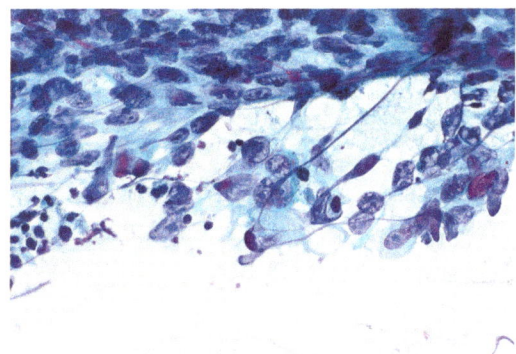

Fig. 13.11 Poorly differentiated squamous cell carcinoma with large cohesive tissue fragments containing cells with dense nonkeratinized sometimes polygonal, often spindle cytoplasm consistent with squamous differentiation. Excision showed a metastatic p16-positive squamous cell carcinoma. Pap ×60

nuclei are pleomorphic and hyperchromatic with variably prominent nucleoli and some perinucleolar clearing. The chromatin can be coarse or fine, which raises a differential diagnosis with neuroendocrine carcinomas from the lung or other sites. Necrosis is usually present in the background. There is no or limited keratinization. Cell block material can be used for ICC confirmation as NPC is strongly positive to cytokeratins AE1/AE3, CAM5.2, CK5/6 and EMA, with strong nuclear positivity to p63 and p40. As the majority of nasopharyngeal carcinomas are associated with Epstein-Barr Virus

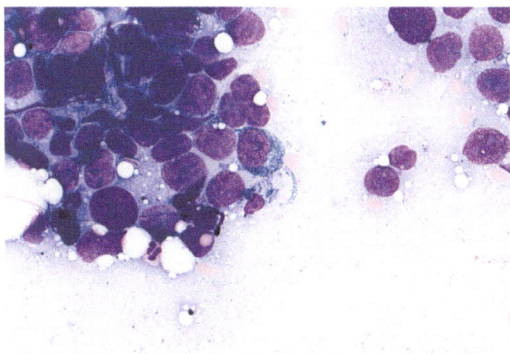

Fig. 13.12 Metastatic melanoma with a tissue fragment and discohesive single cells that are highly plemophic, spindle and contain prominent nucleoli. Occasional cells contain bluish-grey melanin pigment. Giemsa ×60

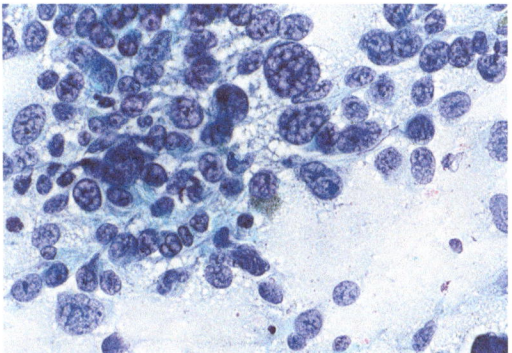

Fig. 13.13 Metastatic melanoma with tissue fragment and discohesive pleomorphic single cells that are polygonal or spindle, containing highly pleomorphic nuclei with prominent nucleoli. Occasional melanoma cells contain khaki melanin pigment. Pap ×60

(EBV), ISH for EBER should be strong and diffusely nuclear positive.

Melanoma usually produces highly cellular smears that show a wide range of patterns from dispersed single cells to small tissue fragments of varying size, consisting of medium to large usually pleomorphic epithelioid cells and occasionally spindle cells (Figs. 13.12 and 13.13). The N:C ratio is variable but polygonal cells with considerable eccentric cytoplasm are present. The nuclei are round to highly pleomorphic with hyperchromatic chromatin, prominent nucleoli and intranuclear pseudoinclusions in some cases. There may be khaki (Pap stain) to bluish-black (Giemsa stain) melanin granules in the cytoplasm

and in macrophages, and this has to be distinguished from hemosiderin pigment in macrophages of nonmelanoma metastases. ICC on cell block material is very useful and melanoma will be MART1, S100, HMB45 and SOX10 positive (Table 13.1).

Merkel cell carcinoma has highly cellular smears with dispersed single cells, small discohesive tissue fragments and rarely rosette formation. The cells are small to intermediate with a high N:C ratio. The nuclei are round to oval often containing finely granular or powdery chromatin. Nuclear moulding may be present as well as nuclear streaking and apoptotic bodies. Often the smears are monomorphous though occasional cells may show moderate nuclear pleomorphism. ICC for neuroendocrine markers such as synaptophysin, chromogranin, CD56 and INSM1 is usually positive, and this carcinoma is positive in pankeratins. CK20 shows a distinctive paranuclear dot-like positivity, which along with a negative TTF-1 may be helpful in differentiating this carcinoma from metastatic small cell carcinoma of the lung.

13.7   Lymphoid Material in Head and Neck Lymph Node FNAB Smears

Once the pattern recognition assessment of the smears shows a dispersed cell population and high power cell assessment confirms the cells as lymphoid, the crucial decision to make is whether the lymphoid cells are predominantly small lymphocytes or a mixed population with small lymphocytes predominating consistent with a reactive process, or a mixed population without small lymphocytes predominating or a monotonous population of small to intermediate or large atypical lymphoid cells, suggesting a lymphoma. Fragments of lymphoid cell cytoplasm ('lymphoglandular bodies') are usually present.

If the lymphoid cells are *predominantly small lymphocytes and mixed with scattered centroblasts and centrocytes* then *germinal centres* should be searched for: at low power the germinal centres will form denser areas of cells with or without small vessels, which actually represent lymphoid tissue fragments held together by dendritic cell processes (Figs. 13.14, 13.15, 13.16, 13.17, 13.18 and 13.19). The dendritic cells are the key cells to define a germinal centre, and have no discernible cytoplasm and oval nuclei with fine even nuclear margins, fine even reticular chromatin and small nucleoli. They are often seen in pairs along with tingible body macrophages, which are the other marker of germinal centres, and mixed with a small number of

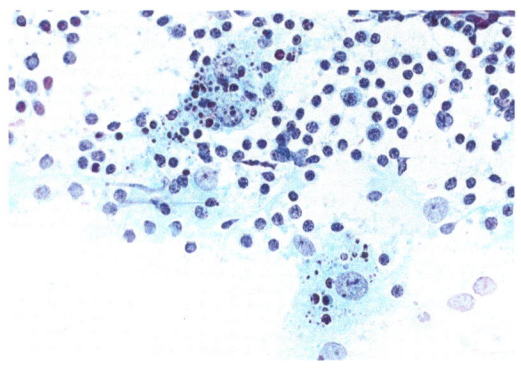

Fig. 13.16 Reactive lymph node with tingible body macrophages seen within a follicular germinal centre with dendritic reticulin cells with stripped oval nuclei, fine even chromatin and small nucleoli. Pap ×60

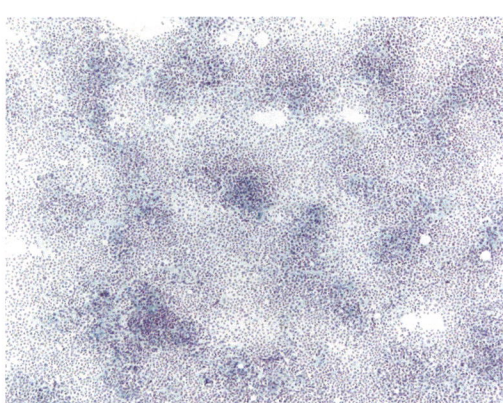

Fig. 13.14 Reactive follicular hyperplasia with low-power nodularity with follicular germinal centre tissue fragments in a dispersed lymphoid cell background. Pap ×20. (Courtesy of Dr. William R Geddie)

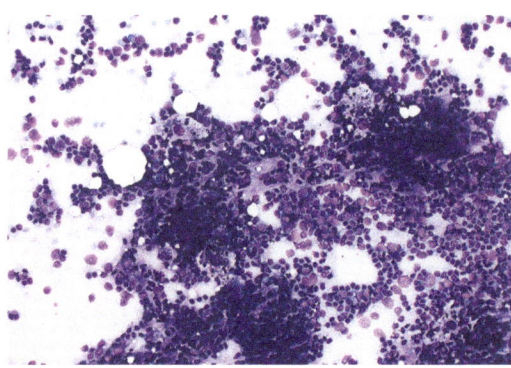

Fig. 13.17 Follicular hyperplasia with follicular germinal centre tissue fragments in a dispersed mixed lymphoid cell background with small lymphocytes predominating. Four tingible body macrophages are seen. Giemsa ×20

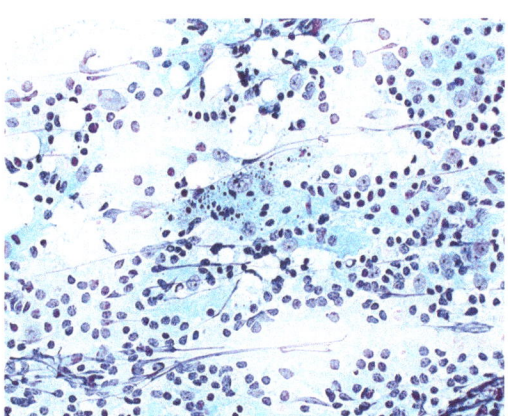

Fig. 13.15 Reactive lymph node with tingible body macrophages seen within a follicular germinal centre with multiple dendritic reticulin cells in a heterogeneous background with small lymphocytes predominating. Pap ×40

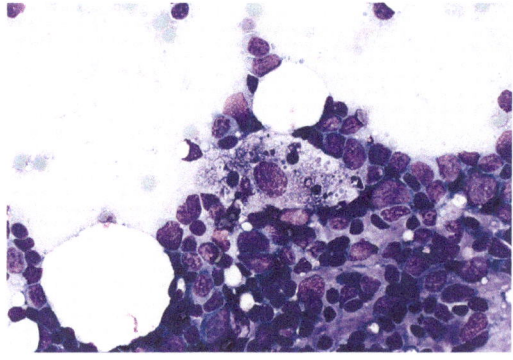

Fig. 13.18 Reactive lymph node with tingible body macrophages seen within a follicular germinal centre. Giemsa ×60

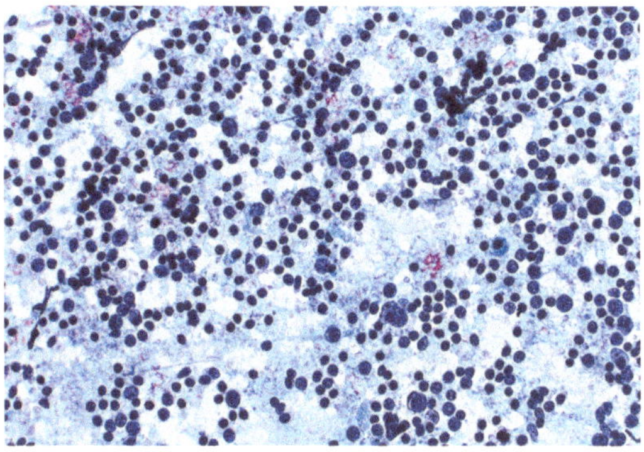

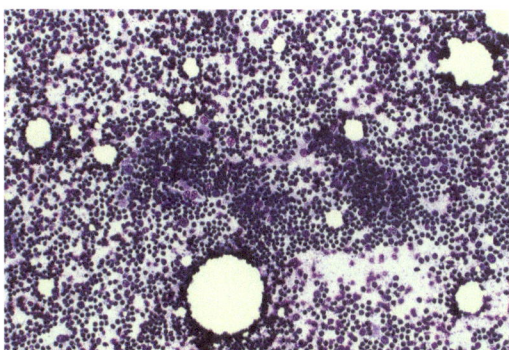

Fig. 13.19 Reactive lymph node showing an immunoblastic pattern with scattered immunoblasts in a background of small mature lymphocytes. Pap ×40

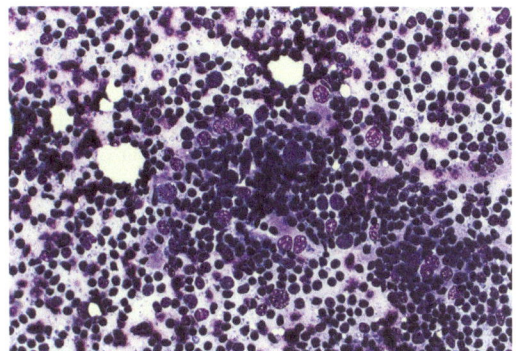

Fig. 13.21 Follicular lymphoma with follicular centre cell tissue fragment including dendritic reticulin cell at 12 o'clock, in a dispersed heterogeneous background that contains centrocytes and centroblasts. Giemsa ×40

Fig. 13.20 Follicular lymphoma with follicular centre cell tissue fragments in dispersed heterogeneous background. Giemsa ×20

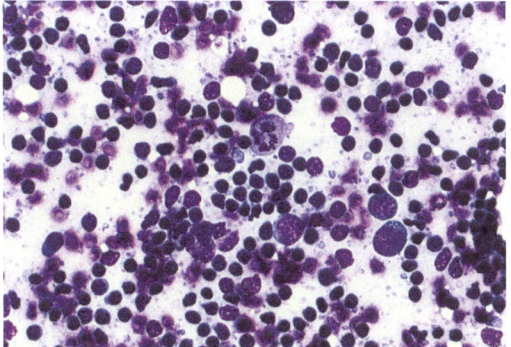

Fig. 13.22 Follicular lymphoma with a mixed population including small to intermediate centrocytes and occasional centroblasts. An atypical mitosis is noted. Giemsa ×60

centroblasts and more plentiful centrocytes. Centroblasts are larger lymphoid cells with round nuclei, one or two nucleoli frequently at the equator of the nuclear margin and a small amount of cytoplasm, and centrocytes vary in size from small to intermediate and occasionally large, with irregular sometimes angular or indented nuclei and inconspicuous nucleoli. Germinal centres may not always be seen in reactive lymph nodes, but their presence in a background of small lymphocytes is evidence of a benign reactive lymph node.

The differential diagnosis of a mixed lymphoid population is *follicular lymphoma* (FL) (Figs. 13.20, 13.21, 13.22 and 13.23). FL of low grade may show a predominantly small centrocyte-like cell in a relatively monotonous

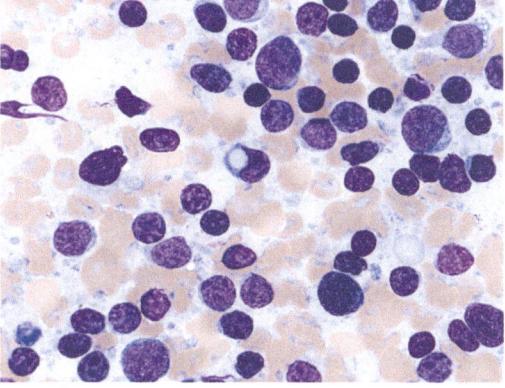

Fig. 13.23 Follicular lymphoma can show occasional lymphoid cells showing signet ring change with eccentric vacuoles impinging into the nuclei, usually filled with wispy immunoglobulin. Giemsa ×60. (Courtesy of Dr. William Geddie, Toronto)

population, but usually FL shows a mixed lymphoid population with no predominance of small lymphocytes. The centrocyte-like cells have angulated or indented or irregular nuclei with inconspicuous nucleoli and are usually small to intermediate or occasionally large. The second cell type in FL is a centroblast-like lymphoid cell with a round nucleus, one or several nucleoli frequently on the cell margin and a small amount of cytoplasm that can be eccentric. High-grade follicular lymphomas have a mixed lymphoid population of centrocyte-like and larger centroblastic cells, and may resemble diffuse large B-cell lymphoma (DLBCL) in FNAB smears. Flow cytometry and excision biopsy is frequently needed to type and grade these lymphomas including FISH for Myc and Bcl2 and Bcl6 rearrangements. In follicular lymphoma, flow cytometry demonstrates CD10 positive B-cells with restricted light chain expression (Table 13.3).

FL is a nodular proliferation in most cases, and the follicular nodules consist of more prominent centroblasts, centrocytes and dendritic cells. There may be small capillaries within these nodules. These nodules can be seen at low power assessment and resemble germinal centres of follicular hyperplasia, and provide a clue to the diagnosis. There are no tingible body macrophages associated with FL nodules and there are no or very few small mature lymphocytes in these smears. This allows for a differentiation from reactive germinal centres which feature dendritic cells, tingible body macrophages and a small number of centrocytes and even fewer centroblasts, within a background of predominantly small lymphocytes, with scattered larger cells and occasional large lymphoid cells with high N:C ratio, round nuclei and a rim of blue cytoplasm (Giemsa stain).

However, the differential diagnosis of follicular hyperplasia with plentiful tingible body macrophages, germinal centres with dendritic cells and predominantly small lymphocytes in the background, from FL can be difficult and leads frequently to an 'Atypical' categorization of 'atypical lymphoid cells of uncertain significance'. Follicular hyperplasia can change over time in the course of a single infection that may

be specific or never specifically diagnosed by culture or PCR studies. Flow cytometry is required if available and is particularly valuable in assessing light chain expression. In follicular hyperplasia, the B-cell kappa: lambda ratio is within normal limits, and there may be a subset of reactive B-cells that are CD10 positive, with brighter than normal CD20 expression, and with dimmer than normal expression of light chains with a normal kappa:lambda ratio. ICC is of less use when applied to cell blocks. In younger patients with a clinical history consistent with an infectious process, a 'watch and wait' approach can be used, but in older patients flow cytometry, core needle biopsy or excision biopsy may be appropriate.

If the lymphoid cells are *predominantly small lymphocytes*, which can be assessed on well smeared and fixed air-dried (Giemsa stained) smears but is often made easier on alcohol fixed (Pap stained) smears which allow assessment of the nuclear membrane for irregularities, then the pattern and cell type assessment can establish a resting or possibly reactive lymph node. The lymphocyte population of a resting lymph node particularly can be monotonous and the differential diagnosis includes chronic lymphocytic leukaemia/small lymphocytic lymphoma (CLL/SLL), mantle cell lymphoma (MCL) and possibly nodal marginal zone lymphoma (MZL). Small lymphocytes may predominate in an immunoblastic reaction with plentiful immunoblasts usually related to a viral infection, or a histiocytic reaction with plentiful histiocytes, or a plasma cell reaction with plentiful plasma cells as seen in syphilitic lymphadenitis. Small lymphocytes may also predominate with plentiful eosinophils in Langerhans cell histiocytosis and allergic conditions. The Langerhans cells have large irregular and grooved nuclei with eccentric cytoplasm and are CD1a positive. Prominent histiocytes can be present in lymph nodes draining chronic skin conditions in dermatopathic lymphadenopathy, where the histiocytes may contain melanin pigment, and massive cervical lymphadenopathy where some of the large histiocytes show emperiopolesis containing engulfed lymphocytes and other inflammatory cells. Clinical history and negative flow cytometry are required.

The other differential diagnosis is that of *Hodgkin lymphoma*. Uninuclear Hodgkin cells and Reed-Sternberg cells with bilobed or binucleated cells usually have abundant pale cytoplasm, best seen in the Giemsa-stained smears, and round to oval to more pleomorphic nuclei with one to several small to prominent nucleoli (Figs. 13.24, 13.25, 13.26, 13.27, 13.28, 13.29 and 13.30). These diagnostic cells should be searched for in any lymph node smears with a predominance of small lymphocytes. Classic Hodgkin lymphoma also has increased eosinophils and to a lesser extent increased plasma cells and histiocytes mixed with the small lymphocytes, and this background is often a clue to the diagnosis. The neoplastic cells in Hodgkin lymphoma are not normally detected by flow cytometry.

T-cell/histiocyte-rich diffuse large B-cell lymphoma can also have large numbers of small T-cells or on occasion histiocytes with scattered large atypical lymphoid cells resembling large centroblasts and immunoblasts, which are monoclonal B-cells. The large atypical lymphoid cells are small in number making diagnosis difficult diagnosis by both FNAB and flow cytometry. CNB or usually excision biopsy should be recommended if this lymphoma is suspected.

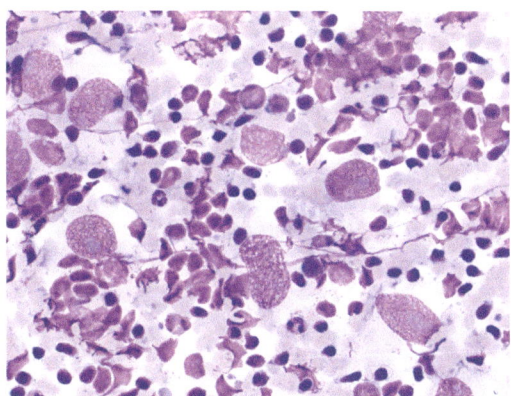

Fig. 13.25 Hodgkin lymphoma. Alien cell pattern with large mononuclear Hodgkin cells with macronucleoli in a background of lymphocytes. Giemsa ×60

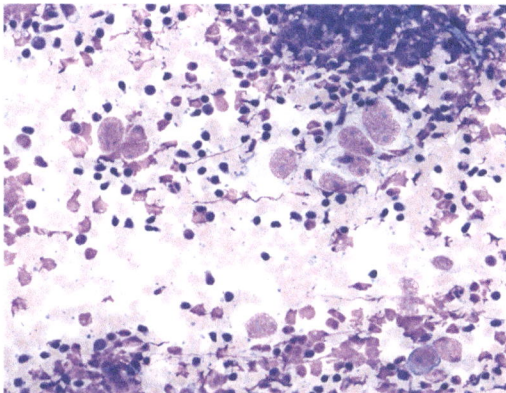

Fig. 13.26 Hodgkin lymphoma. Alien cell pattern with large mononuclear Hodgkin cells in a background of lymphocytes. Many of the nuclei are stripped. Giemsa ×40

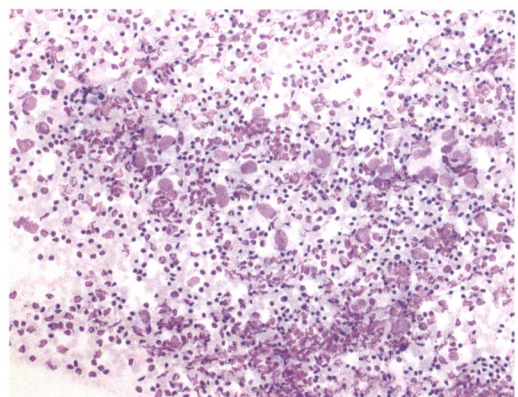

Fig. 13.24 Hodgkin lymphoma with mononuclear Hodgkin cells with macronucleoli in a heterogeneous background of lymphocytes, eosinophils and plasma cells. Giemsa ×20

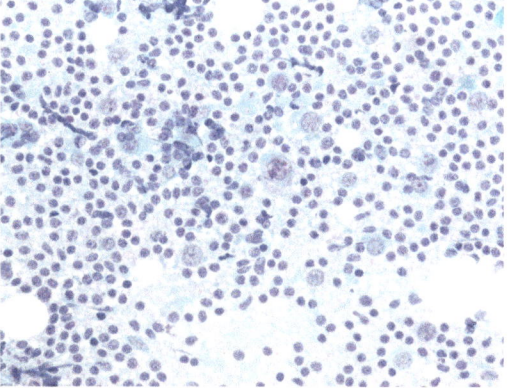

Fig. 13.27 Hodgkin lymphoma. Alien cell pattern with large mononuclear Hodgkin cells in a background of small lymphocytes. Pap ×60

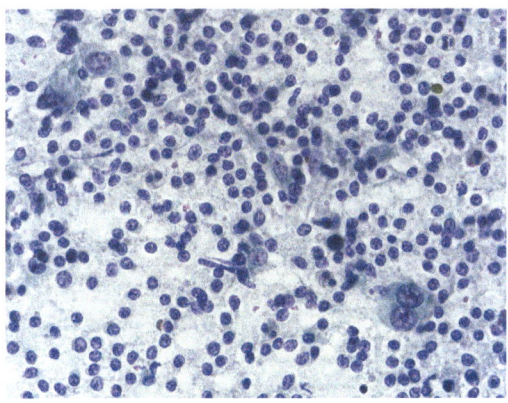

Fig. 13.28 Hodgkin lymphoma with Reed Sternberg cell and mononuclear Hodgkin cells in a background of small lymphocytes ×40

Small-cell lymphomas have a monotonous population of small to intermediate lymphoid cells with varying degrees of nuclear atypia. Though described as 'small', these neoplastic lymphoid cells are still larger than a small benign mature lymphocyte. *CLL/SLL* consists of lymphoid cells with a high N:C ratio, a narrow rim of cytoplasm and round to mildly irregular nuclei with coarse chromatin that tends to form a checkerboard distribution, seen best in the Pap-stained smears (Figs. 13.31, 13.32, 13.33 and 13.34). Nucleoli are inconspicuous. There will be a variable number of para immunoblasts with eccentric cytoplasm and round nuclei with a prominent nucleolus, and prolymphocytes with rounded larger nuclei. In direct Giemsa-stained cellular

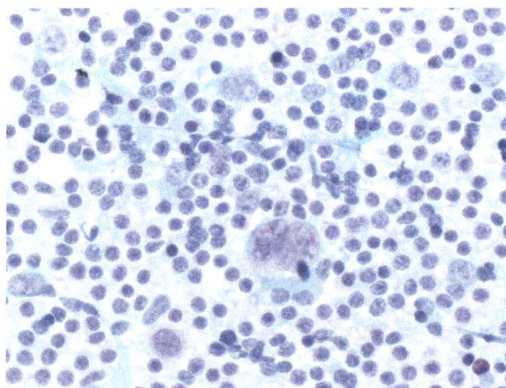

Fig. 13.29 Hodgkin lymphoma with multinucleated Reed Sternberg cell with multiple nucleoli (central) and several mononuclear Hodgkin cells in a background of small lymphocytes. Pap ×60

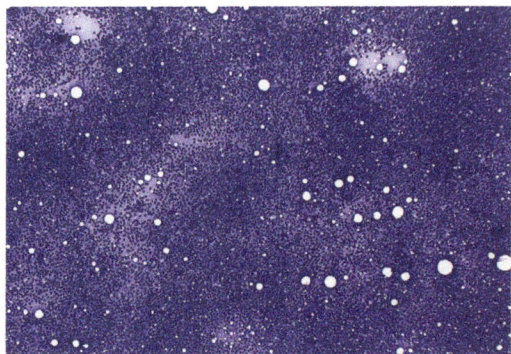

Fig. 13.31 Small lymphocytic lymphoma/chronic lymphocytic leukaemia showing dispersed monotonous pattern with a vague nodularity caused by proliferation centres. Giemsa ×10

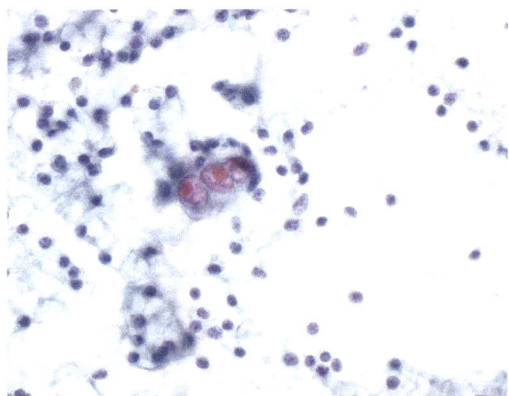

Fig. 13.30 Hodgkin lymphoma with multinucleated Reed Sternberg cell with macronucleoli. Pap ×60

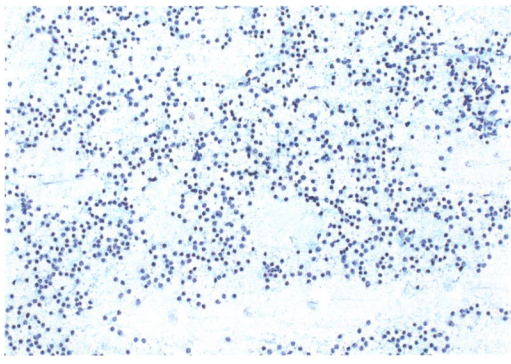

Fig. 13.32 Small lymphocytic lymphoma/chronic lymphocytic lymphoma showing dispersed monotonous pattern. Pap ×20

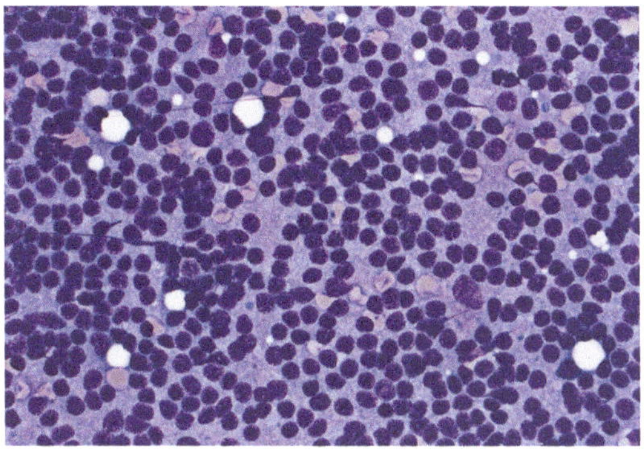

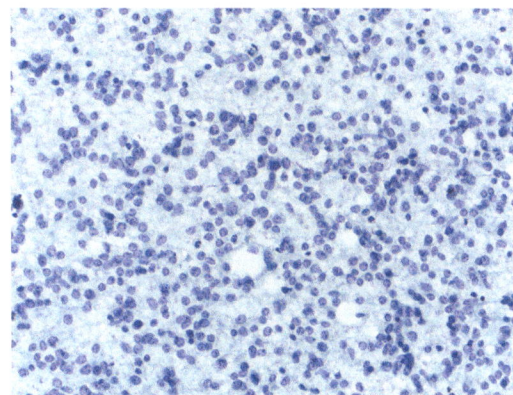

Fig. 13.33 Small lymphocytic lymphoma/chronic lymphocytic lymphoma showing dispersed monotonous pattern with 'soccer ball' clumped chromatin. A prolymphocyte is seen at 3 o'clock. Giemsa ×60

Fig. 13.35 Mantle cell lymphoma with monotonous small lymphoid cell pattern. Pap ×40

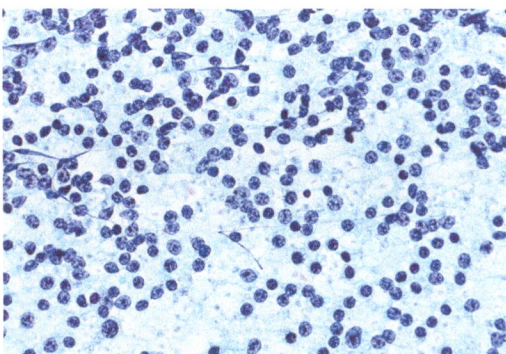

Fig. 13.34 Small lymphocytic lymphoma/chronic lymphocytic lymphoma showing dispersed monotonous pattern with 'soccer ball' clumped chromatin with scattered small lymphocytes with dense chromatin. Pap ×60

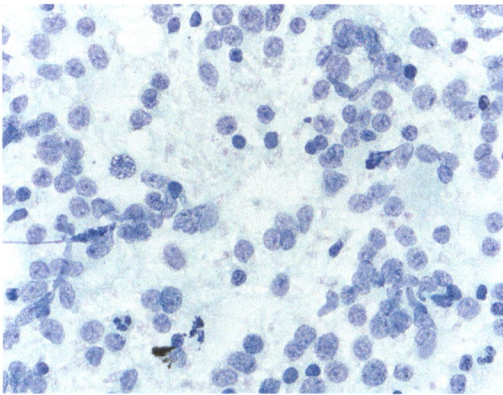

Fig. 13.36 Mantle cell lymphoma with small to intermediate lymphoid cells with mild to moderately irregular nuclear shape and minimal eccentric cytoplasm. An atypical mitotic figure is noted at 6 o'clock. Pap ×60

smears, these larger cells may create pale rounded areas. Tingible body macrophages are not seen and the overall diagnostic feature is the monotonous small-cell population. CLL/SLL cells have a characteristic immunophenotype by flow cytometry. They are typically positive for CD5, CD19, CD23 and CD200, and express restricted kappa or lambda light chains at dim intensity, with CD20 also dimly expressed (Table 13.3).

Mantle cell lymphoma (MCL) shows a variety of cell types but there is a monotonous population of small to intermediate lymphoid cells with indented, angulated, sometimes grooved or 'cleaved' nuclei with occasional small nucleoli and pale cytoplasm that is usually limited and may be eccentric (Figs. 13.35 and 13.36). By flow cytometry, both CLL/SLL and MCL are CD5 and CD19 positive monoclonal B-cell populations expressing restricted light chains. MCL differs from CLL/SLL in that MCL has a brighter light chain and CD20 than CLL/SLL, and MCL is typically negative for CD23 and CD200 (Table 13.3). By ICC, MCL is typically SOX11 and cyclin D1 positive, whereas CLL/SLL is negative for these markers. When MCL is suspected at ROSE, the material should be set aside for a cell block for ICC and not just for flow cytometry. Cytogenetic or FISH studies should be used to confirm the MCL, as it is associated with CCND family rearrangements, most commonly CCND1, and over 95% of cases will contain a

CCND1::IGH translocation t(11;14)(q13;q32). The blastic subtype has finely granular chromatin and larger lymphoid cells in a monotonous population, and although categorizable as malignant, it is a difficult lymphoma to subtype.

Lymphoblastic lymphoma (LBL) either T- or B-cell type often presents in younger patients and may have a distinctive clinical presentation with or without an acute lymphoblastic leukaemia (ALL) component. The smears are usually highly cellular with a monotonous population of intermediate cells with a high N:C ratio, round to indented, 'clover-leaf' nuclei with grooves and limited cytoplasm. Nucleoli are usually inconspicuous. By flow cytometry, B-LBL typically expresses CD10, CD19, CD34 and intracellular CD79a, but is dim or negative for CD20 and light chains (Table 13.3). T-LBL is typically intracellular CD3 positive, with usually negative or weak surface CD3 by flow cytometry. CD7 is positive and CD4 and CD8 are frequently co-expressed along with CD1a (Table 13.3).

Marginal zone lymphoma (MZL) has a mix of small centrocyte-like cells, monocytoid cells with rounded clear pale cytoplasm, small plasmacytic lymphoid cells with eccentric cytoplasm, plasma cells and occasional larger blastic lymphoid cells (Figs. 13.37, 13.38, 13.39 and 13.40). The differential diagnosis includes a reactive pro-

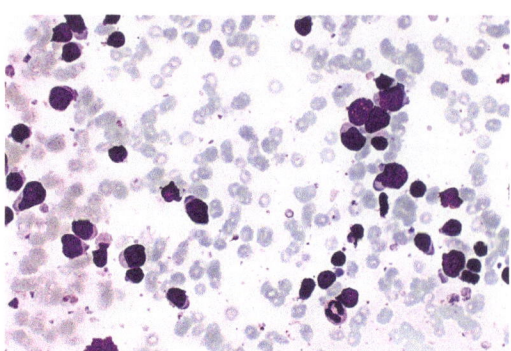

Fig. 13.38 Marginal zone lymphoma with dispersed heterogeneous pattern including monocytoid cells and plasmacytoid cells. Giemsa ×40

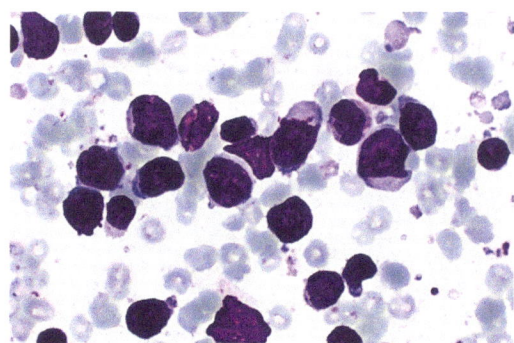

Fig. 13.39 Marginal zone lymphoma with the dispersed heterogeneous pattern including centrocyte-like cells, monocytoid cells and plasmacytoid cells Giemsa ×60

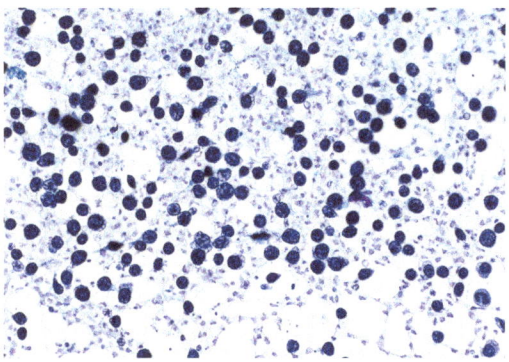

Fig. 13.37 Marginal zone lymphoma with dispersed heterogeneous pattern including centrocyte-like cells and occasional plasmacytoid cells. Pap ×60

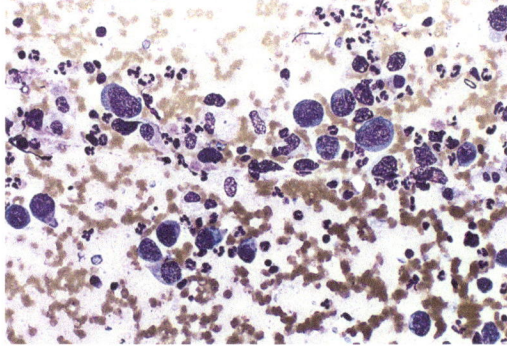

Fig. 13.40 Large B-cell lymphoma showing dispersed monotonous large lymphoid cell pattern. There is dispersed or open chromatin and nucleoli are present. Giemsa ×40

cess. Flow cytometry will show a monoclonal B-cell population by light chain restriction (Table 13.3), but further specific diagnosis often requires excision biopsy.

Lymphoplasmacytic lymphoma (LPL) usually presents with a history of macroglobulinemia in the setting of Waldenstrom macroglobulinemia. LPL has a mix of small lymphoid cells, plasmacytic and plasmacytoid cells with some larger lymphoid cells, and may also show Ducher bodies and Russell bodies, that is, immunoglobulins impinging the nucleus or found in the cytoplasm, respectively, as well as occasionally crystalline immunoglobulins expanding eccentric cytoplasm. Flow cytometry shows a monoclonal B-cell population by light chain restriction, typically accompanied by a monoclonal plasma cell population, which expresses the same light chain intracellularly (Table 13.3).

Peripheral T-cell lymphomas also present with a mixed lymphoid population but virtually all the lymphoid cells present are atypical with irregular nuclear margins, irregular chromatin, one or more nucleoli, a variable but usually small amount of cytoplasm, and a small to more pronounced number of eosinophils. *Nodal T follicular helper cell lymphoma, angio-immunoblastic type* also has a mixed lymphoid population of intermediate to large atypical lymphoid cells but with a smaller number of larger lymphoid cells, small 'monocytoid' lymphoid cells and eosinophils. The smears may also show fragments of small capillaries with large prominent endothelial cells. Flow cytometry of peripheral T-cell lymphomas is complicated by the presence of non-neoplastic T-cells, and a thorough knowledge of such background cells is essential. Peripheral T-cell lymphoma cells often show abnormal expression of one or more of the pan-T-cell markers CD2, CD3, CD5 or CD7 (Table 13.3). Monoclonality can be assessed by flow cytometry by determination of TRBC1 expression, provided the cells express sufficient surface alpha-beta T-cell receptors. T-cell gene rearrangement studies are frequently required, and when T-cell lymphoma or a recurrence is suspected clinically, appropriate ancillary testing is required. Excision biopsy is usually required to make the initial diagnosis.

Diffuse large B-cell lymphoma (DLBCL) provides usually cellular smears with a monotonous population of large cells that can appear immunoblastic, with eccentric cytoplasm and round nuclei with a single nucleolus, or centroblastic with less cytoplasm and several nucleoli in a more pleomorphic nucleus, or pleomorphic with large cells and highly pleomorphic nuclei (Figs. 13.40, 13.41, 13.42 and 13.43). These variants and the other subtypes of LBCL all have very similar features in that they are easily diagnosed as malignant but the subtypes cannot be distinguished on FNAB cytopathology. Clinical and immunophenotyping correlation is then

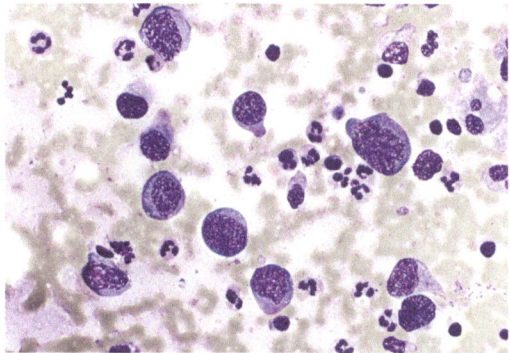

Fig. 13.41 Large B-cell lymphoma showing a dispersed, monotonous large lymphoid cell pattern with cells resembling large centroblasts. There is dispersed granular chromatin and nucleoli are present. Giemsa ×60

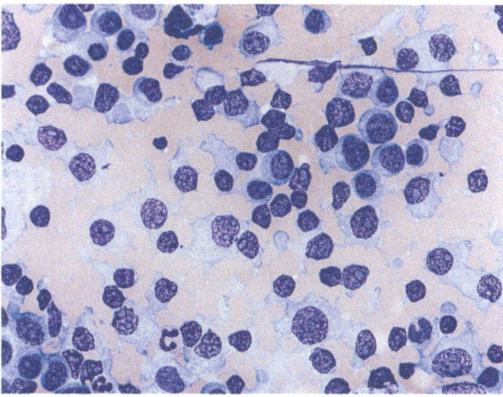

Fig. 13.42 Large-cell lymphoma with predominantly large cells with a high N:C ratio, round to more pleomorphic nuclei and large single nucleoli, resembling immunoblasts. Giemsa ×60. (Courtesy of Dr. William Geddie, Toronto)

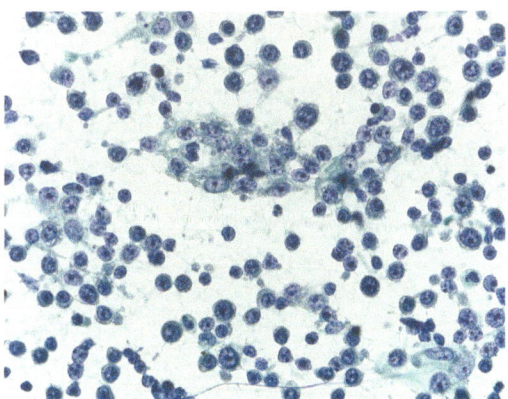

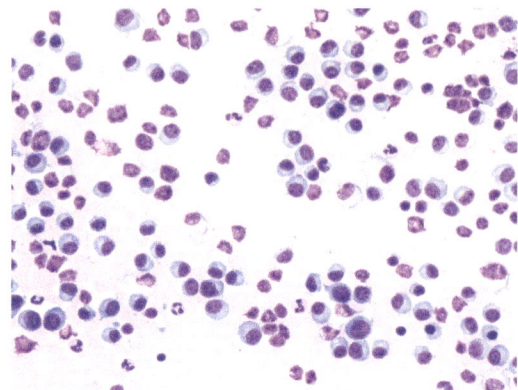

Fig. 13.43 Large-cell lymphoma with predominantly large cells with a high N:C ratio, round to more pleomorphic nuclei and prominent single nucleoli. Pap ×40

Fig. 13.44 Multiple myeloma showing a relatively monotonous pattern of small to intermediate plasmacytoid lymphoid cells with varying degrees of condensed chromatin and eccentric cytoplasm, sometimes showing a perinuclear clearing ('hof'). Giemsa ×40

required. Flow cytometry can demonstrate a monoclonal B-cell population by light chain restriction (Table 13.3), but further classification depends on ICC, IHC or molecular studies.

Reactive lymph nodes, usually related to Epstein Barr virus (EBV) or CMV infection, can show prominent immunoblasts with eccentric cytoplasm, round nuclei and small nucleoli, in a background of small lymphocytes with no spectrum of atypical lymphoid cells. However, some immunoblastic reactions to infections can start with follicular hyperplasia and evolve over time to an immunoblastic pattern and confident diagnosis of a reactive pattern versus immunoblastic LBCL can be difficult. The clinical setting and serology for a viral cause can help. Flow cytometry may be helpful in the evaluation of monoclonal B- or T-cells.

Other lymphomas such as *plasmablastic lymphoma* (PL) and *multiple myeloma* (MM) can present with a monotonous population of large lymphoid cells with varying degrees of plasma cell differentiation. PL has a range of large cells with round to more pleomorphic nuclei, prominent one or more nucleoli, and some eccentric cytoplasm lacking a Golgi apparatus clearing ('hof') in a background of lymphoid cell cytoplasmic fragments. MM has round nuclei that can be pleomorphic and binucleated in some cases, with coarse chromatin, one or sometimes more nucleoli and eccentric cytoplasm, that may con-

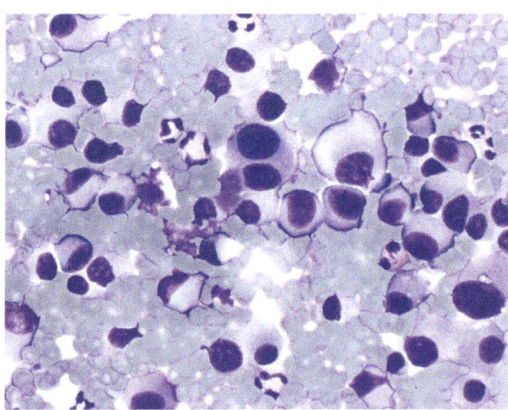

Fig. 13.45 Multiple myeloma showing a relatively monotonous pattern of small to intermediate plasmacytoid lymphoid cells with varying degrees of condensed chromatin and eccentric cytoplasm. Giemsa ×60

tain an hof (Figs. 13.44 and 13.45). Prominent plasma cells can occur in a reactive lymph node related to syphilis or other infections and may be seen in HIV infections, where involution of the lymph node after initial follicular hyperplasia can occur and make diagnosis difficult. Serology and clinical information are of assistance. By flow cytometry, abnormal cells in PL and MM can be identified by the expression of bright CD38 and CD138 (Table 13.3). The cells lack surface immunoglobulin but contain abundant intracellular immunoglobulin and monoclonality can be assessed by intracellular light chain restriction.

Necrosis can occur in a lymph node that is inflammatory or neoplastic. Necrosis can be seen in caseous necrosis due to mycobacterial infection, where an acid-fast stain such as the Ziehl–Neelsen or auramine stain can be diagnostic along with PCR and cultures, or in a lymph node involved by lymphoma or metastatic carcinoma, where shadowy degenerate cells may be recognizable in a background of granular necrosis. There may be residual lymphoid cells or not. Lymph node infarction can occur in reactive and lymphomatous lymph nodes. Amyloidosis has to be distinguished and provides amorphous pale material with or without lymphoid cells and a Congo red stain or ICC can confirm the diagnosis. Kikuchi-Fujimoto disease, which usually occurs in younger patients, shows a background of necrotic karyorrhectic debris often with a mixture of plasmacytoid dendritic cells, histiocytes, small lymphocytes and a few immunoblasts. Usually, the key is recognising the apoptotic nuclear debris, the presence of histiocytes with irregular elongated crescentic nuclei and eccentric cytoplasm, and the absence of neutrophils, plasma cells and eosinophils.

13.8 Conclusion

FNAB of lymph nodes is an efficient, minimally invasive, cost-effective procedure to assess lymphadenopathy in the H&N region, whether under ultrasound direction or by palpation. Assessment of the clinical history and ultrasound findings should take place whenever possible prior to the FNAB. Care should be taken with the FNAB procedure and the making of direct smears, consideration should be given to using the 'needle only' technique, and ROSE is highly recommended. When assessing the direct smear material, the pattern should be assessed at low power to look for tissue fragments which are the hallmark in lymph node FNAB of metastatic carcinoma. Then, a high-power assessment of any cell tissue fragments and the single dispersed cells should take place. If the cells are lymphoid a step-wise assessment has been provided.

Suggested Reading

Texts

1. Field AS, Geddie WR. Cytohistology of lymph nodes and spleen, Toronto, Papanicolaou Society Small Biopsy Monograph Series. Cambridge University Press; 2014.
2. Monaco SE, Teot LA. Pediatric cytopathology: a practical guide. Germany: Springer; 2014.
3. Zeppa P, Cozzolino I. Lymph Node FNC. Cytopathology of lymph nodes and extranodal lymphoproliferative processes. Monogr Clin Cytol. Karger. 2018.
4. Field AS, Zarka M. Practical cytopathology: a diagnostic approach to fine needle aspiration biopsy. Philadelphia: Elsevier; 2017.

Articles

5. Al-Abbadi MA, Barroca H, Bode-Lesniewska B, Calaminici M, Caraway NP, Chhieng DF, Cozzolino I, Ehinger M, Field AS, Geddie WR, Katz RL, Lin O, Medeiros LJ, Monaco SE, Rajwanshi A, Schmitt FC, Vielh P, Zeppa P. A proposal for the performance, classification and reporting of lymph node fine-needle aspiration cytopathology: the Sydney system. Acta Cytol. 2020;64:306–22.
6. Al-Abbadi M, Barroca H, Bode-Lesniewska B, Calaminici M, Chhieng DC, Cozzolino I, Ehinger M, Field AS, et al. Letter to the Editor: Fine needle aspiration cytology and core needle biopsy in the diagnosis of lymphadenopathies: words of endorsement. Eur J Haematology. 2021;107:295–6.
7. Ahuja S, Malviya A. Categorisation of lymph node aspirates using the proposed Sydney system with assessment of risk of malignancy and diagnostic accuracy. Cytopathology. 2022;33:430–8.
8. Auerbach A, Schmieg JJ, Aguilera NS. Pediatric lymphoid and histiocytic lesions in the head and neck. Head Neck Pathol. 2021;15:41–58.
9. Balla A, Hampel KJ, Sharma MK, et al. Comprehensive validation of cytology specimens for next-generation sequencing and clinical practice experience. J Mol Diagn. 2018;20:812–21.
10. Barroca H, Bode-Lesniewska B, Cozzolino I, et al. Management of cytologic material, preanalytic procedures and biobanking in lymph node cytopathology. Cytopathology. 2019;30:17–30.
11. Maddocks K. Update on mantle cell lymphoma. Blood. 2018;132:1647–56.
12. Barroca H, Bode-Lesniewska B, Cozzolino I, Zeppa P. Management of cytologic material, preanalytic procedures and biobanking in lymph node cytopathology. Cytopathology. 2019;30:17–30.
13. Caputo A, Ciliberti V, D'Antonio A, et al. Real-world experience with the Sydney System on 1458 cases of lymph node fine needle aspiration cytology. Cytopathology. 2022;33:166–75.

14. Cozzolino I, Giudice MC, Selleri C, Caputo A, Zeppa P. Lymph node fine-needle cytology in the era of personalized medicine. Is there a role? Cytopathology. 2019;30:348–62.

15. Foshat M, Stewart J, Khoury JD, et al. Accuracy of diagnosing mantle cell lymphoma and identifying its variants on fine-needle aspiration biopsy. Cancer Cytopathol. 2019;127;44–51.

16. Frederiksen JK, Sharma M, Casulo C, Burack WR. Systematic review of the effectiveness of fine-aspiration and/or core-needle biopsy for subclassifying lymphoma. Arch Pathol Lab Med. 2015;139:245–51.

17. Gupta P, et al. Assessment of risk of malignancy by application of the proposed Sydney system for classification and reporting of lymph node cytopathology. Cancer Cytopath. 2021;129:701–18.

18. Jin M, Wakely PE Jr. Lymph node cytopathology: Essential ancillary studies as applied to lymphoproliferative neoplasms. Cancer Cytopathol. 2018;126:615–26.

19. Khanlari M, Daneshbod Y, Yazdi S, et al. Discrepancy of target sites between clinician and cytopathological reports in head and neck FNA: Did I miss the target or did the clinician mistake the organ site? Cancer Med. 2015;4:1374–80.

20. Makarenko VV, DeLelys ME, Hasserjian RP, et al. Lymph node FNA cytology: diagnostic performance and clinical implications of proposed diagnostic categories. Cancer Cytopathol. 2022;130:144–53.

21. Michelow P, Omar T, Field A, Wright C. The cytopathology of mycobacterial infection. Diagn Cytopathol. 2016;44:255–62.

22. Monaco SE, Khalbuss WE, Pantanowitz L. Benign non-infectious causes of lymphadenopathy: a review of cytomorphology and differential diagnosis. Diagn Cytopathol. 2012;40:925–38.

23. Rawstron AC, Kreuzer K-A, Soosapilla A, et al. Reproducible diagnosis of chronic lymphocytic leukemia by flow cytometry: an European Research Initiative on CLL (ERIC) & European Society for Clinical Cell Analysis (ESCCA) Harmonisation project. Cytometry B Clin Cytom. 2018;94:121–8.

24. Rivas A, et al. Ultrasound guided FNA of superficial lymphadenopathoy performed by interventional pathology: the applicability of the Sydney System from two years of experience and 363 cases. Acta Cytol. 2021;21:1–10.

25. Ronchi A, Caputo A, Pagliuca F, et al. Lymph node fine needle aspiration cytology (FNAC) in paediatric patients: why not? Diagnostic accuracy of FNAC in a series of heterogeneous paediatric lymphadenopathies. Pathol Res Pract. 2021;217:153–9.

26. Scott GD, Lau HD, Kurzer JH, et al. Flow immunophenotyping of benign lymph nodes sampled by FNAB: representative with diagnostic pitfalls. Cancer Cytopathol. 2018;126:797–808.

27. Torres Rivas HE, Villar Zarra K, Pérez Pabón LA, et al. Ultrasound-guided fine-needle aspiration of superficial lymphadenopathy performed by interventional pathologists: the applicability of the Sydney system from 2 years of experience and 363 cases. Acta Cytol. 2021;65:453–62.

28. Vigila E, et al. A novel approach to classification and reporting of lymph node FNAC: application of the proposed Sydney System. Diagnostics (Basel). 2021;11:13–4.

29. Wakely PE. Mantle cell lymphoma: a report of 31 nodal and extranodal fine-needle aspirates. J Am Soc Cytopathol. 2015;4:307–12.

30. Zeppa P, Cozzolino I, Caraway N, et al. Announcement: the international system for reporting lymph node cytopathology. Acta Cytol. 2020;64:299–305.

Andrew S. Field is the Director of the Anatomical Pathology Department at St Vincent's Hospital, Sydney, Australia, a Conjoint Professor at the University of New South Wales Sydney, and an Adjunct Professor at the Notre Dame University Medical School. He was the President from 2019 to 2022 and is now the Immediate Past President of the International Academy of Cytology. He is committed to teaching FNAB cytopathology, particularly in LMIC, where he has provided 22 tutorials since 2007 and spoken at 19 IAC and Sydney tutorials. His major interest lies in standardized international reporting systems. He was a co-editor and author of the IAC Yokohama System for Reporting Breast FNAB Cytopathology and is the Co-chair of the IAC WHO IARC Cytopathology Joint Standing Editorial Board, which has led to his involvement in the writing and publication of the WHO Reporting Systems for Lung and Pancreaticobiliary Cytopathology in 2023. He is also a Member of the WHO Classification of Tumours Standing Editorial Board.

Sharron Liang, MBBS, FRCPA. As practicing cytopathologist and anatomical pathologist at St Vincent's Hospital SydPath in Sydney, Australia, she enjoys all aspects of cytopathology and has a keen interest in the growing field of molecular cytopathology. She is passionate about teaching, education, and sharing new knowledge.

William Sewell is an Immunopathologist, St Vincent's Hospital Sydney. He is a Conjoint Associate Professor, School of Clinical Medicine, University of New South Wales Sydney, Australia, and also a Visiting Scientist, Garvan Institute of Medical Research. He has a special interest in clinical flow cytometry and its application to tumors of the hematolymphoid system. His research has focused on cells and molecules of the immune system.

Sydney and WHO Classification and Reporting System for Lymph Nodes Cytopathology

14

Pio Zeppa and Immacolata Cozzolino

14.1 General

The adoption of a codified system for the performance, classification, and reporting of lymph nodes and other lymphoid organs through Fine Needle Aspiration Cytology (FNAC) arose from the need to standardize the sampling technique, the use, and the application of ancillary techniques, the formulation of basic diagnoses and possibly a subsequent, more accurate classification of lymphoproliferative processes and metastases. In this perspective, the Proposal for the Performance, Classification, and Reporting of Lymph Node Fine-Needle Aspiration Cytopathology, called the Sydney System was conceived and proposed in 2020 [1]. The next objective has been the development of a cytological classification along the lines of the latest WHO classifications of lymphomas to provide the basis for the diagnosis and treatment of lymphoid lesions [2]. The rationale for developing these classifications was the recognition that FNAC of lymph nodes and other lymphoid organs having specific diagnostic criteria, which are often ignored in books describing the histopathology of hematolymphoid tissue tumors. Such criteria can be applied to classify different lymphoproliferative processes, according to the last WHO classification. This deficiency still represents a gap in the practice of cytopathology of lymphoid tissues, including the spleen and thymus, causing distrust toward LN-FNAC [3–5]. The near to be published WHO reporting system for the cytology of lymph nodes and other lymphoid organs [6] maintains the 2-diagnostic-level classification system of the Sydney system that can be used as a first-line method for the diagnosis of lymphoid lesions and classifies the specific pathological entities in tight accordance with the last WHO classification [2]. In these systems, the importance of a multiparametric approach using FNAC is emphasized: morphology is combined with ancillary techniques, allowing a basic diagnosis (first diagnostic level) of benign or malignant entity (lymphoma or metastasis) and, when possible, a second diagnostic level in which specific pathological entities are diagnosed (i.e., non-Hodgkin lymphoma (first diagnostic level) and follicular lymphoma (second diagnostic level)).

Cytopathologists dedicated to the pathology of lymphoid tissues, including the spleen, thymus, and other extra nodal organs, have demonstrated that, in expert hands, the diagnosis of lymphoproliferative processes through the application of state-of-the-art diagnostic and ancillary tech-

P. Zeppa (✉)
Department of Pathology, University di Salerno, Salerno, Italy
e-mail: pzeppa@unisa.it

I. Cozzolino
Department of Mental and Physical Health and Preventive Medicine, University of Campania "Luigi Vanvitelli", Naples, Italy

niques can be done with a very high level of accuracy, despite the many challenges. In fact, the combination of rapid on-site evaluation (ROSE), immunophenotyping by multiparametric flow cytometry, immunocytochemistry on different technical supports, and molecular studies such as fluorescence in situ hybridization and PCR in combination with cytological evaluation [7, 8] allow accurate diagnoses of the clonal lymphoproliferative process and numerous specific histotypes. Moreover, cytological samples provide high-quality DNA and RNA as regard the preservation of the expression of biomarkers [9, 10].

Despite all these advantages and potential of LN-FNAC, unjustified criticisms and the objective impossibility to sub-classify all the lymphoproliferative processes and some specific pathological entities cause limitations in the usage of this procedure in different Institutions [3, 4], even for basic diagnoses (i.e., benign, malignant, and metastasis).

This awareness determined the need to establish guidelines to standardize diagnostic criteria and create a uniform reporting system, which cytopathologists around the world can adhere to according to their facilities and specific diagnostic requests. In fact, although some ancillary techniques, such as flow cytometry or molecular facilities, may not be available in all laboratories (especially in low- and middle-income countries), cytopathologists from any country need to diagnose benignity or malignancy based on morphology; they also need to be able to define a cytological sample as insufficient for diagnosis, atypical, or suspicious, while indicating the risk of malignancy (ROM) and providing recommendations to the referring physician for treatment and/or follow-up.

14.2 Workflow: Standardized Reporting System Categories

The categories of the Sydney system [1], subsequently adopted by the WHO reporting system [6], for lymph node and other lymphoid organ cytology are five and represent the first diagnostic level containing basic diagnostic information:

- Insufficient/inadequate/nondiagnostic
- Benign
- Atypical
- Suspicious of malignancy
- Malignant

14.2.1 Insufficient/Inadequate/Nondiagnostic

This category includes cases that cannot be diagnosed due to scant cellularity, extensive necrosis (Fig. 14.1), or technical limitations that cannot be overcome; repeat FNAC or core needle biopsy or excision biopsy should be requested based on the specific clinical context. Only one of the terms "insufficient," "inadequate," or "nondiagnostic" should be consistently used by a single cytopathologist or multiple cytopathologists within a single department.

14.2.2 Benign

This category includes cases with a heterogeneous lymphoid population with small lymphocytes, and often germinal centers with dendritic cells and tingible body macrophages and cases with suppurative and granulomatous inflammation and specific infections (Fig. 14.2). The lym-

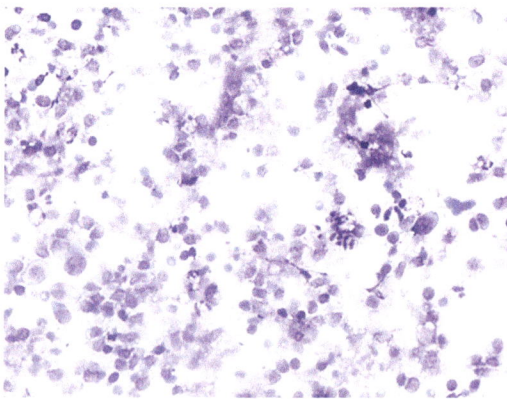

Fig. 14.1 Inadequate lymph node FNAC showing ill-preserved lymphoid cells in a necrotic background. The risk of malignancy in these cases is high (Diff-Quik stain, 270X)

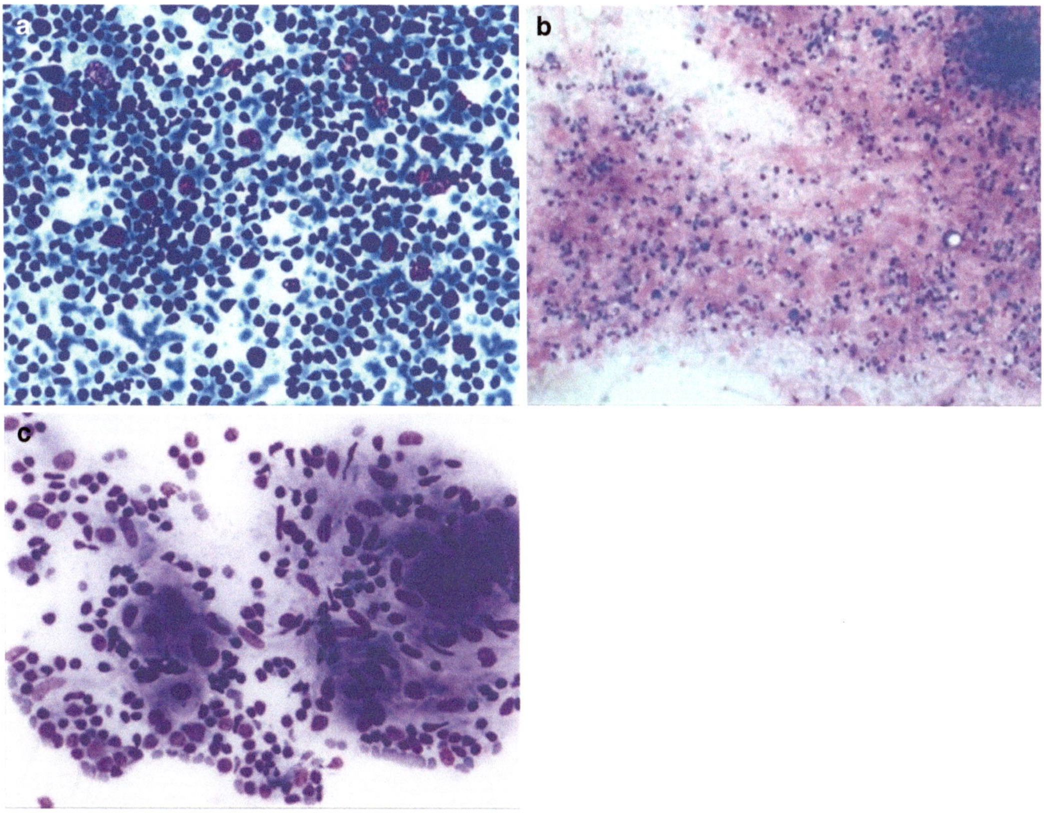

Fig. 14.2 Negative lymph nodes FNAC showing a polymorphous (**a**), suppurative (**b**), and granulomatous (**c**) patterns diagnosed and reported reactive as the first diagnostic level. A second diagnostic level may be achieved and reported when, combining clinical data, cytological features, and ancillary techniques, it is possible to identify the specific agents or processes (Diff-Quik stain, **a**, **b** 270X, **c**: 430X)

phoid proliferations can be diagnosed as reactive with or without flow cytometry or immunocytochemistry and referred for clinical follow-up when the FNAC findings agree with the clinical presentation and ultrasound features. When the clinical or ultrasound features are discrepant or suspicious, lymph node FNAC repetition with immunophenotyping, preferably by flow cytometry, is required.

14.2.3 Atypical

This category includes cases with adequate smears in which the cellular material is insufficient for proper ancillary techniques. This category includes highly cellular lymphoid smears with mainly benign cytopathological features and

features that can increase the possibility of malignancy (Fig. 14.3), for example, a smear with exceeding follicular center cells and lacking macrophages with tingible bodies and small lymphocytes, which raises the differential diagnosis of follicular hyperplasia and follicular lymphoma. Repetition of the FNAC, with flow cytometry, cytogenetics, or biopsy may be required, regardless of clinical and ultrasound findings.

14.2.4 Suspicious

This category includes cases with small and/or medium-sized, monomorphic atypical lymphoid cells suspicious of lymphoma, in which cytomorphology alone is not sufficient for a definitive

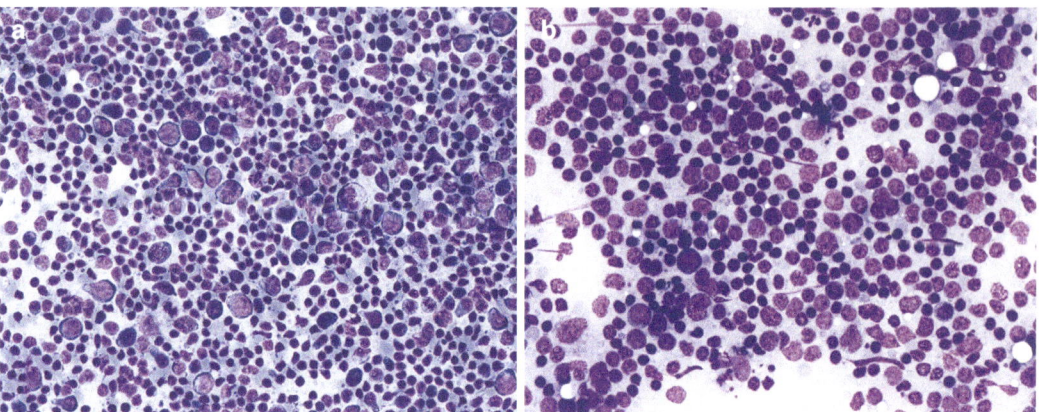

Fig. 14.3 Atypical lymphoid cells of undetermined significance (ALUS) lymph node FNAC showing relative monomorphic smear with immature lymphoid cells. The risk of malignancy of routine-stained smears only is high. Ancillary techniques, namely flow cytometry, may discriminate in reactive cases or low-grade non-Hodgkin lymphoma in most of the cases (Diff-Quik stain, **a**, **b** 270X)

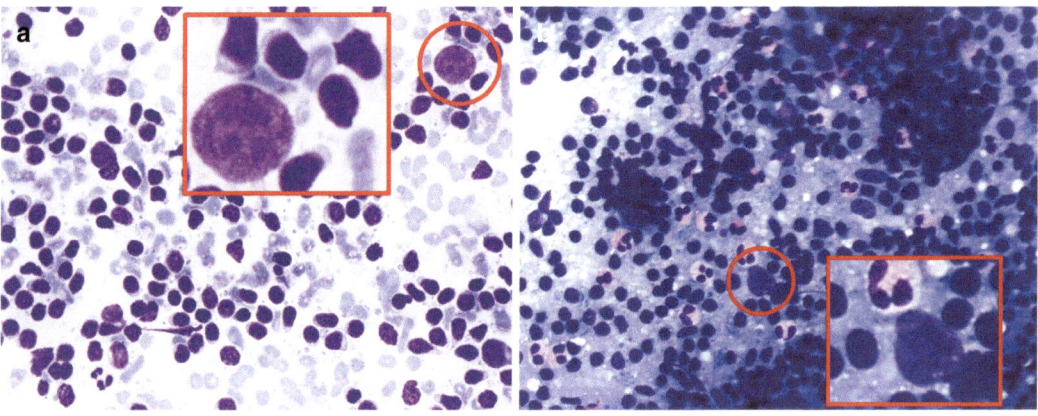

Fig. 14.4 Suspicious for malignancy cases showing rare but clearly atypical, isolated cells (inset) in otherwise reactive lymph node FNAC pattern (**a**), ill-preserved atyp- ical cell in a polymorphous background suspect for Hodgkin lymphoma (**b**) (Diff-Quik stain, **a**, **b** 270X, insets 430X)

diagnosis of malignancy and flow cytometry or immunocytochemistry data are not available or do not demonstrate B-cell monoclonality. The suspicious category also includes polymorphous lymphoid smears in which few large, atypical cells, Hodgkin- or Reed-Sternberg-like cells are detected (Fig. 14.4), but immunocytochemistry cannot be performed or did not lead to diagnosis; large cell lymphomas scantly cellular in which ancillary techniques are not available; smears in which atypical cells suspicious for metastasis are detected but are too scant for diagnosis and again there is no material available to perform immunocytochemistry. Repeating FNAC to obtain additional diagnostic material may be one of the options; core needle biopsy or excisional biopsy may be required.

14.2.5 Malignant

This category includes small to large-sized cells of non-Hodgkin lymphoma (Figs. 14.5, 14.6 and 14.7) possibly supported by evidence of clonality by flow cytometry or molecular testing showing clonal immunoglobulin (IGH or IGK) or T-cell receptor (TRG, TRB) gene rearrangements. This category also includes all the entities in which

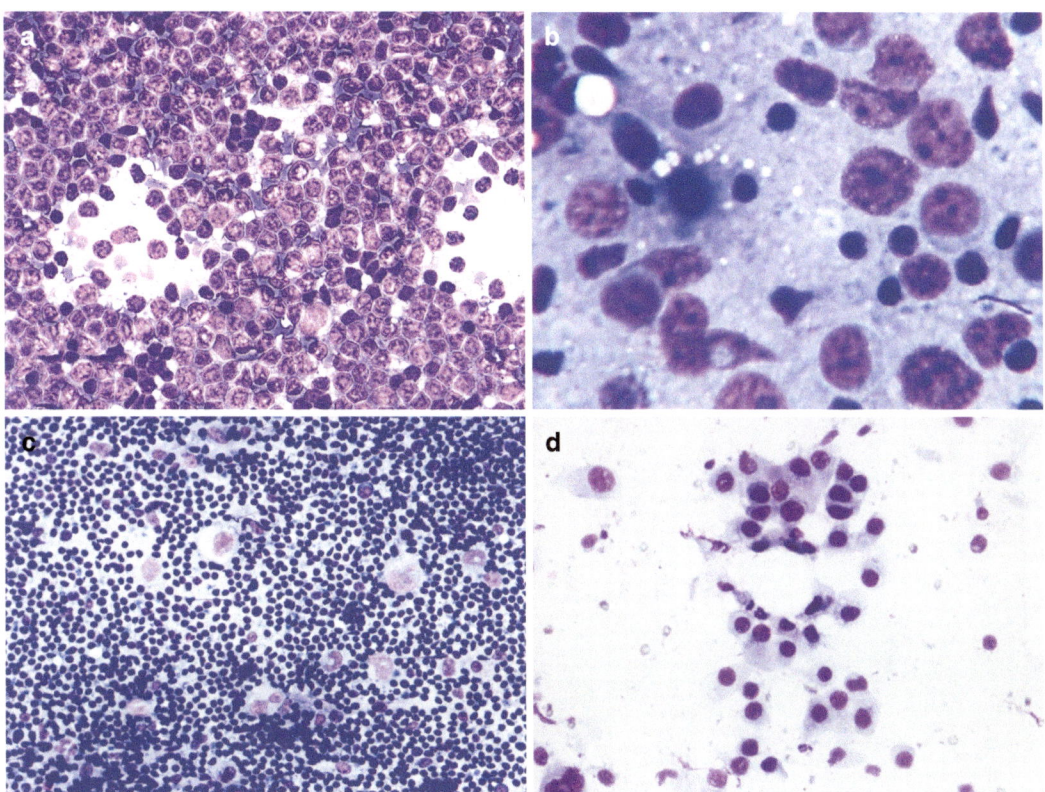

Fig. 14.5 Malignant lymph nodes FNAC showing metastasis, Hodgkin lymphoma, and high-grade non-Hodgkin lymphoma not otherwise specifiable in routinely stained smears(Diff-Quik stain, **a** 270X, **b** 430X, **c** 106X, **d** 270X)

cytopathological features alone are sufficient to identify malignancy as large cell non-Hodgkin lymphoma. This category also includes classical Hodgkin lymphoma with diagnostic Hodgkin and Reed-Sternberg in an appropriate cellular background and cell metastases (Fig. 14.8).

Each of these five categories is associated with a risk of malignancy (ROM) and is linked to recommendations for further tests and specific ancillary techniques to diagnose specific entities or refine the differential diagnoses. Specific processes or tumors that have a similar ROM when diagnosed on cytopathology are placed in the same category, for example, lymphadenopathies and lymphadenitis are placed in the "Benign" category. Notably, the Sydney System [1] and the WHO reporting system [6] use the same diagnostic categories for basic diagnoses and to facilitate the communication of ROM to the physician. Specific diagnoses and differential diagnoses,

which can be further refined by clinical data and ancillary testing, are afterward developed, and reported when possible [1, 6]. Currently, there are a few publications defining the ROM for these categories in lymph node cytopathology and more studies are needed to better define the ROM of each category [11–18].

As for the categorization of single entities: each case should have a specific diagnosis; if this is not possible, a preferred diagnosis should be made, with the possible differential diagnoses. For example, the first diagnostic level of benign diagnosis should be followed by the statement of the basic cytological pattern (follicular, suppurative, and granulomatous). The second diagnostic level for benign reactive diagnosis is deserved in cases in which the specific agent or pathological process is diagnosed. For instance, in granulomatous processes, if Kock acid-fast bacilli are detected by the Ziehl–

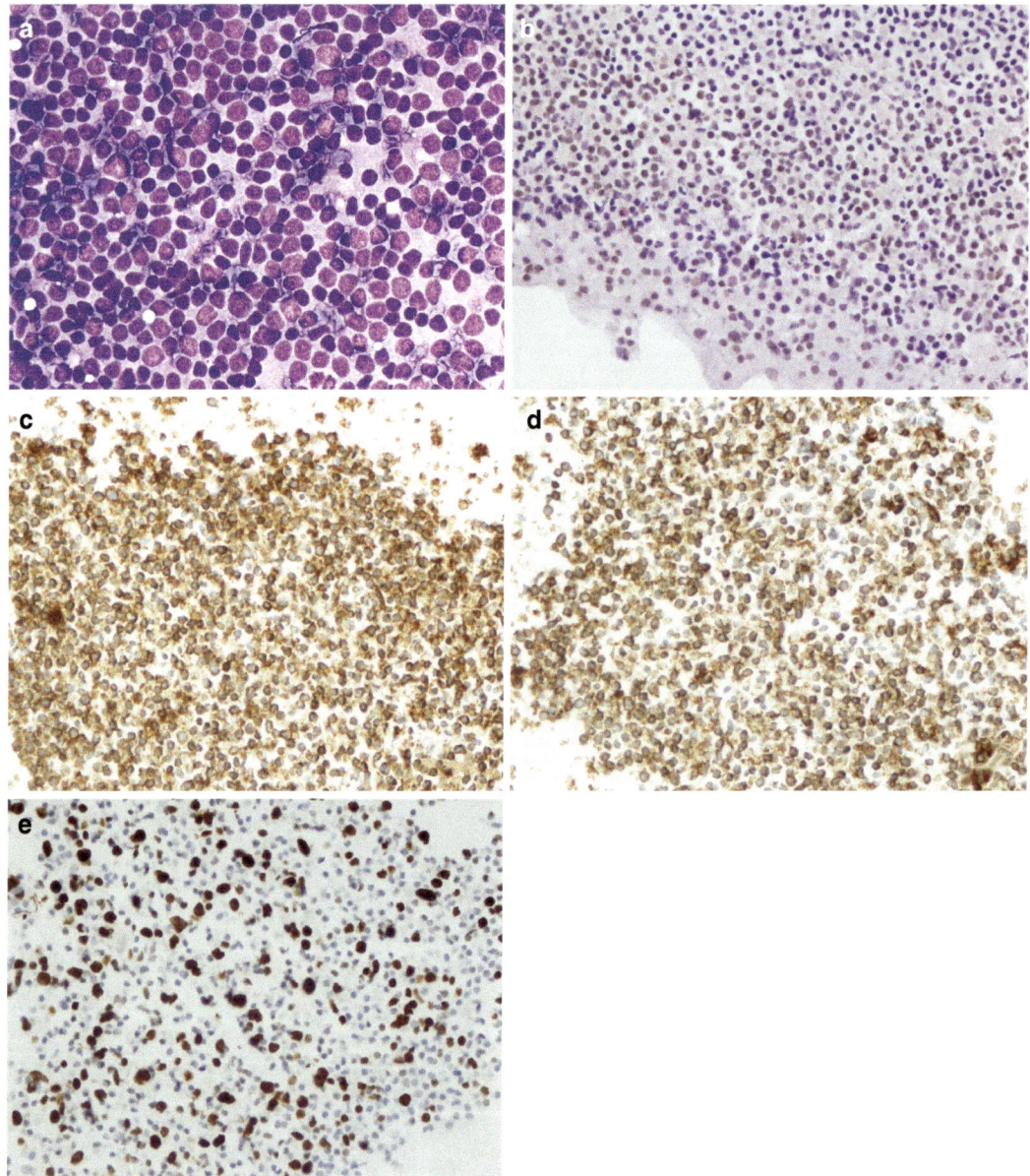

Fig. 14.6 Positive lymph node FNAC showing monomorphic, medium-sized size atypical lymphoid cells (**a**); flow cytometry evidenced light chain restriction assessing the diagnosis of B-cell non-Hodgkin lymphoma. Immunocytochemistry on cell-block (**b**) assessed positivity for CD10 (**c**), Bcl2 (**d**), and a low percentage of Ki67 positivity (Ki67) assessing the diagnosis of follicular lymphoma as a second diagnostic level (**e**) (**a**: Diff-Quik stain 270X, **b, c, d, e**: cell-block 106X)

Neelsen stain or PCR, a tuberculosis diagnosis can be rendered as the second diagnostic level. Malignant examples include cases in which a first diagnostic level of lymphoma is performed and, according to coherent FC or ICC pheno-type, the specific entity is identified (i.e., FL, SLL/CLL, and MCL) (Figs. 14.6 and 14.7). For large-cell non-Hodgkin lymphoma, diagnosed as such at the first diagnostic level, the second diagnostic level, if achievable, provides addi-

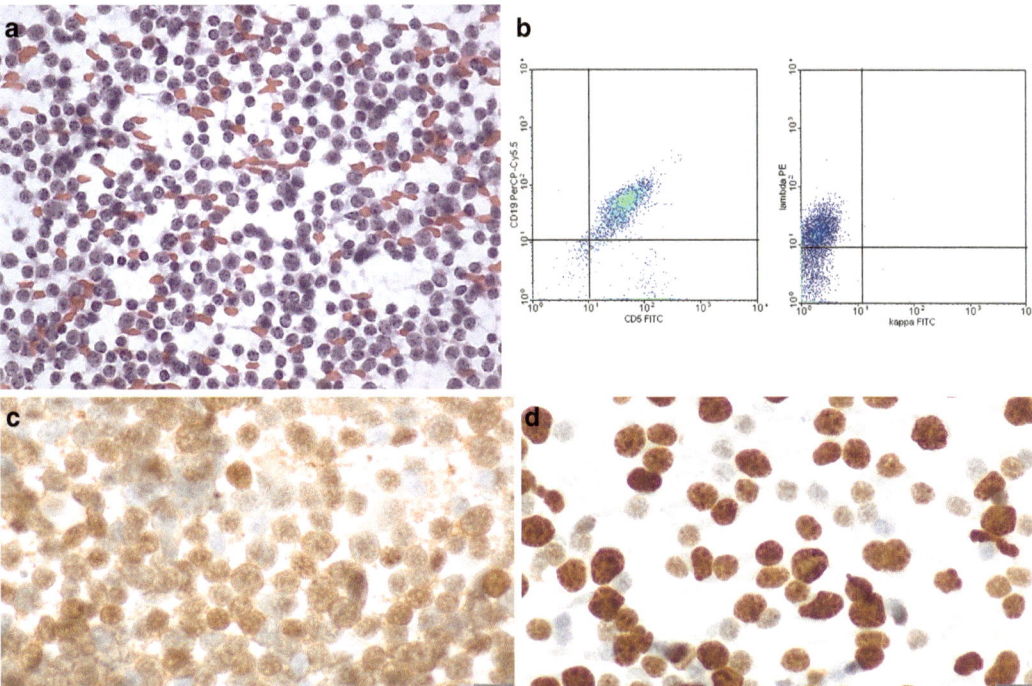

Fig. 14.7 Positive lymph node FNAC showing monomorphic medium-sized atypical lymphoid cells with irregular nuclei assessing the diagnosis of B-cell non-Hodgkin lymphoma (**a**). Flow cytometry evidenced light chain restriction and CD5 positivity (**b**); immunocytochemistry on cell-block showed Cyclin D1 (**c**) and Ki67 (**d**) positivity assessing the diagnosis of mantle-cell lymphoma with high mitotic index, as a second diagnostic level (**a, c, d**, 270X)

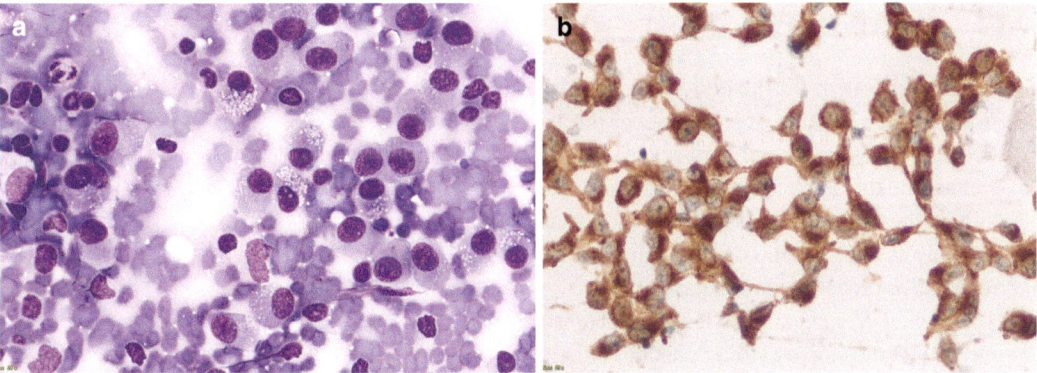

Fig. 14.8 FNAC of lymph node metastasis: metastasis from malignant, dispersed cells with vacuolated cytoplasm (**a**) (first diagnostic level). Immunocytochemical cytoplasmic positivity for HMB45 (**b**) indicative for a metastasis from melanoma (second diagnostic level) (**a, b** 430X, **a**: Diff Quik stain)

tional information and the identification of a specific histotype, such as diffuse, large B-cell lymphoma, and its own variants or follicular lymphoma grade 3. In the case of metastases, the second diagnostic level is achieved when, by ICC the primary tumor is indicated

(Fig. 14.8). Therefore, the goals of the second diagnostic level are:

- Identify specific benign entities, such as specific infections, using PCR, culture, and drug sensitivity results to confirm a mycobacterial infection or by immunocytochemistry or in situ hybridization for EBV infection.

- Diagnose specific non-Hodgkin lymphoma entities as listed in the current WHO hemato-pathology classification [2, 5] using flow cytometry for B-cell monoclonality and specific markers. For example, the diagnosis of mantle cell lymphoma is supported by CD5+ B-cell lineage, best shown by flow cytometry, combined with cyclin D1 and/or SOX11 positivity shown by immunocytochemistry.
- Diagnose the site of origin of a primary tumor in lymph node metastases and any possible prognostic or predictive markers; for example, the estrogen and progesterone receptors and HER2 status in metastatic breast carcinoma.

When the combination of the cytomorphology and ancillary testing findings allows the cytopathologist to achieve the second diagnostic level, the corresponding findings should be reported in one final integrated cytopathology report with the diagnosed specific entity.

14.3 Main Message

- A codified system for the performance, classification, and reporting of lymph nodes through FNAC is necessary to standardize the sampling technique, the application of ancillary techniques, the formulation of basic diagnoses, and possibly an accurate classification of lymphoproliferative processes and metastases.
- The Sydney System and the later WHO reporting system develop a cytological classification along the lines of the latest WHO classifications of lymphomas.
- Basic diagnostic categories are: insufficient/inadequate/nondiagnostic, benign, atypical, suspicious of malignancy, and malignant.
- Each of the five categories is associated with a risk of malignancy (ROM).
- A further diagnostic level for the benign category is deserved for cases in which the spe-

cific agent or a specific pathological process is diagnosed.

- A further diagnostic level for malignant category is deserved for cases in which specific non-Hodgkin lymphoma or primary tumors in case of metastases are diagnosed.
- An integrated FNAC report including clinical data, cytomorphology, and ancillary tests should be provided.

References

1. Al-Abbadi MA, Barroca H, Bode-Lesniewska B, Calaminici M, Caraway NP, Chhieng DF, Cozzolino I, Ehinger M, Field AS, Geddie WR, Katz RL, Lin O, Medeiros LJ, Monaco SE, Rajwanshi A, Schmitt FC, Vielh P, Zeppa P. A proposal for the performance, classification, and reporting of lymph node fine-needle aspiration cytopathology: the Sydney system. Acta Cytol. 2020;64(4):306–22.
2. WHO Classification of Tumours, 5th edition: Haematolymphoid tumours. 2023, in press.
3. Al-Abbadi M, Barroca H, Bode-Lesniewska B, Calaminici M, Chhieng DC, Cozzolino I, Ehinger M, Field A, Geddie W, Hosone M, Katz RL, Lin O, Michelow P, Monaco S, Rajwanshi A, Schmitt F, Vielh P, Zeppa P. Letter to the Editor: fine-needle aspiration cytology and core-needle biopsy in the diagnosis of lymphadenopathies: words of endorsement. Eur J Haematol. 2021;107(2):295–6.
4. Zeppa P. Haematocytopathology: why? Cytopathology. 2012;23(2):73–5.
5. Kroft SH, Sever CE, Bagg A, Billman B, Diefenbach C, Dorfman DM, Finn WG, Gratzinger DA, Gregg PA, Leonard JP, Smith S, Souter L, Weiss RL, Ventura CB, Cheung MC. Laboratory workup of lymphoma in adults: guideline from the American Society for Clinical pathology and the College of American Pathologists. Arch Pathol Lab Med. 2021;145(3):269–90.
6. WHO Reporting System for Lymph Node, Spleen, and Thymus Cytopathology. 2025 in press.
7. Wang H, Hariharan VS, Sarma S. Diagnostic accuracy of fine-needle aspiration cytology for lymphoma: a systematic review and meta-analysis. Diagn Cytopathol. 2021;49(9):975–86.
8. Jin M, Wakely PE Jr. Lymph node cytopathology: essential ancillary studies as applied to lymphoproliferative neoplasms. Cancer Cytopathol. 2018;126(Suppl 8):615–26.
9. Goy A, Stewart J, Barkoh BA. The feasibility of the gene expression profile generated in fine needle aspiration samples from patients with follicular lym-

phoma and diffuse large B cell lymphoma. Cancer. 2006;108(1):10–20.

10. Cozzolino I, Giudice MC, Selleri C, Caputo A, Zeppa P. Lymph node fine-needle cytology in the era of personalized medicine. Is there a role? Cytopathology. 2019;30:348–62.

11. Vigliar E, Acanfora G, Iaccarino A, Mascolo M, Russo D, Scalia G, Della Pepa R, Bellevicine C, Picardi M, Troncone G. A novel approach to classification and reporting of lymph node fine-needle cytology: application of the proposed Sydney system. Diagnostics (Basel). 2021;11(8):1314.

12. Caputo A, Ciliberti V, D'Antonio A, D'Ardia A, Fumo R, Giudice V, Pezzullo L, Sabbatino F, Zeppa P. Real-world experience with the Sydney System on 1458 cases of lymph node fine-needle aspiration cytology. Cytopathology. 2022;33(2):166–75.

13. Bode-Lesniewska B. Neue Aspekte zur Feinnadelpunktion von Lymphknoten [New aspects in fine needle biopsies of the lymph nodes]. Pathologe. 2022;43(2):109–16.

14. Gupta P, Gupta N, Kumar P, Bhardwaj S, Srinivasan R, Dey P, Rohilla M, Bal A, Das A, Rajwanshi A. Assessment of risk of malignancy by application of the proposed Sydney system for classification and reporting lymph node cytopathology. Cancer Cytopathol. 2021;129(9):701–18.

15. Torres Rivas HE, Villar Zarra K, Pérez Pabón LA, González Gutierréz MP, Zapico Ortiz N, Olmo Fernández MDM, Nieto Llanos S, Antoranz Álvarez N, Gómez Martín Á, Fernández Fernández LM. Ultrasound-guided fine-needle aspiration of superficial lymphadenopathy performed by interventional pathologists: the applicability of the Sydney System from 2 years of experience and 363 cases. Acta Cytol. 2021;65(6):453–62.

16. Makarenko VV, DeLelys ME, Hasserjian RP, Ly A. Lymph node FNA cytology: diagnostic performance and clinical implications of proposed diagnostic categories. Cancer Cytopathol. 2022;130(2):144–53.

17. Uzun E, Erkilic S. Diagnostic accuracy of Thinprep® in cervical lymph node aspiration: assessment according to the Sydney system. Diagn Cytopathol. 2022;50(5):253–62.

18. Ahuja S, Malviya A. Categorization of lymph node aspirates using the proposed Sydney system with assessment of risk of malignancy and diagnostic accuracy. Cytopathology. 2022;33(4):430–8.

Pio Zeppa is the Professor of pathology at the University of Salerno, Italy, and Chief of the Pathology Institute. He is the Former Secretary of the Working Group (WG) of the European Society of Pathology (ESP) and author of 220 scientific articles with IF, as well as chapters in books and encyclopedias. His present position is Full Professor of Pathology at the University of Salerno and Chief of the Pathology Institute at the AOU San Giovanni di Dio e Ruggi d' Aragona, Salerno.

Immacolata Cozzolino is the Pathologist at the Vanvitelli University of Naples, Italy. She is a co-author of volume 23, "Lymph Node FNC," of the Monographs in Clinical Cytology and of Lymph Node and Spleen Cytology chapters for Eurocytology website project. She is one of the authors of the Sydney System and the new WHO System for reporting lymph node cytopathology. She has published over 100 articles in various international scientific journals.

Pio Zeppa and Immacolata Cozzolino

15.1   General

The head and neck district is one of the most common sites of lymph node metastasis. Lymph node metastases from loco-regional or distant neoplasms can be an early or late manifestation in patients with a history of cancer or even the onset of a neoplastic disease. The role of Fine Needle Aspiration Cytology (FNAC) is relatively different in these two clinical situations. In the case of known primary tumours, FNAC may confirm the clinical diagnosis and contribute to clinical staging and prognostic-predictive evaluations [1–3]. When the primary tumour is unknown, FNAC, in addition to labelling a given lymph node as metastatic, should identify or suggest the possible origin [4, 5].

Any malignant tumour can metastasize to the head and neck lymph nodes, but the incidence varies greatly depending on the type of tumour. Carcinoma is the most common cause of lymph node metastasis, followed by melanoma and germ cell tumours. In contrast, sarcoma rarely causes lymph node metastases and tumours of

the central nervous system almost never. Furthermore, the time of onset of a lymph nodal metastasis can vary from tumour to tumour. For example, papillary thyroid carcinoma can produce early antero-cervical metastatic lymph node (levels V a and b), while renal cell carcinoma can cause late metastasis in the same region [6–8]. A schematic report of the involved lymph node station and possible primary tumour is reported in Table 15.1.

Therefore, the anatomical level of a metastatic lymph node should be taken into account as it may suggest the possible primary tumour. For instance, lymph node in level Ia. The later-cervical region may be the site of metastases from the oral cavity, anterior nasal cavity, submandibular gland, and midface skin. While carcinoma from oropharynx, larynx, hypopharynx, upper oesophagus, and thyroid may metastasize to nodal group in level IV. Scalene lymph nodes are commonly the recipient of metastases from intrathoracic carcinoma and, on the left of the same station, from abdominal tumours. Cytopathologists dealing with lymph node FNAC should be aware of the specific morphologic aspects, of the clinical-topographical aspects and of the many exceptions to these general rules concerning lymph node stations and the time of onset of lymph node metastases. Finally, the possibility of a second neoplasm is currently not a rare event, especially in elderly or long-surviving patients from treated primary tumours. Metastatic lymph nodes are generally character-

P. Zeppa (✉)
Department of Pathology, University di Salerno, Salerno, Italy
e-mail: pzeppa@unisa.it

I. Cozzolino
Department of Mental and Physical Health and Preventive Medicine, University of Campania "Luigi Vanvitelli", Naples, Italy

J. Klijanienko et al. (eds.), *Diagnostic Procedures in Patients with Neck Masses*,
https://doi.org/10.1007/978-3-031-67675-8_15

Table 15.1 Head and neck metastases: lymph node stations and possible primary tumour

Lymph node level	Involved neck lymph nodes	Possible primary tumour
I a, b	Submandibular	Mouth floor, lips, anterior
II a, b	Jugulodigastric/upper jugular	Epipharynx, tongue, tonsils, larynx
III	Middle jugular	Supraglottic larynx, pyriform sinus
IV	Inferior jugular	Hypopharynx, thyroid, esophagus
V a, b	Supraclavicular	Lung, thyroid, breast, gastrointestinal

ized by widespread involvement, therefore FNAC can generally provide an accurate diagnosis. Usually, the cytological characteristics of a metastatic lymph node differ significantly from the "normal cytology" of the lymph node so the diagnosis of lymph node metastasis vs reactive hyperplasia or lymphoproliferative processes is generally simple and immediate on direct smears, although exceptions can always occur. Therefore, in the majority of metastatic lymph nodes, the lymph node cytology classification and reporting system can be effectively applied [9]. In clinically evident metastatic lymph nodes, metastatic cancer cells outnumber background lymphocytes, if any. The cytological features that favour the diagnosis of lymph node metastases are the presence of cell clusters compared to isolated lymphoid cells and other cytological aspects such as "cell-in-cell", moulding, intranuclear inclusions, cytoplasmic vacuolations, and abundant and clear cytoplasm. In the background, necrosis and fibrosis may be present; the lymphoglandular bodies are missing. These features may also be present in combination. Whereas much of the solid tumours are characterized by cohesive patterns either in their primary localizations or in metastases, others such as melanoma, breast lobular carcinoma, and seminoma are discohesive in their canonical presentations or occasionally (gastric carcinoma and lung adenocarcinoma) creating problems of differential diagnosis with other pathological entities (anaplastic lymphoma and histiocytosis). Sometimes the metastatic cells can be scarce and mixed with or even hidden by the lymphoid cells.

In these cases, the differential diagnosis of metastatic cells with plasma cells, dendritic cells, histiocytes, or large lymphocytes must be made. In some cases, metastatic carcinoma may mimic Hodgkin lymphoma and non-Hodgkin lymphoma. For example, nasopharyngeal lymphoepithelial carcinoma may simulate Hodgkin lymphoma clinically and cytologically, due to its common onset in young adults with unilateral painless cervical enlarged lymph node. FNAC smears generally show few isolated malignant cells in a polymorphic reactive cell population, including eosinophils. Instead, other carcinomas can be confused with non-Hodgkin lymphoma. Lymph node metastases from monomorphic, small cell tumours may be confused with lymphoid cells, for example from lobular carcinoma and neuroendocrine carcinoma of the lung. In these cases attention should be paid to the presence of intracytoplasmic vacuoles which is a specific feature of lobular carcinoma; for neuroendocrine carcinoma, the key cytological features are the dense nuclear chromatin pattern, the absence of nucleoli, nuclear moulding, and focal necrosis. Metastatic lymph node melanoma can also mimic large cell non-Hodgkin lymphoma and plasmacytoma on FNAC smears. In all these cases, the immunocytochemistry identification of diagnostic cells is mandatory for a correct diagnosis. Conversely, some lymphoma, namely Hodgkin lymphoma, diffuse large B-cell lymphoma, ALK+/- anaplastic large cell lymphoma and some histiocytosis may simulate metastatic lymph nodes. True or apparent cohesion, anaplasia of neoplastic cells, and the prevalence of lymphoid background may lead to this misinterpretation. Again, immunocytochemistry (ICC) is mandatory for an accurate FNAC diagnosis. Sometimes the microscopic features in metastatic lymph nodes are completely obscured by abundant necrosis with a few viable cells. In these cases, the morphological diagnosis of metastases and the identification of the primary tumour may be difficult, and ICC may not be helpful. Cystic changes may frequently occur in lymph node metastasis from squamous cell carcinoma and other tumours. When cystic changes are prominent, the FNAC harvesting of neoplastic cells may be scanty and limited to the more superficial and better differentiated cell layers. Therefore, malignant cells may be missed or confused with benign squamous cells, mainly when occurring in the neck, simulating dysembriogenetic cysts. Prominent cystic changes are possible in metastatic papillary thyroid carcinoma. In these cases, the thyroglobulin assay on FNAC wash-out, combined with traditional smears, may be helpful [10].

15.2 Diagnostic Workflow

ICC is the ancillary technique of choice in the case of FNAC lymph node metastasis. ICC may confirm the clinical lymph node metastasis diagnosis in a patient with known primitivity in the staging process or during cancer follow-up or may identify the primary tumour in an unknown neoplasm metastasis. Beyond the identification of primary carcinoma, FNAC differential diagnosis in metastatic lymph node may affect the differentiation between high-grade non-Hodgkin lymphoma and metastatic poorly differentiated carcinoma.

The application of ICC on cytological samples may be hampered by different problems. In fact,

FNAC samples for ICC can be set up on different supports, which include direct smears fixed in alcohol (additional or destained smears), cytocentrifugated, and cell block sections with specific characteristics of fixation and treatment. Sample heterogeneity hampers the reproducibility and evaluation of a single test and has determined the lack of specific guidelines and quality control procedures. Therefore, the heterogeneous and variable nature of tumours and the possible immunophenotypic differences between primary and metastatic tumours have also to be considered. Finally, FANC samples are quantitatively limited when compared to the histological counterpart.

These data should be considered in the choice of antibodies for ICC; furthermore, the corresponding results should be in line with clinical and morphological data. The choice of antibodies for metastatic lymph node ICC should take into account their sensitivity and specificity, the possibility of internal and external controls, the rate of incidence of suspected primary tumours, and antigen specificity.

A basic panel for poorly differentiated tumours is CKAE1AE3, CD45 (LCA), Vimentin, and S100 as markers for epithelial, lymphoid, mesenchymal, and melanocytic tumours, respectively. A second panel of antibodies should be reserved to better differentiated tumours in which cytological features and clinical data suggest the possible primary tumour. This second panel of antibodies includes several antibodies, e.g. CK7, CDX2, CK19, CA19.9, CK20, p63, CK5/6, TTF1, tireoglobulin, PAX8, parathormone, calcitonin, oestrogen, progesterone, CD56, chromogranin, synaptophysin, calretinin, CD30, CD117, Melan A, and SOX10 (Figs. 15.1 and 15.2). When properly applied and interpreted, the evaluation of these markers should lead to the identification of specific entities.

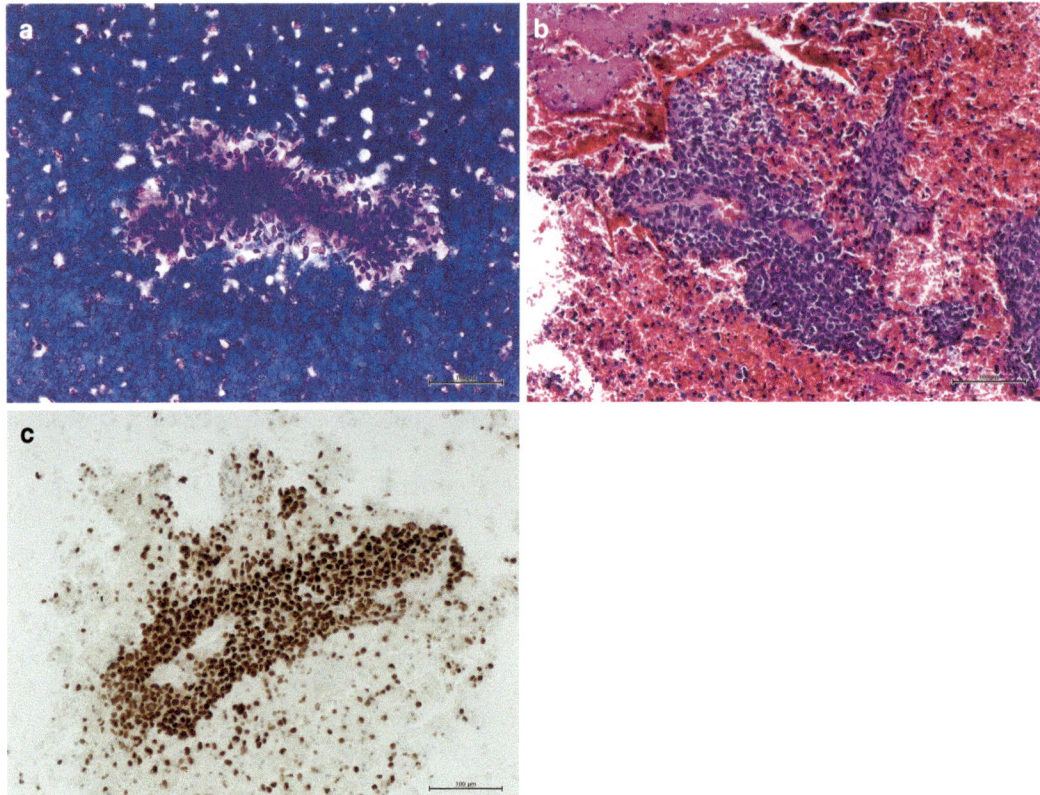

Fig. 15.1 Left Jugulodigastric, IIA lymph node FNAC, in patient with previous diagnosis of melanoma at the right temple. (**a**): cohesive cellular group of medium-sized cells organized around a vascular structure (MGG, 270X). (**b**): cell-block section: a monotonous cellular sheet in a necrotic-proteinaceous background (H&E, 270X), (**c**): immunocytochemical positivity for SOX10 (270X)

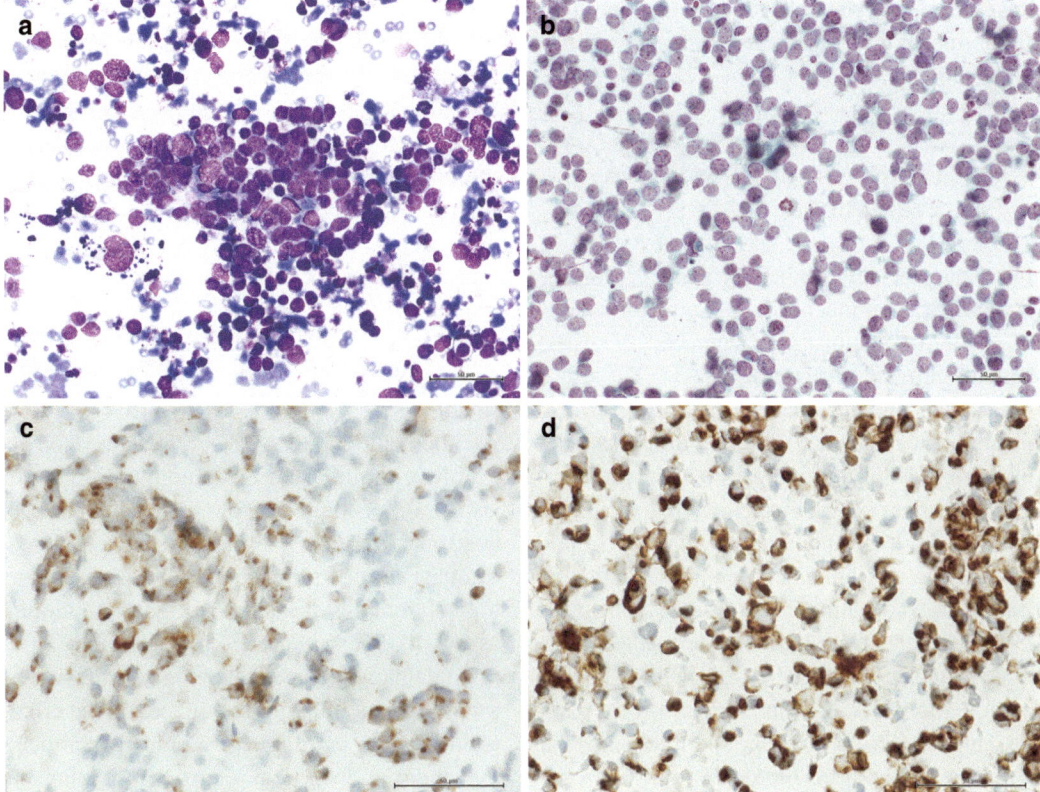

Fig. 15.2 Right Jugulodigastric, IIA lymph node FNAC. (**a**): Metastasis from Merkel cell carcinoma showing undifferentiated, small cells (Diff-Quik, 430X). (**b**): cells in a prevalent dispersed pattern show scanty or absent cytoplasm, nuclei with finely dispersed chromatin and inconspicuous or absent nucleoli (Papanicolaou, 430X). (**c**): chromogranin positivity (APAP immunostaining 430X). (**d**): cytokeratin 20 dot-like positivity (APAP immunostaining 430X)

15.3 Occult Lymph Node Metastasis

The "occult" lymph node metastasis has always been FNAC "Achilles' heel". Generally, metastases arise in the sub capsular sinus as little cellular aggregates or even as isolated cells that may be easily missed by FNAC. However, FNAC is now assisted by sophisticated equipment that allow accurate needle guidance and sampling specific lymph node areas, thus increasing the diagnostic sensitivity in case of partial lymph node involvement [11, 12].

Thanks to the introduction of new technologies, it is now possible to obtain diagnostic information even in the case of micro metastases on cytological samples. The miR-203 and miR-205 determination by qRT-PCR for the detection of micro metastases in cervical lymph nodes has a role in the therapy choice and prognostic evaluation of head and neck squamous cell carcinoma patients. MiR-203 and miR-205 determination has been successfully applied on FNAC of neck lymph nodes at the time of treatment and during the follow-up [13]. A prompt and accurate diagnosis of lymph node metastasis is important for the staging, treatment, and prognosis of melanoma. Occult metastasis in lymph nodes is a relevant problem of melanoma, as it may be easily missed by FNAC as well as on histological sections. Reverse transcriptase-polymerase chain reaction (RT-PCR) analysis of sentinel lymph nodes can detect lymph node micro metastases from melanoma and has been successfully applied on FNAC samples [14–17].

15.4 Prognostic and Predictive Evaluation

In recent years, cytopathology gained increasing credibility as an independent diagnostic method to guide the clinical management of cancer patients in many different contexts. The use of ancillary techniques, such as ICC, in situ hybridization, and molecular tests of cytological samples to identify prognostic and predictive biomarkers has contributed crucially to achieving this goal [17]. Lymph node FNAC of most non-lymphomatous tumours generally yields cell fragments, rather than isolated cells. Therefore, FNAC samples from lymph node metastasis are more suitable for embedding and cell-block preparation. Moreover, ICC on "formalin-fixed paraffin embedded (FFPE) cells" perfectly matches with the standardized protocols of ICC, in particular for prognostic and predictive markers.

Numerous options are currently available for the molecular typing of tumours and the evaluation of prognostic and predictive biomarkers.

A prognostic biomarker provides information on the possible outcome of the tumour regardless of the therapy, while a predictive marker provides information on the effect of a therapeutic intervention. A predictive biomarker can therefore also be a target for therapy. Markers with a similar purpose include the well-known oestrogenic, progesterone, and HER2/neu for breast cancer, c-KIT mutations in GIST tumours, EGFR1 mutations in non-small cell lung cancer (Fig. 15.3), RAS in colorectal carcinoma, BRAF in melanoma, and PD-L1 in squamous cell carcinoma (Fig. 15.4) [18–24]. All these biomarkers can be evaluated on the primitive tumour and on lymph node metastasis, as well as on the cytological samples of the head and neck district. It is currently possible to evaluate single or multiple biomarkers on cytological samples through multigene mutational assays like next generation sequencing (NGS) to guide patient care. The cytopathologist plays a key role in ensuring the success of ancillary techniques in cytological samples by influencing the pre-analytical steps, optimizing the types of preparation, and adequacy requirements in terms of cellularity and tumour fraction and ensuring an optimal extraction of nucleic acid [25–28].

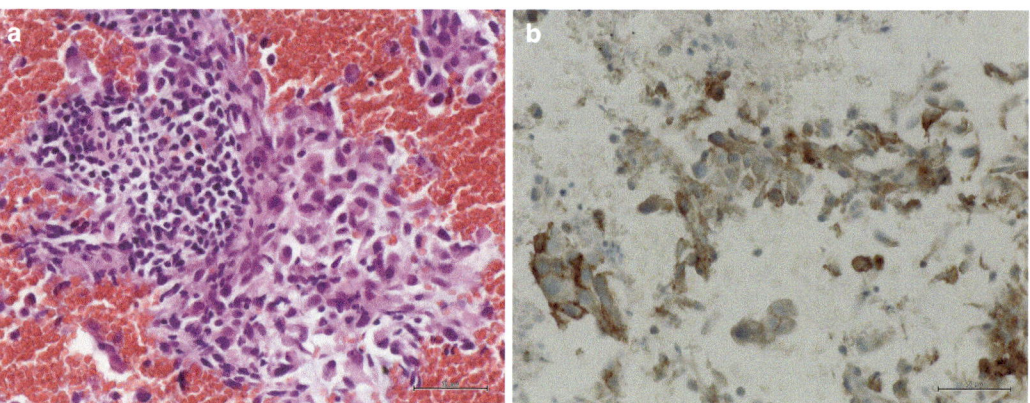

Fig. 15.3 Supraclavicular, V a, lymph node FNAC. (**a**): lymph node metastasis in advanced lung adenocarcinoma (H&E, 40X), (**b**): PDL1 immunocytochemical stain on cell-block section (430X)

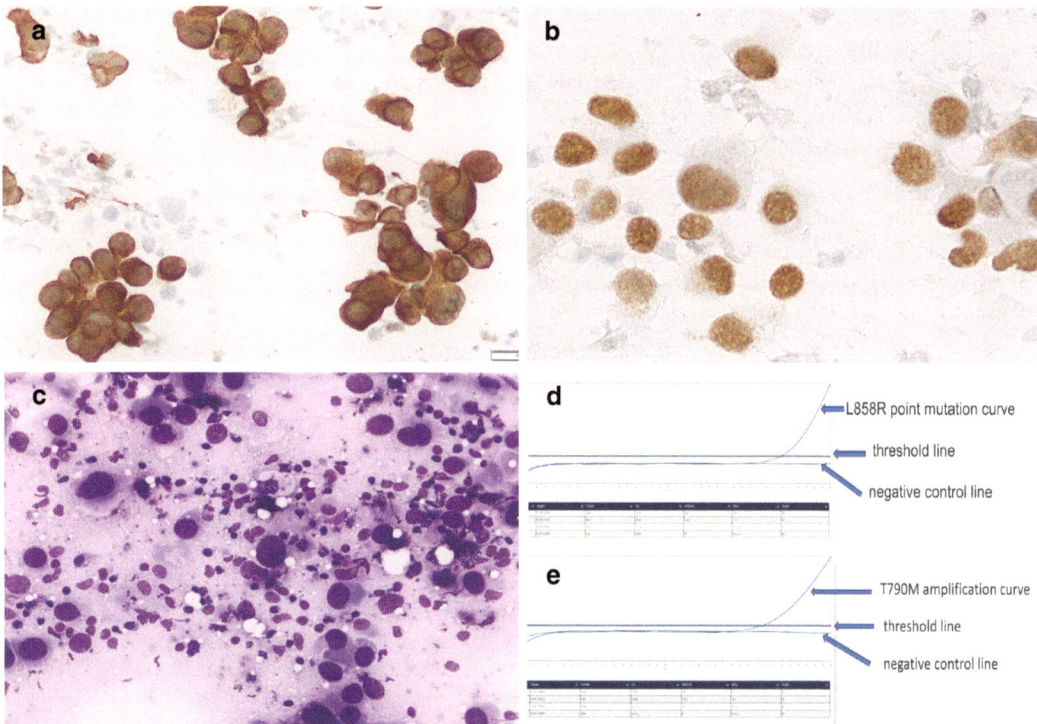

Fig. 15.4 Supraclavicular, V a, lymph node FNAC. (**a**): Epithelial cells, isolated or in small groups, with nuclear atypia and well represented cytoplasm; mature lymphocytes are present in the background. (**b**): Diffuse, cytoplasmic, Cytokeratin 7 positivity (APAP stain, 430X). (**c**): Diffuse nuclear positivity for TTF1, indicating a lung pri-mary tumor. (**d**): EGFR, L858R and T790M point mutations assessed on DNA obtained by cells scraped from a Diff-Quik stained smear (**e**): RT-PCR analysis of EGFR, performed DNA extracted from a smear of the same case, showing the T790M mutation curve

15.5   Main Message

- Fine Needle Aspiration Cytology of lymph node metastases may confirm the clinical diagnosis and may contribute to the staging and prognostic-predictive evaluations in case of known primary tumours. When the primary tumour is unknown, lymph node FNAC may diagnose a lymphadenopathy as metastatic and identify or suggest the possible primary tumour.
- Any malignant tumour can metastasize to the head and neck lymph nodes with specific stations prevalence, but the incidence varies greatly depending on the type of tumour.
- The diagnosis of lymph node metastasis vs reactive hyperplasia or lymphoproliferative processes is generally immediate on direct smears, although exceptions may always occur.
- Main cytological features of lymph node metastases are the presence of cell clusters and moulding, intranuclear inclusions, cytoplasmic vacuolations, and abundant cytoplasm.
- Sometimes the metastatic cells can be scarce and mixed with or hidden by the lymphoid cells: nasopharyngeal lymphoepithelial carcinoma, cells may mimic Hodgkin lymphoma and non-Hodgkin lymphoma; breast lobular carcinoma and neuroendocrine carcinoma can be confused with non-Hodgkin lymphoma. ICC is mandatory for an accurate FNAC diagnosis.
- Microscopic features may be obscured by abundant necrosis that hamper the identification of vital cells and the usage of ICC.

- Cystic changes may occur in lymph node metastasis from papillary thyroid carcinoma and squamous cell carcinoma. In this latter, malignant cells may be missed or confused with benign squamous-simulating dysembriogenetic cysts.
- ICC is the ancillary technique of choice in case of lymph node metastases; ICC can be set up on direct smears fixed or destained smears, cytospins, and cell block sections.
- Basic antibodies panel for lymph node metastasis is CKAE1AE3, CD45 (LCA), Vimentin, S100, and SOX10 as markers for epithelial, lymphoid, mesenchymal, and melanocytic tumours respectively.
- Second panel of antibodies is reserved to tumours in which cytological features and clinical data suggest the possible primary tumour and includes CK20, CK7, CDX2, CK19, CA19.9, p63, CK5/6, TTF1, tireoglobulin, PAX8, parathormone, calcitonin, oestrogen, progesterone, CD56, chromogranin, synaptophysin, Melan A, calretinin, CD30, and CD117.
- Occult lymph node metastasis may be missed by FNAC; an ultrasound guide may assist the needle guidance and the sampling of specific lymph node areas.
- The miR-203 and miR-205 determination by qRT-PCR is effective in the detection of micro metastases and has a role in the therapy choice and the prognostic evaluation of head and neck squamous cell carcinoma. Reverse transcriptase-polymerase chain reaction can detect lymph node micro metastases from melanoma and has been used on FNAC samples.
- Immunocytochemistry, in situ hybridization, and molecular tests may be utilized to identify prognostic and predictive biomarkers on FNAC samples.
- Prognostic and predictive biomarkers include oestrogenic, progesterone, and HER2/neu for breast cancer, c-KIT mutations in GIST tumours, EGFR1 mutations in non-small cell lung cancer, RAS in colorectal carcinoma, BRAF in melanoma, and PD-L1 in lung squamous cell carcinoma.

References

1. Silvestri GA, Gonzalez AV, Jantz MA, Margolis ML, Gould MK, Tanoue LT, Harris LJ, Detterbeck FC. American College of Chest Physicians evidence-based clinical practice guidelines. Chest. 2013;143(5 (Suppl)):e207. Methods for staging non-small cell lung cancer: Diagnosis and management of lung cancer. 3rd ed.
2. Gelberg J, Grondin S, Tremblay A. Mediastinal staging for lung cancer. Can Respir J. 2014;21(3):159–61.
3. Park SH, Kim MJ, Park BW, et al. Impact of preoperative ultrasonography and fine-needle aspiration of axillary lymph nodes on surgical management of primary breast cancer. Ann Surg Oncol. 2011;18:738–44.
4. Koelliker SL, Chung MA, Mainiero MB, et al. Axillary lymph nodes: US-guided fine-needle aspiration for initial staging of breast cancer—correlation with primary tumor size. Radiology. 2008;246:81–9.
5. Jain A, Haisfield-Wolfe ME, Lange J, et al. The role of ultrasoundguided fine-needle aspiration of axillary nodes in the staging of breast cancer. Ann Surg Oncol. 2008;15:462–71.
6. Strojan P, Ferlito A, Medina JE, Woolgar JA, Rinaldo A, Robbins KT, Fagan JJ, Mendenhall WM, Paleri V, Silver CE, Olsen KD, Corry J, Suárez C, Rodrigo JP, Langendijk JA, Devaney KO, Kowalski LP, Hartl DM, Haigentz M Jr, Werner JA, Pellitteri PK, de Bree R, Wolf GT, Takes RP, Genden EM, Hinni ML, Mondin V, Shaha AR, Barnes L. Contemporary management of lymph node metastases from an unknown primary to the neck. A review of diagnostic approaches. Head Neck. 2013;35(1):123–32.
7. Langille G, Taylor SM, Bullock MJ. Metastatic renal cell carcinoma to the head and neck: summary of 21 cases. J Otolaryngol Head Neck Surg. 2008;37(4):515–21.
8. Strojan P, Ferlito A, Langendijk JA, Corry J, Woolgar JA, Rinaldo A, Silver CE, Paleri V, Fagan JJ, Pellitteri PK, Haigentz M Jr, Suárez C, Robbins KT, Rodrigo JP, Olsen KD, Hinni ML, Werner JA, Mondin V, Kowalski P, Devaney KO, de Bree R, Takes RP, Wolf GT, Shaha AR, Genden EM, Barnes. Contemporary management of lymph node metastases from an unknown primary to the neck: II. A review of therapeutic options. Head Neck. 2013;35(2):286–93.
9. Al-Abbadi MA, Barroca H, Bode-Lesniewska B, Calaminici M, Caraway NP, Chhieng DF, Cozzolino I, Ehinger M, Field AS, Geddie WR, Katz RL, Lin O, Medeiros LJ, Monaco SE, Rajwanshi A, Schmitt FC, Vielh P, Zeppa P. A proposal for the performance, classification, and reporting of lymph node fine-needle aspiration cytopathology: the Sydney system. Acta Cytol. 2020;64(4):306–22.
10. Jo K, Kim MH, Lim Y, Jung SL, Bae JS, Jung CK, Kang MI, Cha BY, Lim DJ. Lowered cutoff of lymph node fine-needle aspiration thyroglobulin in thyroid cancer patients with serum anti-thyroglobulin antibody. Eur J Endocrinol. 2015;173(4):489–97.

11. Balu-Maestro C, Ianessi A, Chapellier C, Marcotte C, Stolear S. Ultrasound-guided lymph node sampling in the initial management of breast cancer. Diagn Interv Imaging. 2013;94(4):389–94.

12. Ewing DE, Layfield LJ, Joshi CL, Travis MD. Determinants of false-negative fine-needle aspirates of axillary lymph nodes in women with breast cancer: lymph node size, cortical thickness and hilar fat retention. Acta Cytol. 2015;59(4):311–4.

13. de Carvalho AC, Scapulatempo-Neto C, Maia DC, Evangelista AF, Morini MA, Carvalho AL, Vettore AL. Accuracy of microRNAs as markers for the detection of neck lymph node metastases in patients with head and neck squamous cell carcinoma. BMC Med. 2015;13:108. Erratum in BMC Med. 2015;13:155.

14. Voit C, Kron M, Rademaker J, Schwürzer-Voit M, Sterry W, Weber L, Ozdemir C, Proebstle T, Keilholz U. Molecular staging in stage II and III melanoma patients and its effect on long-term survival. J Clin Oncol. 2005;23(6):1218–27.

15. Scoggins CR, Ross MI, Reintgen DS, Noyes RD, Goydos JS, Beitsch PD, Urist MM, Ariyan S, Davidson BS, Sussman JJ, Edwards MJ, Martin RC, Lewis AM, Stromberg AJ, Conrad AJ, Hagendoorn L, Albrecht J, McMasters KM. Prospective multi-institutional study of reverse transcriptase polymerase chain reaction for molecular staging of melanoma. J Clin Oncol. 2006;24(18):2849–57.

16. Mocellin S, Hoon DS, Pilati P, Rossi CR, Nitti D. Sentinel lymph node molecular ultrastaging in patients with melanoma: a systematic review and meta-analysis of prognosis. J Clin Oncol. 2007;25(12):1588–95.

17. Roy-Chowdhuri S, Pisapia P, Salto-Tellez M, Savic S, Nacchio M, de Biase D, Tallini G, Troncone G, Schmitt F. Invited review-next-generation sequencing: a modern tool in cytopathology. Virchows Arch. 2019;475(1):3–11.

18. Ronchi A, Pagliuca F, Zito Marino F, Accardo M, Cozzolino I, Franco R. Current and potential immunohistochemical biomarkers for prognosis and therapeutic stratification of breast carcinoma. Semin Cancer Biol. 2021;72:114–22.

19. Pagliuca F, Ronchi A, Cozzolino I, Montella M, Zito Marino F, Franco R. Mesenchymal neoplasms: Is it time for cytology? New perspectives for the preoperative diagnosis of soft tissue tumors in the molecular era. Pathol Res Pract. 2020 Jun;216(6):152923.

20. Cozzolino I, Malapelle U, Carlomagno C, Palombini L, Troncone G. Metastasis of colon cancer to the thyroid gland: a case diagnosed on fine-needle aspirate by a combined cytological, immunocytochemical, and molecular approach. Diagn Cytopathol. 2010;38(12):932–5.

21. D'Ardia A, Caputo A, Fumo R, Ciaparrone C, Gaeta S, Picariello C, Zeppa P, D'Antonio A. Advanced non-small cell lung cancer: Rapid evaluation of EGFR status on fine-needle cytology samples using Idylla. Pathol Res Pract. 2021 Aug;224:153547.

22. Caputo A, D'Ardia A, Sabbatino F, Picariello C, Ciaparrone C, Zeppa P, D'Antonio A. Testing EGFR on cytological specimens of lung cancer: a review. Int J Mol Sci. 2021;22(9):4852.

23. Pirker R, Herth FJ, Kerr KM, Filipits M, Taron M, Gandara D, Hirsch FR, Grunenwald D, Popper H, Smit E, Dietel M, Marchetti A, Manegold C, Schirmacher P, Thomas M, Rosell R, Cappuzzo F, Stahel R; European EGFR Workshop Group. Consensus for EGFR mutation testing in non-small cell lung cancer: results from a European workshop. J Thorac Oncol. 2010;5(10):1706–13.

24. Ronchi A, Montella M, Zito Marino F, Caraglia M, Grimaldi A, Argenziano G, Moscarella E, Brancaccio G, Troiani T, Napolitano S, Franco R, Cozzolino I. Predictive evaluation on cytological sample of metastatic melanoma: the role of BRAF immunocytochemistry in the molecular era. Diagnostics (Basel). 2021;11(6):1110.

25. Heymann JJ, Bulman WA, Swinarski D, Pagan CA, Crapanzano JP, Haghighi M, Fazlollahi L, Stoopler MB, Sonett JR, Sacher AG, Shu CA, Rizvi NA, Saqi A. PD-L1 expression in non-small cell lung carcinoma: Comparison among cytology, small biopsy, and surgical resection specimens. Cancer Cytopathol. 2017;125(12):896–907.

26. da Cunha SG, Saieg MA. Preanalytic specimen triage: Smears, cell blocks, cytospin preparations, transport media, and cytobanking. Cancer Cytopathol. 2017;125(S6):455–64.

27. Barroca H, Bode-Lesniewska B, Cozzolino I, Zeppa P. Management of cytologic material, preanalytic procedures and biobanking in lymph node cytopathology. Cytopathology. 2019;30(1):17–30.

28. Zeppa P, Cozzolino I. Fine-needle cytology: technical procedures and ancillary techniques. Monogr Clin Cytol. 2018;23:4–13.

Pio Zeppa is the Professor of pathology at the University of Salerno, Italy, and Chief of the Pathology Institute. He is the Former Secretary of the Working Group (WG) of the European Society of Pathology (ESP) and author of 220 scientific articles with IF, as well as chapters in books and encyclopedias. His present position is Full Professor of Pathology at the University of Salerno and Chief of the Pathology Institute at the AOU San Giovanni di Dio e Ruggi d' Aragona, Salerno.

Immacolata Cozzolino is the Pathologist at the Vanvitelli University of Naples, Italy. She is a co-author of volume 23, "Lymph Node FNC," of the Monographs in Clinical Cytology and of Lymph Node and Spleen Cytology chapters for Eurocytology website project. She is one of the authors of the Sydney System and the new WHO System for reporting lymph node cytopathology. She has published over 100 articles in various international scientific journals.

Fernando Schmitt and Ricella Souza da Silva

16.1 General

The lateral neck (Fig. 16.1) is the region of the posterior triangle of the neck. The neck posterior triangle is defined anatomically as an area between the posterior border of the sternocleidomastoid, the anterior border of the trapezius, and the clavicle [50]. The exact location of the nodule in the neck allows the exclusion of several differential diagnoses. For example, thyroglossal duct cysts, heterotopic or ectopic thyroid gland, and inflamed sub-mental lymph nodes are confined to the anterior neck, and are not considered in the differential diagnosis of the lateral neck lump [27]. The development of the laterocervical region is closely connected with the formation of the branchial apparatus, which occurs within the first month of intrauterine life.

The branchial arches are arranged in pairs on either side of the midline as a succession of folds and grooves corresponding to the branchial clefts and pouches. A "cleft" refers to the ectoblastic furrow in each arch and a "pouch" refers to the endoblastic depression found on each arch. Four arches can be clearly identified on the embryo, and a rudimentary fifth arch appears but quickly regresses [37]. Each arch coalesces with its contralateral counterpart ventrally on the midline. Each merged arch gives rise to a bone and cartilage derivate, one or more striated muscles, a mixed cranial nerve, and a vascular component. The second arch then expands downward to meet and merge with the fifth arch, thus covering the second third and fourth arch and forming the cervical sinus. Malformations of the midline, on the other hand, are unrelated to the development of the branchial apparatus. These anomalies result from either defective closure of the midline or the persistence of remnants after thyroid migration. These embryologic differences explain the distinction that must be made between malformations of the laterocervical region from malformations of the midline [40].

Anatomically, the layers of the lateral neck are filled with multiple lymph nodes. In addition, due to the anatomical locations of the carotid artery and jugular vein, vascular or lymphatic lesions may present as lateral lesions. A neck mass is defined as an abnormal lesion that is visible, palpable, or seen

F. Schmitt (✉)
Department of Pathology and Oncology, Medical Faculty of the University of Porto, Porto, Portugal

RISE (Health Research Network), Porto, Portugal

Molecular Pathology Unit, Institute of Pathology and Molecular Immunology of Porto University, IPATIMUP, Porto, Portugal

International Academy of Cytology, Freiburg im Breisgau, Germany
e-mail: fernando.schmitt@ipatimup.pt

R. S. da Silva
Molecular Pathology Unit, Institute of Pathology and Molecular Immunology of Porto University, IPATIMUP, Porto, Portugal

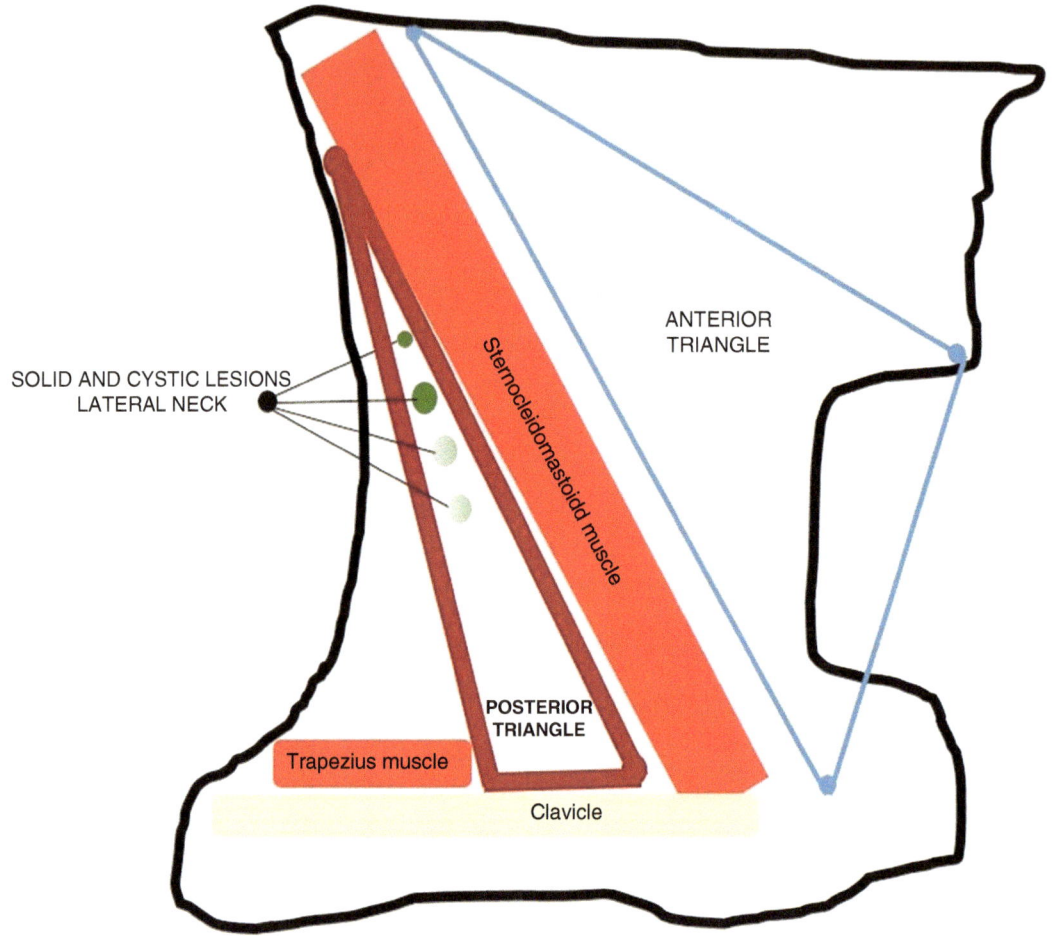

Fig. 16.1 Lateral neck. Region of the posterior triangle of the neck, delimited by the posterior border of the sternocleidomastoid, anterior border of the trapezius, and the clavicle

in an imaging study [42] and can be solid or cystic. These lesions can be derived from infectious, inflammatory, congenital, traumatic, benign, or malignant neoplastic processes [42, 56].

The main cystic lateral neck lesions include: (1) Skin and subcutaneous lesions: epidermal inclusion cyst, dermoid cyst, and teratoid cyst; (2) Developmental masses: branchial cyst, thymic cyst, and lymphagioma. The main solid lateral neck lesions include: (1) Skin and subcutaneous lesions: lipoma; (2) Developmental masses: teratoma (also solid-cystic presentation); (3) Lymph nodes (also solid-cystic presentation): infectious, inflammatory, and neoplastic (discussed in Chap. 14); (4) Neurogenic tumors (also solid-cystic presentation): neurofibroma and schwannoma; (5) Carotid body tumor (also solid-cystic presentation); (6) Metastatic tumors (also solid-cystic presentation); and (7) Salivary glands (discussed in the Chaps. 11 and 12) (Fig. 16.2).

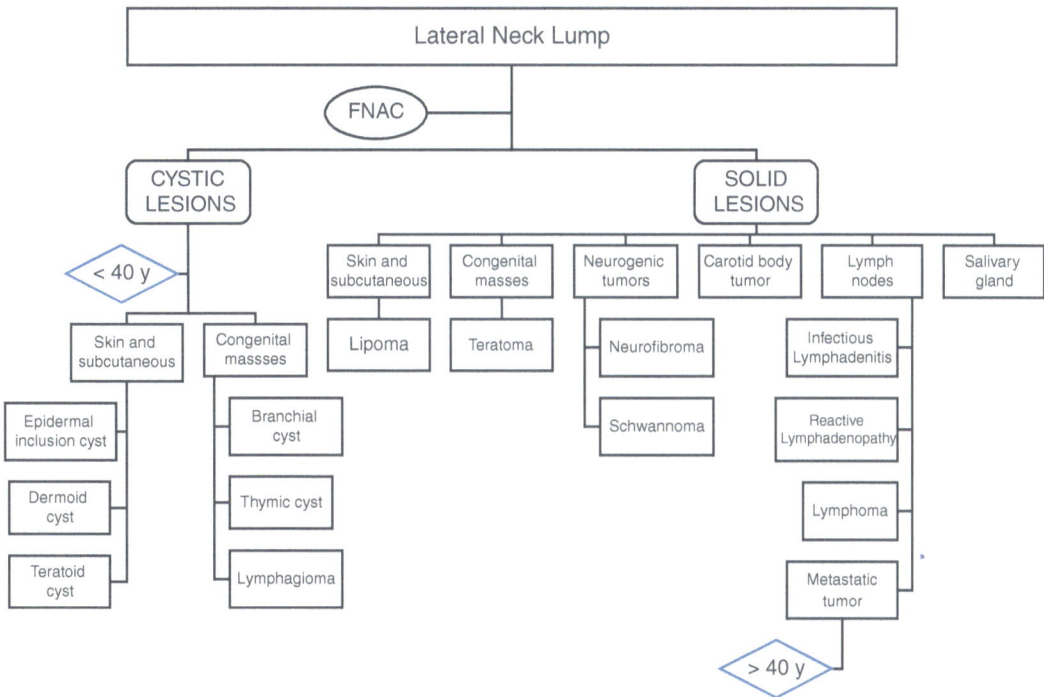

Fig. 16.2 Solid and cystic lesions of the lateral neck in fine-needle aspiration cytology procedure

16.2 Diagnostic Workflow

Masses in the head and neck are especially adequate targets for fine needle aspiration cytology (FNAC) because it is cost-effective, rapid to perform, minimally invasive, well accepted by patients, and associated with low morbidity [4, 7, 53, 56]. FNAC can be performed by palpation or preferentially under image guidance including ultrasound and computed tomography [30, 42, 56]. The main advantage of FNAC is the avoidance of a surgical biopsy and its attendant risks, which include scarring, potential tumor seeding, increased hospital stay, and increased costs. Other risks include discomfort, bruising, and infection [42]. Correlation of clinical, ultrasound, or other imaging modalities with cytological findings is quite important to achieve correct results and to reduce the rates of inadequate samples [7].

The diagnostic accuracy of FNAC is over 90% [4, 53], with sensitivities ranging from 77% to 95% and specificities from 93% to 100% [41, 60]. In a meta-analysis evaluating 3459 aspirates

from head and neck lesions studied by FNAC, the predictive positive value was 96.2% and the negative predictive value was 90.3% [53]. The rate of accuracy is lower in cystic lesions than solid masses [14, 20] and its lower sensitivity (70–75%) warrants caution when a benign diagnosis is rendered [41].

The diagnostic accuracy is dependent on the site of aspiration as well as the skill of the individual performing and interpreting the FNAC [30]. Fine-needle aspirations (FNAs) performed by cytopathologists show significantly better diagnostic accuracy and this advantage is potentially related to the proper application of the technique, the capability for immediate assessment of specimen adequacy, and the maximized use of the material obtained [58].

The main goal of the FNAC is to determine the presence or absence of a neoplasm, assure the clinical benign impression of the mass, and if malignant, to determine the type of malignancy. The age of the patient is often strongly indicative of the likely diagnoses. Information about anatomic site and clinical history can assist with the differential diagnoses [56].

The majority of lateral neck lesions in newborns and infants are benign (congenital or developmental). In children, infectious/inflammatory etiologies are more common [25, 41]. Cystic entities are more common in late childhood or early adulthood. In patients under 40 years old, benign branchial apparatus anomalies are the most common diagnosis of lateral neck masses, with increasing age, differentiating between branchial cleft cysts and solid or cystic lymph node metastasis becomes challenging [55].

Malignancy is an important component that must be considered in a lateral neck lump in patients over 40 years of age [41, 51]. It must be ruled out since metastases arising from head and neck cancers may undergo cystic degeneration, and thus mimic the presentation of benign masses [60]. Notably, an asymptomatic neck mass may be the first or only clinically visible manifestation of a head and neck cancer, such as squamous cell carcinoma, lymphoma, thyroid cancer, or salivary gland cancer [42]. Malignancy has been reported to be as high as 56% in adults over 40 compared to 1.6% for those under the age of 40 years. The proportion of malignancy is greater than 80% in patients over the age of 70 years and is most commonly found in female patients [16].

All the ancillary studies such as flow cytometry, immunocytochemistry, cytogenetic analysis, and molecular studies can be performed on material retrieved by FNA. A parallel scenario goes for the no neoplastic inflammatory conditions where triaging appropriate samples for culture and any other needed studies can be performed successfully on specimens obtained by FNA [26, 48].

16.3   Main Lateral Neck Lesions

16.3.1 Lateral Cystic Lesions

16.3.1.1   Epidermal Inclusion Cysts
Epidermal inclusion cysts (EICs) are also known as epidermoid cysts, infundibular cysts, keratin cysts, inclusion cysts, and epidermal cysts. They can occur everywhere on the body, although the

face, scalp, neck, and trunk are the most typical sites [44]. They occur in young to middle age adults with an incidence ranging from 1.6% to 6.9% in the head and neck. They are usually solitary and connect with the surface by keratin-filled pores [1].

They are likely to be formed by the sequestration of epidermal rests during embryonic life, occlusion of the pilosebaceous unit, or traumatic implantation of epithelial elements [23]. They typically manifest as a small nodule with visible punctum, located in the mid and lower dermis [24]. EICs can remain dormant or swell and/or infect.

Aspirates from EICs (Fig. 16.3) reveal a clear background, with high cellularity, and nucleate and anucleate squames. Keratinous material is seen in some cases, but the amount is usually less compared to cellular elements. Infected EICs show additional features with dense inflammatory cell infiltrate comprising predominantly of neutrophils, lymphocytes, multinucleate foreign body giant cells, in addition to the nucleate and anucleate squame. These lesions can be missed on cytology, largely due to inadequate or unrepresentative sampling liquids [23, 24].

Although the diagnosis of EIC can be easily made on cytological examination, it has to be differentiated from other squamous cell containing lesions such as dermoid cyst, branchial cyst, thyroglossal cyst, and well-differentiated squamous

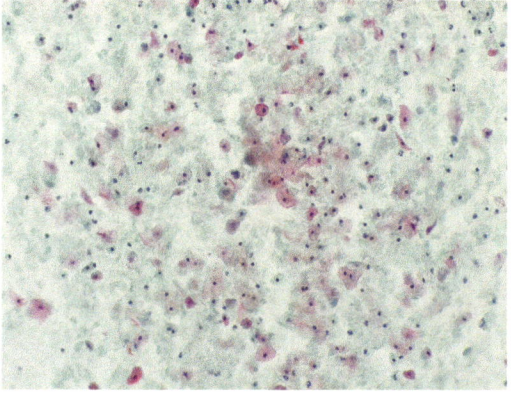

Fig. 16.3 Epidermal inclusion cyst. Aspirates showing high cellularity with nucleate, anucleate squames, and keratinous material with some inflammatory background (Pap)

cell carcinoma. Malignant changes, although extremely rare, have been reported in epidermoid cysts [10].

16.3.1.2 Dermoid Cysts and Teratoid Cysts

Dermoid cysts may occur anywhere in the body, with only 1–3.5% affecting the head and neck region [1]. About 60% of cases occur in children 5 years old or younger or during the second and third decades of life [41]. Dermoid cysts are lined by squamous epithelium and differ from epidermoid cysts in that they contain dermal appendages, such as hair, hair follicles, sebaceous, and sweat glands [44].

The smears display moderate-high cellular samples, sheets of keratinaceous cellular material, benign-appearing, anucleated and nucleated squamous cells, and sometimes degenerated inflammatory cells [5].

Teratoid cysts include tissue components from all three germ layers—ectoderm, mesoderm, and endoderm—in contrast to dermoid cysts. The presence of other differentiated types of cells including skin appendages along with mature cartilage, enteric, and/or respiratory epithelium leads to the definition of teratoid cysts [5, 44]. The presence of these components in cytological samples is infrequent and FNA interpretation can be difficult when sampling occurs in cystic areas without yielding enough diagnostic material

16.3.1.3 Branchial Cysts

Branchial cleft anomalies arise from the incomplete obliteration of any branchial tract, resulting in either a cyst (75%) or a sinus or fistulous tract (25%) [41]. The majority of cases arise in young patients between 20 and 40 years of age [60], occur equally in both males and females, and frequently become symptomatic in the second and third decades [20]. The masses are typically soft, slow-growing, and painless. It is usual to have a history of

an infection, a spontaneous discharge, or an incision and drainage [49].

Branchial fissures giving rise to sinuses and fistulas are located in the anterior triangle of the neck and present earlier in childhood. While branchial cleft cysts appear more laterally in the neck [12]. The cysts, by definition, do not physically connect with the skin or aerodigestive tract, situated beneath the deep cervical fascia [18]. Branchial cleft cysts are clinically divided into first, second, third, or fourth branchial cleft cysts, depending on the anatomical location of the lesion. First branchial cleft cysts can occur anywhere from the external auditory canal. Second branchial anomalies are present along the anterior border of the sternocleidomastoid muscle and comprise 80–95% of all branchial cleft cysts. Third/fourth branchial cleft represents 1–8% of branchial cysts and emerge predominantly left-sided (97%) [41].

Lateral neck branchial cyst (Fig. 16.4) aspirates appear as a straw-colored or pus-like fluid that microscopically may exhibit a matrix of amorphous debris, squamous epithelial cells of variable maturity, columnar and ciliated cells, or also the presence of mucinous cells. Depending on the degree of infection, those cysts present inflammatory features with neutrophils, abundant lymphocytes, macrophages, and plasmocytes on a clean background [7, 12, 18]. Cholesterol crystals can also be found in 3–50% of the branchial cysts aspirates [60]. These features are nonspecific.

Differential diagnoses include epidermal cyst, dermoid cyst, thyroglossal duct cyst, thymic cyst, metastatic squamous cell carcinoma, and papillary thyroid carcinoma metastasis. The location and cytomorphology of branchial cysts are important factors to yield the correct diagnosis. Atypical features such as high nuclei-cytoplasmic ratio, irregular nuclear membranes, and small cell clusters raise the possibility of a malignant process [31] (Fig. 16.5).

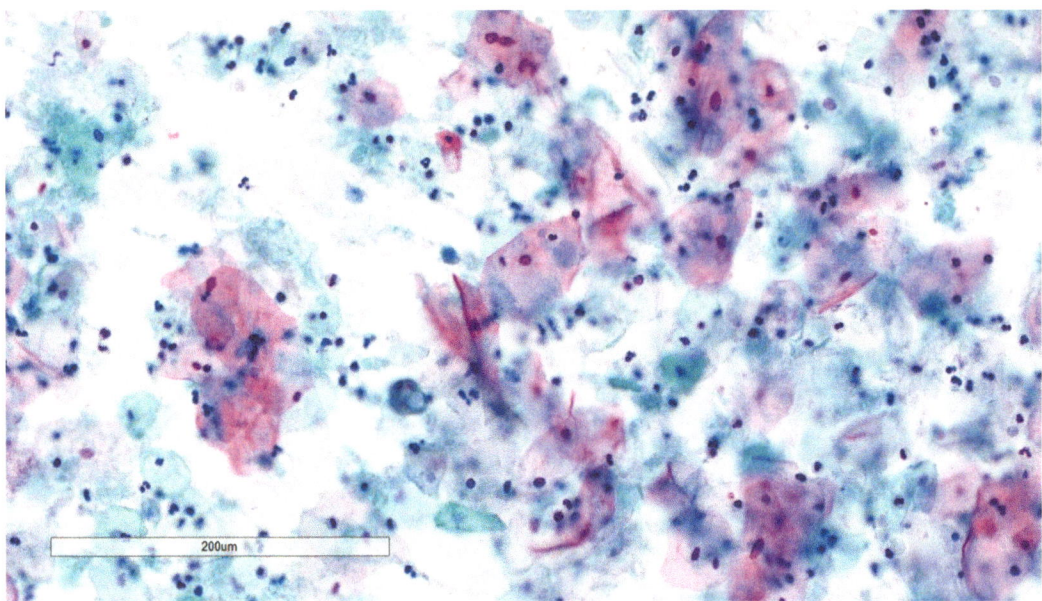

Fig. 16.4 Branchial cyst. Aspirates exhibit a matrix of amorphous debris, squamous epithelial cells of variable maturity, and mucinous cells surrounded by inflammatory cells (Pap)

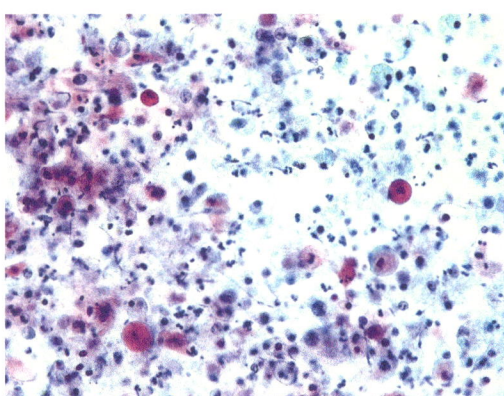

Fig. 16.5 Metastatic cystic squamous cell carcinoma with slight atypia. In some cases, the differential diagnosis of branchial cysts can be difficult (Pap)

16.3.1.4 Thymic Cysts

Thymic cysts are very rare causes of benign neck masses in adults, more common in males, and are usually not diagnosed before surgery. Their prevalence is less than 1% of all cervical masses, and they are usually noted in childhood, generally 2–13 years [36]. The most common cervical topography is anterolateral with/without extension into the mediastinum, but occasionally it may be located in the left neck [12].

They remain asymptomatic and alarm the patient with cervical swelling when spontaneous hemorrhage occurs within these cysts [38]. This entity is often diagnosed by its well-demarcated margins on ultrasound guide, chest x-ray, or computed tomography in which the size is usually reduced after FNA.

Aspirates reveal a straw-colored fluid, abundant mature lymphocytes, loosely scattered benign-looking epithelial cells (squamous or ciliated, cuboid, and columnar) with round to oval nuclei, regular nuclear margin and a moderate amount of cytoplasm, foamy macrophages, and proteinaceous debris in a hemorrhagic background.

Surgical excision shows that the thymic tissue consists of cuboidal or flat epithelium and Hassall's corpuscle. The differential diagnoses of a cervicomediastinal cystic lesion are lymphangioma, thymoma, thymic carcinoma, and very rarely lymphoma [38].

16.3.1.5 Lymphangioma and Cystic Hygroma

Lymphangiomas occur from the early sequestration of embryonic lymphatic vessels, most frequently along the jugular chain. They are infrequent lesions of lymphatic channels that are often present at birth and usually diagnosed during childhood, mostly (90%) before the age of two years [3]. Very often these lesions composed of dilated lymphatic channels are associated with chromosomal defects, such as Turner's syndrome, Trisomy 13, 18, and 21, as well as Noonan syndrome [2]. Two-thirds of all reported cases are in the head and neck region, with occasional extension to the mediastinum [41].

Four types of lymphangioma are described based on the microscopic size of the dilated lymphatic channel: cystic hygroma, cavernous lymphangioma, capillary lymphangioma, and vasculolymphatic malformation [29].

Cystic hygromas are the most common form of lymphangioma; 75% of these occur in the neck. The cytological characteristic of cystic hygroma is the presence of clear fluid with red blood cells, lymphocytes, histiocytes, and a proteinaceous debris [8, 41].

16.3.2 Lateral Solid Lesions

16.3.2.1 Lipoma

Lipomas may present in the neck as large isolated masses present for long periods of time without change over the years [41], constituting the most common soft tissue benign neoplasm in the cervical region. Clinically, they can be misdiagnosed as epidermal cysts due to the same isoechoic presentation on ultrasound [57].

The cytomorphology of lipomas includes a poor cellular sample showing dispersed fragments of collagen fibers and mature adypocytes with wide empty cytoplasm, single lipid large vacuole, and small eccentric dark nuclei.

Lipoblastomas are rare and present mostly during infancy and in men. They are characterized by the presence of moderately or poor cellular smears containing lipocytes, lipoblasts (cells with cytoplasmic vacuoles indenting the nucleus and nuclei small), and spindle cells in various proportions. Naked oval nuclei with fine ramified vessels mixed and occasional myxoid matrix can also be observed. No necrosis, atypia,

or mitoses are present. In about 70% of cases, these tumors carry abnormalities in chromosome 8, mainly leading to rearrangements of the PLAG1 gene [13, 28].

Pleomorphic lipoma smears reveal hypocellular specimens with atypical large and floret cells (large cells with multiple hyperchromatic nuclei arranged in a circle or semicircle) with fragments of mature adipocytic cells and collagen fibers and myxoid background with occasional mast cells. Mitotic activity and nuclear pleomorphism are absent. CD34 staining by immunocytochemistry further supports the diagnosis [6, 46, 54]. These lesions usually affect middle-aged to elderly men.

16.3.2.2 Teratoma (Also Solid-Cystic Presentation)

Cervical teratomas are extremely rare neoplasms, with an incidence of 1 in 20,000 to 40,000 live births; they account for approximately 5% of all neonatal teratomas [41]. Teratomas contain mature and/or immature somatic elements derived from ectodermal, mesenchymal, or endodermal cells. This entity is distinguished from teratoid cysts by the presence of recognizable organic structures such as teeth or skin [5].

Cytomorphologically, smears can be very variable, with diverse combinations of mature and/or immature elements. Mature elements include tissues from the skin and adnexal structures, cartilage, bone, all types of epithelial lining, and stromal components. Some respiratory-type ciliated columnar cells or mature intestinal elements such as goblet cells with vacuolated cytoplasm and hyaline cartilage might be present in the smears [59].

Immature elements include immature neuroepithelium characterized by spindled primitive cells with scant cytoplasm and hyperchromatic nuclei forming rosette, pseudorosette, or primitive tubule. The use of immunocytochemistry seems to be limited to the evaluation of the immature neuroectodermal component [45]. The most important differential diagnoses include a bronchogenic cyst and in cases with abundant squamous cell component the possibility of a metastatic squamous cell carcinoma [7].

16.3.2.3 Neurogenic Tumors (Also Solid-Cystic Presentation)

Neurogenic tumors, schwannomas and neurofibromas, are found in the head and neck region particularly in the carotid space (vagus nerve or sympathetic chain) or in the posterior cervical space (spinal nerve or brachial plexus). Schwannomas and neurofibromas may occur in patients with neurofibromatosis type 1 and type 2 [41].

Cytomorphology of these entities has considerable overlap, showing a hypocellular smear exhibiting bundles of fibrous tissue composed of large fragments of cohesive cells with indistinct cytoplasmic borders, giving a syncytial appearance. These cells are elongated with hook-shaped extremities (comma-shaped cells), and most nuclei appear small, bland, and monotonous with pointed ends [57]. An inconstant amount of fibril-

lar, occasionally collagenous, and/or myxoid matrix is often associated with tumor cells, and focal nuclear pleomorphism can be occasionally seen. Fragments of necrotic tissue and prominent nucleoli must raise the suspicion of a malignant nerve sheath tumor [32].

Schwannomas (Fig. 16.6) aspirates can demonstrate more characteristically hypercellular regions with elongated cells and palisading nuclei that are tightly packed together—Antoni A pattern. Antoni B pattern is characterized by regions of loosely organized tissue with myxomatous found adjacent to Antoni A regions, with immunoexpression for S100, CD68, and SOX10, and negativity for cytokeratin [11, 56].

It is not uncommon for cystic areas to develop within schwannomas and neurofibromas, either due to mucinous degeneration, hemorrhage, or necrosis [41].

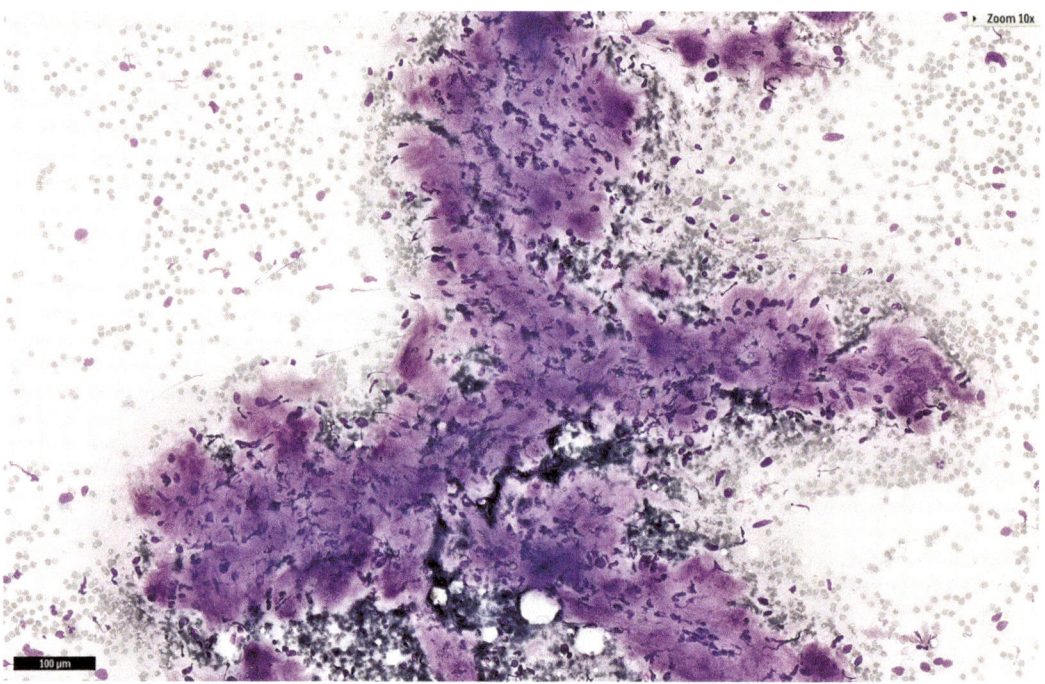

Fig. 16.6 Schwannoma. Aspirates showing hypercellular regions with elongated cells on a myxomatous background (MGG)

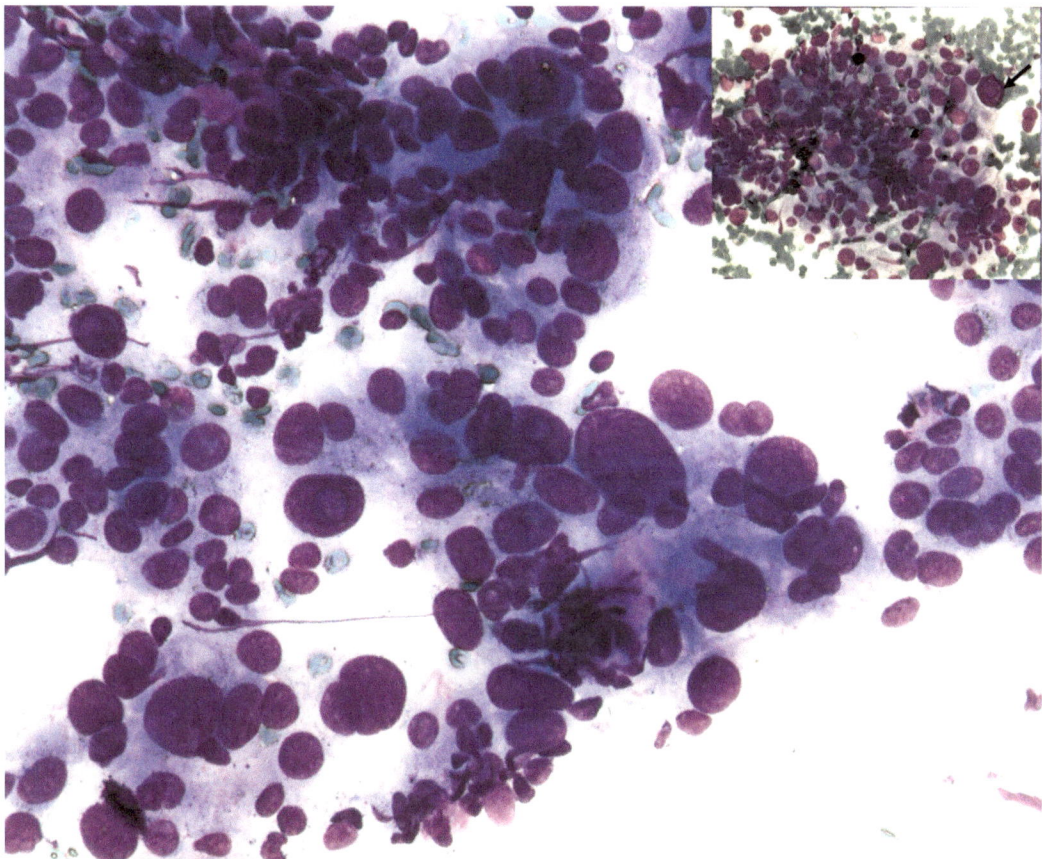

Fig. 16.7 Carotid body tumor. Moderate cellularity of a round to oval cell irregular group with rare acinar formation, vacuolated cytoplasm, pleomorphic nuclei, and intranuclear inclusion (arrow-inset) (MGG)

16.3.2.4 Carotid Body Tumor

A carotid body tumor (Fig. 16.7) is a paragangli-oma that develops from the chief cells of the carotid body, which are located at the bifurcation of the common carotid artery. FNA is rarely performed due to the risk of hemorrhage [22].

The analysis of cytological features reveals blood-rich aspirate with poor to moderate cellularity, loosely arranged irregular groups and acinar formation by round to oval cells, delicate, ill-defined, vacuolated cytoplasm, cytoplasmic granulations, pleomorphic nuclei with distinct nucleoli, sporadic binucleation, rare intranuclear, and cytoplasmic inclusions [15, 39]. In some cases, giant bare nuclei, spindle-shaped tumor cells, and moderate anisokaryosis can be observed [9].

16.3.2.5 *Lymph Nodes* (Also Solid-Cystic Presentation)

The enlarged lymph nodes may present as a solid or solid-cystic mass. Lymphadenopathy can be the clinical presentation of a group of benign and malignant conditions [34]. The most common cytological diagnoses from cervical lymph nodes are reactive lymphadenopathy, infectious diseases, metastatic carcinoma, and lymphoma. FNAC of cervical lymph nodes has an accuracy of 85%, sensitivity of 88–94.2%, and specificity of 96.9% [41].

Persistent unilateral adenopathy can include acquired etiologies such as *Mycobacterium tuberculosis*, the atypical mycobacterium spectrums such as *Mycobacterium avium intracellulare*, *Mycobacterium scrofulaceum*, granulomatous processes, or cat scratch disease [55]. Persistence of lymph node enlargement beyond a few weeks, and/or after an empiric course of antibiotics, often prompts clinical suspicion regarding the possibility of a malignancy [3]. Furthermore, age, gender, and site of lymphadenopathy also provide useful information in predicting the cause of lymphadenopathy, as reactive lymphadenitis is more common in the younger age group, tuberculosis lymphadenitis in middle age, and metastatic carcinoma in the older age group.

16.3.2.6 Reactive Lymphadenopathy

The size and activity of lymph nodes increase in response to various stimuli. Patients under the age of 2 years are most likely to have reactive lymphadenopathy, which may occasionally progress to a cervical abscess due to bacterial infection. Patients aged between 2 and 6 years also may present with reactive lymphadenopathy, but this is less common than in the first 2 years of life [3]. Morphologically, this response is characterized by hyperplasia of the lymphoid follicles with the activation of germinal centers.

Cytological analysis of the reactive lymph node (Fig. 16.8a) reveals mixed lymphoid population with variable maturation, increased numbers of larger lymphocytes, lymphohistiocytic aggregate from germinal center intermixed, lymphoplasmacytoid cells, plasma cells, with vari-

able number of immunoblasts, centroblasts, occasional follicular dendritic cells, and tingible body macrophages may contain apoptotic debris.

Certain findings may indicate suspicion for more specific disorders. Large and some atypical immunoblasts present may indicate infectious mononucleosis or viral and post-vaccinal lymphadenitis (Fig. 16.8b). Recent studies have shown this presentation in a series of COVID-19 post-vaccination lymphadenomegaly [17, 21, 52]. In autoimmune diseases, like lupus erythematosus or rheumatoid arthritis, there may be a correlation between the presence of numerous plasma cells and Russell bodies. Interdigitating dendritic cells with pale, unclear cytoplasm, and macrophages with dark melanin pigment are suggestive of dermatopathic lymphadenopathy, especially if the patient has a history of a persistent skin condition. Suspected HIV infection can be pointed out in the presence of exuberant follicular hyperplasia with many immunoblasts.

Sinus histiocytosis or Rosai-Dorfman disease is a rare illness that, particularly in black children and adolescents, results in massive cervical lymph node growth. The cytology is distinguished by the presence of numerous lymphocytes and large pale histiocytes with an abundance of vacuolated cytoplasm, vesicular nuclei, and small nucleoli. Emperipolesis is frequently observed (lymphocytes and other inflammatory

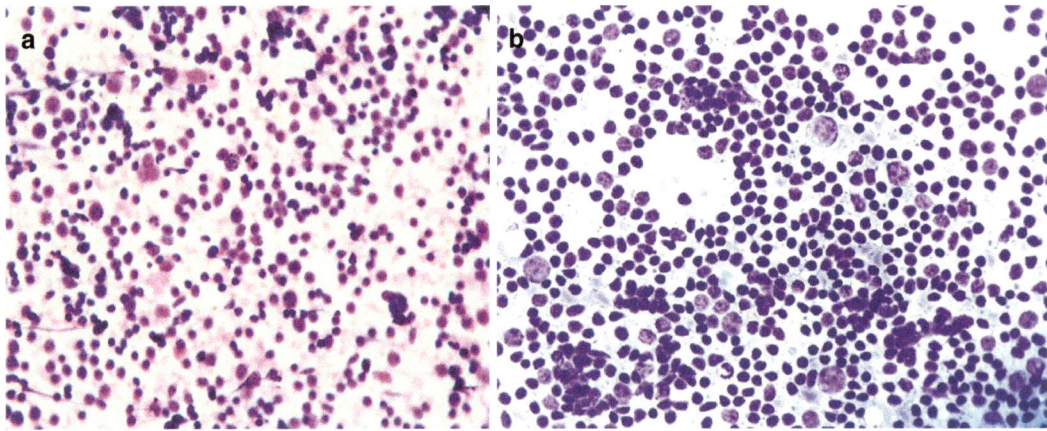

Fig. 16.8 Reactive lymphadenopathy. Twenty-year-old man; right-sided cervical adenopathy. (**a**) Reactive lymph node showing mixed lymphoid population with variable maturation, increased numbers of larger lymphocytes. (**b**)

Infectious mononucleosis. Twenty-seven-year-old man; fever and cervical lymphadenomegaly. Reactive lymphoid hyperplasia is characterized by lymphoid cells with large and some atypical immunoblasts (MGG)

cells reside undisturbed in their cytoplasm) and S100 is positive.

FNAC should be used in conjunction with immunological characterization in lymphadenopathy patients. This diagnostic strategy will significantly affect the accuracy of the diagnosis and, as a result, the clinical care of the patients.

16.3.2.7 Infectious Lymphadenitis

Usually, the nodes are not greater than 2 cm in diameter by the time of infectious presentation. Viral etiologies (adenovirus, rhinovirus, and parainfluenza) are responsible for the majority of cases of cervical lymphadenitis, and may be seen

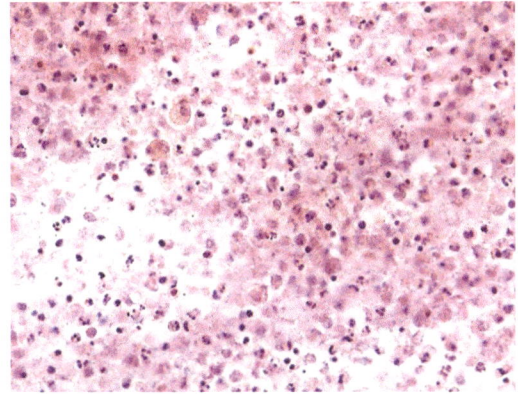

Fig. 16.9 Suppurative lymphadenitis. High concentration of degenerative neutrophils and sparse mature lymphocytes in a background rich in cell debris (H&E)

with concomitant upper respiratory tract infections. Viral lymphadenopathy is usually bilateral, with multiple small nodes involved. Bacterial causes include tonsillitis, pharyngitis, and sinusitis, and usually affect one particular node or several adjacent nodes [34]. A major cause of a lateral neck lump is mycobacterial lymphadenitis. Bartonellosis (caused by *Bartonella henselae*), Tularemia (*Francisella tularensis*), and fungal infection (such histoplasmosis, cryptococcosis, actinomycosis, and paracoccidioidomycosis) are examples of uncommon infectious agents [41]. For accurately identifying the infectious agent, polymerase chain reaction (PCR) or microbiological culture is a frequently very helpful technique.

The presence of a proteinaceous background with cell debris, mature lymphocytes, and sparse granulocytes is seen in the early stages of acute suppurative lymphadenitis (Fig. 16.9). Later, the aspirate becomes purulent, with a high concentration of degenerative neutrophils in a background rich in cell debris.

In granulomatous lymphadenitis, the primary cause in Europe is sarcoidosis, while tuberculosis is the main cause in underdeveloped and developing countries (endemic areas—up to 40% of cervical masses). Aspirates from granulomatous lymphadenitis (Fig. 16.10) have clusters of epithelioid cells with imprecise outline cytoplasm

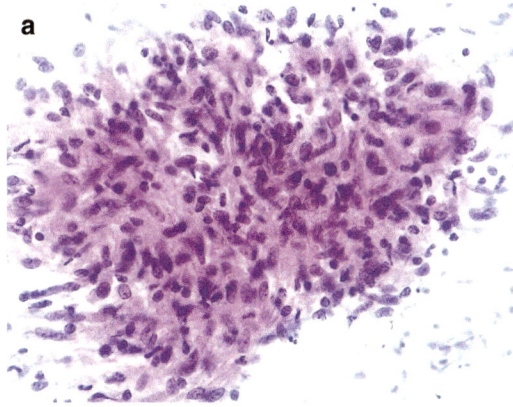

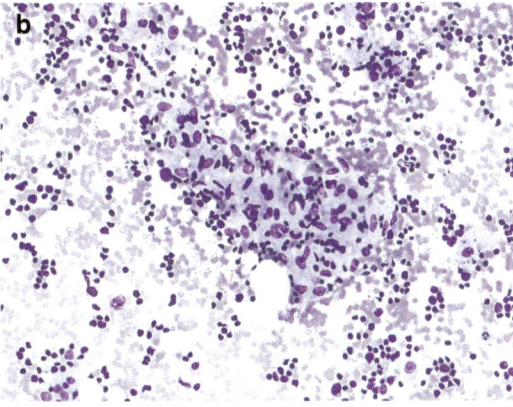

Fig. 16.10 Granulomatous lymphadenitis. Clusters of epithelioid cells with imprecise outline cytoplasm, elongated nuclei in a syncytial pattern. (**a**) Necrotizing chronic granulomatous lymphadenitis: *M. tuberculosis*. Fifty-

seven-year-old woman; multiple cervical nodules (H&E). (**b**) Chronic granulomatous lymphadenitis. Sarcoidosis. Thirty-five-year-old woman; fever, cough, and cervical adenopathy (MGG)

and elongated nuclei that are organized in a syncytial pattern. There may be one or more multinucleated Langhans large cells with the nuclei polarized at the cell border.

The diagnosis can be aided by the presence or absence of background necrosis, characterized by a pale stained amorphous material. Necrosis is a common occurrence in tuberculosis, but absent in sarcoidosis. It is important to note that tuberculosis smears can occasionally be predominantly suppurative.

In patients with immune deficiencies, including AIDS, atypical mycobacterial infection can lead to swelling of the head and neck lymph nodes. The smears are distinguished by a large number of histiocytes with pale cytoplasm.

Mycobacteria appear as cylindrical "negative images" at the cytoplasm of the cells in Giemsa-stained preparations and are positive for Ziehl-Neelsen. The Ziehl-Neelsen stain can be used to identify acid-fast bacilli for a conclusive diagnosis in cell blocks. Currently, PCR methods are used in place of this stain to identify *Mycobacterium tuberculosis*.

16.3.2.8 Metastasis in Cervical Lymph Nodes

FNAC is an important tool for metastatic workup. A mass that has been present for more than two weeks; reduced mobility; size greater than 1.5 cm; firm consistency; and overlying skin ulceration constitute red flag symptoms for head and neck cancer. Depending on parameters including age, sex, clinical history, place of metastatic node, and cytological features, this examination will concentrate on different organs. The most frequent metastatic sites for lymph nodes in the neck are the oral cavity, pharynx, larynx, salivary glands, thyroid, lung, and breast.

Metastatic lymph node involvement is often diffuse, resulting in a cell-rich and therefore diagnostic aspirate. Immunocytochemistry analysis of the aspirated cells can aid in the search for a primary tumor. Cytokeratin profile can frequently be useful in focusing on potential areas of the primary tumor in metastases from epithelial malignancies. CK7-/CK20+ suggests the gastrointestinal tract, while CK7+/CK20- suggests

lung, thyroid, or breast as major sites in head and neck metastases. It is frequently possible to get accurate information about the primary location by using an extra panel of antibodies, however in some cases the primary site may remain unknown (discussed in Chap. 19).

16.3.2.9 Squamous Cell Carcinomas

Squamous cell carcinoma (SCC) is the most common metastasis, nonthyroid, to cervical lymph nodes [30]. All aspirates of lateral neck cysts need to be diligently searched for these atypical elements indicative of metastatic squamous cell carcinoma. A typical debut of head and neck SCC could be in the form of a cystic metastasis on the lateral neck [20].

Malignant tumors of the neck are rare in patients younger than 40 years of age; however, among young nonsmokers, an increasing incidence of human papillomavirus (HPV)-related head and neck squamous cell carcinomas (HNSCC) arising from the lymphatic tissue of the Waldeyers ring has been reported. More specifically, cystic neck metastases are usually considered the hallmark of HPV-related SCC of the oropharynx [19]. It is important to consider the possibility of an HPV-related tumor, mainly in patients with cancer of unknown primary.

The cytomorphology of SCC (Fig. 16.11) includes keratinized epithelial cells with atypia,

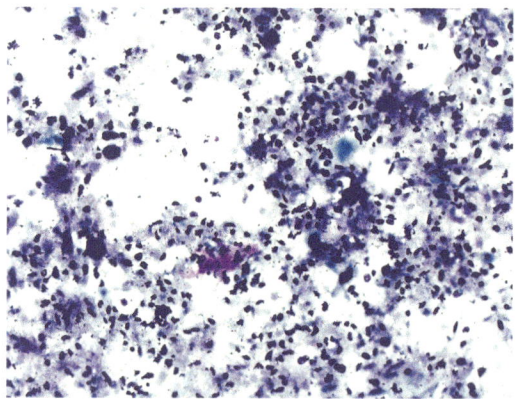

Fig. 16.11 Metastatic squamous cell carcinoma. Sixty-one-year-old female; swelling in the left cervical region. Smears reveal large epithelial cells, isolated and in three-dimensional clusters permeated by necrotic materials. These cells have preserved cytoplasm, signs of squamous differentiation, and irregular nuclei (Pap)

small cell cluster, increased cellular nuclear/cytoplasmic ratio, irregular nuclear membranes, and nuclei hyperchromatic. Even when inflamed, cystic squamous cell carcinomas have a higher number of atypical squamous elements and, in most cases, at least occasional squamous cells with hyperchromatic and irregular nuclei are present [30].

16.3.2.10 HPV-Associated HNSCC: Basaloid Pattern

Basaloid squamous cell carcinoma is an aggressive variant of squamous cell carcinoma with poorer survival rate that has a predilection for the upper aerodigestive tract and frequently metastasizes to cervical lymph nodes [43, 61]. FNA features characteristic of basaloid squamous cell carcinoma include a smear pattern with a predominance of tightly cohesive tumor cell clusters, small- to medium-sized nuclei, single small nucleoli, nuclear molding, and scant cytoplasm. Mitoses and single cell necrosis are common, indicating that the aspirate is from a high-grade tumor. Immunostaining of squamous differentiation markers may help diagnosis (CK5/6 and p63). Adenoid cystic-like features and the presence of single keratinized cells are more specific for basaloid squamous cell carcinoma [35].

16.3.2.11 Metastatic Adenocarcinoma

Papillary thyroid carcinoma (discussed in Chap. 17), gastrointestinal, lung, and breast carcinoma constitute the main primary sites with cervical lymph node metastasis. The aspirated fluid can be of low to moderate cellularity, composed of epithelial pattern cells with varied architecture, organized in acini or sheets or papillary structures; indistinct cytoplasmic borders; pale cytoplasm; eccentric, round/oval nuclei; and granular chromatin and large nucleoli. The main difficulty in diagnosing metastatic adenocarcinoma in cervical lymph nodes is determining the primary site. Additional characteristics may indicate, but an immunocytochemistry analysis is recommended.

On Giemsa staining, some cells in metastases from lobular breast carcinomas may have cytoplasmic lumina with pinkish purple inclusions and magenta bodies. FNA smears of metastatic colon carcinoma regularly exhibit fragments of palisading atypical cells on a necrotic background. Mucin production is common in gastrointestinal and lung cancers. Cells with pale gray vacuolated large cytoplasm and a nucleus with a central nucleolus suggest renal cell carcinoma.

The immunocytochemical panel includes the evaluation of cytokeratins, CK 7 and CK20, TTF-1 (favor lung cancer or thyroid); TRPS1, GATA-3, ER, and PR (favor breast cancer); and CDX-2, SATB2, and vilin (favor the gastrointestinal tract).

16.3.2.12 Metastatic Small Cell Carcinoma

Small cell lung cancer metastases are characterized by dense clusters of tumor cells with molding, sparse cytoplasm, coarse chromatin, numerous mitoses, and a background of necrosis. Although they may look like lymphoma cells, the presence of molding in cohesive tumor cell clumps and cytokeratin positive is a significant evidence against a lymphoma diagnosis. Small cell carcinoma cytokeratin-stained smears frequently exhibit paranuclear spots. Additionally, the immunoexpression of CD56, chromogranin, and synaptophysin is found.

16.3.2.13 Metastatic Melanoma

The smearing pattern from metastatic melanoma usually shows poorly cohesive cells. In direct smears that contain large tissue fragments, the architecture of the lesions can vary widely. Most fragments comprise three-dimensional syncytial clusters of tumor cells without distinct cell borders. A clearly malignant pattern with pleomorphic, spindled, and epithelioid cell shapes may be present. Despite being a high-grade malignancy, apoptosis, and necrosis in melanoma are not a frequent features in FNAs, occurring in less than 20% of cases [47].

Melanin, present as fine pigment granules staining darkly on Giemsa staining, is only present in 50% of cases [33]. Polygonal cells are often dominant; they have a moderate to abundant amount of granular or clear cytoplasm and relatively distinct cytoplasmic borders. Melanoma cells can show microvacuoles in the cytoplasm, better seen in Romanowsky-stained smears. Classic nuclear cytological characteristics of melanoma cells include the presence of multinucle-ation, eccentric nuclei, and prominent nucleoli. Intranuclear inclusions and binucleated cells with each nucleus apart from the other are accessory features for the cytological interpretation.

Numerous morphologic patterns of melanoma are potentially seen to resemble carcinoma, sarcoma, or even lymphoma. Even if the patient has a history of melanoma, cytomorphology alone

can be inconclusive. Vimentin, S-100, SOX-10, Melan A, and HMB-45 positivity will definitively identify a metastatic melanoma. However, HMB-45 positivity is absent in approximately 20% of melanomas.

Table 16.1 provides a summary of the main clinical features, cytomorphology, and differential diagnoses for lateral cystic and solid lesions.

Table 16.1 Lesions with cystic and solid presentations in the lateral neck: clinical features, cytological findings, and differential diagnosis

Lateral neck lesions	Clinical features	FNA cytology	Differential diagnosis
Epidermoid cyst	Young to middle-age Solitary Small nodule with visible punctum	High cellularity Nucleate and anucleate squames Keratinous material Clear background	Dermoid cyst Branchial cyst Thyroglossal cyst Squamous cell carcinoma
Dermoid cyt	Children 5 years old or younger 2nd and 3rd decades of life Solitary	Moderate-high cellularity Keratinaceous cellular material Anucleated and nucleated squamous cells Degenerated inflammatory cells	Epidermoid cyst Teratoid cyst Teratoma
Branchial cyst	20 and 40 years 2nd and 3rd decades of life: symptomatic Solitary	Straw-colored or pus-like fluid Amorphous debris Squamous, columnar, ciliated, and/ or mucinous cells Inflammatory features Cholesterol crystals Clean background	Epidermoid cyst Dermoid cyst Teratoma Bronchogenic cyst Lymphadenitis Lymphoma
Thymic cyst	Childhood, generally 2–13 years More common in males Solitary Well-demarcated margins on ultrasound Asymptomatic or cervical swelling when spontaneous hemorrhage	Straw colored fluid Abundant mature lymphocytes Scattered epithelial cells (squamous or ciliated, cuboid, and columnar) Round to oval nuclei Foamy macrophages Proteinaceous debris Hemorrhagic background	Lymphangioma Thymoma Thymic carcinoma Thyroid tumors Lymphoma(rarely)
Cystic hygroma	Childhood, before 2 years Associated with chromosomal defects Solitary	Clear fluid Red blood cells Lymphocytes and histiocytes Proteinaceous debris	Thymic cyst Hemangioma
Lipoma	Isolated masses Isoechoic presentation on ultrasound	Hypocellularity Mature adipocytes Wide empty cytoplasm Small eccentric dark nuclei	Pleomorphic lipoma Atypical lipomatous tumor Liposarcoma
Lipoblastoma	Infancy More common in males	Moderate–poor cellularity Lypocytes, lipoblasts, spindle cells Naked oval nuclei Branching vessels Myxoid background	Lipoma Lipofibromatosis Atypical lipomatous tumor Liposarcoma

Table 16.1 (continued)

Lateral neck lesions	Clinical features	FNA cytology	Differential diagnosis
Pleomorphic lipoma	Middle aged to elderly More common in males Solitary	Hypocellularity Floret cells Mature adipocytic cells Myxoid background with mast cells	Lipoma Atypical lipomatous tumor Liposarcoma
Teratoma	Rare Solitary	Respiratory-type ciliated, columnar cells, goblet cells with vacuolated cytoplasm, and hyaline cartilage	Bronchogenic cyst Epidermoid cyst Dermoid cyst Teratoid cyst Squamous cell carcinoma
Neurogenic tumors	Associated with neurofibromatosis type 1 and type 2 Solitary	Hypocellularity Bundles of fibrous tissue Cohesive cells, indistinct cytoplasmic borders, and syncytial appearance Elongated cells (comma-shaped cells) Nuclei small, bland with pointed ends Focal nuclear pleomorphism Fibrillar, collagenous, and/or myxoid matrix	Neuroma Leiomyoma Malignant peripheral nerve sheath tumor Melanoma
Carotid body tumor	Complication of hemorrhage Solitary	Poor–moderate cellularity Acinar formation Delicate and vacuolated cytoplasm Cytoplasmic granulations Pleomorphic nuclei with distinct nucleoli Intranuclear and cytoplasmic inclusions Hemorrhagic background	Branchial cyst Neurogenic tumors Hemangioma Lymphadenopathy Malignant diseases
Reactive Lymphadenopathy	More common: <2 year Solitary or multiples History of post-vaccination or autoimmune disease	Lymphoid population with variable maturation, increased numbers of larger lymphocytes Lymphohistiocytic aggregate, lymphoplasmacytoid cells Follicular dendritic cells Tingible body macrophages Apoptotic debris	Atypical lymphoid hyperplasia Lymphoma
Suppurative Lymphadenitis	Nodes <2 cm diameter Solitary or multiples Concomitant upper respiratory tract infections Viral: bilateral and multiples	Cell debris Mature lymphocytes Degenerative neutrophils Proteinaceous background	Cat scratch disease Tuberculosis
Granulomatous lymphadenitis	Middle age Persistent and unilateral	Clusters of epithelioid cells with imprecise outline cytoplasm and elongated nuclei Multinucleated Langhans cells Necrosis: Tuberculosis No necrosis: Sarcoidosis	Bartonellosis Tularemia Fungal infection Malignant diseases
Lymph node metastasis	Older age Persistent lymph node enlargement	Diagnoses based on cytomorphology and immunophenotype	Squamous cell carcinoma Adenocarcinomas Small cell carcinoma Melanoma

Acknowledgments The authors would like to thank Drs. Carlos Alberto Ribeiro, Sueli Maeda, and Jerzy Klijanienko, who provided some of the figures illustrated in this chapter.

References

1. Al-Khateeb TH, Al-Masri NM, Al-Zoubi F. Cutaneous cysts of the head and neck. J Oral Maxillofacial Surg. 2009;67(1):52–7.
2. Alqahtani A, Nguyen LT, Flageole H, Shaw K, Laberge JM. 25 years' experience with lymphangiomas in children. J Pediatr Surg. 1999;34(7):1164–8.
3. Anne S, Teot LA, Mandell DL. Fine needle aspiration biopsy: role in diagnosis of pediatric head and neck masses. Int J Pediatr Otorhinolaryngol. 2008;72(10):1547–53.
4. Arabi H, Yousef N, Bandyopadhyay S, Feng J, Yoo GH, Al-Abbadi MA. Fine needle aspiration of head and neck masses in the operating room: accuracy and potential benefits. Diagn Cytopathol. 2008;36(6):369–74.
5. Babuccu O, Işiksaçan Ozen O, Hoşnuter M, Kargi E, Babuccu B. The place of fine-needle aspiration in the preoperative diagnosis of the congenital sublingual teratoid cyst. Diagn Cytopathol. 2003;29(1):33–7.
6. Bala N, Gupta N, Sachdeva M, Singh Y, Kumar M. A diagnostic dilemma in fine-needle aspiration cytology: spindle cell/pleomorphic lipoma. Cureus. 2022;14(1):e20919.
7. Cardesa A, Slootweg PJ, Gale N, Franchi A, editors. Pathology of the head and neck [Internet]. Berlin/Heidelberg: Springer; 2016. Available from: http://link.springer.com/10.1007/978-3-662-49672-5
8. Damaskos C, Garmpis N, Manousi M, Garmpi A, Margonis GA, Spartalis E, et al. Cystic hygroma of the neck: single center experience and literature review. Eur Rev Med Pharmacol Sci. 2017;21(21):4918–23.
9. Das DK, Gupta AK, Chowdhury V, Satsangi DK, Tyagi S, Mohan JC, et al. Fine-needle aspiration diagnosis of carotid body tumor: report of a case and review of experience with cytologic features in four cases. Diagn Cytopathol. 1997;17(2):143–7.
10. Debaize S, Gebhart M, Fourrez T, Rahier I, Baillon JM. Squamous cell carcinoma arising in a giant epidermal cyst: a case report. Acta Chir Belg. 2002;102(3):196–8.
11. Domanski HA, Akerman M, Engellau J, Gustafson P, Mertens F, Rydholm A. Fine-needle aspiration of neurilemoma (schwannoma). A clinicocytopathologic study of 116 patients. Diagn Cytopathol. 2006;34(6):403–12.
12. Fanous A, Morcrette G, Fabre M, Couloigner V, Galmiche-Rolland L. Diagnostic approach to congenital cystic masses of the neck from a clinical and pathological perspective. Dermatopathology (Basel). 2021;8(3):342–58.
13. Ferreira J, Esteves G, Fonseca R, Martins C, André S, Lemos MM. Fine-needle aspiration of lipoblastoma: cytological, molecular, and clinical features. Cancer Cytopathol. 2017;125(12):934–9.
14. Firat P, Ersoz C, Uguz A, Onder S. Cystic lesions of the head and neck: cytohistological correlation in 63 cases. Cytopathology. 2007;18(3):184–90.
15. Fleming MV, Oertel YC, Ren Rodríguez EÉ, Fidler WJ. Fine-needle aspiration of six carotid body paragangliomas. Diag Cytopathol. 1993;9(5):510–5.
16. Franzen A, Günzel T, Buchali A, Coordes A. Cystic lateral neck lesions: etiologic and differential diagnostic significance in a series of 133 patients. Anticancer Res. 2019;39(9):5047–52.
17. García-Molina F, Cegarra-Navarro MF, Andrade-Gonzales RJ, Martinez-Díaz F. Cytologic and histologic features of COVID-19 post-vaccination lymphadenopathy. Cyto J. 2021;18:34.
18. Glosser JW, Pires CAS, Feinberg SE. Branchial cleft or cervical lymphoepithelial cysts: Etiology and management. J Am Dental Assoc. 2003;134(1):81–6.
19. Goldenberg D, Begum S, Westra WH, Khan Z, Sciubba J, Pai SI, et al. Cystic lymph node metastasis in patients with head and neck cancer: an HPV-associated phenomenon. Head Neck. 2008;30(7):898–903.
20. Grønlund S, Mey K, Andersen E, Rasmussen ER. The true malignancy rate in 135 patients with preoperative diagnosis of a lateral neck cyst. Laryngoscope Investig Otolaryngol. 2016;1(4):78–82.
21. Hagen C, Nowack M, Messerli M, Saro F, Mangold F, Bode PK. Fine needle aspiration in COVID-19 vaccine-associated lymphadenopathy. Swiss Med Wkly. 2021;151:w20557.
22. Handa U, Bal A, Mohan H, Dass A. Parapharyngeal paraganglioma: diagnosis on fine-needle aspiration. Am J Otolaryngol. 2005;26(5):360–1.
23. Handa U, Chhabra S, Mohan H. Epidermal inclusion cyst: cytomorphological features and differential diagnosis. Diagn Cytopathol. 2008;36(12):861–3.
24. Hoang VT, Trinh CT, Nguyen CH, Chansomphou V, Chansomphou V, Tran TTT. Overview of epidermoid cyst. Eur J Radiol Open. 2019;6:291–301.
25. Hsieh YY, Hsueh S, Hsueh C, Lin JN, Luo CC, Lai JY, et al. Pathological analysis of congenital cervical cysts in children: 20 years of experience at Chang Gung Memorial Hospital. Chang Gung Med J. 2003;26(2):107–13.
26. Kanber Y, Pusztaszeri M, Auger M. Immunocytochemistry for diagnostic cytopathology-A practical guide. Cytopathology. 2021;32(5):562–87.
27. King SK. Lateral neck lumps: a systematic approach for the general paediatrician. J Paediatr Child Health. 2017;53(11):1091–5.
28. Kloboves-Prevodnik VV, Us-Krasovec M, Gale N, Lamovec J. Cytological features of lipoblastoma: a report of three cases. Diagn Cytopathol. 2005;33(3):195–200.
29. Kraus J, Plzák J, Bruschini R, Renne G, Andrle J, Ansarin M, et al. Cystic lymphangioma of the neck in

adults: a report of three cases. Wien Klin Wochenschr. 2008;120(7–8):242–5.

30. Layfield LJ. Fine-needle aspiration in the diagnosis of head and neck lesions: a review and discussion of problems in differential diagnosis. Diagn Cytopathol. 2007;35(12):798–805.

31. Layfield LJ, Esebua M, Schmidt RL. Cytologic separation of branchial cleft cyst from metastatic cystic squamous cell carcinoma: a multivariate analysis of nineteen cytomorphologic features. Diagn Cytopathol. 2016;44(7):561–7.

32. Lee J, Kazmi S, VandenBussche CJ, Ali SZ. Mesenchymal neoplasms of the head and neck: a cytopathologic analysis on fine needle aspiration. J Am Soc Cytopathol. 2017;6(3):105–13.

33. Lindsey KG, Ingram C, Bergeron J, Yang J. Cytological diagnosis of metastatic malignant melanoma by fine-needle aspiration biopsy. Semin Diagn Pathol. 2016;33(4):198–203.

34. Liu ES, Bernstein JM, Sculerati N, Wu HC. Fine needle aspiration biopsy of pediatric head and neck masses. Int J Pediatr Otorhinolaryngol. 2001;60(2):135–40.

35. Marks RA, Cramer HM, Wu HH. Fine-needle aspiration cytology of basaloid squamous cell carcinoma and small cell carcinoma-a comparison study. Diagn Cytopathol. 2013;41(1):81–4.

36. Michalopoulos N, Papavramidis TS, Karayannopoulou G, Cheva A, Pliakos I, Triantafilopoulou K, et al. Cervical thymic cysts in adults. Thyroid. 2011;21(9):987–92.

37. Mirilas P. Lateral congenital anomalies of the pharyngeal apparatus: Part I. Normal developmental anatomy (embryogenesis) for the surgeon. Am Surg. 2011;77(9):1230–42.

38. Mohakud S, Sethy M, Naik S, Mohapatra PR. Giant cervicomediastinal thymic cyst in an elderly: diagnosis by multimodality imaging and fine-needle aspiration cytology with immunocytochemistry. BMJ Case Rep. 2020;13(7):e235425.

39. Naniwadekar MR, Jagtap SV, Kshirsagar AY, Shinagare SA, Tata HR, Sahoo K. Fine needle aspiration diagnosis of carotid body tumor in a case of multiple paragangliomas presenting with facial palsy: a case report. Acta Cytol. 2010;54(4):635–9.

40. Nicollas R, Guelfucci B, Roman S, Triglia JM. Congenital cysts and fistulas of the neck. Int J Pediatr Otorhinolaryngol. 2000;55(2):117–24.

41. Pelt GV, Tollenaar R, Mesker W. Filling the gap between microscopic and automated analysis of the tumor-stroma ratio. Ann Colorectal Res. 2020;8(1):29–32.

42. Pynnonen MA, Gillespie MB, Roman B, Rosenfeld RM, Tunkel DE, Bontempo L, et al. Clinical practice guideline: evaluation of the neck mass in adults. Otolaryngol Head Neck Surg. 2017;157(2_suppl):S1–30.

43. Rahimi S. HPV-related squamous cell carcinoma of oropharynx: a review. J Clin Pathol. 2020;73(10):624–9.

44. Ranabhat S, Tiwari M, Maharjan S. Teratoid cyst of the postauricular region: the first ever case report. Case Rep Pathol. 2017;2017:9235925.

45. Reynolds JP, Liu S. Fine needle aspiration of mediastinal germ cell tumors. Sem Diag Pathol. 2020;37(4):174–8.

46. Sakhadeo U, Mundhe R, DeSouza MA, Chinoy RF. Pleomorphic lipoma: a gentle giant of pathology. J Cytol. 2015;32(3):201–3.

47. Saqi A, McGrath CM, Skovronsky D, Yu GH. Cytomorphologic features of fine-needle aspiration of metastatic and recurrent melanoma. Diag Cytopathol. 2002;27(5):286–90.

48. Schmitt FC, editor. Molecular applications in cytology. Springer International Publishing; 2018.

49. Schwetschenau E, Kelley DJ. The adult neck mass. Am Fam Physician. 2002;66(5):831–8.

50. Sinnatamby CS. Last's anatomy, International Edition: Regional and applied. Elsevier Health Sciences; 2011.

51. Sira J, Makura ZGG. Differential diagnosis of cystic neck lesions. Ann Otol Rhinol Laryngol. 2011;120(6):409–13.

52. Tan NJH, Tay KXJ, Wong SBJ, Nga ME. COVID-19 post-vaccination lymphadenopathy: report of cytological findings from fine needle aspiration biopsy. Diagn Cytopathol. 2021;49(12):E467–70.

53. Tandon S, Shahab R, Benton JI, Ghosh SK, Sheard J, Jones TM. Fine-needle aspiration cytology in a regional head and neck cancer center: comparison with a systematic review and meta-analysis. Head Neck. 2008;30(9):1246–52.

54. Thirumala S, Desai M, Kannan V. Diagnostic pitfalls in fine needle aspiration cytology of pleomorphic lipoma. A case report. Acta Cytol. 2000;44(4):653–6.

55. Tracy TF, Muratore CS. Management of common head and neck masses. Semin Pediatr Surg. 2007;16(1):3–13.

56. Vazquez Salas S, Pedro K, Balram A, Syed S, Kotaka K, Kadivar A, et al. Head and neck cystic lesions: a cytology review of common and uncommon entities. Acta Cytol. 2022;1–12

57. Wilbur DC, Bibbo M. Comprehensive Cytopathology. 4th ed. Philadelphia: Saunders; 2021.

58. Wu M, Burstein DE, Yuan S, Nurse LA, Szporn AH, Zhang D, et al. A comparative study of 200 fine needle aspiration biopsies performed by clinicians and cytopathologists. Laryngoscope. 2006;116(7):1212–5.

59. Xu H, Fan F, Gong Y, Jing X, Lin X, Wang H, et al. Diagnostic challenges in fine-needle aspiration cytology of mediastinal tumors and lesions. Arch Pathol Lab Med. 2021;146(8):960–74.

60. Yehuda M, Schechter ME, Abu-Ghanem N, Golan G, Horowitz G, Fliss DM, et al. The incidence of malignancy in clinically benign cystic lesions of the lateral neck: our experience and proposed diagnostic algorithm. Eur Arch Otorhinolaryngol. 2018;275(3):767–73.

61. Zbären P, Nuyens M, Stauffer E. Basaloid squamous cell carcinoma of the head and neck. Curr Opin Otolaryngol Head Neck Surg. 2004;12(2):116–21.

Fernando Schmitt, Professor of Pathology at the University of Porto, Director of RISE (Clinical and Translational Research Network of the Medical Faculty) and Head of Molecular Pathology Unit at IPATIMUP, President of the International Academy of Cytology (IAC). Co-editor 3rd Ed *The Bethesda System for Reporting Thyroid Cytology*. Standing member of the WHO-IAC Classification of Tumours

Ricella Souza da Silva, Assistant pathologist and preceptor at the Federal University of Paraíba, Brazil and Research Trainee in Molecular Pathology at IPATIMUP. Professor of Pathology at the Faculty of Medicine of the Federal University of Paraíba, and official forensic doctor in the State of Paraíba, Brazil.

Ivana Kholová and David Kalfert

17.1 General

17.1.1 The Median Neck Cyst (Thyroglossal Duct Cyst)

The median neck cyst (thyroglossal duct cyst; TGDC) is the most common congenital neck mass, with the population prevalence estimated at 7%. It is caused by incomplete obliteration of the thyroglossal duct. During embryonic development, TGDC originates from the thyroid gland and is typically involuted after migration of the primitive thyroid to its final position in the inferior neck [1]. Failure of involution results in persistence of a remnant of the thyroglossal duct [1].

The aberrant persistence of the thyroglossal duct leads to a median neck cyst, which occurs predominantly in children and is usually recognized by the age of five years. TGDC is rarely diagnosed in adult patients, with a mean age of 26 to 55 years, with the same distribution between sexes [2–4].

The most common presentation of TGDC is a mobile cervical mass of the upper midline (Fig. 17.1); less commonly it is localized in the left or right paramidline. The most common location of TGDC is infrahyoid area [4].

Although most TGDCs are asymptomatic (painless and non-tender) with a diameter of 0.5 to 6 cm, with most between 1.5 and 3 cm, they can occasionally be associated with dysphagia [1]. Growth is typically indolent, although associated infection can result in rapid cyst enlarge-

I. Kholová (✉)
Department of Pathology, Fimlab Laboratories,
Tampere, Finland

Faculty of Medicine and Health Technology, Tampere
University, Tampere, Finland
e-mail: ivana.kholova@tuni.fi

D. Kalfert
Department of Otorhinolaryngology and Head and
Neck Surgery, University Hospital Motol,
Prague, Czechia

First Faculty of Medicine, Charles University,
Prague, Czechia
e-mail: david.kalfert@fnmotol.cz

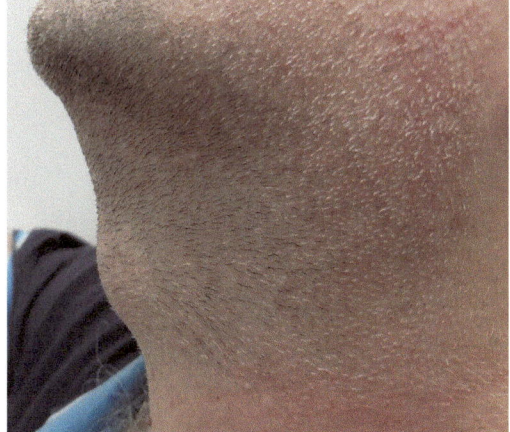

Fig. 17.1 Visible mass located in the middle of the neck

ment [3]. Complications include abscess and fistula/drainage sinus formation. Large cysts at the base of the tongue can cause dyspnea, dysphagia, or even sore throat symptoms.

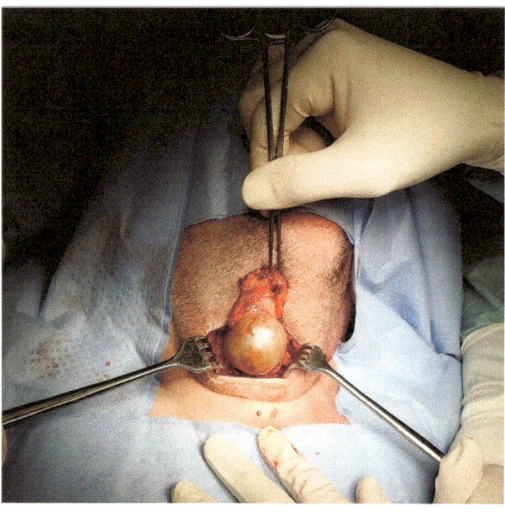

Fig. 17.2 Intraoperative finding. The median neck cyst removal

TGDCs are benign lesions; however, carcinomas of the thyroglossal duct occur in <1% of cases, with papillary thyroid carcinoma being the most common pathologic diagnosis [3, 4].

The recommended surgical approach to TGDC is a Sistrunk procedure with removal of the central portion of the hyoid bone, along with the cyst and the accompanying tract (Fig. 17.2), with a recurrence rate of 3–5% [5].

Ultrasonography (Fig. 17.3), computed tomography (CT), or magnetic resonance imaging (MRI) can be all applied to imagine TGDC. On ultrasound, it is an oval and well-circumscribed anechoic lesion with hyperechoic enhancement of the posterior wall. Such a typical finding is present only in about half of the cases. Hypoechoic obscuration in the part of the cyst is caused by repeated inflammations and hemorrhages. On CT, TGDCs are depicted as well-circumscribed lesions with mucoid attenuation, typically with thin walls. Similarly, in MRI, TGDCs demonstrate low signal intensity with T1-weighted sequences, high signal intensity

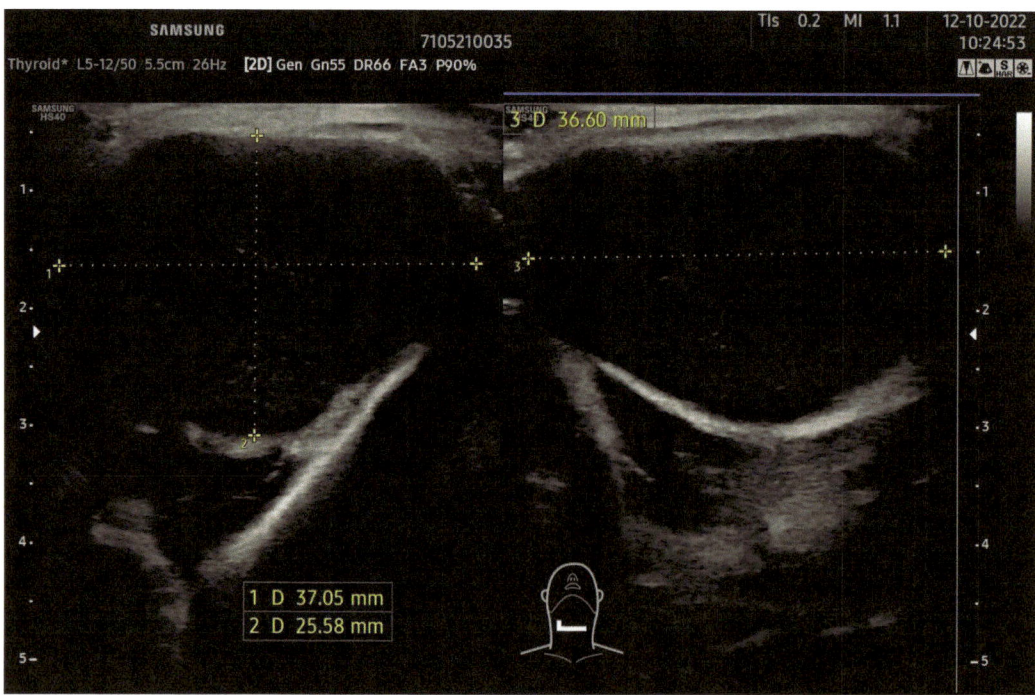

Fig. 17.3 Sonographic image. The thyroglossal cyst is located below the hyoid bone. The cyst is anechoic, with a hyperechoic enhancement of the posterior wall

with T2-weighted sequences, and do not restrict diffusion [6].

Microscopically, the lining epithelial component is predominantly ciliated columnar, i.e., respiratory epithelium, mature and immature squamous epithelium with parakeratotic squamous cells. Rarely, thyroid follicular cells are present. The thyroid tissue may be normal, hyperplastic, or neoplastic. Both wall and cyst content can feature inflammatory cells, namely lymphocytes, neutrophils, macrophages, and multinucleated giant cells. The cyst material may be watery, granular, proteinaceous, mucinous, or colloid. Cholesterol crystals can be detected in rare cases. Fine-needle aspiration material contains mainly macrophages with other inflammatory cells, predominantly respiratory epithelium, and variable background material [2].

17.1.2 Cervical Bronchogenic Cysts

Cervical bronchogenic cysts are extremely rare, resulting from an abnormal development of the foregut. They are usually located in the thyroid or paratracheal region, rarely in the suprasternal or supraclavicular location. The definitive diagnosis of bronchogenic cyst requires histopathological confirmation. Morphologically, the cysts are unilocular lined by the respiratory epithelium [7].

17.1.3 Dermoid Cyst

Dermoid cysts belong to midline cervical developmental anomalies that originate from the ectoderm and mesoderm. Dermoid cysts usually appear as superficial, painless subcutaneous masses in the anterior neck, but can also occur in other locations outside the head and neck area. Cyst enlargement may be due to the accumulation of sebaceous content over time. Cyst rupture can occur due to trauma or enlargement that results in granulomatous inflammation in the surrounding skin and soft tissues. The treatment of choice for all symptomatic dermoid cysts is surgical excision with complete resection. Dermoid cysts located near the hyoid bone may not differentiate from TGDC intraoperatively, but histologically [8, 9].

In imaging, the sonographic findings tend to be diverse. Most often a well-defined anechoic lesion is found with enhancement of the dorsal signal; however, the frequent presence of fragments of fat, bone, or teeth causes a heterogeneous, granular character of the lesion. On CT, the rim of the cyst may show contrast enhancement. On non-contrast CT, the dermoid cyst usually appears as a low-density, unilocular, well-circumscribed mass. Fat, mixed-density fluid, and calcification may also be seen. There may be a coalescence of fat in small nodules within the cystic lesion, giving a "sac of marbles" appearance. Epidermoid cysts usually show fluid-density material [7].

Microscopically, dermoid cysts are lined with the stratified squamous epithelium and contain cutaneous adnexal structures, such as hairs, hair follicles, sebaceous, eccrine, and apocrine glands within the fibroconnective wall.

17.1.4 Thymic Cyst

Thymic cysts rarely occur in the neck area. The thymus develops from the third branchial arch in the sixth week of fetal life and subsequently descends into the mediastinum. Thymic cysts arise as a result of the implementation of thymic tissue during descent. They affect women more frequently than men in the first decade of life. Only a few cases were reported in adults [10]. Thymic cyst is a slow growing mainly asymptomatic neck mass. Due to secondary infection, the thymic cyst may be painful. Thymic cysts can rarely manifest as faster growth accompanied by dysphagia, odonyphagia, dyspnea, hoarseness, and sore throat [2]. It is typically located between the thyroid lobe and the common carotid artery, commonly on the left side. The choice of treatment is surgical complete excision [11].

Radiologically, cystic lesions are associated with large vessels (carotid sheath) (Figs. 17.4 and 17.5).

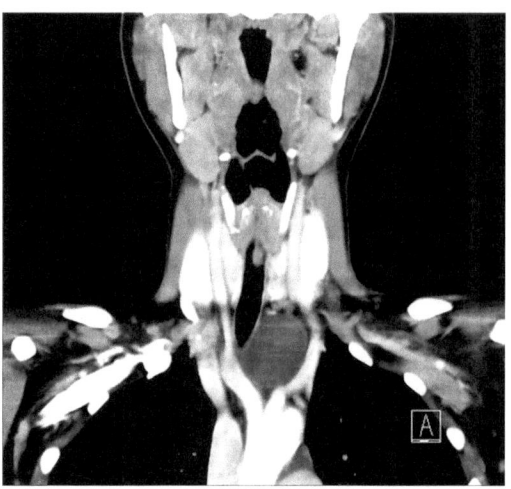

Fig. 17.4 Contrast CT of the neck and upper mediastinum, coronal projection. Cystic mass (thymus cyst) is localized in the anterior mediastinum

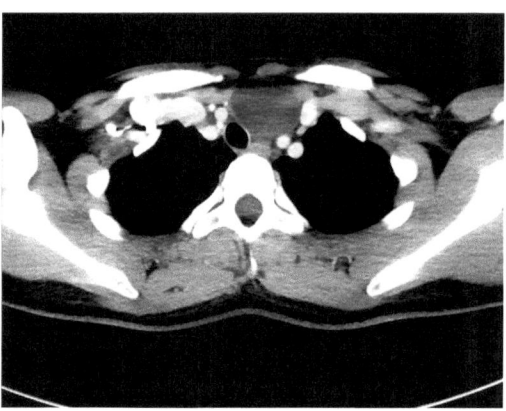

Fig. 17.5 Contrast CT of the neck and upper mediastinum, axial projection. Cystic mass (thymus cyst) is localized in the anterior mediastinum

Thymic cysts are unilocular or multilocular and contain brownish fluid. Microscopically, the lining of the cyst wall ranges from flattened cuboidal epithelium to columnar and multilayered stratified squamous epithelium. Thymic lobulated lympho-epithelial tissue in the cyst wall contains Hassall's corpuscles [10]. By definition, thymic tissue is pathognomic for thymic cysts. In addition, foreign body giant cell reaction with or without cholesterol crystals is observed in some cases. Thyroid tissue may be rarely found.

17.1.5 Parathyroid Cyst

Parathyroid cysts are a rare finding and occur more frequently in women. Parathyroid cysts are located paratracheally and, in some cases, can be mistaken for thyroid cysts. Cysts range in size from a few millimeters to a few centimeters. It usually presents as an asymptomatic neck mass. An elevation in parathyroid hormone level is determined in the cytological aspirate [2].

The sonographic characteristic is typical; it is an anechoic mass with dorsal enhancement and reverberations.

Microscopically, parathyroid cells are variably organized in sheets, rosettes, or groups. The cells vary in size and shape. Macrophages represent cystic component.

17.2 Diagnostic Workflow

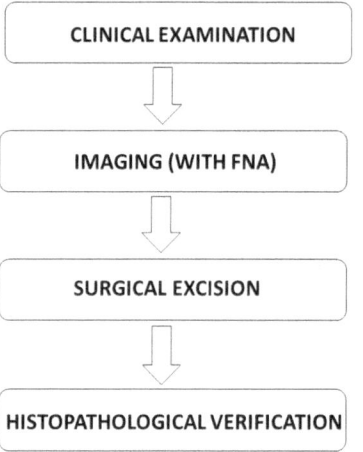

17.3 Framed Text with the Main Massage

Median cystic and solid lesions are mainly asymptomatic developmental disorders in neck midline: median neck cyst (thyroglossal duct cyst), bronchogenic/bronchial cyst, dermoid cyst, thymic cyst, and parathyroid cyst. The final diagnosis is performed histologically after surgical excision.

References

1. Koeller KK, Alamo L, Adair CF, Smirniotopoulos JG. Congenital cystic masses of the neck: radiologic-pathologic correlation. Radiographics. 1999;19(1):121–46; quiz 52–3.
2. Vazquez Salas S, Pedro K, Balram A, Syed S, Kotaka K, Kadivar A, et al. Head and neck cystic lesions: a cytology review of common and uncommon entities. Acta Cytol. 2022;66(5):359–70.
3. Anderson JL, Vu K, Haidar YM, Kuan EC, Tjoa T. Risks and complications of thyroglossal duct cyst removal. Laryngoscope. 2020;130(2):381–4.
4. Thompson LD, Herrera HB, Lau SK. A clinicopathologic series of 685 thyroglossal duct remnant cysts. Head Neck Pathol. 2016;10(4):465–74.
5. Cheng J, Lerebours R, Lee HJ. Current trends and 30-day surgical outcomes for thyroglossal duct cyst excision in children. Int J Pediatr Otorhinolaryngol. 2020;128:109725.
6. Zander DA, Smoker WR. Imaging of ectopic thyroid tissue and thyroglossal duct cysts. Radiographics. 2014;34(1):37–50.
7. Mittal MK, Malik A, Sureka B, Thukral BB. Cystic masses of neck: a pictorial review. Indian J Radiol Imaging. 2012;22(4):334–43.
8. Foley DS, Fallat ME. Thyroglossal duct and other congenital midline cervical anomalies. Sem Pediatr Surg. 2006;15(2):70–5.
9. Godinho GV, Da Silva EJ, Da Silva CAL, Volpato LER. Epidermoid cyst mimicking a thyroglossal duct cyst in a pediatric patient: a case report. Gen Dent. 2022;70(1):61–4.
10. Alzahrani HA, Iqbal JM, Abu Shaheen AK, Al Harthi BN. Cervical thymic cyst in an adult. Case Rep Surg. 2014;2014:1–4.
11. Sturm JJ, Dedhia K, Chi DH. Diagnosis and management of cervical thymic cysts in children. Cureus. 2017.

Ivana Kholová is the Adjunct Professor of pathology at the Tampere University, Faculty of Medicine and Health Technology, Finland. She is the President of Finnish Society for Clinical Cytology. She also serves as Secretary-Treasurer of the Association for European Cardiovascular Pathology. She is a co-author of *The Milan System for Reporting Salivary Gland Cytopathology* and *The Bethesda System for Reporting Thyroid Gland Cytopathology*. She is an expert member of the Executive Editorial Board of The WHO System for Reporting Cytopathology of the Lung. She has authored and co-authored 122 PubMed-indexed papers.

David Kalfert, ENT surgeon at the University Hospital Motol, First Faculty of Medicine, Charles University, Prague, Czechia. Author and co-author of more than 70 articles and book chapters.

Management of a Thyroid Nodule in 2023 (Adults Only)

18

Zahra Maleki and Beatrix Cochand-Priollet

18.1 Introduction

A quick look over the past 25-year period, nothing has changed in the United States (USA) as well as in Europe concerning the thyroid nodule assessment. All the nodules have to be investigated in order to detect the malignant nodules which are rare but with an increasing incidence higher than 2% in the United States and in Europe. With a wide consensus, the diagnosis of these nodules is usually based on a fine-needle aspiration (FNA) with a very thin needle, a gauge 25–27 wide, preferably under ultrasonography (US). In 70–75% of the cases, a definitive diagnosis of benign or malignant nodule is rendered; however, in 25–30% of the nodules called the "indeterminate cases," a specific diagnosis cannot be proposed. In the past, the aim of all the tests performed in medicine was to detect the malignant cases and to avoid any false-negative, with the "ipso facto" acceptance of some false-positive cases. The main objective was to obtain a high sensitivity. Therefore, concerning the thyroid, the option of some total thyroidectomies for finally some benign nodules was acceptable for the clinicians as well as for the patients in these doubtful "indeterminate" cases.

Currently, essentially because the patients do not accept unnecessary surgical resection anymore, a high sensitivity has to be "coupled" with a high specificity as well. In other terms, a very specific diagnosis has to be made before any clinical decision-making and surgery is an option accepted only if its necessity has been really demonstrated. During the last 25 years, tremendous technical improvements have occurred especially for imaging techniques. Therefore, ultrasound (US) is no more used to only monitoring if the tip of the needle is well located into the nodule. It is a part of the diagnosis scheme with a classification of the nodules in five categories whatever the applied terminology, the American or the European ones both linked with a risk of malignancy (ROM) for each category. Since the global accuracy of the thyroid cytology remains higher than those for the United States, the combination of these two techniques together is recommended.

Due to the technical improvements in our labs, the pathology has entered in a new era of molecular pathology. Therefore, the so-called cytological indeterminate cases now have the benefit of implementing molecular testings or immunocytochemistry (ICC) leading toward a more refined assessment.

Z. Maleki
Department of Pathology, Johns Hopkins Hospital,
The Johns Hopkins Medical Institution,
Baltimore, MD, USA
e-mail: zmaleki1@jhmi.edu

B. Cochand-Priollet (✉)
Department of Pathology, Cochin AP-HP-Paris
Centre, University Paris-Cité, Paris, France
e-mail: beatrix.cochand-priollet@aphp.fr

In parallel and in order to homogenize thyroid cytological diagnosis based on very well-defined criteria, a terminology was proposed by the American Society of Cytopathology (ASC) called "The Bethesda System for Reporting Thyroid Cytology (TBSRTC)," the first one in 2010 [1], followed by the second edition in 2017 [2] taking into account some of the above-described improvements. In 2023, the third edition is published in order to be correlated with the new 2022 WHO classification [3] which has introduced most of the more recent molecular data concerning the thyroid. Concerning the cytology, some other terminologies have been proposed in countries like the United Kingdom [4], Italy [5], and Japan [6]. Nevertheless, a recent survey proposed by the EFCS has shown that with a great majority, the European National Societies of Cytology/Pathology was involved in the terminology implementations as well as translations, especially in Southern and Western European countries (80 to 100%) and that the TBSRTC is well known and widely used throughout Europe (75 to 100%).

Therefore, it is now obvious that the management of the thyroid nodules has been totally modified for all the above-mentioned reasons. The management of these nodules is now based on "triplex" quite complex algorithms taking into account the clinical data and especially the US findings, the cytological categorization, and, when available, the ancillary testings. Should we add the "patients' preference," then we could speak about "quadriplex algorithms"!

18.2   Clinical Data

The American Thyroid Association (ATA) published clinical guidelines for primary care physicians in the evaluation and management of patients with thyroid nodules or differentiated thyroid cancers in 1996 [7, 8]. The ATA guidelines were developed based on the expert opinion of the committee participants and previously published information [8]. The aim of the guidelines is to inform clinicians, patients, researchers, and health policymakers about the best available evidence (and its limitations), relating to the diagnosis and treatment of adult patients with thyroid nodules and differentiated thyroid cancer [7, 9]. A main goal of the guidelines is to minimize potential harm from overtreatment in a majority of patients at low risk for disease-specific mortality and morbidity, while appropriately treating and monitoring those patients at higher risk. The guidelines are intended to inform clinical decision-making without replacement for clinical judgment for each individual patient [7]. Discovering a thyroid nodule or a multinodular thyroid gland includes, first of all, a very precise clinical assessment that encompasses: age; gender (male sex, nodules that appear in patients younger than 20 years, or older than 60 years, are additional risk factors for malignancy); symptoms or not (fullness or discomfort); history of neck radiation; thyroid cancer in the family; context of another personal cancer; and solitary or multiple nodules disease. A clinical examination is required including a thyroid gland palpation as well as a neck palpation for the lymph nodes. In 2006, ATA revised the guidelines including the algorithm for the evaluation of patients with one or more thyroid nodules [9]. In 2015, The ATA developed evidence-based recommendations for clinical decision-making in the management of thyroid nodules and differentiated thyroid cancer. The revised ATA guidelines include recommendations regarding initial evaluation, clinical and ultrasound criteria for FNA, interpretation of FNA results, application of molecular markers, and management of benign thyroid nodules [7]. For the ATA and the recent 2022 SFE (Societe Française d'Endocrinologie) consensus [10], it is recommended to measure the serum thyrotropin (TSH) level since the nodule assessment should widely differ depending on the result. In case of a low TSH level, the FNA is usually not recommended. Routine calcitonin testing has not been recommended by the SFE [10] recommendations; the ATA task force [7] could not recommend for or against this routine testing due to controversial arguments. On the other hand, calcitonin testing should be performed in cases of suggestive symptoms or in case of personal or family history of medullary thyroid carcinoma

(MTC) or multiple endocrine neoplasms type 2 (MEN2). Routine measurement of serum thyroglobulin (TG) for the initial assessment of thyroid nodules is not useful. Recommendations related to the initial management of thyroid cancer include those relating to screening for thyroid cancer, staging and risk assessment, surgical management, radioiodine remnant ablation and therapy, and thyrotropin suppression therapy using levothyroxine. Recommendations regarding long-term management of differentiated thyroid cancer include those related to surveillance for recurrent disease using imaging and serum thyroglobulin, thyroid hormone therapy, management of recurrent and metastatic disease, consideration for clinical trials and targeted therapy, as well as directions for future research [7].

18.3 Radiology

18.3.1 Ultrasonography

Ultrasonography is the modality of choice for the evaluation of thyroid lesions. Ultrasound imaging is a safe, noninvasive, quick, cost-effective, and relatively simple technology. The main purpose of initial assessment of thyroid nodules by ultrasound is to distinguish between benign nodules that can be managed conservatively from those that possess malignant or suspicious features which require further work-up by fine-needle aspiration and even surgical excision in some circumstances [11]. In fact, ultrasound of thyroid nodules can prevent unnecessary aggressive treatment. The normal thyroid gland appears homogenous and of an intermediate gray scale. Thyroid ultrasound is mainly used to evaluate thyroid nodules and to determine any associated risk of malignancy. Moreover, ultrasound is a helpful tool to assess autoimmune and inflammatory diseases of the thyroid. Cystic nodule, colloid nodule, follicular neoplasms, papillary thyroid carcinoma, Hashimoto's thyroiditis, and Grave's disease are characterized by their typical ultrasound findings [12–14]. Thyroid ultrasound is most useful in assessing for thyroid malignancies. Ultrasound is also the most accurate tool for

measuring thyroid nodules, and it is the most sensitive radiographic modality for detecting thyroid carcinoma, with sensitivity of 80%, when it is done by an experienced radiologist [12–14]. Ultrasound examination should evaluate thyroid parenchyma (homogeneous or heterogeneous), thyroid gland size, size (in three dimensions), location, and sonographic features of any nodules, the presence or absence of any suspicious cervical lymph nodes in the central or lateral compartment, nodules sonographic features and compositions (solid, cystic, spongiform), echogenicity, margins, presence and type of calcifications, and shape if taller than wide, and vascularity [15, 16]. The sonographic features of a thyroid nodule can predict risk of malignancy and along with nodule size guide FNA decision-making [17, 18]. In patients with low serum TSH, if radionuclide scintigraphy studies suggest thyroid nodules, ultrasound should be performed to evaluate the hyperfunction area and the presence of nodules. The hyperfunction area does not require FNA, and nodules may require FNA if they meet the criteria for performing FNA [19]. While there is no pathognomonic feature in sonography for detecting thyroid carcinoma, there are features suggestive of malignancy including macrocalcifications (intranodular intrinsic and not peripheral), increased vascularity, extrathyroid extension, irregular or microlobulated margins, and dimensions that are more tall than wide on transverse imaging and absent "halo sign." The presence of these features raises the likelihood of malignancy 70% up to 90% in a suspicious thyroid nodule. Nodules that are completely cystic are considered benign with less than 1% associated risk of malignancy, which do not require fine-needle aspiration. Spongiform or mixed solid and cystic nodules are associated with less than 3% risk of malignancy. Nodules with both cystic and solid components are associated with 5% risk of malignancy. Solid isoechoic or hyperechoic nodules are considered low risk (5% to 10% risk of malignancy), while solid hypoechoic nodules have an estimated 10% to 20% risk of malignancy. Thyroid nodules, solitary or multinodular, need to be evaluated carefully, since thyroid carcinoma may arise in both settings. The nodule with suspicious features for malignancy is evaluated by fine-needle aspiration [20, 21]. The only disadvantage of thyroid ultrasound is that it is operator-dependent [22].

18.3.1.1　EU-TIRADS 2017: Principles; ROM; Management; Algorithms for the Thyroid Gland

By definition, a thyroid nodule is a discrete mass within the thyroid gland that is radiologically distinct from the surrounding parenchyma [23]. There are palpable lesions that do not meet the criteria for a thyroid nodule on radiologic imaging, and also, there are distinct nodules on ultrasound that are nonpalpable called "incidentaloma." Palpable and nonpalpable nodules of the same size share the same risk of malignancy [24]. In general, nodules greater than 1 cm require further evaluation since they are more likely to be malignant with potential of distant metastasis [7]. Nodules less than 1 cm should be evaluated if there are associated clinical symptoms or lymphadenopathy. Fine-needle aspiration plays a pivotal role in further work-up of thyroid nodules. However, it is not practical to perform fine-needle aspiration on all thyroid nodules since it may lead unnecessary aggressive treatment [22, 25, 26]. Therefore, a subset of thyroid nodules is selected for fine-needle aspiration based upon their clinical risk factors and risk of malignancy stratification on ultrasound imaging. The European Thyroid Association convened a panel of international experts' taskforce to work on ultrasound risk stratification of thyroid nodules. The panel reviewed the literature, and based on the American Association of Clinical Endocrinologists, American Thyroid Association, and Korean guidelines, they created the novel European Thyroid Imaging and Reporting Data System, called EU-TIRADS. The EU-TIRADS is a standardized reporting system of thyroid ultrasound findings with the estimated risk of malignancy for each category. It defines thyroid nodules as benign, low, intermediate, and high risk for malignancy based on their ultrasound features and provides indications for fine-needle aspiration [22]. The aim of EU-TIRADS is to enhance interob-

server reproducibility of thyroid ultrasound descriptions, to improve and simplify communication of the results, and to serve physicians in their clinical practice [22].

There are features of thyroid nodules on ultrasound that are associated with high risk for malignancy and are used as criteria for FNA performance [22, 26–29]. Several meta-analysis studies investigated ultrasound accuracy in the prediction of thyroid cancer [18, 30, 31]. Brito et al conducted a meta-analysis on 31 studies comprising a total of 18,288 thyroid nodules, of which 20% were malignant. The features associated with the highest diagnostic odd ratio (DOR) for predicting malignancy were a "taller-than-wide" shape (11.1; 95% CI: 6.6–18.9) and internal calcifications (6.8; 95% CI: 4.5–10.2), while a spongiform (12; 95% CI: 0.6–234.3) and a cystic appearance (6.8; 95% CI: 2.3–20.3) were features most associated with a benign nodule [18]. Their analysis found that nodule size is a poor predictor for malignancy. The absence of elasticity, microcalcifications, irregular margins, and a "taller-than-wide" shape (86.2, 87.8, 83.1, and 96.6%, respectively) were found to be associated with the highest specificities by Remonti et al [30]. Campanella et al reported "taller-than-wide" shape (DOR of 10.2; 95% CI: 6.7–15.3), an absent halo sign (7.1; 95% CI: 3.7–13.7), microcalcifications (6.8; 95% CI: 4.7–9.7), and irregular margins (6.1; 95% CI: 3.1–12.0) as features associated with highest risk of malignancy [31]. Considering that there is no single diagnostic ultrasound feature to predict a malignant thyroid nodule, a pattern-based ultrasound classification system, known as the Thyroid Imaging Reporting and Data System (TIRADS), was introduced by Horvath et al [32] in 2009. The TIRADS is a 6-point scale for risk stratification, the higher point means the greater risk of malignancy [22, 32]. In 2011, it was endorsed by the French Society of Endocrinology, and subsequently, the Initial TIRADS was modified into a more user-friendly version and validated by a large prospective study [33]. The aim of European Thyroid Association (ETA) task force was to: 1) create guidelines and a standardized risk stratification system to assess features suspicious for thyroid malignancy, 2) establish a standard US description lexicon, 3) provide ultrasound criteria for performing FNA, 4) provide a structured ultrasound reporting template, and 5) provide a practical image guide for clinical use [22, 34–39]. Nodular shape, margin, echogenicity, hyperechoic foci, and composition are the fundamental features for TIRADS scoring system.

EU-TIRADS 1 category refers to thyroid ultrasound examination when no nodule is identified. The thyroid is considered benign and FNA should be avoided unless there is a clinical justification. Thyroid scintigraphy can be performed if the serum thyroid-stimulating hormone level (TSH) is low to normal, particularly in iodine-deficient countries. FNA should be avoided on hot thyroid nodules [40].

EU-TIRADS 2 category includes two patterns on ultrasound purely cystic/anechoic nodules and spongiform nodules. Purely cystic nodules are devoid of solid component of wall thickening. A few traversing septa separating a cyst into compartments can be seen. The presence of echogenic material inside the cyst can be due to a fibrin clot or a solid component, which can be further characterized by the application of Doppler ultrasound. Spongiform nodules composed of tiny cystic spaces occupying the entire nodule by numerous isoechoic septa. Purely cystic nodules and entirely spongiform nodules should be considered benign. The risk of malignancy is almost null. FNA is not indicated, unless for therapeutic purposes, in patients with compressive symptoms [28, 40].

EU-TIRADS 3 comprises oval-shaped, isoechoic or hyperechoic nodules with smooth margins and no features of high-risk malignancy. Grouped or coalescing nodules are also included in this category. FNA should be considered only if the nodule is greater than 20 mm. Minimal cystic changes are in favor of a benign condition. In contrast, entirely isoechoic nodules are diagnosed as follicular carcinoma or follicular variant of papillary thyroid carcinoma in less than 4% of cases on surgical excision. The risk of malignancy is estimated to be 2–4% [41–44].

EU-TIRADS 4 category refers to oval-shaped, mildly hypoechoic thyroid nodules with smooth margins without any features of malignancy. FNA is performed on nodules greater than 15 mm. All hypoechoic nodules are considered intermediate risk. The presence of a thin halo, comet-tail artifacts, partially cystic nodule, peripheral vascularity, and low stiffness decreases risk of malignancy. In contrast, a thick halo, discontinuous peripheral/ rim microcalcifications, and high stiffness raises the possibility of malignancy. The risk of malignancy is 6–17% [33, 35].

EU-TIRADS 5 category includes thyroid nodules with at least one of following ultrasound features: non-oval shape, microcalcifications, marked hypoechogenicity, and irregular margins. These features are highly specific (83–84%), but they are not very sensitive (26–59%). The composition of these features is of paramount importance. FNA should be performed on all nodules greater than 10 mm unless the patient is not a candidate for surgery due to other comorbidities. Subcentimeter nodules with features of malignancy in ultrasound are candidates for FNA procedure or active surveillance if the patient is willing to have regular ultrasound scanning and if there are no abnormal lymph nodes. In order to avoid false-negative FNA results, it is recommended to repeat FNA within 3 months if the first FNA diagnosis is benign. This category is considered a high-risk category with an estimated ROM of 26–87% [29, 33, 39, 45–47].

Ultrasound in Multinodular Thyroid Disease

EU-TIRADS scoring system is also applicable in multinodular thyroid disease. Here are the recommendations:

1. Look for high-risk nodules and describe their ultrasound features regardless of their size, and perform FNA on the nodule greater than 10 mm.
2. Continue by looking for nodules with intermediate risk and describe those greater than 5 mm and perform FNA if they are larger than 15 mm.
3. Look for low-risk nodules and describe those greater than 10 mm and perform FNA if they are great than 20 mm.

4. If there are numerus nodules, describe at least the three most important ones according to the size and risk.

There are other additional ultrasound features that are considered helpful in risk assessment of thyroid nodules.

18.3.1.2   Cervical Lymph Nodes

Ultrasound assessment of the lymph nodes of all thyroid nodules is advised. However, it is mandated to evaluate cervical lymph nodes on all patients with intermediate- to high-risk thyroid nodules. An FNA on lymph nodes with suspicious features on ultrasound provides material for cytology evaluation and washout for thyroglobulin or calcitonin measurement. In the presence of a suspicious thyroid nodule and a suspicious lymph node of a possible thyroid origin, FNA of both the suspicious lymph node and the most suspicious thyroid nodule should be performed [48].

18.3.1.3   Extrathyroid Extension

Capsular bulging, protrusion into the adjacent structures, or disruption of the capsular margin by the thyroid nodule is indicative of extrathyroidal invasion, and it should be described in the report. Macrocalcifications are defined as echogenic foci greater than 1 mm in size with posterior shadowing. Central intranodular, isolated, and rim, peripheral, curvilinear, or eggshell calcifications are three different patterns of macrocalcifications that should be described in the report. A distributed eggshell calcification at the margin of the nodule may be associated with increased risk of malignancy [49–52].

18.3.1.4   Macrocalcifications and Hyperechoic Spots

Macrocalcifications are echogenic foci greater than 1 mm in size with posterior shadowing. Three patterns can be described as follows: (1) central intranodular macrocalcifications (not consistently associated with malignancy), (2) isolated macrocalcification, occupying an entire calcified nodule (low risk), and (3) rim, eggshell or peripheral or curvilinear calcifications at the margin of the nodule (can increase the risk of malignancy if disrupted. Hyperechoic spots are another feature on ultrasound that need to be described and reported. They correspond to: (1) colloid crystals or fibrin debris that generate comet-tail artifacts or reverberations and they are always benign, (2) posterior acoustic enhancement of the back wall of a microcystic area, which are suggestive of a benign condition and it can be better visualized with high-frequency probes, (3) true microcalcifications which are multiple round echogenic foci around 1 mm in size without posterior shadowing located in the solid component of a nodule, corresponding to psammoma bodies and is highly suggestive of malignancy especially when it is associated with macrocalcifications, and (4) hyperechoic spots of uncertain significance that are linear than round, with no comet-tail artifacts or microcystic cavities. Macrocalcifications are non-specific findings, and they should be interpreted in the context of other features in ultrasound. Nodules with true microcalcifications must undergo FNA [53–57].

18.3.1.5   Halo

A halo may correspond to the capsule of a thyroid nodule, or to the surrounding capsular vessels, or even to the adjacent compressed parenchyma. A thick halo or absence of a halo is associated with increased risk of malignancy, while a thin halo is associated with low risk of malignancy [30, 31, 45, 58].

18.3.2   Vascularity on Doppler Ultrasound

The blood flow of thyroid nodules can be evaluated with different ultrasound imaging modalities including color Doppler, power Doppler, high-resolution studies of microvascularity, and pulsed wave Doppler, either with color imaging or plot velocities over time. Real-time Doppler ultrasound is widely used in clinical practice. The blood flow can be classified into types I-III using color-derived techniques as follows:

Type I: absence of intranodular or perinodular flow

Type II: presence of perinodular and/or slight intranodular flow

Type III: presence of marked intranodular and slight perinodular flow

Malignant nodules tend more to have type III vascularity, and benign nodules show type I or type II vascularity. The use of Doppler ultrasound is not recommended for risk stratification of thyroid nodules due to variable ultrasound equipment and setting and low interobserver agreements [59, 60].

18.3.3 Stiffness: Elastography

The stiffness of a nodule is analyzed by ultrasound elastography either by strain elastography or shear wave elastography. Strain elastography measures the amount of distortion of the nodule in response to an external pressure, while shear wave elastography measures the speed of the shear wave produced by an ultrasound pulse. Both methods have limitations and are not reliable in evaluation of large nodules (>30 mm), cystic nodules, nodules with macrocalcifications, deeply located or isthmic nodules, and coalescent nodules. Moreover, the results of elastography can be variable due to interobserver variability, differences in pressure level, scoring method, type of used software, imaging plane, and data acquisition. Grayscale ultrasound is used to differentiate benign form malignant nodules, and elastography is not recommended for the risk stratification of thyroid nodules; however, it can be applied as additional tool for assessment of thyroid nodules for FNA, due to its high NPV [22, 61–65].

18.3.4 Nodule Growth

Nodular growth cannot predict thyroid cancer since nodule growth cannot delineate benign from malignant nodules. Therefore, serial thyroid assessment for nodular growth for purpose of cancer detection is not recommended [22, 66].

18.3.5 Others

18.3.5.1 Radioiodine Scintigraphy

Nuclear scintigraphy is a diagnostic tool that provides important information about thyroid gland function. The radionuclide used to image the gland is utilized in hormone synthesis. The primary role of scintigraphy is to detect whether a thyroid mass is "hot" or "cold," which hot thyroid nodules are associated with low risk of malignancy and cold thyroid nodules carry a higher risk of malignancy. Gamma scintillation camera is used for imaging of the thyroid gland. The patient is placed in a hyperextended supine position, and the images are obtained from the chin to the sternal notch in multiple views [67]. Subsequently, findings on imaging are correlated with those on palpation of the gland. Technetium (Tc-99 m) pertechnetate, iodine 123 (I-123), and iodine 131 (I-131) are used to visualize the thyroid mass. Imaging is performed approximately 20 minutes following administration of Tc-99 m pertechnetate, 4 to 24 hours following oral ingestion of I-123, and 24 to 72 hours following administration of I-131. The normal thyroid gland demonstrates homogeneous radionuclide uptake and distribution, and the isthmus shows slightly less uptake than the right and left lobes.

18.3.5.2 Dual Isotope 123iodine/99mTc-MIBI Scintigraphy

Both European and American guidelines suggest FNA for evaluation of thyroid nodules that meet the criteria for FNA performance based on their size and ultrasound features [7, 22, 68, 69]. Although FNA has high sensitivity (65% to 98%), specificity (72% to 100%), and overall diagnostic accuracy (75% to 90%) [70], FNA cytology can be nondiagnostic in 2% -16% of cases and indeterminate in 5% to 20% of cases. The risk of malignancy was estimated to be 5–10% for nondiagnostic category and 6% to 40% for intermediate category [71]. Histology follow-up was benign in 60% to 95% of patients who underwent thyroidectomy due to a nondiagnostic or indeterminate cytology [72, 73]. Different modalities such as molecular testing, nuclear medicine scan alone, or in combination of both have been utilized to prevent unnecessary thyroidectomies. 99mTc-MIBI scintigraphy has been reported to be highly accurate in differential diagnosis of indeterminate cytology [74–76]. In euthyroid patients, a study conducted quantitative dual isotope 123iodine/99mTc-MIBI scintigraphy on a series of solid thyroid nodules greater than 1 cm that underwent ultrasound and FNA procedures with diagnosis of nondiagnostic or indeterminate. Dual isotope scintigraphy was performed in the same day. Radioiodine 123 was injected first, and 99mTc-MIBI was injected 90 minutes later. In 123Iodine scintigraphy, thyroid nodules were categorized as 1) hyperfunctioning or hot (uptake in the nodule is greater than uptake in normal thyroid tissue); 2) indifferent or warm (uptake in the nodule is equal to uptake in normal thyroid tissue); or 3) hypofunctioning or cold (uptake in the nodule is less than uptake in normal thyroid tissue). 99mTc-MIBI scintigraphy was always interpreted comparatively with 123Iodine scintigraphy to exclude indifferent and hot nodules. Mean uptake values were lower in benign than in malignant nodules at both time points: early, 8.7 ± 4.1 versus 12.9 ± 3.5 (P = 0.005); and late, 5.3 ± 2.7 versus 7.7 ± 1.1 (P = 0.008). Interobserver reproducibility was excellent. The intraclass correlation coefficient was 0.86 in benign and 0.92 in malignant lesions for early uptake result (ER) and 0.94 and 0.85, respectively, for late uptake result (LR). The optimal LR cut-off to exclude a diagnosis of malignancy was set at 5.9. The sensitivity, specificity, positive predictive value, negative predictive value, and accuracy of this cut-off were, respectively, 100%, 65.2%, 60%, 100%, and 77.1% [77]. The study concluded that quantitative analysis of 99mTc-MIBI thyroid scintigraphy is a helpful tool to rule out malignancy in cold nodules with indeterminate or nondiagnostic FNA diagnosis, which may reduce the number of the number of unnecessary thyroidectomies whenever LR is below 5.9 [77].

18.3.5.3 18F-FDG PET/CT

[^{18}F] fluorodeoxyglucose positron emission tomography (^{18}FDG-PET) is increasingly per-

formed to evaluate thyroid in both malignant and nonmalignant conditions. ^{18}FDG-PET is not recommended for the routine evaluation of patients with newly detected thyroid nodules or thyroid illness. However, an abnormal thyroid uptake detected incidentally should be encountered. The pattern of ^{18}FDG-PET uptake can be focal (1–2%) or diffuse (2%) [78–80]. Focal ^{18}FDG-PET uptake within a confirmed nodule by ultrasound is associated with an increased risk of malignancy, and FNA is recommended for those nodules of 1 cm or greater in size. ^{18}FDG-PET-positive thyroid nodules less than 1 cm do not meet FNA criteria and should be monitored similar to those thyroid nodules with high-risk sonographic pattern. A meta-analysis demonstrated that approximately 35% of focally ^{18}FDG-PET-positive thyroid nodules proved to be cancer [78]. A study assessed the role of [^{18}F] FDG PET/CT, fine-needle aspiration (FNA) cytology and ultrasound in patients with focally positive thyroid nodules on FDG PET/CT. Malignancy was confirmed in 38.2% of the cases including primary thyroid carcinoma, parathyroid carcinoma, metastatic carcinoma, and lymphoma. Interestingly, approximately 30% of focally 18F-FDG-positive nodules were Hurthle cell/oncocytic nodules including infarcted Hürthle cell follicular adenoma, follicular adenoma with variable oncocytic change, a noninvasive follicular thyroid neoplasm with papillary-like nuclei (NIFTP) but with background oncocytic change, and multiple benign adenomatoid nodules focally with oncocytic appearances [81].

In contrast, diffuse ^{18}FDG-PET uptake mostly represent benign conditions and it is associated with an inflammatory uptake in Hashimoto thyroiditis or other diffuse thyroid diseases. Diffuse ^{18}FDG-PET uptake requires ultrasound evaluation to rule out any evidence of clinically relevant nodularity. Diffuse ^{18}FDG-PET uptake corresponds to diffuse heterogeneity of ultrasound. Diffuse ^{18}FDG-PET uptake does not require further imaging or FNA in cases of chronic lymphocytic thyroiditis proven by ultrasound and clinical evidence. The thyroid function needs to be evaluated in these patients. The accuracy of ^{18}FDG-PET is reported to be higher than qualitative

^{99m}Tc-MIBI-scan and ultrasound [76]. A negative ^{18}FDG-PET correctly detects a benign nodule confirmed on histology. A positive ^{18}FDG-PET is highly associated with malignancy, and it becomes more specific when it is combined with ultrasound [76].

18.4 FNA

18.4.1 Techniques

Whatever the chosen technique is, it has to be applied following the recommendations of the individual labs as well as the quality assurance rules. Several techniques are available and can be used. Their choice has to be based on a consensus between the sampler and the cytopathologist.

18.4.1.1 Direct Smears
This is the oldest and most likely the most often used technique in the world, especially in the United States. After removing the needle, a drop of the material contained in the needle has to be put on one end of a slide which is usually a ground-glass slide with a depolished glass part. The drop, placed close to this depolish glass side, is then spread with another glass slide along its surface. Immediately after, the spread material has to be shaken for 5–10 sec in order to be stained with a Giemsa technique. It is also possible to prepare slides for a Papanicolaou staining; an immediate fixation is then required (via an alcoholic liquid fixative). Another technique consists of placing the drop in the middle of a glass slide, to cover it with a second glass slide and then to pull the two slides in reverse order. For all these techniques, some experience and training are required especially for dosing the pressure on the slides. In case of hemorrhagic material, it is recommended to share the cytological material on several slides and not to push all the punctured material on a unique slide in order to avoid thick smears which are very difficult to evaluate under the microscope [82, 83].

18.4.1.2 Centrifugation
This technique is applied only in case of a fluid aspiration (large cystic nodule) [82].

18.4.1.3 Liquid-Based Cytology
This technique is mostly used in European countries [84, 85]. Once more, the choice of the liquid-based material is made by the cytopathologist and the radiologist together. The choice of the cytopathologist is often the decisive one since he is the owner of the material and is used with a given technique. Regardless of the choice, it is required to choose a FDA technique validated for the thyroid FNA. The sampling is easy to prepare since the sampler simply has to push the cytological material inside the needle into the vial containing the chosen liquid.

The advantages of this technique are the following:

(a) avoiding smears "less than satisfying" in case of untrained people for the conventional smear technique;
(b) to obtain well-preserved cells;
(c) to keep some additional material for ancillary techniques (ICC or molecular techniques).

The cons are:

(a) the cost of this technique being more expensive than the conventional one;
(b) that only a Papanicolaou staining is feasible due to the alcoholic fixative usually included in the liquid.

18.4.1.4 Cell Blocks
This technique is progressively becoming the choice for more and more pathologists since it offers some advantages especially for applying the ancillary techniques extensively used since the solely morphological diagnosis is often not sufficient in a context of targeted therapies. Several techniques are available [86–90]. Nevertheless, and concerning the thyroid gland, some studies have reported the lack of sufficient

cytological material for rendering this method. Like for the conventional smears, working with trained samplers as well as trained cytotechnicians aware of the technique is a requirement.

The most frequently used techniques are the following:

(a) fixation of the FNA material in formalin; centrifugation 10 min at 2500 rpm; and then inclusion of the pellets into the paraffine
(b) Shandon Cytoblock technique including two reagents: reagent 1 (colorless) and reagent 2 (colored in blue): put 2 or 3 drops of reagent 2 on the pellet after centrifugation through the supernatant; when solidifying put 2 or 4 drops of reagent 1 on the pellet trough the supernatant once again
(c) Histogel (Thermo Fisher) technique with the FNA material fixation obtained in formalin or alcoholic fixation or in CytoLyt (Hologic) and centrifugation before clotting with the Hydroxyethyl Agarose liquid
(d) Other techniques; plasma-thrombin cell block; albumin cell block; agar cell block; etc......

Considering the many techniques available, it is now recommended in Europe to follow some recommendations. A cell block method validation study is underway at the EFCS (European Federation of Cytological Societies) in partnership with the UK NEQAS (National External Quality Assessment Site). The recommendations that will be published should serve as a reference.

18.4.1.5 Microbiopsy (CNB)

Microbiopsy is a controversial technique. Since it is performed with a needle with the same gauge or almost the same gauge as the needles used for the FNA and since the puncture can be performed only in one site and not in the whole nodule like for the FNA, it is easy to understand that the cytological material is more representative of the entire nodule than the microbiopsy. Nevertheless, thyroid CNB is reported as decreasing the rate of inconclusive results and showing a higher category IV diagnostic rate than FNA [91] Other

studies have proposed similar conclusions for the nondiagnostic (ND) nodules as well as for the indeterminate nodules [92, 93]. Many pathologists are more comfortable with histological features, and it is easier to perform some immunohistochemistry or molecular testing on this type of material. As reported by two EFCS studies concerning ICC conducted first in 2011 [94] and then in 2020 [95] in the great majority of the laboratories, ICC is performed by a non-cytology staff at a non-cytology department, such as immunohistochemistry, while there are only 13% laboratories where ICC is performed at the cytology laboratory by a cytology staff. Concerning the molecular techniques, they are more often performed on histological material than on a cytological one—especially in Europe—since the molecular tests are either not available or very expensive. Few laboratories in Europe and the United States have developed these techniques on cytology. Therefore, microbiopsies are performed and recommended for the ancillary techniques. Currently, with the opportunity to propose a mere follow-up or new management like thermoablation for the benign nodules in case of solid nodules with a low-risk of malignancy on the United States and 2 nondiagnostic samples, performing a microbiopsy is usually recommended [84]. For some teams, it is also recommended in case of nodules or mass suspicious for anaplastic carcinoma, metastasis, or lymphoma since these diagnoses usually need some additional techniques [84]. On the other hand, CNB is more invasive and may have more significant complications [96]. Finally, in cases of follicular lesions no precise diagnosis may be done without a visible nodular capsule and the percentage of its presence on the biopsies is usually not reported in the published studies [92, 93, 97, 98]. Furthermore and even when the capsule has been sampled on the biopsy, considering the small size of this biopsy and since the majority of these nodules are currently minimally invasive cancers the chance to have caught the focally located capsular invasion is quite rare. For all these above-cited studies, CNB was not beneficial in the diagnosis of follicular thyroid lesions.

18.4.2 Rapid On-Site Evaluation (ROSE)

It is well established that ultrasound guidance is a valuable tool in improving diagnostic yield of fine-needle aspiration biopsy (FNA) of thyroid nodules [99–101]. FNA under ultrasound guidance is the best test to evaluate thyroid nodules pre-operatively [102]. Ultrasound-guided FNA can be performed by a radiologist, an endocrinologist, an otolaryngologist, or a pathologist in an ultrasound unit or an office setting. It is of paramount importance to collect adequate mate-

rial for rendering a cytology diagnosis. However, benign (Bethesda II) (Figs. 18.1a–d, 18.2a–d, 18.3a, b and 18.4) and malignant (Bethesda VI) (Figs. 18.5a–j, 18.6a–f, 18.7a–c, 18.8) are the only two categories with a definitive cytology diagnosis. Nondiagnostic and AUS categories require additional work-up steps such as repeat FNA in both scenarios and maybe molecular studies in AUS cases [103]. Approximately, 5% to 20% of thyroid FNA cases are nondiagnostic due to insufficient material for cytologic evaluation [104–106]. Nondiagnostic results on thyroid FNA cytology can be frustrating for clinician and

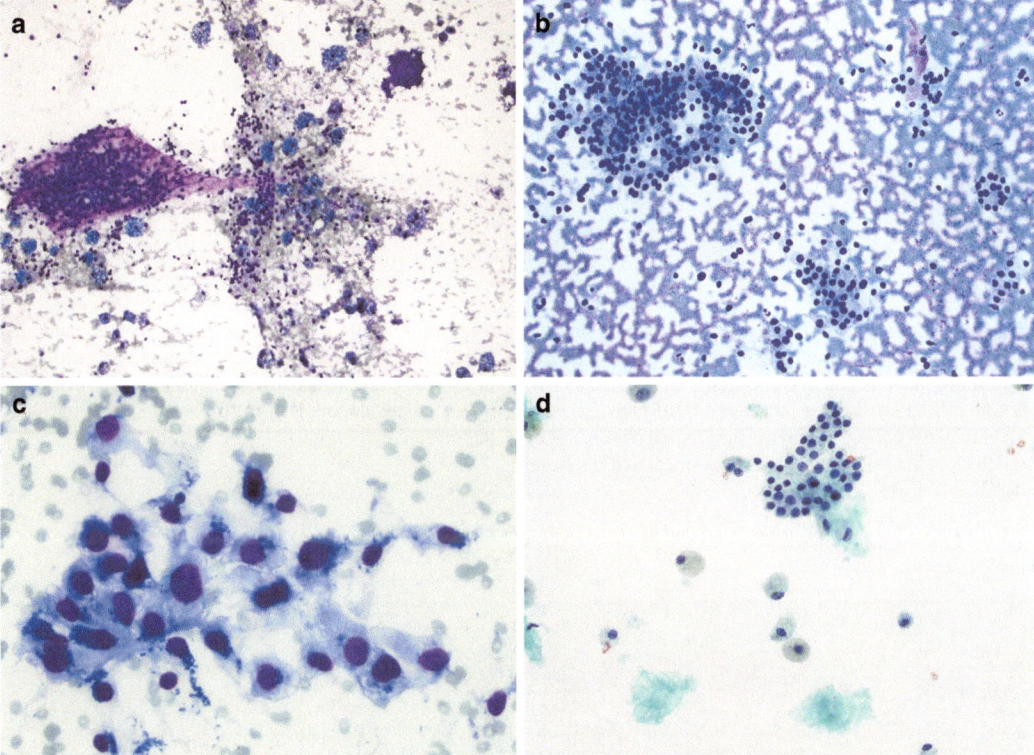

Fig. 18.1 Adenomatoid nodule of the thyroid. (**a**) Numerous thyroid follicular cells are arranged in mainly macrofollicles. Multiple macrophages are recognized with their large size, abundant cytoplasm, and small round nuclei. Some thick colloid is seen on the top right (Diff-Quik, smear) in a background of red blood cells. (**b**) Follicular cells are seen mostly in macrofollicles (the left side) and a few microfollicles (the right side) on higher magnification. All nuclei are small, relatively round, and uniform (Diff-Quik stain, smear). (**c**) Follicular cells are seen with slight elongation and wispy cytoplasm, features associated with cystic changes. Note: A few cells contain intracytoplasmic lysosomes, an additional finding (Diff-Quik, smear). (**d**) A large follicle, a few macrophages, and colloid are seen in a clear background (Papanicolaou stain, ThinPrep). Adenomatoid nodule is categorized Bethesda II

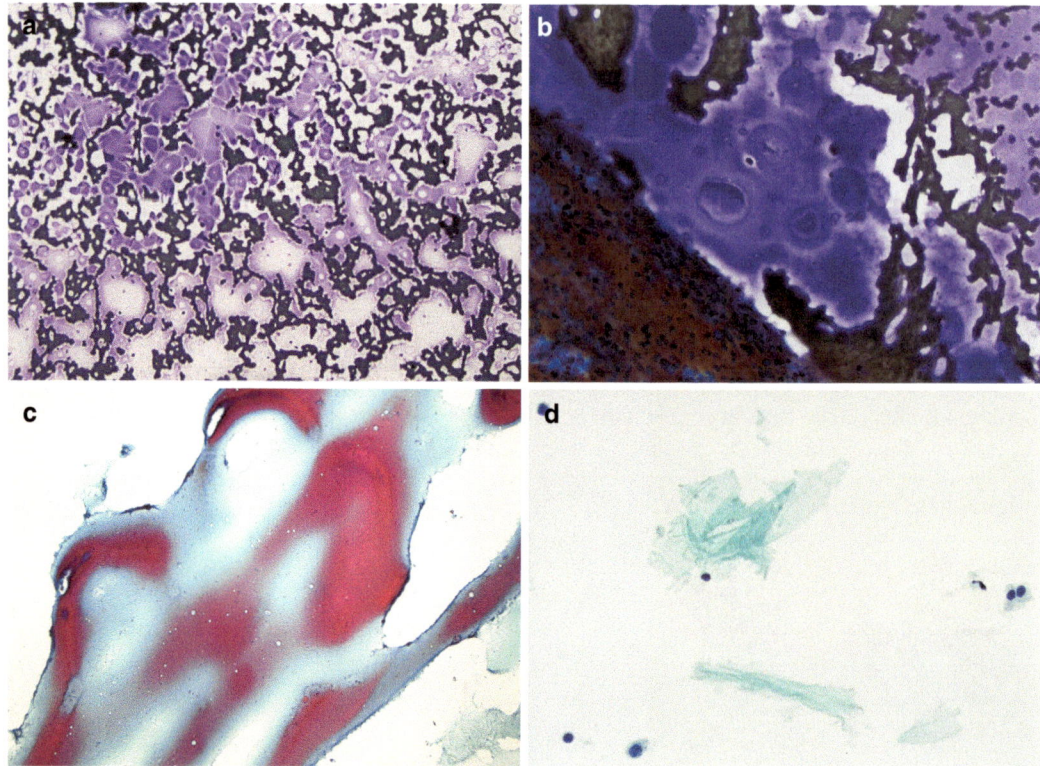

Fig. 18.2 Colloid in adenomatoid nodule with variable presentations. (**a**) Colloid appears in small particles resembling the cracked dry clay (Diff-Quik, Smear). (**b**) Dense colloid covering a large area (Diff-Quik, smear). (**c**) Very dense colloid giving the impression of very sticky and thick colloid (Papanicolaou stain, smear). (**d**) Delicate fragments of colloid resembling tissue paper (Papanicolaou stain, ThinPrep). Abundant colloid in the absence of follicular cells is consistent with colloid nodule, which falls in benign or category II of the Bethesda system for reporting thyroid cytology

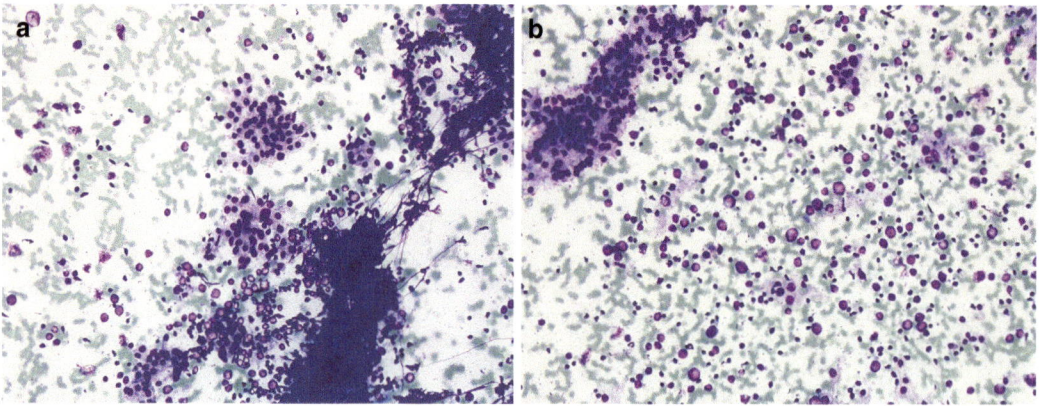

Fig. 18.3 Lymphocytic thyroiditis. (**a**) A few follicles are seen comprised follicular cells with Hurthle/oncocytic change in a background of numerous lymphocytes (Diff-Quik, smear). (**b**) Follicular cells demonstrate Hurthle/oncocytic changes characterized by abundant cytoplasm in lymphocytic thyroiditis. Numerous lymphocytes and epithelioid histiocytes are present in the background (Diff-Quik, smear). Lymphocytic thyroiditis is categorized Bethesda II

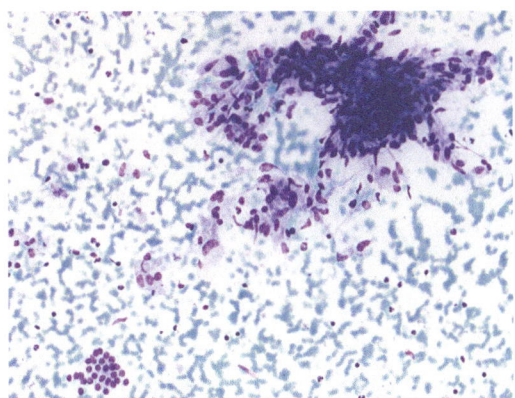

Fig. 18.4 Granulomatous thyroiditis. A large granuloma is seen comprised histiocytes with elongated nuclei (carrot shape or bare foot shape) and syncytial cytoplasm. A macrofollicle is seen on the lower left (Diff-Quik, smear). Granulomatous thyroiditis is categorized Bethesda II

patient since it requires repeat biopsy or surgery [14]. If the nodule is solid or has solid component and repeat FNA is also nondiagnostic, then lobectomy is considered a diagnostic approach [14]. Factors contributing to a nondiagnostic result are cystic nature of the nodule and the experience of the aspirator, or the posterior location of the nodule [14, 104]. Risk of malignancy for nondiagnostic category is approximately 8.9% [107]. Therefore, it is important to become familiar with criteria for nondiagnostic specimen and also adequate specimen. By definition, at least six well-preserved follicles, each containing of ten follicular cells or more is required for a thyroid FNA specimen to be considered sufficient for evaluation [108]. Specimens consisting of blood only, cystic contents with macrophages (Fig. 18.9) scant colloid with or without few follicular cells in the absence, or any other types of diagnostic cells such as lymphocytes are considered nondiagnostic. ROSE is a method of assessment of the aspirated material for adequacy in real time aiming to decrease the rate of nondiagnostic cases [14, 99, 105, 106]. ROSE improves specimen adequacy and decreases the rate of nondiagnostic cases [109]. Moreover, ROSE may

improve diagnosis by triage of specimen for ancillary studies such as PTH assessment or flow cytometry studies [110]. Some practices may implement rapid on-site evaluation only if the previous FNA result was nondiagnostic [14].

AUS or category III (Fig. 18.10) in Bethesda system is defined by the presence of cytologic and or architectural atypia that is insufficient for a more definitive diagnosis and also the atypia cannot be ignored to diagnose these cases benign [108, 111]. Sparse cellularity, artifacts of sample preparation such as drying artifact and focal atypia are among contributing factors to this diagnosis [108, 111]. AUS constitutes 4–15% of the thyroid samples, although it is recommended to be limited to 7% and associated risk of malignancy is variable between 5% and 48% [111]. A few studies have suggested that ROSE decreases the rate of nondiagnostic [112] and AUS categories and increases the rate of Bethesda category II and category VI, and improves diagnostic accuracy. The experience of aspirator and particularly in a high-volume center is another factor improving specimen adequacy [112]. ROSE also improves diagnostic accuracy by improving sparse cellularity and artifact [103]. Rapid on-site evaluation is performed by a cytotechnologist or a pathologist who is pathologist is present on-site during performance of the procedure. The results for accuracy of ROSE rendered by cytotechnologist are comparable with that of cytopathologists [113]. A routine protocol is to perform two FNA passes from two different areas of a nodule for an immediate assessment [110] and take a pause. Subsequently, the FNA performer deposits one drop of the aspirated material on one slide for ROSE and the cytologist makes a smear by using a slide. A variety of quick stains are utilized depending on the preference of the laboratory such as Diff-Quik, rapid Papanicolaou stain, toluidine blue, and hematoxylin and eosin stain [105, 106]. The rest of the material either collected in PreservCyt solution, which a methanol-based transport medium for ThinPrep preparation or it

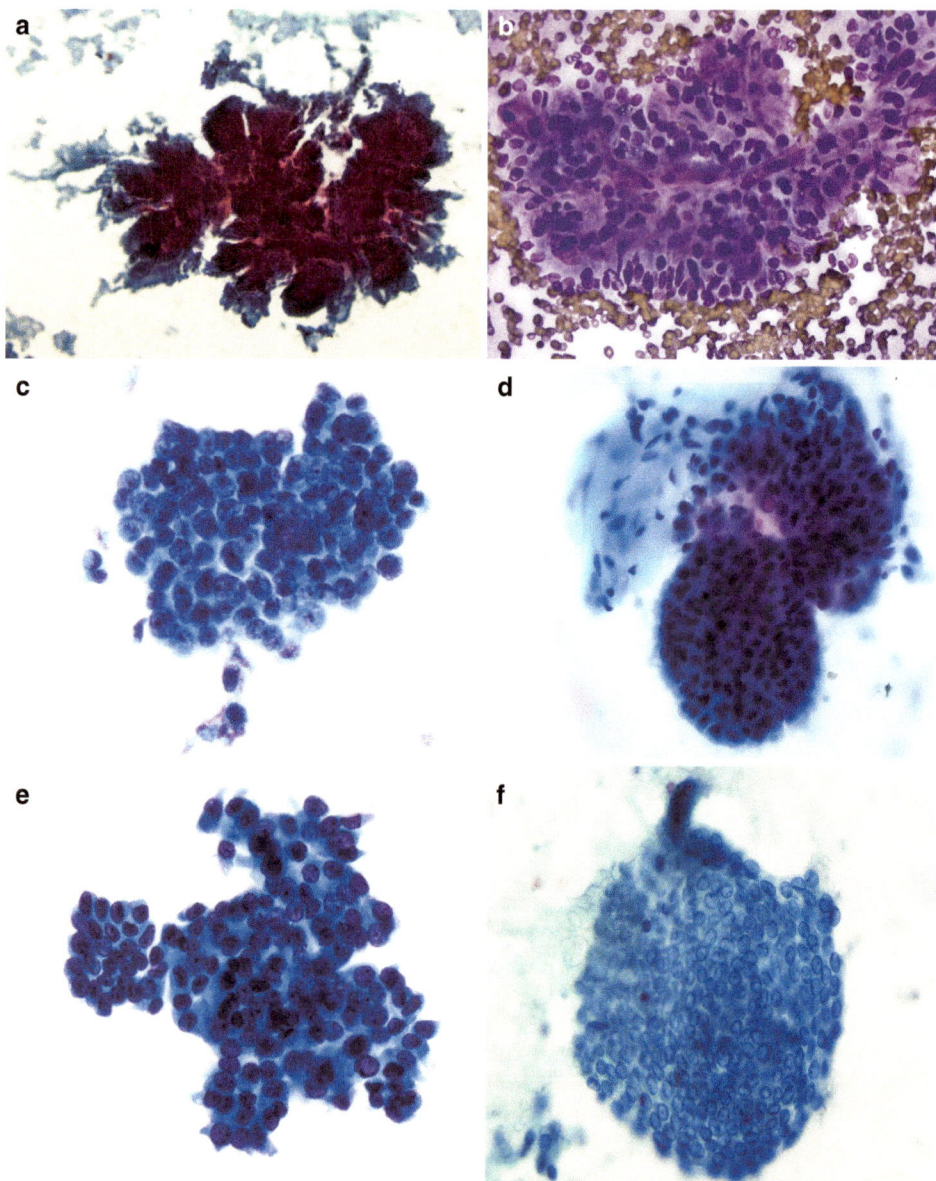

Fig. 18.5 Papillary thyroid carcinoma.(**a**) A large, 3-dimentional, papillary fragment is seen (Papanicolaou stain, smear). (**b**) A papillary structure comprised a central fibrovascular core surrounded by malignant follicular cells. Note: cytoplasmic intranuclear inclusions, nuclear elongation, enlargement, and overlapping (Diff-Quik stain, Smear). (**c**) A large, 3-dimentional fragment of malignant follicular cells are seen. The nuclei are enlarged and contain small nucleoli (Papanicolaou stain, ThinPrep). (**d**) Cytoplasmic intranuclear inclusion is a helpful finding in diagnosis of papillary thyroid carcinoma (Papanicolaou stain, ThinPrep). (**e**) A fragment of malignant follicular cells displaying nuclear features of malignancy including nuclear enlargement, nuclear grooves, nuclear inclusions, and small nucleoli (Papanicolaou stain, ThinPrep). (**f**) A round, whorl shape fragment of cohesive cells. Nuclei contain pale, powdery chromatin with numerous nuclear grooves, and small nucleoli (Papanicolaou stain, ThinPrep). (**g**) Bubble gum colloid is seen with round, homogenous, dense, structure in papillary thyroid carcinoma (Diff-Quik stain, Smear). (**h**) Ropey colloid is another feature of abnormal colloid in papillary thyroid carcinoma displaying strings of magenta colloid (Diff-Quik stain, Smear). (**i**) A papillary structure is seen with central fibrovascular core, surrounded by malignant follicular cells. Note nuclear clearing of the follicular cells (H&E stain, Cell block). (**j**) Histology section shows papillary formation and diffuse nuclear clearing (H&E stain, Histology section). It is an example of malignant, Bethesda category VI

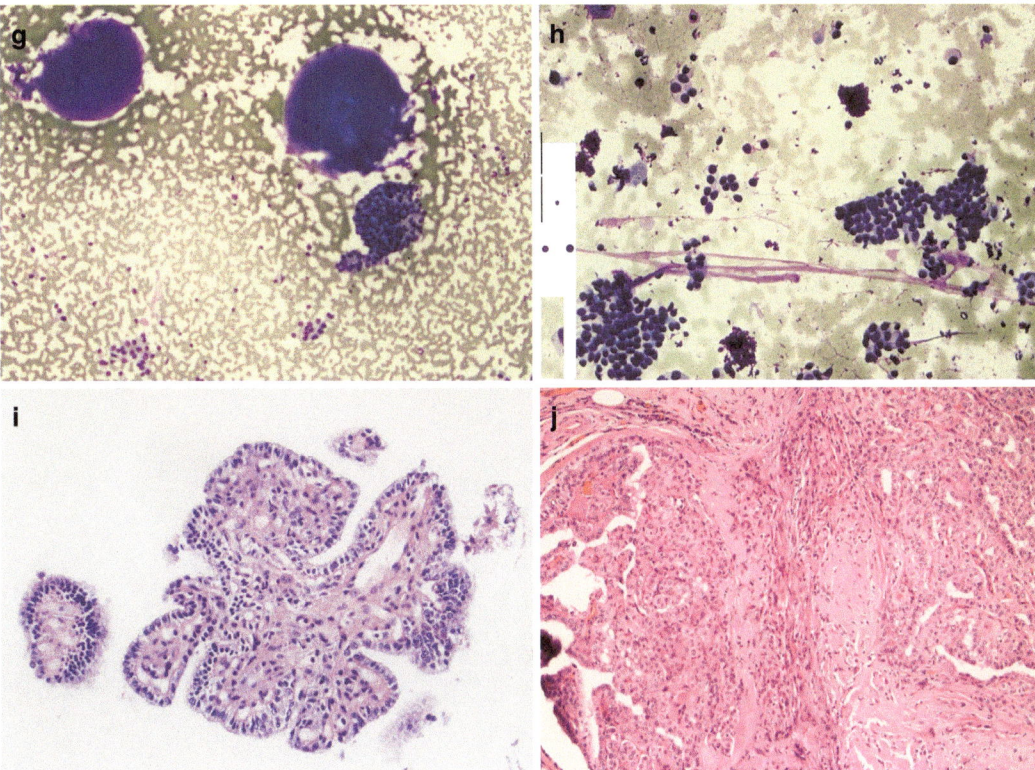

Fig. 18.5 (continued)

is deposited on the second slide and smeared, and it is immersed in ethanol in Kaplon jar. Additional FNA passes are required if there is a residual solid component in a cystic mass, or the cellularity is insufficient, or additional material is needed for a cell block preparation or ancillary studies [110]. Sometimes, additional passes are performed if there is inadequate material for Papanicolaou stains. After assessment of aspirated material, separate or dedicated passes may be collected for ancillary studies. Dedicated passes can be utilized for thyroid molecular studies in cases with AUS cytology on ROSE, flow cytometry, PTH, or microbiology. The disadvantages of rapid on-site evaluation are scheduling and coordination in a busy practice. ROSE will add to the cost; however, a few studies have shown that overall cost of ROSE is less than repeat FNA or performing molecular studies [103, 114]. It has been shown that ROSE will improve specimen adequacy; however, there were no statistical differences observed with regard to the risk of malignancy for each TBSRTC category when the two groups of thyroid FNA cases with ROSE compared with those thyroid FNA cases without ROSE [109]. Six passes are considered maximum number of passes for each nodule regardless of specimen adequacy [7].

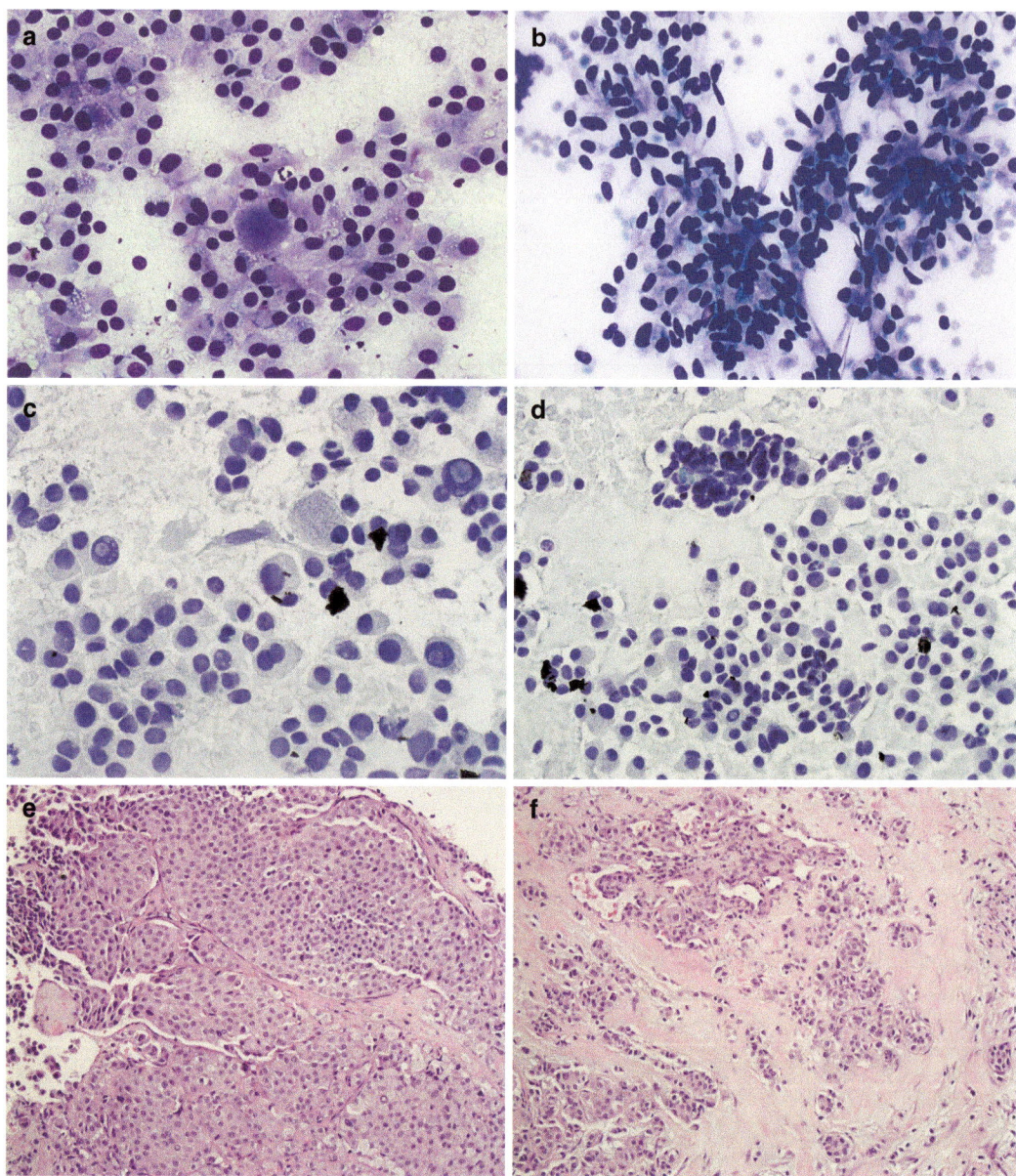

Fig. 18.6 Medullary thyroid carcinoma. (**a**) Loosely cohesive malignant cells of C cell /parafollicular cell origin are seen with abundant, finely granular cytoplasm, and round eccentric nuclei with minimal atypia (Diff-Quik, Smear). (**b**) Loosely cohesive malignant cells appear as spindle cells, displaying oval to elongated nuclei, a helpful diagnostic feature (Diff-Quik, smear). (**c**) Cytoplasmic intranuclear inclusion is seen in a subset of medullary thyroid carcinomas (Papanicolaou stain, Smear). (**d**) Nuclei are eccentric, round to oval with coarse chromatin, and focal nuclear molding (Papanicolaou stain, Smear). (**e**) The cells are relatively uniform with abundant cytoplasm and round nuclei, arranged in nests (H&E stain, Histology section). (**f**) Variable amount of amyloid can be seen in medullary thyroid carcinoma (H&E stain, Histology section). It is an example of malignant, Bethesda category VI

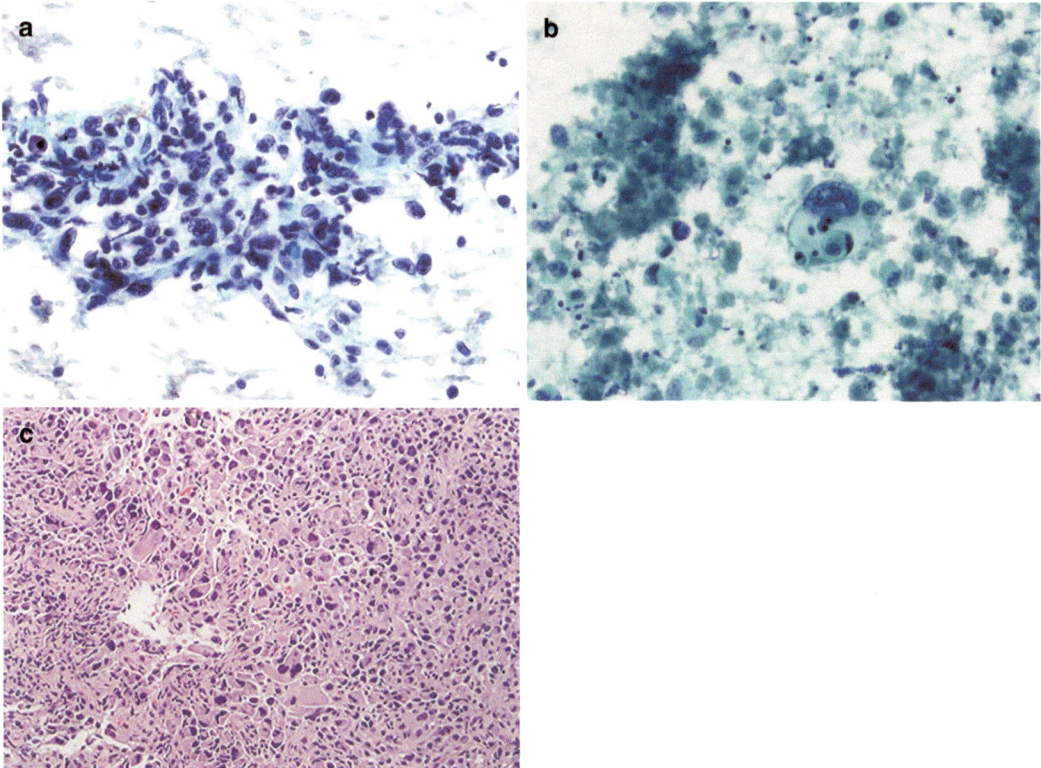

Fig. 18.7 Anaplastic thyroid carcinoma. (**a**) A large fragment of malignant cells is seen with pleomorphic nuclei, anisonucleosis, and coarse chromatin (Papanicolaou stain, Smear). (**b**) Extensive necrosis with rare viable malignant cells is a common finding in FNA of anaplastic thyroid carcinoma. The small cluster in the center shows a huge, eccentrically located nucleus (Papanicolaou stain, Smear). (**c**) The malignant cells display abundant eosinophilic cytoplasm and large nuclei (H&E stain, Histology section). It is an example of malignant, Bethesda category VI

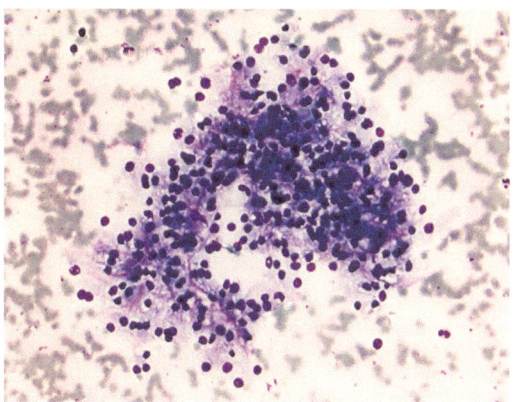

Fig. 18.8 Metastatic clear cell renal cell carcinoma. A large fragment of malignant cells is seen. The cells contain moderate to abundant delicate, finely vacuolated cytoplasm and relatively uniform, round nuclei. Note the capillary vasculature. It is an example of malignant, Bethesda category VI

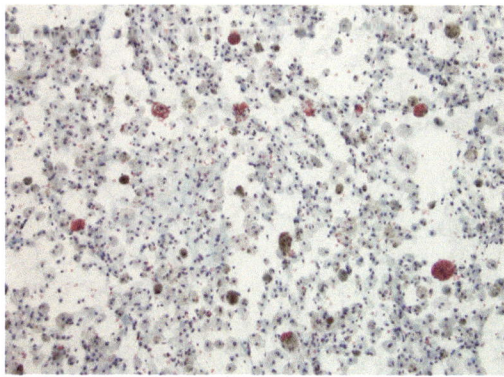

Fig. 18.9 Cyst content. Numerous macrophages are seen, some hemosiderin-laden and a few containing fresh red blood cells. No follicular cells are present. The specimen is considered inadequate, category I, applying the Bethesda System for reporting Thyroid Cytology

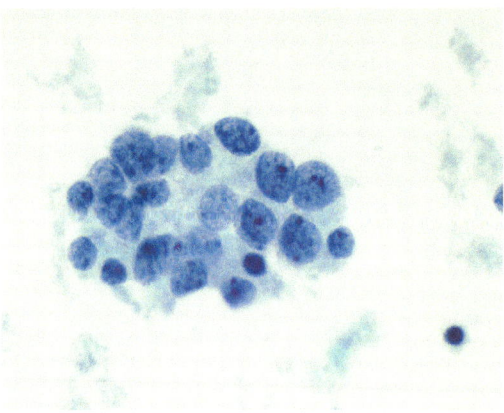

Fig. 18.10 Atypical follicular cells. A follicle is seen and consists of cells with nuclear atypia. The nuclei are slightly enlarged, with mild overlapping. A few nuclei contain very small nucleoli (Papanicolaou stain, ThinPrep). This is an example of AUS-other category, Bethesda III

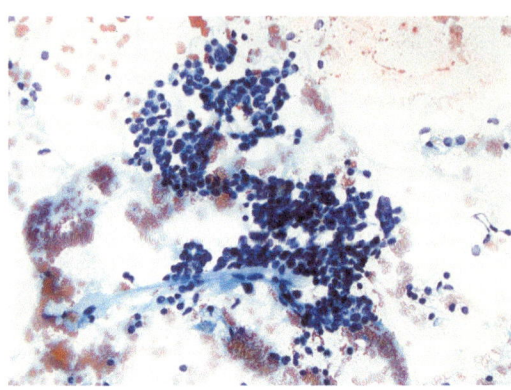

Fig. 18.11 Poorly differenced carcinoma. Malignant cells are characterized by high nuclear to cytoplasmic ratio, focal nuclear molding, and coarse chromatin (Papanicolaou stain, Smear). It is an example of malignant, Bethesda category VI

18.4.3 Cytological Diagnosis

18.4.3.1 TBS 2023

In the third edition of The Bethesda System for Reporting Thyroid Cytology [115] (TBSRTC under press), the main objectives have been

(a) to simplify the terminology;
(b) to propose a more precise assessment of the ROM;
(c) to include all the data available for a better management of the patient.

Therefore, the new items to retain are the following:

(a) The new TBSRTC has taken in account the new 2022 WHO classification of thyroid neoplasms and tried to use the same terms. In that way, all the high-grade follicular-derived carcinomas, including poorly differentiated thyroid carcinoma (PDTC) (Fig. 18.11) as well as differentiated high-grade thyroid carcinoma (DHGTC), are described and discussed

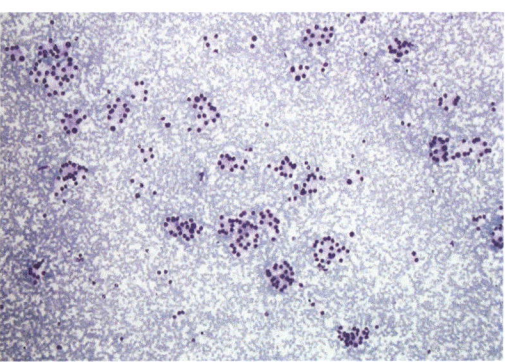

Fig. 18.12 Follicular neoplasm. A cellular smear shows numerous microfollicles with no colloid in the background (Diff-Quik, Smear). It is an example of follicular neoplasm, Bethesda category IV

(b) For the categories with the possibility to choose between two names, now only one name is recommended: "Nondiagnostic" instead of "Nondiagnostic/Unsatisfactory"; "Atypia of Undetermined Significance (AUS)" instead of category "Atypia of Undetermined Significance/Follicular Lesion of Undetermined Significance (AUS /FLUS)" and "Follicular Neoplasm (FN)" (Figs. 18.12 and 18.13a, b) instead of the category "Follicular Neoplasm / Suspicious For a Follicular Neoplasm (FN/SFN)"

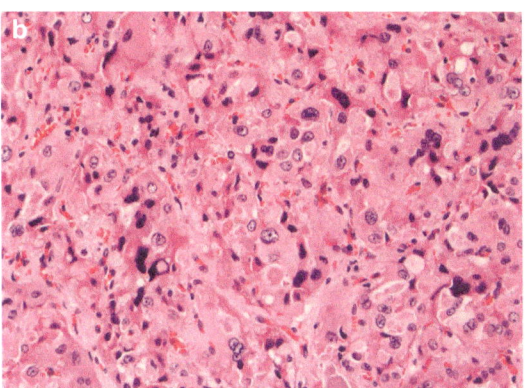

Fig. 18.13 (**a**) Follicular neoplasm, Hurthle/oncocytic type. Large and small clusters of loosely cohesive Hurthle/oncocytic cells are seen characterized by abundant finely granular cytoplasm and round, relatively uniform nuclei (Diff-Quik stain, Smear). It is an example of follicular neoplasm, Hurthle/oncocytic type, Bethesda category IV. (**b**) Hurthle/oncocytic cell adenoma consists of large cells with abundant eosinophilic cytoplasm and nuclei with variable degree of pleomorphism and anisonucleosis (H&E stain, Histology section)

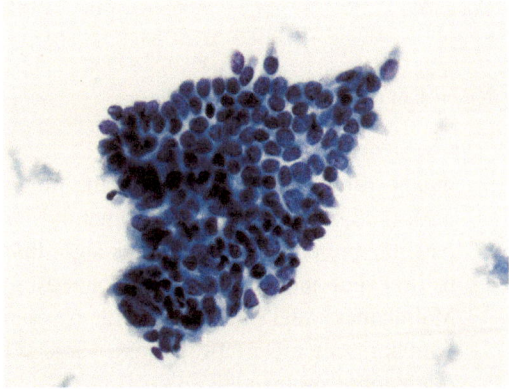

Fig. 18.14 Suspicious for papillary thyroid carcinoma A large fragment of follicular cells is seen. The nuclei are enlarged with focal overlapping and hyperchromatic chromatin. Multiple nuclei are elongated. The features are suspicious for papillary thyroid carcinoma. However, nuclear inclusions or nuclear grooves are not seen (Papanicolaou stain, ThinPrep). It is an example of suspicious for malignancy, Bethesda category V

(c) Nevertheless, the category AUS is now divided into two subcategories: AUS-nuclear atypia or AUS-other. The AUS-nuclear atypia subcategory concerns all the cases with nuclear atypia suggestive for a PTC but insufficient to propose a diagnosis of "suspicious for malignancy" (Fig. 18.14); this division into two categories is based on the ROM twofold higher for the AUS-nuclear atypia than for the AUS-other.

In the AUS-nuclear atypia subcategory are now included the following previous subcategories of the TBSRTC 2017, i.e.,

(a) Focal nuclear atypia
(b) Extensive but mild nuclear atypia
(c) Atypical cyst lining cells
(d) "Histiocytoid" cells
(e) Nuclear and architectural atypia

The AUS-other subcategory concerns all the cases with architectural changes as well as the oncocytic nodules in a context of a MNTD or of a Hashimoto thyroïditis. In the AUS-other sub category are now included the following previous subcategories of the TBSRTC 2017, i.e.,

(a) Architectural atypia
(b) Oncocytic/oncocyte atypia
(c) Atypia, not otherwise specified (NOS)
(d) Atypical lymphoid cells, rule-out lymphoma

Information concerning the ROM of each category has been widely refined taking into account all the recent studies but also the possible bias encountered for some categories especially for the AUS one since most of the surgical controls are performed on AUS nodules with some other data suspicious for malignancy and since the other AUS nodules are not surgically controlled;

therefore, the surgical control is no longer the only one "gold standard" and different ROM are proposed considering all the available data, the follow-up, the ancillary techniques, and the NIFTP entity which is a very indolent tumor.

(a) Standard and different ROM are proposed considering all the available data, the follow-up, the ancillary techniques, and the NIFTP entity which is a very indolent tumor.

(b) New chapters including clinical data, US imaging, other imaging studies if required, and ancillary testing leading to very specific "almost personalized" algorithms for the management of the patients

(c) Many new cytological pictures in order to improve our interobserver reproducibility

(d) A chapter for pediatric population since TBSRTC is now recommended for children and since the ROM is higher for them

18.4.3.2 Usual Management of the Patients Based on Cytology Exclusively

At a first glance, this table (Table 18.1) does not appear very different from the previous one published in the TBSRTC second edition; nevertheless, many footnotes have been added to this table. We are trying to summarize most of them.

(a) The ROM for the categories "Nondiagnostic" as well as "AUS" is relatively high, 13% and 22%, directly linked with the surgical bias; in these two categories, only the large or rapidly growing nodules or the nodules with high EU-TIRADS classification will undergo a surgical control. The ROM also depends on the structure of the nodule since this ROM is lower in a widely cystic nodule than in a solid one; as explained above, the ROM for the AUS is higher for the AUS-nuclear atypia as for the AUS-other. Finally, a decrease of the ROM percentage varying from 6.4% to 9.1% has been estimated for the "indeterminate categories" when excluding the NIFTP from the malignant nodules

(b) Concerning the management of the nodules, especially when different options are proposed, the choice is based on the cytological

Table 18.1 Standard management of thyroid nodules based on their diagnostic category and associated risk of malignancy

Diagnostic category	ROM Ave% (range)	Usual management
Nondiagnostic	13 (5–20)	Repeat FNA with ultrasound guidance
Benign	4 (2–7)	Clinical and sonographic follow-up
Atypia of undetermined significance	22 (13–30)	Repeat FNA, molecular testing, diagnostic lobectomy, or surveillance
Follicular neoplasm	30 (23–34)	Molecular testing, diagnostic lobectomy
Suspicious for malignancy	74 (67–83)	Molecular testing, lobectomy, or near-total thyroidectomy
Malignant	97 (97–100)	Lobectomy or near-total thyroidectomy

ROM risk of malignancy, *Ave* average

diagnosis but also correlated with the clinical data, the US appearance, and sometimes the patients' preference (see complex algorithms below). For the categories "Suspicious for Malignancy" and "Malignant," in cases of lymphoma or metastatic tumors, surgery is often not recommended

(c) In all the categories (except the AUS one), it is necessary to specify a more precise diagnosis: for instance, in the category "Benign" specify if it is a follicular nodule or a thyroïditis; in the category "Malignant" specify the type of cancer. The category "Follicular Neoplasm" includes the oncocytic variant, and this variant has to be specified (Table 18.2).

18.4.3.3 Specific Context of MNT

Benign solitary nodules and follicular nodules in a multinodular thyroid gland are not considered different from a cytological approach; the term proposed is "consistent with follicular nodular disease." This term may be used regardless of the hyperplastic or clonal nature of the nodule. The challenge is for the radiologist who has to select

Table 18.2 More specific diagnoses or cytomorphologic findings for each diagnostic category

I. Nondiagnostic
Cyst fluid only
Virtually acellular specimen
Other (obscuring blood, clotting artifact, drying artifact, etc.)
II. Benign
Consistent with follicular nodular disease (includes adenomatoid nodule, colloid nodule, etc.)
Consistent with chronic lymphocytic (Hashimoto) thyroiditis in the proper clinical context
Consistent with granulomatous (subacute) thyroiditis
Other
III. Atypia of undetermined significance
Specify if AUS-nuclear atypia or AUS-other
IV. Follicular neoplasm
Specify if oncocytic (Hürthle cell) type
V. Suspicious for malignancy
Suspicious for papillary thyroid carcinoma
Suspicious for medullary thyroid carcinoma
Suspicious for metastatic carcinoma
Suspicious for lymphoma
Other
VI. Malignant
Papillary thyroid carcinoma
High-grade follicular-derived carcinoma
Medullary thyroid carcinoma
Undifferentiated (anaplastic) carcinoma
Squamous cell carcinoma
Carcinoma with mixed features (specify)
Metastatic malignancy
Non-Hodgkin lymphoma
Other

the nodule(s) requiring an FNA, i.e., the largest one and those with suspicious ultrasonographic features

18.4.4 Ancillary Techniques

18.4.4.1 Immunocytochemistry (ICC)

Considering the thyroid nodules, it is usually accepted that immunohistochemistry is a valuable technique for some diagnosis like Medullary carcinoma (calcitonin) or metastases/lymphoma and some rare primitive tumors like a paraganglioma but not useful and therefore not recommended to better classify some follicular cells-derived indeterminate tumors into a benign or a malignant tumor. In the United States, the molecular testing is considered more discriminative (see paragraph below). Nevertheless, in Europe, where these tests are either not available or too expensive, several studies have shown that panels of antibodies, including 2 or 3 antibodies, could increase our diagnostic accuracy especially with a very high negative predictive value (NPV) of 97–99%. The highest positive predictive value (PPV) combined with a very high NPV was achieved using the following antibody combinations—CK19/HBME1/Gal 3, CK19/HBME1/TPO, and Gal 3/HBME1/TPO [116–124]. The most efficient two antibody panel achieves the same NPV as the three antibody panel seems to be HBME1/TPO. Furthermore, since the BRAF V600E antibody (clone.VE1) is also available, many studies have been published using this antibody. An unequivocal positivity is characteristic for a papillary carcinoma, excluding NIFTP and benign nodules, but is not very sensitive since around 50% of the PTC, especially the follicular variants are not BRAF V600E-mutated [125–129].

Nevertheless, the limits of ICC are first of all the occasional low number of cells available, allowing a morphological diagnosis but not additional slides for ICC. Furthermore, if ICC is a daily routine technique in most of the labs, a recent inquiry conducted under the auspices of the EFCS [95] has shown that in Europe for more than half of the laboratories (65%), ICC is performed by a non-cytology staff at a non-cytology department very often without rigorous quality assurance measures [130, 131].

18.4.4.2 Molecular Tests

In the era of personalized medicine, molecular profiling of the malignant neoplasms has gained significant attention due to diagnostic, therapeutic, predictive, or prognostic implications [132]. Thyroid carcinomas have also been an area of interest and investigated for their molecular alterations. In fact, molecular alterations in papillary thyroid carcinoma have been extensively investigated by the Cancer Genome Atlas (TCGA) and multiple research laboratories [133]. Prior studies reported high frequency (70%) of alterations in the mitogen-activated protein kinase (MAPK) signaling pathway such as point mutations of BRAF and the RAS genes, and fusion of RET and NTRK1 tyrosine kinases [133–135]. In addition, there are low frequency molecular alterations such as PIK3CA, AKT1, and PTEN, which are members of the phosphoinositide 3-kinases (PI3K) pathway [133].

Several studies have demonstrated that papillary thyroid carcinomas harboring BRAF-V600E differ from papillary thyroid carcinomas with wild-type BRAF [69, 136]. The incidence rate for BRAF is estimated to be 40–45% [7]. A study showed that 61.7% (248/402) of BRAF mutations were BRAF-V600E and 12.9% of those had additional RAS mutations. There was a strong association between BRAF and RAS mutation status at histology. BRAF-V600E mutation is associated with classic papillary thyroid carcinoma and tall cell variant, while RAS mutations are associated with follicular variant of papillary thyroid carcinoma like the follicular thyroid carcinoma [133]. Papillary thyroid carcinomas with BRAF-V600E mutations are associated with higher risk of mortality in the setting of higher risk of recurrence, extrathyroidal extension, lymph node metastasis and distant metastasis, AJCC stage IV disease, and age equal or greater than 55 years [137, 138]. Moreover, papillary thyroid carcinomas with BRAF-V600E mutations exhibit more aggressive histologic features and clinical behavior. BRAF-V600E-mutated papillary thyroid carcinomas were associated with higher rate of recurrence (8%) compared with those papillary thyroid carcinomas with wild-type BRAF (1%) [7, 139]. A meta-analysis of 2167 patients showed that BRAF-V600E mutation has a sensitivity of 65% in predicating tumor recurrence and a PPV of 25% in identifying the risk of recurrence [137]. Interestingly, BRAF-V600E mutation has a small impact on overall tumor recurrence in intrathyroid unifocal papillary microcarcinomas less than 1 cm, estimated 1% to 6%, while it is found in 30% to 67% of microcarcinomas [140, 141]. Recent studies suggest that thyroid carcinomas harboring a combination of BRAF mutation and other mutations

such as TP53, AKT1, PIK3CA, and a TERT promotor behave more aggressively and are more likely to recur [142–145]. TERT and TP53 mutations are associated with increased rate of tumor recurrence and tumor-related mortality. TERT mutations have been reported in both well-differentiated thyroid carcinomas including papillary thyroid carcinomas (7–22%), follicular thyroid carcinoma (14–17%) as well as oncocytic carcinoma and poorly differentiated carcinomas, and it is a molecular marker associated with unfavorable outcome [146–148]. Tumors harboring a combination of BRAF and TERT have an increased rate of recurrence [142]. TP53 mutation was seen in a subset of well-differentiated papillary thyroid carcinoma (3.5%) and follicular thyroid carcinoma (11%), which can be in combination with BRAF mutations [149]. Thyroid carcinomas with a combination of several mutations comprise a small fraction of all papillary thyroid carcinomas, and they are associated with an unfavorable outcome. Whole genome DNA sequencing of 402 pairs of tumor and normal thyroid revealed valuable information about thyroid carcinomas. This study suggests that age should be considered a continuous variable in risk stratification [150]. A small fraction of papillary thyroid carcinoma (4.2%, 18/402) harbors mutations in the PI3K and PPARy pathways including PTEN, AKT2/, and PAX8/PPARG. Rare cases (4/484, 0.8%) revealed fusions involving ALK including EML4/ALK, which may suggest targeted therapy with ALK inhibitors [151]. ETV6/NTRK3 and RBPMS/NTRK3 fusions were seen in a small fraction of cases (1.2%, 6/484), and they were more prevalent in radiation-induced thyroid cancers [152]. BRAF-V600E mutation is highly specific (99%); however, it is not very sensitive. Therefore, a panel of multiple genes including BRAF, NRAS, HRAS, KRAS, RET/PTC1, and RET/PTC3 and PAX8/PPARY has been proposed in order to improve the sensitivity.

The National Comprehensive Cancer Network (NCCN) guidelines suggest that diagnostic molecular testing can be utilized for further reclassification of thyroid FNA specimens with indeterminate cytology including AUS, and follicular neoplasm [153] whenever the diagnosis becomes more or less likely to be benign or malignant based on the molecular profiling of the cells. The AUS diagnostic category in the Bethesda system refers to those thyroid FNA specimens that display cytological or architectural atypia that is not qualified for higher category, and meanwhile, the atypia cannot be ignored and they cannot be diagnosed benign. Risk of malignancy associated with AUS is 6–48% [154] and 20–30% (TBSRTC third edition 2023). It was recommended to limit the AUS diagnosis to 7% [108]. Since 2017 and the second edition of TBSRTC, a 10% limit was accepted. After reviewing clinical findings and sonographic features, the AUS category requires further work-up such as repeat FNA or molecular studies prior to a clinical decision-making for diagnostic surgery or surveillance. A second opinion of reviewing slides by an expert in a center with high-volume thyroid cases may reclassify a subset of these cases with AUS diagnosis [155].

If molecular diagnostics are suggestive of malignancy, it may have impact on patient treatment plan, for instance, AUS cases with BRAF-V600E mutations may be considered for lobectomy of total thyroidectomy. Medullary thyroid carcinomas may possess diagnostic challenges on FNA cytology, and it may be reported in categories III VI in Bethesda system. Molecular diagnostics specifically for medullary thyroid carcinoma may identify these malignancies. Molecular testing either should have either a high negative predictive value (NPV) or a high positive predictive value (PPV). Two more common molecular testing in the United States are Afirma testing and Thyroseq testing, which their clinical validity, clinical utility, and analytical validity have been assessed [7, 156–158]. The Afirma Xpression Atlas (XA) (Veracyte, South San Francisco, California) was launched in 2018 [156] using RNA sequencing of material collected via FNA to detect molecular variants and fusions. In 2019, they expanded the molecular panel of the Afirma Genomic Sequencing Classifier (GSC) and XA to evaluate 593 genes including 905 variants and 235 fusions [156].

The Afirma XA is utilized for thyroid nodules with Bethesda categories V/VI (suspicious for malignancy/ malignant) diagnoses, and Afirma GSC is introduced for molecular characterization of indeterminate diagnosis (Bethesda III/IV). The Afirma GSC is a molecular panel to rule out cancer with high negative predictive value (NPV). Therefore, a thyroid nodule with indeterminate diagnosis (Bethesda III/IV) with a benign result on Afirma GSC can be considered benign and clinically observed, which reduces diagnostic surgery [156]. In a prospective, multicenter cohort study on thyroid nodules with Bethesda III/IV cytology diagnosis, Afirma GSC showed 91% sensitivity, 68% specificity, 47% PPV, 96% NPV, and 24% cancer prevalence [156, 159]. However, Afirma XA is not a cancer rule-out testing. The molecular findings of Afirma XA performed on FNA samples from thyroid nodules with cytology diagnosis of suspicious for malignancy or malignant provide valuable information which can be utilized in clinical decision-making [156]. Afirma XA testing identifies genomic variants using methods of targeted DNA and RNA sequencing [158]. The Afirma XA demonstrated high PPV with targeted DNA sequencing (74% and 88% at 5% and 20% variant allele frequency, respectively) and targeted RNA sequencing (89%). Furthermore, validating RNA fusions, Afirma XA showed 82% positive predictive agreement with targeted RNA sequencing. The patient's sample obtained via FNA (2 dedicated passes per biopsied nodule) is collected into a tube containing FNA protect (QIAGEN, Valencia, California), which is provided by Veracyte, and shipped to Veracyte with frozen bricks. The same sample is used for both Afirma GSC and Afirma XA molecular testing. The PPV is very high for some molecular alterations, for instance, it is >95% for BRAF-V600E, RET fusions, and NTRK fusions and >99% for medullary thyroid cancer [156, 160]. Noninvasive follicular thyroid neoplasm with papillary-like nuclear features (NIFTP) is a diagnosis made on histology and reported commonly as Bethesda III/IV on FNA cytology [161]. The current recommendation for a definitive diagnosis and treatment of NIFTP is surgical resection, which is usually just a lobectomy. Therefore, NIFTP is considered a true positive entity and it is imperative to pre-operatively diagnose NIFTP. Afirma testing provides a PPV for NIFTP [156, 159]. Medullary thyroid cancer (MTC) classifier predicts MTC with RET or RAS variants [160, 162, 163]. The PAX8/GLIS3 fusion is associated with hyalinizing trabecular tumor [164]. The Afirma XA may identify molecular alterations that are associated with hereditary thyroid cancers including RET (multiple endocrine neoplasia type 2), PTEN (PTEN hamartoma tumor syndrome; Cowden syndrome), APC (APC-associated polyposis; familial adenomatous polyposis), and DICER1 (DICER1 syndrome). The genetic alterations are reported in these cases, and a recommendation for genetic counseling is included in the patient report [165]. In addition to thyroid molecular panel, Afirma testing includes parathyroid classifier, which positive samples can distinguish parathyroid hyperplasia, parathyroid adenoma, or parathyroid carcinoma [156, 166].

ThyroSeq v3 is another molecular testing validated for clinical use for thyroid nodules with indeterminate diagnosis (Bethesda III/IV) on FNA specimens, and the results are reported as positive or negative[167]. ThyroSeq v3 is a DNA- and RNA-based next-generation sequencing assay that analyzes 112 genes [168] requiring minimal nucleic acid input of 2.5 ng. The ThyroSeq v3 genomic classifier analyzes a variety of genetic alterations including point mutations, gene fusions, insertions/deletions, copy number alterations, and abnormal gene expressions. The ThyroSeq v3 uses a genomic classifier to distinguish malignant lesions from benign lesions (high PPV). It has detected over 100 genetic alterations including BRAF, RAS, TERT, and DICER1 mutations, NTRK1/3, BRAF, and RET fusions, 22q loss, and gene expression alterations [168]. The ThyroSeq v3 has a 90.9% diagnostic accuracy, 98.0% sensitivity, and 81.8% specificity to distinguish cancer from a benign thyroid nodule on FNA specimens [168]. The NPV of Thyroseq v3 is significantly higher for AUS than for FN/SFN (99.5% vs 95.4%) [167]. It can correctly classify most carcinoma of follicular origin such as papillary thyroid carci-

noma, medullary thyroid carcinoma, and parathyroid lesions [168]. NIFTP is classified malignant in ThyroSeq v3 analyses considering that NIFTP diagnosis requires surgical excision.

Moreover, molecular tests that are intended for clinical use should be validated and performed in certified molecular laboratories. The cost of molecular testing is still relatively high, and there are limitations of testing results. Therefore, the patients should be consulted about potential benefits or possible uncertainties of the molecular testing. NCCN guidelines recommend that the results of all molecular markers should be interpreted with caution and in the context of clinical, radiologic, and cytologic findings for each patient [153]. NCCN Tumor Marker Task Force has indicated that molecular testing should be utilized clinically when there is strong evidence that use of the marker adequately improves patient outcome that justifies its use into routine clinical practice [7, 153]. In conclusion, there is no single molecular test that can be reliably used to rule in or rule out malignancy in thyroid nodules with indeterminate cytology.

Further studies and progress in identifying mutations of thyroid cancer are underway, which may significantly improve accurate diagnosis of cancer in thyroid nodules. Moreover, it is expected future molecular testing decreases the rate of indeterminate category of FNA cases. Currently, the cost of molecular testing is still relatively high. The molecular testing will be more utilized in the future as its costs become more affordable [7].

18.5 Management of the Patients

18.5.1 Algorithms Based on the Triplex [10]

18.5.1.1 Surgery
Management of thyroid nodules can be conservative or surgical [169–171]. Conservative options include a) watchful observation in benign nodule, nondiagnostic nodule with low-risk EU-TIRADS score, or indeterminate- or low-risk malignant nodules in select patients, b) needle drainage in

cystic nodules causing moderate structural or cosmetic concerns, and c) radiofrequency ablation, high-intensity focused ultrasound, cryoablation, ethanol sclerotic therapy, laser thermal ablation, or microwave thermal ablation in benign nodule causing structural or cosmetic concerns, and cystic nodule causing structural or cosmetic concerns.

Recommendations for TT or Lobectomy

Surgical management of the thyroid nodules includes lobectomy (hemithyroidectomy) and near-total thyroidectomy.

Lobectomy is considered in (a) large benign nodules (>4 cm) causing structural or cosmetic concerns, (b) nodules with indeterminate cytology (e.g., Bethesda IV, follicular neoplasm, Hurthle cell neoplasm) or abnormal molecular findings, and (c) intrathyroid papillary thyroid carcinoma of 1–4 cm in diameter, without aggressive histology or abnormal lymph adenopathy [7, 172].

Total thyroidectomy is indicated if (a) benign bilateral multinodular goiter causing structural or cosmetic concerns, (b) bilateral confirmed or suspected carcinoma, and (c) unilateral confirmed or suspected large carcinomas or metastasis to lymph nodes, for which [^{131}I] is planned as adjuvant therapy, and (d) poorly differentiated, anaplastic, or medullary carcinoma.

18.6 Role of the Histological Diagnosis in Case of Cancer (TNM; Prognostic; HGDTC; PDC; Subtypes; Molecular Tests)

18.6.1 WHO Classifications

18.6.1.1 THE Fourth Edition 2017

Histologic evaluation of lobectomy or thyroidectomy specimen establishes the diagnosis and provides information that are essential for risk stratification of cancer and post-surgical patient management [7]. AJCC/UICC TNM staging is recommended for all patients with differentiated thyroid cancer. TNM postoperative staging is used for thyroid cancer to provide prognostic information and risk stratification, which facilitates communication among healthcare professionals [7]. The pathology report must provide characteristics required for AJCC/UICC TNM staging including tumor histology, size, number of nodules (unifocal vs multifocal), presence of extrathyroidal extension, presence of vascular invasion, and number of invaded vessels, status of margin, total number of lymph nodes examined and involved with tumor, size of the largest metastatic focus to the lymph node, and presence or absence of extranodal extension of the metastatic tumor. Histologic features of tumor provide information about the tumor prognosis. Histologically, papillary thyroid carcinoma and follicular carcinoma are well-differentiated. Encapsulated follicular variant of papillary thyroid carcinoma without invasion and minimally invasive follicular thyroid carcinoma are associated with more favorable outcomes. Encapsulated follicular variant of papillary thyroid carcinoma more commonly harbors RAS mutations, whereas non-encapsulated follicular variant of papillary thyroid carcinoma frequently harbors BRAF-600E mutations [173]. Other histologic variants of papillary thyroid carcinoma such as tall cell, columnar cell, and hobnails, widely invasive follicular thyroid carcinoma, and poorly differentiated carcinoma are associated with less favorable outcomes [7]. The tall cell variant is characterized by predominance of tall cells (height at least three times of width) comprising >50% of tumor volume. The columnar cell variant shows prominent nuclear stratification. Hobnail variant displays hobnail cells with bulging of apical cell surface and apically placed nuclei. These variants of tall cell, columnar, and hobnail cells more frequently harbor BRAF-V600 E mutation [174–177]. The solid variant and diffuse sclerosing variant may be associated with less favorable outcome [7, 178]. Moreover, histologic variants of thyroid carcinoma associated familial syndromes should be identified and reported such as cribriform-morular variant of papillary thyroid carcinoma associated with familial adenomatous polyposis (FAP) or follicular or papillary thyroid carcinoma associated with PTEN-hamartoma tumor syndrome [7]. Poorly differentiated carcinoma, used to be called insular carcinoma, is an aggressive thyroid tumor with less favorable outcome. Diagnostic features by Turin proposal are: (1) solid, trabecular, and insular growth pattern, (2) lack of nuclear features of papillary thyroid carcinoma, (3) convoluted nuclei, (4) necrosis, and (5) three or more mitoses per 10 high-power fields [179].

Anaplastic thyroid carcinoma is a rare, aggressive tumor with very poor prognosis [180, 181]. The diagnosis of anaplastic thyroid carcinoma is based on clinical, imaging, and histomorphologic findings. Anaplastic thyroid carcinoma is suspected when there is a large, rapidly growing neck mass in an old patient. FNA and core biopsy are the initial diagnostic approaches. A cell block or core biopsy provides additional material for immunohistochemistry [182, 183]. The diagnosis of anaplastic thyroid carcinoma can be challenging due to a wide spectrum of morphologic features including spindle cell or sarcomatoid, giant cell, and squamoid cells, presence of abundant mixed chronic inflammatory cells, and necrosis. Rhabdoid, angiomatoid, lymphoepithelial, and paucicellular are rare variants[180, 184]. However, it is essential to render a definitive diagnosis prior to surgical resection of the tumor [180]. All anaplastic thyroid carcinomas are characterized by infiltration of adjacent soft tissue, blood vessel, and lymphatic invasion. Atypical mitotic figures are common, and Ki-67 immunostain shows high proliferation index (at least 30%) [180, 184]. The tumor cells are immunoreactive for PAX-8 in 40–60% of anaplastic thyroid carcinomas [185]. However, lack of TTF-1 and TGB expression is expected in most cases [184]. BRAF immunostain expression is detected in 40–70% of anaplastic thyroid carcinomas [184]. It is of paramount importance to differentiate anaplastic thyroid carcinoma from other malignant neoplasms due to significant differences in their prognoses and management. The most important differential diagnoses are poorly differentiated thyroid carcinoma, primary squamous cell carcinoma of the thyroid, medullary thyroid carcinoma, metastatic spindle cell melanoma, and lymphoma (large B-cell lymphoma and anaplastic large cell lymphoma). There are growing evidence that anaplastic thyroid carcinoma can arise in patients with a history of differentiated (e.g., tall cell variant of papillary thyroid carcinoma, follicular carcinoma, Hurthle cell carcinoma), or poorly differentiated thyroid carcinoma [186]. BRAF mutation should be assessed in all cases of anaplastic thyroid carcinoma by immunostaining and molecular testing [180]. Overall, molecular alterations are more commonly detected in anaplastic thyroid carcinoma than other thyroid carcinomas [187]. TP53 (65%) and TERT (65%) are the most common mutated genes followed by BRAF (41%) and RAS (27%) mutations [187]. A subset of anaplastic thyroid carcinomas (11–28%) express programmed death ligand-1 (PD-L1) in the tumor cells or the inflammatory cells in the background, making them potentially benefit of immunotherapies [188]. Molecular profiling should be performed at the time of diagnosis in order to detect mutations amenable to FDA-approved targeted therapies [180].

Medullary thyroid carcinoma is a rare malignancy of thyroid, derived from C cells. It can be sporadic or familial. A diagnosis of medullary thyroid carcinoma on FNA is followed by ultrasound of neck, measurement of serum levels of calcitonin, and CEA and DNA analysis for RET germline mutation [162]. Detection of RET germline mutation triggers additional testing for hereditary medullary thyroid carcinoma. All patients with MEN2A and MEN2B harbor germline RET mutations. In patients with sporadic medullary thyroid carcinoma, nearly half of them have somatic RET mutations and RAS mutations are detected in 18–80% of patients without somatic RET mutations [162]. Medullary thyroid carcinomas often overexpress vascular endothelial growth factor (VEGF) receptors (VEGFR-1 and VEGFR-2) in both tumor cells and in the supporting vascular endothelium [189]. Interestingly, many agents such as tyrosine kinase inhibitors (TKIs) that target VEGF-2 kinase also target RET kinase. This observation and subsequent clinical trials resulted in approval of the U.S. Food and Drug Administration (FDA) and the European Medicines Agency (EMA) of two orally administered TKIs, vandetanib and cabozantinib in patients with advanced medullary thyroid carcinoma [190, 191]. For both patients with sporadic and hereditary medullary thyroid carcinoma, total thyroidectomy and cervical lymph node dissection is the standard treatment, depending on serum calcitonin level and ultrasound findings [162]. The histologic features of medullary thyroid carcinoma are very variable. The classical pattern is the most common pattern, comprised sheets and solid nests of round to polygonal and elongated cells with ill-defined cell borders. The stroma can be vascular and fibrotic containing amyloid in almost half of the cases. Other histologic variants are spindle cell, pseudopapillary, paraganglioma-like, angio-sarcoma-like, and oncocytic follicular variant [192]. Medullary thyroid carcinomas express calcitonin and CEA, the most important diagnostic markers, in the absence of thyroglobulin. Medullary thyroid carcinomas also express CK7, CK18, TTF-1, and chromogranin A [162]. Insulinoma-associated protein 1 (INSM-1) is a reliable marker for detection of neuroendocrine differentiation of medullary thyroid carcinoma. Nuclear expression of INSM-1 in medullary thyroid carcinoma can discriminate medullary thyroid carcinoma from other primary and secondary thyroid carcinomas [193, 194]. Congo red stain highlights amyloid.

18.6.1.2 The Fifth Edition 2022

This new WHO classification of thyroid neoplasms has undergone changes that reflect our better understanding of their cell of origin, morphologic features, molecular profile, and biological behavior [3, 195]. The current classification emphasizes the value of biomarkers that may assist with a diagnosis and provide prognostic information [3]. Here is summary of the major changes [3]:

1. Follicular neoplasms are divided into benign, low risk, and malignant.
   (A) Benign follicular tumors include follicular adenoma, variants of adenoma including those with papillary architecture, and oncocytic adenomas. For the first time, the term thyroid follicular nodular disease (FND) is used to describe the multifocal hyperplastic/neoplastic lesions that commonly occur in the clinical setting of multinodular goiter.
   (B) Low-risk follicular tumors include non-invasive follicular thyroid neoplasm with papillary-like nuclear features (NIFTP), thyroid tumors of uncertain malignant potential, and hyalinizing trabecular tumor.
   (C) Malignant follicular cell-derived neoplasms are re-classified based on molecular profiles and aggressiveness. Papillary thyroid carcinomas with many morphological variants represent the BRAF-like malignancies, while follicular thyroid carcinoma and invasive encapsulated follicular variant of papillary thyroid carcinoma represent the RAS-like malignancies. In the new classification, papillary microcarcinomas are not considered a subtype of papillary thyroid carcinoma and it requires subtyping similar to their counterparts that exceed 1.0 cm. Cribriform-morular thyroid carcinoma is not classified as a subtype of papillary thyroid carcinoma anymore.
2. The term "Hurthle cell" is discouraged and "oncocyte" is the term used. Oncocytic carcinoma is recognized as a distinct entity that it refers to oncocytic follicular cell–derived neoplasms (composed of >75% oncocytic cells) that lack characteristic nuclear features of papillary thyroid carcinoma (also known as oncocytic PTCs) and high-grade features (necrosis and $\geq$5 mitoses per 2 mm^2).
3. Both the traditional poorly differentiated carcinoma and high-grade differentiated thyroid carcinomas are classified as high-grade follicular cell-derived malignancies since both are characterized by increased mitotic activity, tumor necrosis, and similar clinical behavior without anaplastic histology.

4. Squamous cell carcinoma of the thyroid is now recognized as a subtype of anaplastic carcinoma, while anaplastic thyroid carcinoma remains the most undifferenced form.

5. Medullary thyroid carcinomas derived from thyroid C cells retain their separate section. Based on mitotic count (mitoses per 2 mm^2), tumor necrosis, and Ki67 proliferation index, a grading system for medullary thyroid carcinoma is introduced.

6. Mixed tumor malignancies of both follicular cell-derived and C cells are classified in a separate section.

7. Unusual neoplasms of the thyroid have been placed into new section based on their cytogenesis. For instance. salivary gland–type carcinomas of the thyroid including mucoepidermoid carcinoma and secretory carcinoma of the salivary gland type are now in one section or thymomas, thymic carcinomas and spindle epithelial tumor with thymus-like elements are classified as "thymic tumors within the thyroid." There are few neoplasms with uncertain cell lineage, and they are listed as such, sclerosing mucoepidermoid carcinoma with eosinophilia and cribriform-morular thyroid carcinoma.

8. An important new addition is thyroblastoma, which is an unusual embryonal tumor associated with DICER1 mutations.

9. Mesenchymal and stromal tumors, hematolymphoid neoplasms, germ cell tumors, and metastatic malignancies are discussed separately as in all the WHO books in the fifth edition.

10. Thyroid cancer staging in TNM (T=tumor, N=nodes, M= metastasis) system has undergone significant changes due to better understanding of thyroid cancers [196]. The age cut-off from 45 to 55 years of age and excluding microscopic extrathyroid extension from T3 are two major elements in lowering the tumor staging in a large number of patients with thyroid cancer [181, 197, 198]. The definition of nodal metastasis has been modified for neck lymph nodes. Metastasis to the central lymph nodes (levels VI and VII) is staged as N1a and to the lateral neck is staged as N1b. Anaplastic thyroid carcinoma was considered

T4 in the previous edition. It is now classified using the same definition for T category as differentiated thyroid cancer [196].

In 2009, the ATA proposed a three-tiered clinic-pathologic risk stratification system that classified the patients as having low risk, intermediate risk, and/or high risk for recurrence. Based on histological diagnosis, the ATA initial risk stratification system was modified in 2015 including additional prognostic variables such as the extent of lymph node involvement, the degree of vascular invasion, and mutational status [7].

ATA low risk of recurrence is defined as:

(A) Papillary thyroid carcinoma with:
   1. no local or distant metastasis
   2. no tumor invasion of loco-regional tissues or structures
   3. all macroscopic tumor has been resected
   4. no features of aggressive histology (e.g., tall cell, hobnail variant, and columnar cell)
   5. no vascular invasion
   6. if radioactive iodine (^{131}I) is given, there are no RAI-avid metastatic foci outside the thyroid bed on the first post-treatment whole-body RAI scan
   7. Clinical N0 or less than or equal 5 pathologic N1 micrometastases (less than 0.2 cm in greatest dimension)
(B) Intrathyroid, encapsulated follicular variant of papillary thyroid carcinoma
(C) Intrathyroid well-differentiated follicular thyroid carcinoma with capsular invasion and no or minimal (<4 foci) vascular invasion
(D) Intrathyroid, papillary thyroid microcarcinoma, unifocal or multifocal, including BRAF -V600E mutated (if known)

ATA intermediate risk:

(A) Microscopic invasion of tumor into the perithyroidal soft tissue
(B) Aggressive histology (e.g., tall cell, hobnail variant, and columnar cell)
(C) Papillary thyroid carcinoma with vascular invasion

(D) RAI-avid metastatic foci outside the thyroid bed on the first post-treatment whole-body RAI scan

(E) Clinical N1 or >5 pathologic N1 with all metastatic lymph nodes (0.2–3 cm in greatest dimension)

(F) Multifocal papillary microcarcinoma with minor extrathyroid extension, and mutated BRAF-V600E

ATA high risk:

(A) Macroscopic (gross) invasion of tumor into the perithyroidal soft tissue

(B) Incomplete tumor resection

(C) Distant metastasis

(D) Postoperative serum TGB suggestive of distant metastasis

(E) Pathologic N1 with any metastatic lymph node greater or equal to 3 cm in greatest dimension

(F) Follicular thyroid carcinoma with extensive vascular invasion (>4 foci of vascular invasion)

18.7 Main Message: The Diagnosis Has to Be Made Before the Decision of Surgery (or Follow-Up)

Main Messages

2022: The new WHO classification including new entities: NIFTP, differentiated high-grade follicular carcinoma (DHGFC), and a molecular histopathological approach of the tumors leading to a better histomolecular prognosis and tumor characterization

2023: The new TBSRTC taking in account all the clinical, radiological, histological, and molecular data for a precise ROM assessment and a personalized management of the patients

A diagnosis as accurate as possible has to be done before the decision of follow-up or of surgery for a thyroid nodule following very detailed American and European algorithms

References

1. Ali SZ, Cibas EC, editors. The Bethesda system for reporting thyroid cytopathology. Definitions, criteria, and explanatory notes. 1st ed. New York: Wiley; 2010.
2. Ali SZ, Cibas ES. The Bethesda system for reporting thyroid cytopathology. Definitions, criteria, and explanatory notes. 2nd ed. New York: Wiley; 2010.
3. Baloch ZW, Asa SL, Barletta JA, Ghossein RA, Juhlin CC, Jung CK, LiVolsi VA, Papotti MG, Sobrinho-Simoes M, Tallini G, Mete O. Overview of the 2022 WHO classification of thyroid neoplasms. Endocr Pathol. 2022;33(1):27–63.
4. Cross P, Chandra A, Giles T, et al. Guidance on the reporting of thyroid cytology specimens. 2nd ed. London/UK: Royal College of Pathologists; 2016.
5. Fadda G, Basolo F, Bondi A, Bussolati G, Crescenzi A, Nappi O, Nardi F, Papotti M, Taddei G, Palombini L, S.-I.I.C.W. Group. Cytological classification of thyroid nodules. Proposal of the SIAPEC-IAP Italian Consensus Working Group. Pathologica. 2010;102(5):405–8.
6. Kakudo K, Kameyama K, Hirokawa M, Katoh R, Nakamura H. Subclassification of follicular neoplasms recommended by the Japan thyroid association reporting system of thyroid cytology. Int J Endocrinol. 2015;2015:938305.
7. Haugen BR, Alexander EK, Bible KC, Doherty GM, Mandel SJ, Nikiforov YE, Pacini F, Randolph GW, Sawka AM, Schlumberger M, Schuff KG, Sherman SI, Sosa JA, Steward DL, Tuttle RM, Wartofsky L. 2015 American Thyroid Association Management guidelines for adult patients with thyroid nodules and differentiated thyroid cancer: The American Thyroid Association guidelines task force on thyroid nodules and differentiated thyroid cancer. Thyroid. 2016;26(1):1–133.
8. Singer PA, Cooper DS, Daniels GH, Ladenson PW, Greenspan FS, Levy EG, Braverman LE, Clark OH, McDougall IR, Ain KV, Dorfman SG. Treatment guidelines for patients with thyroid nodules and well-differentiated thyroid cancer. American Thyroid Association, Arch Intern Med. 1996;156(19):2165–72.
9. Cooper DS, Doherty GM, Haugen BR, Kloos RT, Lee SL, Mandel SJ, Mazzaferri EL, McIver B, Sherman SI, Tuttle RM, T. American Thyroid Association Guidelines, Management guidelines for patients with thyroid nodules and differentiated thyroid cancer. Thyroid. 2006;16(2):109–42.
10. Borson-Chazot F, Buffet C, Decaussin-Petrucci M, Cao CD, Drui D, Leboulleux S, Leenhardt L, Menegaux F, Pattou F, Lussey-Lepoutre C, Consensus S-A-S. SFE-AFCE-SFMN 2022 consensus on the management of thyroid nodules: synthesis and algorithms. Ann Endocrinol (Paris). 2022;83(6):440–53.
11. Russ G, Leboulleux S, Leenhardt L, Hegedus L. Thyroid incidentalomas: epidemiology, risk strat-

ification with ultrasound and workup. Eur Thyroid J. 2014;3(3):154–63.

12. Shimura H, Haraguchi K, Hiejima Y, Fukunari N, Fujimoto Y, Katagiri M, Koyanagi N, Kurita T, Miyakawa M, Miyamoto Y, Suzuki N, Suzuki S, Kanbe M, Kato Y, Murakami T, Tohno E, Tsunoda-Shimizu H, Yamada K, Ueno E, Kobayashi K, Kobayashi T, Yokozawa T, Kitaoka M. Distinct diagnostic criteria for ultrasonographic examination of papillary thyroid carcinoma: a multicenter study. Thyroid. 2005;15(3):251–8.

13. Chammas MC, Gerhard R, de Oliveira IR, Widman A, de Barros N, Durazzo M, Ferraz A, Cerri GG. Thyroid nodules: evaluation with power Doppler and duplex Doppler ultrasound. Otolaryngol Head Neck Surg. 2005;132(6):874–82.

14. Flint PW. Cummings otolaryngology: head and neck surgery. 7th ed. Philadelphia: Elsevier; 2021.

15. Hall TL, Layfield LJ, Philippe A, Rosenthal DL. Sources of diagnostic error in fine needle aspiration of the thyroid. Cancer. 1989;63(4):718–25.

16. Alexander EK, Heering JP, Benson CB, Frates MC, Doubilet PM, Cibas ES, Marqusee E. Assessment of nondiagnostic ultrasound-guided fine needle aspirations of thyroid nodules. J Clin Endocrinol Metab. 2002;87(11):4924–7.

17. Smith-Bindman R, Lebda P, Feldstein VA, Sellami D, Goldstein RB, Brasic N, Jin C, Kornak J. Risk of thyroid cancer based on thyroid ultrasound imaging characteristics: results of a population-based study. JAMA Intern Med. 2013;173(19):1788–96.

18. Brito JP, Gionfriddo MR, Al Nofal A, Boehmer KR, Leppin AL, Reading C, Callstrom M, Elraiyah TA, Prokop LJ, Stan MN, Murad MH, Morris JC, Montori VM. The accuracy of thyroid nodule ultrasound to predict thyroid cancer: systematic review and meta-analysis. J Clin Endocrinol Metab. 2014;99(4):1253–63.

19. Langer JE, Agarwal R, Zhuang H, Huang SS, Mandel SJ. Correlation of findings from iodine 123 scan and ultrasonography in the recommendation for thyroid fine-needle aspiration biopsy. Endocr Pract. 2011;17(5):699–706.

20. Alexander EK, Marqusee E, Orcutt J, Benson CB, Frates MC, Doubilet PM, Cibas ES, Atri A. Thyroid nodule shape and prediction of malignancy. Thyroid. 2004;14(11):953–8.

21. Jun P, Chow LC, Jeffrey RB. The sonographic features of papillary thyroid carcinomas: pictorial essay. Ultrasound Q. 2005;21(1):39–45.

22. Russ G, Bonnema SJ, Erdogan MF, Durante C, Ngu R, Leenhardt L. European Thyroid Association guidelines for ultrasound malignancy risk stratification of thyroid nodules in adults: The EU-TIRADS. Eur Thyroid J. 2017;6(5):225–37.

23. Marqusee E, Benson CB, Frates MC, Doubilet PM, Larsen PR, Cibas ES, Mandel SJ. Usefulness of ultrasonography in the management of nodular thyroid disease. Ann Intern Med. 2000;133(9):696–700.

24. Hagag P, Strauss S, Weiss M. Role of ultrasound-guided fine-needle aspiration biopsy in evaluation of nonpalpable thyroid nodules. Thyroid. 1998;8(11):989–95.

25. Ross DS. Nonpalpable thyroid nodules—managing an epidemic. J Clin Endocrinol Metab. 2002;87(5):1938–40.

26. Burman KD, Wartofsky L. Thyroid nodules. N Engl J Med. 2016;374(13):1294–5.

27. Papini E, Guglielmi R, Bianchini A, Crescenzi A, Taccogna S, Nardi F, Panunzi C, Rinaldi R, Toscano V, Pacella CM. Risk of malignancy in nonpalpable thyroid nodules: predictive value of ultrasound and color-Doppler features. J Clin Endocrinol Metab. 2002;87(5):1941–6.

28. Bonavita JA, Mayo J, Babb J, Bennett G, Oweity T, Macari M, Yee J. Pattern recognition of benign nodules at ultrasound of the thyroid: which nodules can be left alone? AJR Am J Roentgenol. 2009;193(1):207–13.

29. Kim EK, Park CS, Chung WY, Oh KK, Kim DI, Lee JT, Yoo HS. New sonographic criteria for recommending fine-needle aspiration biopsy of nonpalpable solid nodules of the thyroid. AJR Am J Roentgenol. 2002;178(3):687–91.

30. Remonti LR, Kramer CK, Leitao CB, Pinto LC, Gross JL. Thyroid ultrasound features and risk of carcinoma: a systematic review and meta-analysis of observational studies. Thyroid. 2015;25(5):538–50.

31. Campanella P, Ianni F, Rota CA, Corsello SM, Pontecorvi A. Quantification of cancer risk of each clinical and ultrasonographic suspicious feature of thyroid nodules: a systematic review and meta-analysis. Eur J Endocrinol. 2014;170(5):R203–11.

32. Horvath E, Majlis S, Rossi R, Franco C, Niedmann JP, Castro A, Dominguez M. An ultrasonogram reporting system for thyroid nodules stratifying cancer risk for clinical management. J Clin Endocrinol Metab. 2009;94(5):1748–51.

33. Russ G, Royer B, Bigorgne C, Rouxel A, Bienvenu-Perrard M, Leenhardt L. Prospective evaluation of thyroid imaging reporting and data system on 4550 nodules with and without elastography. Eur J Endocrinol. 2013;168(5):649–55.

34. Wei X, Li Y, Zhang S, Gao M. Meta-analysis of thyroid imaging reporting and data system in the ultrasonographic diagnosis of 10,437 thyroid nodules. Head Neck. 2016;38(2):309–15.

35. Yoon JH, Lee HS, Kim EK, Moon HJ, Kwak JY. Malignancy risk stratification of thyroid nodules: comparison between the thyroid imaging reporting and data system and the 2014 American Thyroid Association Management Guidelines. Radiology. 2016;278(3):917–24.

36. Su HK, Dos Reis LL, Lupo MA, Milas M, Orloff LA, Langer JE, Brett EM, Kazam E, Lee SL, Minkowitz G, Alpert EH, Dewey EH, Urken ML. Striving toward standardization of reporting of ultrasound features of thyroid nodules and lymph nodes: a

multidisciplinary consensus statement. Thyroid. 2014;24(9):1341–9.

37. Andrioli M, Carzaniga C, Persani L. Standardized Ultrasound Report for Thyroid Nodules: The Endocrinologist's Viewpoint. Eur Thyroid J. 2013;2(1):37–48.

38. Grant EG, Tessler FN, Hoang JK, Langer JE, Beland MD, Berland LL, Cronan JJ, Desser TS, Frates MC, Hamper UM, Middleton WD, Reading CC, Scoutt LM, Stavros AT, Teefey SA. Thyroid ultrasound reporting lexicon: white paper of the ACR Thyroid Imaging, Reporting and Data System (TIRADS) Committee. J Am Coll Radiol. 2015;12(12 Pt A):1272–9.

39. Kwak JY, Han KH, Yoon JH, Moon HJ, Son EJ, Park SH, Jung HK, Choi JS, Kim BM, Kim EK. Thyroid imaging reporting and data system for US features of nodules: a step in establishing better stratification of cancer risk. Radiology. 2011;260(3):892–9.

40. Virmani V, Hammond I. Sonographic patterns of benign thyroid nodules: verification at our institution. AJR Am J Roentgenol. 2011;196(4):891–5.

41. Machens A, Holzhausen HJ, Dralle H. The prognostic value of primary tumor size in papillary and follicular thyroid carcinoma. Cancer. 2005;103(11):2269–73.

42. Yoon JH, Kim EK, Hong SW, Kwak JY, Kim MJ. Sonographic features of the follicular variant of papillary thyroid carcinoma. J Ultrasound Med. 2008;27(10):1431–7.

43. Yoon JH, Kwon HJ, Kim EK, Moon HJ, Kwak JY. The follicular variant of papillary thyroid carcinoma: characteristics of preoperative ultrasonography and cytology. Ultrasonography. 2016;35(1):47–54.

44. Sillery JC, Reading CC, Charboneau JW, Henrichsen TL, Hay ID, Mandrekar JN. Thyroid follicular carcinoma: sonographic features of 50 cases. AJR Am J Roentgenol. 2010;194(1):44–51.

45. Russ G, Bigorgne C, Royer B, Rouxel A, Bienvenu-Perrard M. The Thyroid Imaging Reporting and Data System (TIRADS) for ultrasound of the thyroid. J Radiol. 2011;92(7-8):701–13.

46. Na DG, Baek JH, Sung JY, Kim JH, Kim JK, Choi YJ, Seo H. Thyroid imaging reporting and data system risk stratification of thyroid nodules: categorization based on solidity and echogenicity. Thyroid. 2016;26(4):562–72.

47. Brito JP, Ito Y, Miyauchi A, Tuttle RM. A clinical framework to facilitate risk stratification when considering an active surveillance alternative to immediate biopsy and surgery in papillary microcarcinoma. Thyroid. 2016;26(1):144–9.

48. Leenhardt L, Erdogan MF, Hegedus L, Mandel SJ, Paschke R, Rago T, Russ G. 2013 European thyroid association guidelines for cervical ultrasound scan and ultrasound-guided techniques in the postoperative management of patients with thyroid cancer. Eur Thyroid J. 2013;2(3):147–59.

49. Rim JH, Chong S, Ryu HS, Chung BM, Ahn HS. Feasibility study of ultrasonographic criteria for microscopic and macroscopic extra-thyroidal extension based on thyroid capsular continuity and tumor contour in patients with papillary thyroid carcinomas. Ultrasound Med Biol. 2016;42(10):2391–400.

50. Kwak JY, Kim EK, Youk JH, Kim MJ, Son EJ, Choi SH, Oh KK. Extrathyroid extension of well-differentiated papillary thyroid microcarcinoma on US. Thyroid. 2008;18(6):609–14.

51. Moon SJ, Kim DW, Kim SJ, Ha TK, Park HK, Jung SJ. Ultrasound assessment of degrees of extrathyroidal extension in papillary thyroid microcarcinoma. Endocr Pract. 2014;20(10):1037–43.

52. Lee CY, Kim SJ, Ko KR, Chung KW, Lee JH. Predictive factors for extrathyroidal extension of papillary thyroid carcinoma based on preoperative sonography. J Ultrasound Med. 2014;33(2):231–8.

53. Kim BM, Kim MJ, Kim EK, Kwak JY, Hong SW, Son EJ, Kim KH. Sonographic differentiation of thyroid nodules with eggshell calcifications. J Ultrasound Med. 2008;27(10):1425–30.

54. Na DG, Kim DS, Kim SJ, Ryoo JW, Jung SL. Thyroid nodules with isolated macrocalcification: malignancy risk and diagnostic efficacy of fine-needle aspiration and core needle biopsy. Ultrasonography. 2016;35(3):212–9.

55. Malhi H, Beland MD, Cen SY, Allgood E, Daley K, Martin SE, Cronan JJ, Grant EG. Echogenic foci in thyroid nodules: significance of posterior acoustic artifacts. AJR Am J Roentgenol. 2014;203(6):1310–6.

56. Beland MD, Kwon L, Delellis RA, Cronan JJ, Grant EG. Nonshadowing echogenic foci in thyroid nodules: are certain appearances enough to avoid thyroid biopsy? J Ultrasound Med. 2011;30(6):753–60.

57. Chammas MC, de Araujo Filho VJ, Moyses RA, Brescia MD, Mulatti GC, Brandao LG, Cerri GG, Ferraz AR. Predictive value for malignancy in the finding of microcalcifications on ultrasonography of thyroid nodules. Head Neck. 2008;30(9):1206–10.

58. Zhang JZ, Hu B. Sonographic features of thyroid follicular carcinoma in comparison with thyroid follicular adenoma. J Ultrasound Med. 2014;33(2):221–7.

59. Lyshchik A, Moses R, Barnes SL, Higashi T, Asato R, Miga MI, Gore JC, Fleischer AC. Quantitative analysis of tumor vascularity in benign and malignant solid thyroid nodules. J Ultrasound Med. 2007;26(6):837–46.

60. Moon HJ, Kwak JY, Kim MJ, Son EJ, Kim EK. Can vascularity at power Doppler US help predict thyroid malignancy? Radiology. 2010;255(1):260–9.

61. Rago T, Santini F, Scutari M, Pinchera A, Vitti P. Elastography: new developments in ultrasound for predicting malignancy in thyroid nodules. J Clin Endocrinol Metab. 2007;92(8):2917–22.

62. Asteria C, Giovanardi A, Pizzocaro A, Cozzaglio L, Morabito A, Somalvico F, Zoppo A. US-elastography in the differential diagnosis of benign and malignant thyroid nodules. Thyroid. 2008;18(5):523–31.

63. Sun J, Cai J, Wang X. Real-time ultrasound elastography for differentiation of benign and malignant thyroid nodules: a meta-analysis. J Ultrasound Med. 2014;33(3):495–502.

64. Sebag F, Vaillant-Lombard J, Berbis J, Griset V, Henry JF, Petit P, Oliver C. Shear wave elastography: a new ultrasound imaging mode for the differential diagnosis of benign and malignant thyroid nodules. J Clin Endocrinol Metab. 2010;95(12):5281–8.

65. Bhatia KS, Tong CS, Cho CC, Yuen EH, Lee YY, Ahuja AT. Shear wave elastography of thyroid nodules in routine clinical practice: preliminary observations and utility for detecting malignancy. Eur Radiol. 2012;22(11):2397–406.

66. Singh Ospina N, Maraka S, Espinosa DeYcaza A, O'Keeffe D, Brito JP, Gionfriddo MR, Castro MR, Morris JC, Erwin P, Montori VM. Diagnostic accuracy of thyroid nodule growth to predict malignancy in thyroid nodules with benign cytology: systematic review and meta-analysis. Clin Endocrinol (Oxf). 2016;85(1):122–31.

67. Som PM, Curtin HD. Head and neck imaging. St. Louis: Mosby; 2011.

68. Paschke R, Cantara S, Crescenzi A, Jarzab B, Musholt TJ, Sobrinho Simoes M. European Thyroid Association guidelines regarding thyroid nodule molecular fine-needle aspiration cytology diagnostics. Eur Thyroid J. 2017;6(3):115–29.

69. Haugen BR, Sawka AM, Alexander EK, Bible KC, Caturegli P, Doherty GM, Mandel SJ, Morris JC, Nassar A, Pacini F, Schlumberger M, Schuff K, Sherman SI, Somerset H, Sosa JA, Steward DL, Wartofsky L, Williams MD. American Thyroid Association guidelines on the management of thyroid nodules and differentiated thyroid cancer task force review and recommendation on the proposed renaming of encapsulated follicular variant papillary thyroid carcinoma without invasion to noninvasive follicular thyroid neoplasm with papillary-like nuclear features. Thyroid. 2017;27(4):481–3.

70. Singh Ospina N, Iniguez-Ariza NM, Castro MR. Thyroid nodules: diagnostic evaluation based on thyroid cancer risk assessment. BMJ. 2020;368:l6670.

71. Cibas ES, Ali SZ. The 2017 Bethesda system for reporting thyroid cytopathology. Thyroid. 2017;27(11):1341–6.

72. Bongiovanni M, Bellevicine C, Troncone G, Sykiotis GP. Approach to cytological indeterminate thyroid nodules. Gland Surg. 2019;8(Suppl 2):S98–S104.

73. Wang CC, Friedman L, Kennedy GC, Wang H, Kebebew E, Steward DL, Zeiger MA, Westra WH, Wang Y, Khanafshar E, Fellegara G, Rosai J, Livolsi V, Lanman RB. A large multicenter correlation study of thyroid nodule cytopathology and histopathology. Thyroid. 2011;21(3):243–51.

74. Campenni A, Siracusa M, Ruggeri RM, Laudicella R, Pignata SA, Baldari S, Giovanella L. Differentiating malignant from benign thyroid nodules with indeterminate cytology by (99m)Tc-MIBI scan: a new quantitative method for improving diagnostic accuracy. Sci Rep. 2017;7(1):6147.

75. Riazi A, Kalantarhormozi M, Nabipour I, Eghbali SS, Farzaneh M, Javadi H, Ostovar A, Seyedabadi M, Assadi M. Technetium-99m methoxyisobutyl-isonitrile scintigraphy in the assessment of cold thyroid nodules: is it time to change the approach to the management of cold thyroid nodules? Nucl Med Commun. 2014;35(1):51–7.

76. Piccardo A, Puntoni M, Treglia G, Foppiani L, Bertagna F, Paparo F, Massollo M, Dib B, Paone G, Arlandini A, Catrambone U, Casazza S, Pastorino A, Cabria M, Giovanella L. Thyroid nodules with indeterminate cytology: prospective comparison between 18F-FDG-PET/CT, multiparametric neck ultrasonography, 99mTc-MIBI scintigraphy and histology. Eur J Endocrinol. 2016;174(5):693–703.

77. Benderradji H, Beron A, Wemeau JL, Carnaille B, Delcroix L, Do Cao C, Baillet C, Huglo D, Lion G, Boury S, Cussac JF, Caiazzo R, Pattou F, Leteurtre E, Vantyghem MC, Ladsous M. Quantitative dual isotope (123)iodine/(99m)Tc-MIBI scintigraphy: a new approach to rule out malignancy in thyroid nodules. Ann Endocrinol (Paris). 2021;82(2):83–91.

78. Soelberg KK, Bonnema SJ, Brix TH, Hegedus L. Risk of malignancy in thyroid incidentalomas detected by 18F-fluorodeoxyglucose positron emission tomography: a systematic review. Thyroid. 2012;22(9):918–25.

79. Nishimori H, Tabah R, Hickeson M, How J. Incidental thyroid "PETomas": clinical significance and novel description of the self-resolving variant of focal FDG-PET thyroid uptake. Can J Surg. 2011;54(2):83–8.

80. Chen W, Parsons M, Torigian DA, Zhuang H, Alavi A. Evaluation of thyroid FDG uptake incidentally identified on FDG-PET/CT imaging. Nucl Med Commun. 2009;30(3):240–4.

81. Poller DN, Megadmi H, Ward MJA, Trimboli P. Hurthle cells on fine-needle aspiration cytology are important for risk assessment of focally PET/CT FDG. Avid Thyroid Nodules, Cancers (Basel). 2020;12(12):3544.

82. Filie AC, Asa SL, Geisinger KR, Logani S, Merino M, Nikiforov YE, Clark DP. Utilization of ancillary studies in thyroid fine needle aspirates: a synopsis of the National Cancer Institute Thyroid Fine Needle Aspiration State of the Science Conference. Diagn Cytopathol. 2008;36(6):438–41.

83. Rollins SD. Teaching FNA techniques and ultrasound guided FNA. Cancer Cytopathol. 2019;127(1):7–8.

84. Decaussin-Petrucci M, Albarel F, Leteurtre E, Borson-Chazot F, Cochand Priollet B, SFE-AFCE-SFMN. Consensus on the management of thyroid nodules: recommendations in thyroid cytology: from technique to interpretation. Ann Endocrinol (Paris). 2022;83(6):389–94.

85. Bode-Lesniewska B, Cochand-Priollet B, Straccia P, Fadda G, Bongiovanni M. Management of thyroid cytological material, preanalytical procedures and bio-banking. Cytopathology. 2019;30(1):7–16.

86. Torous VF, Chen Y, VanderLaan PA. Comparison of plasma-thrombin, HistoGel, and CellGel cell block preparation methods with paired ThinPrep slides in the setting of mediastinal granulomatous disease. J Am Soc Cytopathol. 2019;8(2):52–60.

87. Rekhtman N, Buonocore DJ, Rudomina D, Friedlander M, Dsouza C, Aggarwal G, Arcila M, Edelweiss M, Lin O. Novel modification of histogel-based cell block preparation method: improved sufficiency for molecular studies. Arch Pathol Lab Med. 2018;142(4):529–35.

88. Shidham VB, Layfield LJ. Cell-blocks and immuno-histochemistry. CytoJournal. 2021;18:2.

89. Shidham VB. Specimen-specific cell-blocking approaches. CytoJournal. 2020;17:28.

90. Krogerus L, Kholova I. Cell block in cytological diagnostics: review of preparatory techniques. Acta Cytol. 2018;62(4):237–43.

91. Kim K, Bae JS, Kim JS, Jung SL, Jung CK. Diagnostic performance of thyroid core needle biopsy using the revised reporting system: comparison with fine needle aspiration cytology. Endocrinol Metab. 2022;37(1):159–69.

92. Nasrollah N, Trimboli P, Guidobaldi L, Cicciarella Modica DD, Ventura C, Ramacciato G, Taccogna S, Romanelli F, Valabrega S, Crescenzi A. Thin core biopsy should help to discriminate thyroid nodules cytologically classified as indeterminate. A new sampling technique. Endocrine. 2013;43(3):659–65.

93. Chen BT, Jain AB, Dagis A, Chu P, Vora L, Maghami E, Salehian B. Comparison of the efficacy and safety of ultrasound-guided core needle biopsy versus fine-needle aspiration for evaluating thyroid nodules. Endocr Pract. 2015;21(2):128–35.

94. Schmitt F, Cochand-Priollet B, Toetsch M, Davidson B, Bondi A, Vielh P. Immunocytochemistry in Europe: results of the European Federation of Cytology Societies (EFCS) inquiry. Cytopathology. 2011;22(4):238–42.

95. Srebotnik Kirbis I, Rodrigues Roque R, Bongiovanni M, Strojan Flezar M, Cochand-Priollet B. Immunocytochemistry practices in European cytopathology laboratories-Review of European Federation of Cytology Societies (EFCS) online survey results with best practice recommendations. Cancer Cytopathol. 2020;128(10):757–66.

96. Pantanowitz L, Thompson LDR, Jing X, Rossi ED. Is thyroid core needle biopsy a valid compliment to fine-needle aspiration? J Am Soc Cytopathol. 2020;9(5):383–8.

97. Hakala T, Kholova I, Sand J, Saaristo R, Kellokumpu-Lehtinen P. A core needle biopsy provides more malignancy-specific results than fine-needle aspiration biopsy in thyroid nodules suspicious for malignancy. J Clin Pathol. 2013;66(12):1046–50.

98. Trimboli P, Guidobaldi L, Amendola S, Nasrollah N, Romanelli F, Attanasio D, Ramacciato G, Saggiorato E, Valabrega S, Crescenzi A. Galectin-3 and HBME-1 improve the accuracy of core biopsy

in indeterminate thyroid nodules. Endocrine. 2016;52(1):39–45.

99. Baloch ZW, Tam D, Langer J, Mandel S, LiVolsi VA, Gupta PK. Ultrasound-guided fine-needle aspiration biopsy of the thyroid: role of on-site assessment and multiple cytologic preparations. Diagn Cytopathol. 2000;23(6):425–9.

100. Sabel MS, Haque D, Velasco JM, Staren ED. Use of ultrasound-guided fine needle aspiration biopsy in the management of thyroid disease. Am Surg. 1998;64(8):738–41; discussion 741–2.

101. Cochand-Priollet B, Guillausseau PJ, Chagnon S, Hoang C, Guillausseau-Scholer C, Chanson P, Dahan H, Warnet A, Huy PTTB, Valleur P. The diagnostic value of fine-needle aspiration biopsy under ultrasonography in nonfunctional thyroid nodules: a prospective study comparing cytologic and histologic findings. Am J Med. 1994;97(2):152–7.

102. Gharib H, Papini E, Garber JR, Duick DS, Harrell RM, Hegedus L, Paschke R, Valcavi R, Vitti P. A.A.A.T.F.o.T. Nodules, American Association of Clinical Endocrinologists, American College of Endocrinology, and Associazione Medici Endocrinologi Medical Guidelines for Clinical Practice for the Diagnosis and Management of Thyroid Nodules—2016 Update. Endocr Pract. 2016;22(5):622–39.

103. Muri R, Trippel M, Borner U, Weidner S, Trepp R. The impact of rapid on-site evaluation on the quality and diagnostic value of thyroid nodule fine-needle aspirations. Thyroid. 2022;32(6):667–74.

104. Houlton JJ, Sun GH, Fernandez N, Zhai QJ, Lucas F, Steward DL. Thyroid fine-needle aspiration: does case volume affect diagnostic yield and interpretation? Arch Otolaryngol Head Neck Surg. 2011;137(11):1136–9.

105. Michael CW, Kameyama K, Kitagawa W, Azar N. Rapid on-site evaluation (ROSE) for fine needle aspiration of thyroid: benefits, challenges and innovative solutions. Gland Surg. 2020;9(5):1708–15.

106. Nasuti JF, Gupta PK, Baloch ZW. Diagnostic value and cost-effectiveness of on-site evaluation of fine-needle aspiration specimens: review of 5,688 cases. Diagn Cytopathol. 2002;27(1):1–4.

107. Jo VY, Stelow EB, Dustin SM, Hanley KZ. Malignancy risk for fine-needle aspiration of thyroid lesions according to the Bethesda System for Reporting Thyroid Cytopathology. Am J Clin Pathol. 2010;134(3):450–6.

108. Nayar R, Krane JF, Renshaw AA. Atypia of undetermined significance/follicular lesion of undetermined significance. In: Ali SZ, Cibas ES, editors. The Bethesda system for reporting thyroid cytopathology. Springer; 2010. p. 37–49.

109. Pastorello RG, Destefani C, Pinto PH, Credidio CH, Reis RX, Rodrigues TA, Toledo MC, De Brot L, Costa FA, do Nascimento AG, Pinto CAL, Saieg MA. The impact of rapid on-site evaluation on thyroid fine-needle aspiration biopsy: a 2-year cancer

center institutional experience. Cancer Cytopathol. 2018;126(10):846–52.

110. Layfield LJ, Cibas ES, Gharib H, Mandel SJ. Thyroid aspiration cytology: current status. CA Cancer J Clin. 2009;59(2):99–110.

111. Geramizadeh B, Bos-Hagh S, Maleki Z. Cytomorphologic, imaging, molecular findings, and outcome in thyroid follicular lesion of undetermined significance/atypical cell of undetermined significance (AUS/FLUS): a mini-review. Acta Cytol. 2019;63(1):1–9.

112. Houdek D, Cooke-Hubley S, Puttagunta L, Morrish D. Factors affecting thyroid nodule fine needle aspiration non-diagnostic rates: a retrospective association study of 1975 thyroid biopsies. Thyroid Res. 2021;14(1):2.

113. Olson MT, Tatsas AD, Ali SZ. Cytotechnologist-attended on-site adequacy evaluation of thyroid fine-needle aspiration: comparison with cytopathologists and correlation with the final interpretation. Am J Clin Pathol. 2012;138(1):90–5.

114. Schmidt RL, Walker BS, Cohen MB. When is rapid on-site evaluation cost-effective for fine-needle aspiration biopsy? PLoS One. 2015;10(8):e0135466.

115. Ali SZ, VanderLaan PA, editors. The Bethesda system for reporting thyroid cytopathology. definitions, criteria, and explanatory notes. 3rd ed. New York: Wiley; 2023. In press.

116. Cochand-Priollet B, Dahan H, Laloi-Michelin M, Polivka M, Saada M, Herman P, Guillausseau PJ, Hamzi L, Pote N, Sarfati E, Wassef M, Combe H, Raulic-Raimond D, Chedin P, Medeau V, Casanova D, Kania R. Immunocytochemistry with cytokeratin 19 and anti-human mesothelial cell antibody (HBME1) increases the diagnostic accuracy of thyroid fine-needle aspirations: preliminary report of 150 liquid-based fine-needle aspirations with histological control. Thyroid. 2011;21(10):1067–73.

117. Dunderovic D, Lipkovski JM, Boricic I, Soldatovic I, Bozic V, Cvejic D, Tatic S. Defining the value of CD56, CK19, Galectin 3 and HBME-1 in diagnosis of follicular cell derived lesions of thyroid with systematic review of literature. Diagn Pathol. 2015;10:196.

118. Das DK, Al-Waheeb SK, George SS, Haji BI, Mallik MK. Contribution of immunocytochemical stainings for galectin-3, CD44, and HBME1 to fine-needle aspiration cytology diagnosis of papillary thyroid carcinoma. Diagn Cytopathol. 2014;42(6):498–505.

119. De Micco C, Kopp F, Vassko V, Grino M. In situ hybridization and immunohistochemistry study of thyroid peroxidase expression in thyroid tumors. Thyroid. 2000;10(2):109–15.

120. Lacoste-Collin L, d'Aure D, Berard E, Rouquette I, Delisle MB, Courtade-Saidi M. Improvement of the cytological diagnostic accuracy of follicular thyroid lesions by the use of the Ki-67 proliferative index in addition to cytokeratin-19 and HBME-1 immuno-

markers: a study of 61 cases of liquid-based FNA cytology with histological controls. Cytopathology. 2014;25(3):160–9.

121. Margari N, Giovannopoulos I, Pouliakis A, Mastorakis E, Gouloumi AR, Panayiotides IG, Karakitsos P. Application of Immunocytochemistry on Cell Block Sections for the Investigation of Thyroid Lesions. Acta Cytol. 2018;62(2):137–44.

122. Ratour J, Polivka M, Dahan H, Hamzi L, Kania R, Dumuis ML, Cohen R, Laloi-Michelin M, Cochand-Priollet B. Diagnosis of follicular lesions of undetermined significance in fine-needle aspirations of thyroid nodules. J Thyroid Res. 2013;2013:250347.

123. Fadda G, Rossi ED, Raffaelli M, Pontecorvi A, Sioletic S, Morassi F, Lombardi CP, Zannoni GF, Rindi G. Follicular thyroid neoplasms can be classified as low- and high-risk according to HBME-1 and Galectin-3 expression on liquid-based fine-needle cytology. Eur J Endocrinol. 2011;165(3):447–53.

124. Arcolia V, Journe F, Renaud F, Leteurtre E, Gabius HJ, Remmelink M, Saussez S. Combination of galectin-3, CK19 and HBME-1 immunostaining improves the diagnosis of thyroid cancer. Oncol Lett. 2017;14(4):4183–9.

125. Rossi ED, Bizzarro T, Martini M, Capodimonti S, Fadda G, Larocca LM, Schmitt F. Morphological parameters able to predict BRAF(V600E) -mutated malignancies on thyroid fine-needle aspiration cytology: Our institutional experience. Cancer Cytopathol. 2014;122(12):883–91.

126. Pusztaszeri MP, Krane JF, Faquin WC. BRAF testing and thyroid FNA. Cancer Cytopathol. 2015;123(12):689–95.

127. Poller DN, Glaysher S, Agrawal A, Caldera S, Kim D, Yiangou C. BRAF V600 co-testing in thyroid FNA cytology: short-term experience in a large cancer centre in the UK. J Clin Pathol. 2014;67(8):684–9.

128. Rossi ED, Martini M, Capodimonti S, Cenci T, Bilotta M, Pierconti F, Pontecorvi A, Lombardi CP, Fadda G, Larocca LM. Morphology combined with ancillary techniques: An algorithm approach for thyroid nodules. Cytopathology. 2018;29(5):418–27.

129. Smith AL, Williams MD, Stewart J, Wang WL, Krishnamurthy S, Cabanillas ME, Roy-Chowdhuri S. Utility of the BRAF p.V600E immunoperoxidase stain in FNA direct smears and cell block preparations from patients with thyroid carcinoma. Cancer Cytopathol. 2018;126(6):406–13.

130. Fischer AH, Schwartz MR, Moriarty AT, Wilbur DC, Souers R, Fatheree L, Booth CN, Clayton AC, Kurtyz DF, Padmanabhan V, Crothers BA. Immunohistochemistry practices of cytopathology laboratories: a survey of participants in the College of American Pathologists Nongynecologic Cytopathology Education Program. Arch Pathol Lab Med. 2014;138(9):1167–72.

131. Kirbis IS, Maxwell P, Flezar MS, Miller K, Ibrahim M. External quality control for immunocytochemis-

try on cytology samples: a review of UK NEQAS ICC (cytology module) results. Cytopathology. 2011;22(4):230–7.

132. Febbo PG, Ladanyi M, Aldape KD, De Marzo AM, Hammond ME, Hayes DF, Iafrate AJ, Kelley RK, Marcucci G, Ogino S, Pao W, Sgroi DC, Birkeland ML. NCCN Task Force report: evaluating the clinical utility of tumor markers in oncology. J Natl Compr Canc Netw. 2011;9(Suppl 5):S1–32. quiz S33

133. Agrawal N. Cancer Genome Atlas Research, Integrated genomic characterization of papillary thyroid carcinoma. Cell. 2014;159(3):676–90.

134. Cohen Y, Xing M, Mambo E, Guo Z, Wu G, Trink B, Beller U, Westra WH, Ladenson PW, Sidransky D. BRAF mutation in papillary thyroid carcinoma. J Natl Cancer Inst. 2003;95(8):625–7.

135. Xing M. Molecular pathogenesis and mechanisms of thyroid cancer. Nat Rev Cancer. 2013;13(3):184–99.

136. Xing M, Alzahrani AS, Carson KA, Viola D, Elisei R, Bendlova B, Yip L, Mian C, Vianello F, Tuttle RM, Robenshtok E, Fagin JA, Puxeddu E, Fugazzola L, Czarniecka A, Jarzab B, O'Neill CJ, Sywak MS, Lam AK, Riesco-Eizaguirre G, Santisteban P, Nakayama H, Tufano RP, Pai SI, Zeiger MA, Westra WH, Clark DP, Clifton-Bligh R, Sidransky D, Ladenson PW, Sykorova V. Association between BRAF V600E mutation and mortality in patients with papillary thyroid cancer. JAMA. 2013;309(14):1493–501.

137. Tufano RP, Teixeira GV, Bishop J, Carson KA, Xing M. BRAF mutation in papillary thyroid cancer and its value in tailoring initial treatment: a systematic review and meta-analysis. Medicine (Baltimore). 2012;91(5):274–86.

138. Xing M, Westra WH, Tufano RP, Cohen Y, Rosenbaum E, Rhoden KJ, Carson KA, Vasko V, Larin A, Tallini G, Tolaney S, Holt EH, Hui P, Umbricht CB, Basaria S, Ewertz M, Tufaro AP, Califano JA, Ringel MD, Zeiger MA, Sidransky D, Ladenson PW. BRAF mutation predicts a poorer clinical prognosis for papillary thyroid cancer. J Clin Endocrinol Metab. 2005;90(12):6373–9.

139. Elisei R, Viola D, Torregrossa L, Giannini R, Romei C, Ugolini C, Molinaro E, Agate L, Biagini A, Lupi C, Valerio L, Materazzi G, Miccoli P, Piaggi P, Pinchera A, Vitti P, Basolo F. The BRAF(V600E) mutation is an independent, poor prognostic factor for the outcome of patients with low-risk intrathyroid papillary thyroid carcinoma: single-institution results from a large cohort study. J Clin Endocrinol Metab. 2012;97(12):4390–8.

140. Mazzaferri EL. Long-term outcome of patients with differentiated thyroid carcinoma: effect of therapy. Endocr Pract. 2000;6(6):469–76.

141. Kim TY, Kim WB, Rhee YS, Song JY, Kim JM, Gong G, Lee S, Kim SY, Kim SC, Hong SJ, Shong YK. The BRAF mutation is useful for prediction of clinical recurrence in low-risk patients with conventional papillary thyroid carcinoma. Clin Endocrinol (Oxf). 2006;65(3):364–8.

142. Xing M, Liu R, Liu X, Murugan AK, Zhu G, Zeiger MA, Pai S, Bishop J. BRAF V600E and TERT promoter mutations cooperatively identify the most aggressive papillary thyroid cancer with highest recurrence. J Clin Oncol. 2014;32(25):2718–26.

143. Nikiforova MN, Kimura ET, Gandhi M, Biddinger PW, Knauf JA, Basolo F, Zhu Z, Giannini R, Salvatore G, Fusco A, Santoro M, Fagin JA, Nikiforov YE. BRAF mutations in thyroid tumors are restricted to papillary carcinomas and anaplastic or poorly differentiated carcinomas arising from papillary carcinomas. J Clin Endocrinol Metab. 2003;88(11):5399–404.

144. Ricarte-Filho JC, Ryder M, Chitale DA, Rivera M, Heguy A, Ladanyi M, Janakiraman M, Solit D, Knauf JA, Tuttle RM, Ghossein RA, Fagin JA. Mutational profile of advanced primary and metastatic radioactive iodine-refractory thyroid cancers reveals distinct pathogenetic roles for BRAF, PIK3CA, and AKT1. Cancer Res. 2009;69(11):4885–93.

145. Henderson YC, Shellenberger TD, Williams MD, El-Naggar AK, Fredrick MJ, Cieply KM, Clayman GL. High rate of BRAF and RET/PTC dual mutations associated with recurrent papillary thyroid carcinoma. Clin Cancer Res. 2009;15(2):485–91.

146. Melo M, da Rocha AG, Vinagre J, Batista R, Peixoto J, Tavares C, Celestino R, Almeida A, Salgado C, Eloy C, Castro P, Prazeres H, Lima J, Amaro T, Lobo C, Martins MJ, Moura M, Cavaco B, Leite V, Cameselle-Teijeiro JM, Carrilho F, Carvalheiro M, Maximo V, Sobrinho-Simoes M, Soares P. TERT promoter mutations are a major indicator of poor outcome in differentiated thyroid carcinomas. J Clin Endocrinol Metab. 2014;99(5):E754–65.

147. Liu X, Bishop J, Shan Y, Pai S, Liu D, Murugan AK, Sun H, El-Naggar AK, Xing M. Highly prevalent TERT promoter mutations in aggressive thyroid cancers. Endocr Relat Cancer. 2013;20(4):603–10.

148. Landa I, Ganly I, Chan TA, Mitsutake N, Matsuse M, Ibrahimpasic T, Ghossein RA, Fagin JA. Frequent somatic TERT promoter mutations in thyroid cancer: higher prevalence in advanced forms of the disease. J Clin Endocrinol Metab. 2013;98(9):E1562–6.

149. Nikiforova MN, Wald AI, Roy S, Durso MB, Nikiforov YE. Targeted next-generation sequencing panel (ThyroSeq) for detection of mutations in thyroid cancer. J Clin Endocrinol Metab. 2013;98(11):E1852–60.

150. Bischoff LA, Curry J, Ahmed I, Pribitkin E, Miller JL. Is above age 45 appropriate for upstaging well-differentiated papillary thyroid cancer? Endocr Pract. 2013;19(6):995–7.

151. Kelly LM, Barila G, Liu P, Evdokimova VN, Trivedi S, Panebianco F, Gandhi M, Carty SE, Hodak SP, Luo J, Dacic S, Yu YP, Nikiforova MN, Ferris RL, Altschuler DL, Nikiforov YE. Identification of the transforming STRN-ALK fusion as a potential therapeutic target in the aggressive forms of thyroid cancer. Proc Natl Acad Sci U S A. 2014;111(11):4233–8.

152. Ricarte-Filho JC, Li S, Garcia-Rendueles ME, Montero-Conde C, Voza F, Knauf JA, Heguy A, Viale A, Bogdanova T, Thomas GA, Mason CE, Fagin JA. Identification of kinase fusion oncogenes in post-Chernobyl radiation-induced thyroid cancers. J Clin Invest. 2013;123(11):4935–44.

153. NCCN. https://www.nccn.org/professionals/physician_gls/pdf/thyroid.pdf

154. Bongiovanni M, Crippa S, Baloch Z, Piana S, Spitale A, Pagni F, Mazzucchelli L, Di Bella C, Faquin W. Comparison of 5-tiered and 6-tiered diagnostic systems for the reporting of thyroid cytopathology: a multi-institutional study. Cancer Cytopathol. 2012;120(2):117–25.

155. Davidov T, Trooskin SZ, Shanker BA, Yip D, Eng O, Crystal J, Hu J, Chernyavsky VS, Deen MF, May M, Artymyshyn RL. Routine second-opinion cytopathology review of thyroid fine needle aspiration biopsies reduces diagnostic thyroidectomy. Surgery. 2010;148(6):1294–9. discussion 1299-301

156. Krane JF, Cibas ES, Endo M, Marqusee E, Hu MI, Nasr CE, Waguespack SG, Wirth LJ, Kloos RT. The Afirma Xpression Atlas for thyroid nodules and thyroid cancer metastases: insights to inform clinical decision-making from a fine-needle aspiration sample. Cancer Cytopathol. 2020;128(7):452–9.

157. Teutsch SM, Bradley LA, Palomaki GE, Haddow JE, Piper M, Calonge N, Dotson WD, Douglas MP, Berg AO, E.W. Group. The Evaluation of Genomic Applications in Practice and Prevention (EGAPP) Initiative: methods of the EGAPP Working Group. Genet Med. 2009;11(1):3–14.

158. Angell TE, Wirth LJ, Cabanillas ME, Shindo ML, Cibas ES, Babiarz JE, Hao Y, Kim SY, Walsh PS, Huang J, Kloos RT, Kennedy GC, Waguespack SG. Analytical and clinical validation of expressed variants and fusions from the whole transcriptome of thyroid FNA samples. Front Endocrinol (Lausanne). 2019;10:612.

159. Patel KN, Angell TE, Babiarz J, Barth NM, Blevins T, Duh QY, Ghossein RA, Harrell RM, Huang J, Kennedy GC, Kim SY, Kloos RT, LiVolsi VA, Randolph GW, Sadow PM, Shanik MH, Sosa JA, Traweek ST, Walsh PS, Whitney D, Yeh MW, Ladenson PW. Performance of a genomic sequencing classifier for the preoperative diagnosis of cytologically indeterminate thyroid nodules. JAMA Surg. 2018;153(9):817–24.

160. Randolph G, Angell T, Babiarz J, Barth N, Blevins T, Duh Q. Clinical validation of the afirma genomic sequencing classifier for medullary thyroid cancer (Clinical Oral Abstract 29). Thyroid. 2017;27(S1):A105.

161. Geramizadeh B, Maleki Z. Non-invasive follicular thyroid neoplasm with papillary-like nuclearfeatures (NIFTP): a review and update. Endocrine. 2019;64(3):433–40.

162. Wells SA Jr, Asa SL, Dralle H, Elisei R, Evans DB, Gagel RF, Lee N, Machens A, Moley JF, Pacini F, Raue F, Frank-Raue K, Robinson B, Rosenthal MS, Santoro M, Schlumberger M, Shah M, Waguespack SG, C. American Thyroid Association guidelines task force on medullary thyroid, revised american thyroid association guidelines for the management of medullary thyroid carcinoma. Thyroid. 2015;25(6):567–610.

163. Wirth LJ, Tahara M, Robinson B, Francis S, Brose MS, Habra MA, Newbold K, Kiyota N, Dutcus CE, Mathias E, Guo M, Sherman SI, Schlumberger M. Treatment-emergent hypertension and efficacy in the phase 3 Study of (E7080) lenvatinib in differentiated cancer of the thyroid (SELECT). Cancer. 2018;124(11):2365–72.

164. Marchio C, Da Cruz Paula A, Gularte-Merida R, Basili T, Brandes A, da Silva EM, Silveira C, Ferrando L, Metovic J, Maletta F, Annaratone L, Pareja F, Rubin BP, Hoschar AP, De Rosa G, La Rosa S, Bongiovanni M, Purgina B, Piana S, Volante M, Weigelt B, Reis-Filho JS, Papotti M. PAX8-GLIS3 gene fusion is a pathognomonic genetic alteration of hyalinizing trabecular tumors of the thyroid. Mod Pathol. 2019;32(12):1734–43.

165. Green RC, Berg JS, Grody WW, Kalia SS, Korf BR, Martin CL, McGuire AL, Nussbaum RL, O'Daniel JM, Ormond KE, Rehm HL, Watson MS, Williams MS, Biesecker LG, G. American College of Medical, Genomics. ACMG recommendations for reporting of incidental findings in clinical exome and genome sequencing. Genet Med. 2013;15(7):565–74.

166. Sosa J, Angell T, Barbiarz J, Barth N, Blevins T, Duh Q, Ghossein R, Harrell R, Huang J, Imtiaz U. Clinical validation of the afirma genomic sequencing parathyroid classifier (poster 168). Thyroid. 2017;27(S1):A50–1.

167. Desai D, Lepe M, Baloch ZW, Mandel SJ. ThyroSeq v3 for Bethesda III and IV: An institutional experience. Cancer Cytopathol. 2021;129(2):164–70.

168. Nikiforova MN, Mercurio S, Wald AI, Barbi de Moura M, Callenberg K, Santana-Santos L, Gooding WE, Yip L, Ferris RL, Nikiforov YE. Analytical performance of the ThyroSeq v3 genomic classifier for cancer diagnosis in thyroid nodules. Cancer. 2018;124(8):1682–90.

169. Leboulleux S, Lamartina L, Lecornet Sokol E, Menegaux F, Leenhardt L, Russ G, SFE-AFCE-SFMN. Consensus on the management of thyroid nodules: follow-up: how and how long? Ann Endocrinol (Paris). 2022;83(6):407–14.

170. Ben Hamou A, Ghanassia E, Muller A, Ladsous M, Paladino NC, Brunaud L, Leenhardt L, Russ G. SFE-AFCE-SFMN 2022 consensus on the management of thyroid nodules: thermal ablation. Ann Endocrinol (Paris). 2022;83(6):423–30.

171. Menegaux F, Baud G, Chereau N, Christou N, Deguelte S, Frey S, Guerin C, Marciniak C, Paladino NC, Brunaud L, Caiazzo R, Donatini G, Gaujoux S, Goudet P, Hartl D, Lifante JC, Mathonnet M, Mirallie E, Najah H, Sebag F, Tresallet C, Pattou

F. SFE-AFCE-SFMN 2022 consensus on the management of thyroid nodules: Surgical treatment. Ann Endocrinol (Paris). 2022;83(6):415–22.

172. Haddad RI, Bischoff L, Ball D, Bernet V, Blomain E, Busaidy NL, Campbell M, Dickson P, Duh QY, Ehya H, Goldner WS, Guo T, Haymart M, Holt S, Hunt JP, Iagaru A, Kandeel F, Lamonica DM, Mandel S, Markovina S, McIver B, Raeburn CD, Rezaee R, Ridge JA, Roth MY, Scheri RP, Shah JP, Sipos JA, Sippel R, Sturgeon C, Wang TN, Wirth LJ, Wong RJ, Yeh M, Cassara CJ, Darlow S. Thyroid Carcinoma, Version 2.2022, NCCN Clinical Practice Guidelines in Oncology. J Natl Compr Canc Netw. 2022;20(8):925–51.

173. Rivera M, Ricarte-Filho J, Knauf J, Shaha A, Tuttle M, Fagin JA, Ghossein RA. Molecular genotyping of papillary thyroid carcinoma follicular variant according to its histological subtypes (encapsulated vs infiltrative) reveals distinct BRAF and RAS mutation patterns. Mod Pathol. 2010;23(9):1191–200.

174. Ghossein RA, Leboeuf R, Patel KN, Rivera M, Katabi N, Carlson DL, Tallini G, Shaha A, Singh B, Tuttle RM. Tall cell variant of papillary thyroid carcinoma without extrathyroid extension: biologic behavior and clinical implications. Thyroid. 2007;17(7):655–61.

175. Chen JH, Faquin WC, Lloyd RV, Nose V. Clinicopathological and molecular characterization of nine cases of columnar cell variant of papillary thyroid carcinoma. Mod Pathol. 2011;24(5):739–49.

176. Lubitz CC, Economopoulos KP, Pawlak AC, Lynch K, Dias-Santagata D, Faquin WC, Sadow PM. Hobnail variant of papillary thyroid carcinoma: an institutional case series and molecular profile. Thyroid. 2014;24(6):958–65.

177. Asioli S, Erickson LA, Sebo TJ, Zhang J, Jin L, Thompson GB, Lloyd RV. Papillary thyroid carcinoma with prominent hobnail features: a new aggressive variant of moderately differentiated papillary carcinoma. A clinicopathologic, immunohistochemical, and molecular study of eight cases. Am J Surg Pathol. 2010;34(1):44–52.

178. Nikiforov YE, Erickson LA, Nikiforova MN, Caudill CM, Lloyd RV. Solid variant of papillary thyroid carcinoma: incidence, clinical-pathologic characteristics, molecular analysis, and biologic behavior. Am J Surg Pathol. 2001;25(12):1478–84.

179. Volante M, Landolfi S, Chiusa L, Palestini N, Motta M, Codegone A, Torchio B, Papotti MG. Poorly differentiated carcinomas of the thyroid with trabecular, insular, and solid patterns: a clinicopathologic study of 183 patients. Cancer. 2004;100(5):950–7.

180. Bible KC, Kebebew E, Brierley J, Brito JP, Cabanillas ME, Clark TJ Jr, Di Cristofano A, Foote R, Giordano T, Kasperbauer J, Newbold K, Nikiforov YE, Randolph G, Rosenthal MS, Sawka AM, Shah M, Shaha A, Smallridge R, Wong-Clark CK. 2021 American Thyroid Association guidelines for management of patients with anaplastic thyroid cancer. Thyroid. 2021;31(3):337–86.

181. Filetti S, Durante C, Hartl D, Leboulleux S, Locati LD, Newbold K, Papotti MG, Berruti A, E.G.C.E.a. clinicalguidelines@esmo.org. Thyroid cancer: ESMO Clinical Practice Guidelines for diagnosis, treatment and follow-updagger. Ann Oncol. 2019;30(12):1856–83.

182. Greenblatt DY, Woltman T, Harter J, Starling J, Mack E, Chen H. Fine-needle aspiration optimizes surgical management in patients with thyroid cancer. Ann Surg Oncol. 2006;13(6):859–63.

183. Giard RW, Hermans J. Use and accuracy of fine-needle aspiration cytology in histologically proven thyroid carcinoma: an audit using a national nathology database. Cancer. 2000;90(6):330–4.

184. Deeken-Draisey A, Yang GY, Gao J, Alexiev BA. Anaplastic thyroid carcinoma: an epidemiologic, histologic, immunohistochemical, and molecular single-institution study. Hum Pathol. 2018;82:140–8.

185. Bishop JA, Sharma R, Westra WH. PAX8 immunostaining of anaplastic thyroid carcinoma: a reliable means of discerning thyroid origin for undifferentiated tumors of the head and neck. Hum Pathol. 2011;42(12):1873–7.

186. Wiseman SM, Loree TR, Rigual NR, Hicks WL Jr, Douglas WG, Anderson GR, Stoler DL. Anaplastic transformation of thyroid cancer: review of clinical, pathologic, and molecular evidence provides new insights into disease biology and future therapy. Head Neck. 2003;25(8):662–70.

187. Pozdeyev N, Gay LM, Sokol ES, Hartmaier R, Deaver KE, Davis S, French JD, Borre PV, LaBarbera DV, Tan AC, Schweppe RE, Fishbein L, Ross JS, Haugen BR, Bowles DW. Genetic analysis of 779 advanced differentiated and anaplastic thyroid cancers. Clin Cancer Res. 2018;24(13):3059–68.

188. Zwaenepoel K, Jacobs J, De Meulenaere A, Silence K, Smits E, Siozopoulou V, Hauben E, Rolfo C, Rottey S, Pauwels P. CD70 and PD-L1 in anaplastic thyroid cancer—promising targets for immunotherapy. Histopathology. 2017;71(3):357–65.

189. Capp C, Wajner SM, Siqueira DR, Brasil BA, Meurer L, Maia AL. Increased expression of vascular endothelial growth factor and its receptors, VEGFR-1 and VEGFR-2, in medullary thyroid carcinoma. Thyroid. 2010;20(8):863–71.

190. Wells SA Jr, Gosnell JE, Gagel RF, Moley J, Pfister D, Sosa JA, Skinner M, Krebs A, Vasselli J, Schlumberger M. Vandetanib for the treatment of patients with locally advanced or metastatic hereditary medullary thyroid cancer. J Clin Oncol. 2010;28(5):767–72.

191. Elisei R, Schlumberger MJ, Muller SP, Schoffski P, Brose MS, Shah MH, Licitra L, Jarzab B, Medvedev V, Kreissl MC, Niederle B, Cohen EE, Wirth LJ, Ali H, Hessel C, Yaron Y, Ball D, Nelkin B, Sherman SI. Cabozantinib in progressive medullary thyroid cancer. J Clin Oncol. 2013;31(29):3639–46.

192. Moura MM, Cabrera RA, Esteves S, Cavaco BM, Soares P, Leite V. Correlation of molecular data with

histopathological and clinical features in a series of 66 patients with medullary thyroid carcinoma. J Endocrinol Invest. 2021;44(9):1837–46.

193. Maleki Z, Nadella A, Nadella M, Patel G, Patel S, Kholova I. INSM1, a novel biomarker for detection of neuroendocrine neoplasms: cytopathologists' view. Diagnostics (Basel). 2021;11(12):2172.

194. Maleki Z, Abram M, Dell'Aquila M, Kilic I, Lu R, Musarra T, Barkan G, Rajakorpi E, Rossi ED, Kholova I. Insulinoma-associated protein 1 (INSM-1) expression in medullary thyroid carcinoma FNA: a multi-institutional study. J Am Soc Cytopathol. 2020;9(3):185–90.

195. Cochand-Priollet B, Maleki Z. Cytology and histology of thyroid nodules: exploring novel insights in the molecular era for enhanced patient management. Curr Oncol. 2023;30(8):7753–72.

196. Zanoni DK, Patel SG, Shah JP. Changes in the 8th Edition of the American Joint Committee on Cancer (AJCC) staging of head and neck cancer: rationale and implications. Curr Oncol Rep. 2019;21(6):52.

197. Nixon IJ, Wang LY, Migliacci JC, Eskander A, Campbell MJ, Aniss A, Morris L, Vaisman F, Corbo R, Momesso D, Vaisman M, Carvalho A, Learoyd D, Leslie WD, Nason RW, Kuk D, Wreesmann V, Morris L, Palmer FL, Ganly I, Patel SG, Singh B, Tuttle RM, Shaha AR, Gonen M, Pathak KA, Shen WT, Sywak M, Kowalski L, Freeman J, Perrier N, Shah JP. An international multi-institutional validation of age 55 years as a cutoff for risk stratification in the AJCC/UICC staging system for well-differentiated thyroid cancer. Thyroid. 2016;26(3):373–80.

198. Tuttle RM, Haugen B, Perrier ND. Updated American Joint Committee on Cancer/tumor-node-metastasis staging system for differentiated and anaplastic thyroid cancer (eighth edition): what changed and why? Thyroid. 2017;27(6):751–6.

Z. Maleki, Associate Professor of pathology at the Johns Hopkins University School of Medicine, at the Johns Hopkins Hospital, Division of Cytopathology, Baltimore, MD, USA. Director of the Johns Hopkins Medical School Scientific Foundations of Medicine, Histology and Pathobiology course. Member of Cancer Registry Committee, co-chair of the Membership Committee at the American Society of Cytopathology and an active committee member at the American Society of Cytopathology and the United States and Canadian Academy of Pathology.

B. Cochand-Priollet, Pathologist at Cochin Hospital, University Paris Cité, Paris, France. Funding Member of the National Agency for Quality Assurance, responsible for the Pap Smear Committee and later Committee for Cytopathology. Past General Secretary of the European Federation of Cytological Societies and Past president of the Société Française de Cytologie Clinique. Currently Editor-in-Chief of Eurocytology. Authoring 152 publications; 2 books and some chapters and co-editor for the new version 2023 of *The Bethesda System for Reporting Thyroid Cytology*.

Zahra Maleki

19.1 General

The parathyroid glands were first identified by Sir Richard Owen in 1852 [1]. Later on, Ivar Sandstrom, a Swedish medical student, identified parathyroid glands in humans in 1880. The first parathyroidectomy was performed by Felix Mandi in 1929 and 30 years later, human parathyroid hormone (PTH) was isolated [2].

19.1.1 Parathyroid Anatomy

The parathyroid glands arise from the third and fourth branchial pouches. The superior or upper parathyroid glands arise from the fourth branchial pouches along with the lateral anlages of the thyroid gland. The positions of the superior parathyroid glands are relatively constant in relation to the dorsal aspect of the upper thyroid with less than 2% of the superior parathyroid glands in ectopic locations. The inferior or lower parathyroid and thymus are derived from the third branchial pouch. In contrary to the upper parathyroid glands, lower parathyroid glands descend with a variable distance from the thymic anlage [3]. Therefore, the anatomic site of lower parathyroid glands can be variable from the neck as far as the mediastinum and pericardium. The parathyroid glands are symmetrical and there are four glands in majority (80%) of the individuals. However, the number of parathyroid glands varies from 1 to 12. A small subset of people may have three glands (%3). Interestingly, a small fraction of cases may have supernumerary glands (13%), which is often found in the thymus. The most common anatomic location of the upper parathyroid gland is posterior to the middle one third of the thyroid gland (75%). The less common locations include behind the upper or lower one third of the thyroid, or behind the pharynx or esophagus. The most common anatomic location of the inferior parathyroid glands is lateral to the lower pole of the thyroid gland (50%). The less common areas are 1 cm below the lower thyroid pole (15%), and anywhere along the thyrothymic tract from the angle of the mandible to the lower anterior mediastinum. Intrathyroid parathyroid (Fig. 19.1) are uncommon comprising 2% of cases [4]. Intrathyroid parathyroid can be detected by ultrasound imaging during work up of hyperparathyroidism or evaluation of thyroid nodules [5]. An intrathyroid parathyroid neoplasm can further be confirmed by Technetium-99 m-sestamibi scintigraphy [6], particularly when thyroid lobectomy is planned and there is concurrent unilateral thyroid nodule and parathyroid nodule [5, 7–9].

Z. Maleki (✉)
Department of Pathology Division of Cytopathology,
Johns Hopkins Hospital Pathology,
Baltimore, MD, USA
e-mail: zmaleki1@jhmi.edu

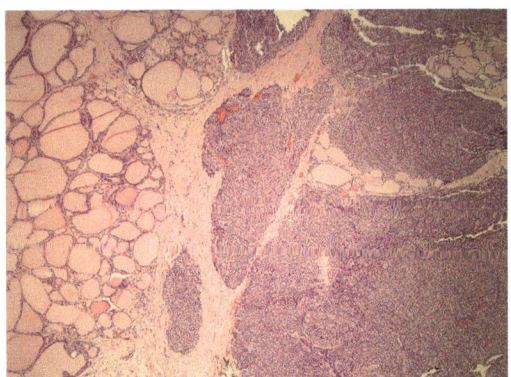

Fig. 19.1 Intrathyroid parathyroid: Thyroid follicles containing colloid are seen mainly on the left side of the image and two small foci on the right, while parathyroid tissue is mainly seen on the right side. The parathyroid cells might be misinterpreted as atypical thyroid follicular cells on cytology material (H&E)

The superior parathyroid glands are located above the intersection between the recurrent laryngeal nerve and the inferior thyroid artery [10]. The inferior parathyroids are located more ventrally, close to the lower thyroid pole or in the upper thymus or thyrothymic ligament [3]. Of note, parathyroid size does not necessarily predict parathyroid function on ultrasound. Other tissues including thymic tissue, lymph nodes, ectopic thyroid, and fat may be masquerading features of an enlarged parathyroid [6, 11]. Normal parathyroid glands weigh 30 to 50 mg and are yellow to brown in color [12]. It is darker in younger patients and yellow in older patients, which is due to gradual accumulation of fat with age [13].

19.1.2 Parathyroid Physiology

Halsted found the parathyroid blood supply on his experience with patients after thyroidectomy [1, 14]. Gley described the correlation between tetany after parathyroidectomy [1, 15]. In 1959, Rusmussen and Craig isolated parathyroid hormone [1, 16]. Later on, Berson and Yalo received Nobel prize for developing an assay to measure PTH levels in serum [1, 2].

The parathyroid glands produce parathyroid hormone (PTH), an 84-amino-acid single-chain peptide, which is the primary regulator of calcium metabolism pathway [17]. Calcium exists in the blood in two forms, bound to protein (55%) (mainly albumin) and free ionized (45%). The normal range for serum calcium is 8.5 to 10.2 mg/dL and normal range for ionized calcium is 4.5 to 5.0 mg/dL. Serum PTH levels are negatively regulated by ionized calcium level. PTH secretion increases sharply in response to decrease in calcium concentration, particularly ionized calcium, from normal to 1.9–2.0 mmol/L.

PTH increases serum calcium level by inducing calcium release by its direct act on bones, enhancing calcium reabsorption in the distal tubules of the kidney, and in the proximal renal tubules by conversion of 25-hydroxyvitamin D3 (calcifediol) to 1,25-dihydroxyvitamin D3 (calcitriol) and decreases phosphorus reabsorption, which in turn increases calcium absorption in the gastrointestinal tract. Intact PTH has a half-life of a few minutes and it is cleared from the blood circulation in the kidney and liver.

Calcitonin is a hormone secreted by the parafollicular C cells in the thyroid, which has a small role in serum calcium regulation. Calcitonin is secreted in response to high calcium levels and it inhibits bone resorption [17].

19.1.3 Hyperparathyroidism

The earliest report about clinical symptoms of hyperparathyroidism was published by von Recklinghausen describing bone disease or osteitis fibrosa cystica [1, 18]. Hyperparathyroidism is characterized by pathologic overproduction of parathyroid hormone. Hyperparathyroidism can be primary or secondary [1]. Primary hyperparathyroidism has the incidence of one per 1000 and it is more common in women than men (3–4:1) [19, 20]. The diagnosis of hyperparathyroidism is primarily based on measurement of serum PTH and calcium level. Both PTH and calcium are elevated in majority of the cases. A small subset of primary hyperparathyroidism is normocalcemic and the diagnosis is made when the PTH level is elevated and total and ionized calcium are normal in the absence of secondary cause of hyperparathyroidism [20, 21]. Primary hyperparathyroidism has the potential to cause clinical symptoms and signs including recurrent nephrolithiasis, peptic ulcers, and osteoporosis presented as broken bones in the absence of major trauma, constipation, insomnia, muscle and joint pain, depression, anxiety, excessive fatigue, difficulty concentrating, hypercalcemia, hypercalciuria, hypophosphatemia, and an elevated serum PTH level [22–25]. However, due to screening test of serum calcium and awareness of the disease, most patients are diagnosed when they are asymptomatic or have minimal symptoms [19, 26]. In addition to sporadic form of primary hyperparathyroidism, there are syndromic types of hyperparathyroidism including Multiple Endocrine Neoplasia (MEN) Type 1 (autosomal dominant disorder associated with *MEN1* gene), MEN2A (autosomal dominant associated with *RET* gene), hyperparathyroidism-jaw tumor syndrome (autosomal dominant associated with *HRPT2* (CDC73) gene), autosomal dominant mild hyperparathyroidism (*CASR* gene), familial hypercalcemic hypocalciuria, and familial isolated hyperparathyroidism [27, 28]. Parathyroid adenoma of a single gland is the most common cause of primary hyperparathyroidism, accounting for 80% to 85% of all primary hyperparathyroidism [29]. Four-gland hyperfuctional glands is the second most common cause of primary hyperparathyroidism (10% to 15%) [30].

Secondary hyperthyroidism is due to an underlying disease such as vitamin D deficiency, primary hypercalciuria, renal insufficiency, malabsorption syndrome, lithium, and thiazide diuretics [24]. Chronic kidney disease is a common cause of secondary hyperparathyroidism [31]. Chronic kidney disease leads to disorders in metabolism including low calcium, high phosphate, and vitamin D deficiency, which subsequently contributes to vascular calcification [31].

A prolonged chronic kidney disease occasionally transforms into a hypercalcemic state resembling hyperparathyroidism, which is known as tertiary hyperparathyroidism [32].

Parathyroid glands can be assessed by sestamibi scintigraphy (Tc99 m-MIBI), cervical ultrasound (US), computed tomography (CT),

magnetic resonance imaging (MRI), and/or positron emission tomography (PET). However, the Technetium 99 m sestamibi scintigraphy (Tc99 m-MIBI) study is the gold standard in evaluation of parathyroid glands [33]. Parathyroid adenomas are characterized by their hypoechoic appearance, extrathyroid location, and one or two vascular pedicles [34]. However, it is difficult to distinguish parathyroid lesions from thyroid nodules on ultrasound. Parathyroid adenomas may not be detected by ultrasound or sestamibi scintigraphy in up to one quarter of cases. Therefore, imaging studies are not used for diagnostic purposes. They are used to localize the lesion [33]. Both ultrasound or sestamibi scintigraphy studies show that the detection of adenomas is highly dependent on their specific location. Both methods are more sensitive in detecting lower left adenomas than upper right ones. Overall, the positive predictive value for all parathyroid gland sites is approximately 54% for sestamibi scintigraphy and 59% for ultrasound, respectively [35].

Primary hyperparathyroidism can be cured by surgical removal of parathyroid adenoma/adenomas [24]. In patients with secondary hyperparathyroidism, parathyroidectomy should be considered when hypercalcemia is refractory to medical therapy [31].

Imaging studies such as ultrasound or CT scan are performed to localize the parathyroid glands prior to potential surgical treatment [33]. Parathyroid adenoma can be preoperatively evaluated by ultrasound-guided FNA [34]. An aspirated PTH washout to serum ratio of 0.5 has been reported as positive results [33]. PTH assay on ultrasound-guided FNA samples are performed in patients with primary hyperparathyroidism or suspicious for parathyroid adenoma [36]. PTH-FNA equal or greater than 100 pg/mL is considered diagnostic for hyperparathyroidism with a sensitivity of 93.7%, a specificity of 100%, a positive predictive value of 100%, and a negative predictive value of 71.4% [36]. The studies suggest that ultrasound-guided parathyroid FNA with PTH measurement in washout is more sensitive than technetium 99 m sestamibi scintigraphy (Tc99 m-MIBI), 95.6% vs 52.2%, respectively [33, 37]. Parathyroid FNA with washout (84%

sensitivity, 100% specificity, 100% PPV, 84% accuracy) is also superior to cytology alone (68% sensitivity, 100% specificity, 100% PPV) or ultrasound imaging alone (78% sensitivity, 6% specificity, 62% PPV, 53% accuracy) [37]. Potential complications of FNA are hematoma, possible dense fibrotic reaction to the needle, and parathyroid abscess. FNA-related changes may rarely convert a minimally invasive surgical procedure to a standard surgical approach [37].

19.1.4 Biochemical Testing

Hypercalcemia can be discovered during screening tests in asymptomatic or mildly symptomatic patients, which warrants further work up in order to find the etiology of its underlying condition. The serum calcium and PTH levels are measured in symptomatic patients with suspicion for parathyroid enlargement, adenoma, or carcinoma to rule out primary hyperparathyroidism [2].

The standard care of primary hyperparathyroidism is preoperatively identification of all 4 parathyroid glands and subsequent surgical removal of the affected gland or glands [34]. Therefore, preoperative localization of parathyroid nodule if crucial. FNA is a useful tool in the diagnosis of parathyroid tissue including the intrathyroid parathyroid gland [38]. FNA procedure can provide material for PTH assessment on an aliquot, or a cell block can be created from needle rinses for immunohistochemistry. For each nodule, needles 23-guage to 27-guage are used and making four to six passes [39]. The FNA needle is rinsed with a small volume (0.1 to 0.5 mL) of Hank's balanced salt solution immediately after a drop of the specimen is expelled from the needle on a glass slide for making a smear. The washes from the same nodule are pooled and collected in one container [39]. PTH levels of the aspirated nodules or washouts suspected for parathyroid adenoma or carcinoma are measured. The PTH washout greater than 436.5 pg/mL has been reported to be 90% sensitive and 89% specific in localizing parathyroid

tissue [40]. Some studies have reported that even a PTH value over 245 pg/mL is associated with parathyroid tissue [41]. The serum PTH level correlates with the PTH level of the needle washings in most cases [34]. The same study reports a sensitivity of 91% and specificity of 89% for FNA washout/serum PTH levels greater than 3.05 [40]. Moreover, intraoperative serum PTH assay after removal of abnormal parathyroid tissue is a useful tool to assist the surgeon during parathyroidectomy. A decrease of PTH greater than 50% of the highest pre-excision value five minutes after removal of the enlarged gland/s is considered as the operative success [42].

Immunohistochemistry is an indispensable tool in differential diagnosis of parathyroid from thyroid and parathyroid lesions from each other [43]. It can be performed on histology sections or on cell blocks to detect parathyroid tissue. A panel of PTH, TTF-1, calcitonin, chromogranin, and CD56 is helpful to differentiate parathyroid tissue from thyroid [43]. Parathyroid cells are immunoreactive for PTH, GATA-3, and chromogranin (98%) and negative for TTF-1, INSM1, and thyroglobulin [44, 45]. A small subset of parathyroid tissue is immunoreactive for synaptophysin [45]. Parafibromin is a tumor suppressor protein coded by *Cell Division Cycle 73* (*CDC73*) gene, and the immunostain detects parathyroid tissue with pathology [43]. Normal parathyroid tissue retains nuclear stain with parafibromin and loss of parafibromin is seen mainly in parathyroid carcinoma (33–100%) and a small subset of atypical adenomas (0–17.6%) [43]. Ki-67 is a useful stain to evaluate the cellular proliferation index in parathyroid tissue. Currently, a cut-off level of 5% is accepted to distinguish parathyroid carcinoma from benign parathyroid tumors [43].

19.1.5 Parathyroid Cyst

Parathyroid mass may present as a cystic lesion. The aspirates show clear fluid and it is virtually acellular on microscopic examination. Measurement of the PTH level should be considered if there is a possibility of a parathyroid cyst, which is markedly elevated [46, 47]. Cystic lesions of the thyroid such as cystic papillary thyroid carcinoma and adenomatoid nodule with cystic degeneration can be mistaken for parathyroid cysts and PTH level of FNA fluid can be useful to differentiate the parathyroid vs thyroid origin. Moreover, parathyroid adenoma and parathyroid carcinoma may be associated with partial cystic changes [48].

19.1.6 Parathyroid Hyperplasia

Parathyroid hyperplasia is defined as an increase in number of parathyroid parenchymal cells (chief cells, oncocytes, and transitional oncocytes) in all four parathyroid glands [30, 49]. It accounts for 15% of primary hyperparathyroidism cases and it usually affects all four glands [30]. There are cytomorphologic overlaps between parathyroid hyperplasia, parathyroid adenoma, and parathyroid carcinoma. However, some features are more common in one entity and less common in others. Parathyroid hyperplasia FNA samples comprised of predominantly loosely and tightly cohesive cells, and dispersed cells (Fig. 19.2a, b). The nuclei display stippled chromatin. Nucleoli, nuclear grooving, and anisonucleosis are rarely seen. The cytoplasm is granular and background may contain macrophages and naked nuclei [50]. PTH immunostain of the cell block confirms the parathyroid tissues, while the cells are negative for TGB immunostain (Fig. 19.3a, d). On gross examination, they are round to oval and appear red to brown and slightly nodular on cut surface [30]. Histologic examination reveals sheets, cords, or an acinar arrangement of parenchymal cells with reduced stromal fat. The chief cells may display mild to marked nuclear atypia and pleomorphism. The nodule may be surrounded by fibrous tissue resembling a fibrous capsule and the nodule may be septated [30]. Parathyromatosis is referred to as a condition when the hyperplastic parathyroid involves the surrounding tissue and lacks distinct circumscription [30]. This phenomenon usually results from prior trauma [51]. Degenerative changes may occur in hyperplastic nodules including hemorrhage, cystic changes, hemosiderin deposition, and fibrosis [51].

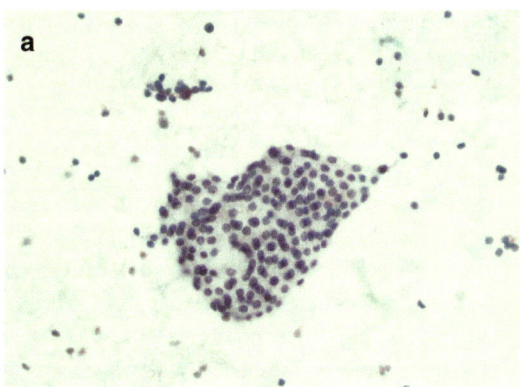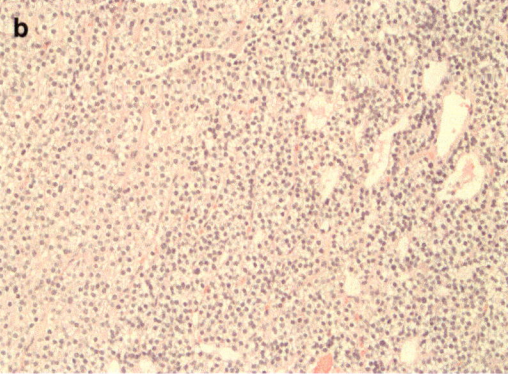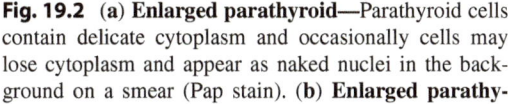

Fig. 19.2 (a) **Enlarged parathyroid**—Parathyroid cells contain delicate cytoplasm and occasionally cells may lose cytoplasm and appear as naked nuclei in the background on a smear (Pap stain). (b) **Enlarged parathyroid:** Parathyroid cells contain clear cytoplasm and mainly arranged in trabecular pattern on surgical excision (H&E)

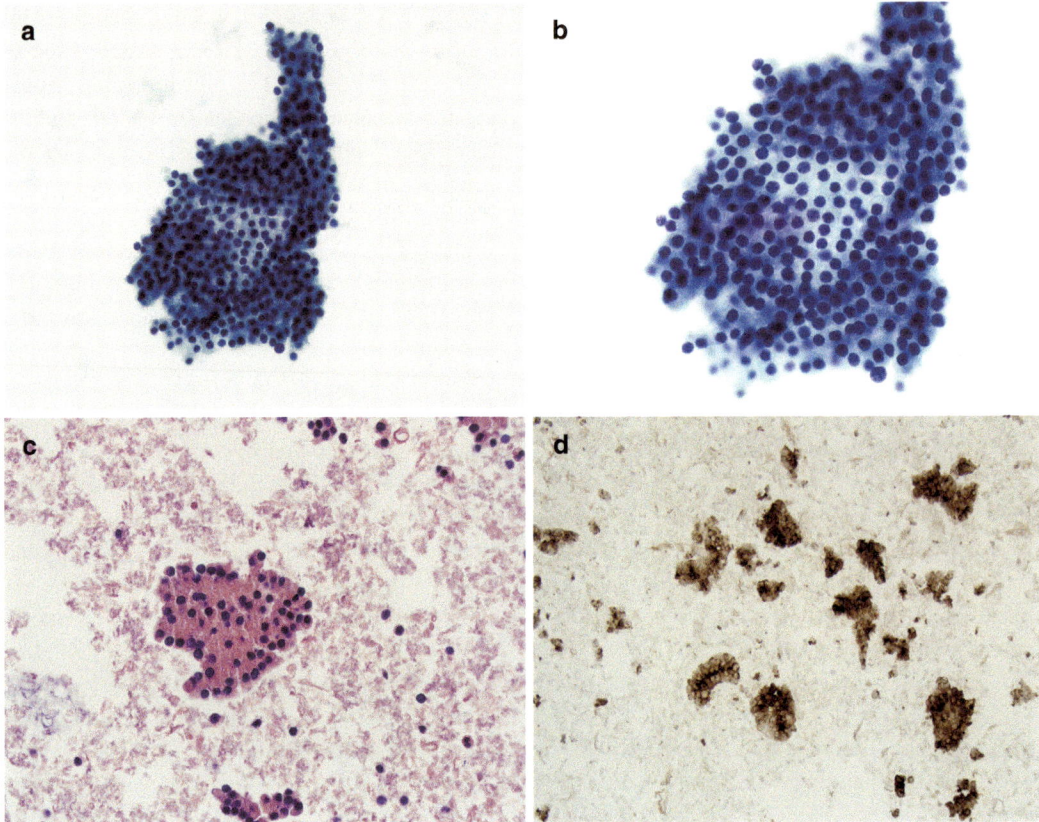

Fig. 19.3 (**a**) **Enlarged parathyroid:** A large sheet of cohesive parathyroid cells characterized by round uniform nuclei and moderate amount of pale cytoplasm (Pap, ThinPrep). (**b**) **Enlarged parathyroid:** Higher magnification shows distinct cell borders, delicate pale cytoplasm, and relatively round uniform nuclei (Pap, ThinPrep). (**c**) **Enlarged parathyroid:** Clusters of cells with moderate amount of finely granular eosinophilic cytoplasm and small round nuclei and scattered single cells in cell block preparation (H&E). (**d**) **Enlarged parathyroid:** PTH immunostaining on the cell block highlights parathyroid cells, confirming the diagnosis (immunostain)

19.1.7 Parathyroid Adenoma

Parathyroid adenomas account for 85% of cases of primary hyperparathyroidism. It can occur in any age groups, with a peak incidence in the fifth and sixth decades with a female predilection (female: male, 2:1) [49, 52]. Parathyroid adenomas tend to occur more frequently in the lower glands than in the upper glands [53]. Parathyroid adenomas may arise in ectopic sites such thymus, thyroid, mediastinum, retroesophageal space, and vestigial aortopulmonary window [3, 30]. Parathyroid adenomas are variable in weight and size, ranging from 300 mg to several grams and a few millimeters to more than 10 cm [54, 55].

FNA of parathyroid masses can be very variable in architecture and cytomorphologic features and multiple patterns can be seen in one aspirated specimen (Fig. 19.5). The aspirated smears are highly to moderately cellular comprised of numerous clusters and fragments of three-dimensional cohesive cells with nuclear overlapping [47]. Disorganized sheets, branched fragments with frayed edges, papillary fragments with a fibrovascular cores, and microfollicles are other patterns seen in parathyroid aspirates [47]. A less common pattern is a single cell pattern mimicking lymphoid cells.

Round cells are the most predominant cell types, which may be arranged in trabecular, insular, tissue fragments, cribriform, or less commonly microfollicular pattern. Isolated cells and numerous naked nuclei are relatively common features seen in parathyroid adenomas [47]. The nuclei are round to oval with regular nuclear membrane and hyperchromatic, coarsely granular chromatin [47]. The cells display stippled chromatin in most cases, and oxyphilic cytoplasm is seen in half of the cases. Anisonucleosis may be seen in a quarter of the cases [46, 47, 56]. Rarely, mast cells are reported in parathyroid aspirates [47]. Nuclear grooves, nuclear molding, nuclear prominent nucleoli, and nuclear inclusions are less common features seen in parathyroid adenoma aspirated specimens [46, 47, 50]. The cells have moderate to high nuclear to cytoplasmic ratio (1:1 to 1:2) with eccentric nuclei, pale to finely granular cytoplasm, and well-defined cytoplasmic membrane [47]. Cytoplasmic vacuoles, oxyphilic cytoplasm, and paravacoular granulation are less common features seen in parathyroid cytology [47]. Follicular structures, papillary-like fragments with vascular cores, macrophages, lymphocytes, colloid-like material, loose and cohesive clusters are less common features seen in parathyroid adenoma, which can be mistaken for thyroid follicles [50]. No significant cytomorphologic differences are found between parathyroid hyperplasia and parathyroid adenoma.

Thyroid aspirates and parathyroid FNA can be mistaken one for the other one. Cytomorphologic features of follicular cells in adenomatoid nodule, follicular adenoma, papillary thyroid carcinoma, and even a reactive lymph node may overlap with parathyroid cells and misinterpreted as parathyroid cells [40]. Three-dimensional fragments with overlapping nuclei is more common in parathyroid aspirates, while flat honeycomb sheets are more common in thyroid FNA. Microfollicles and papillary features are seen in both thyroid and parathyroid aspirates. Macrofollicles are seen in thyroid aspirates and naked nuclei admixed with cohesive cells are seen in parathyroid FNA, respectively [47]. FNA of parathyroid adenoma is useful when it is done in conjunction with imaging studies such as ultrasound or CT scan and PTH level assessment [46].

On gross examination, they are occasionally encapsulated, and well-circumscribed and the cut surface is red-brown. The nodule may show areas of hemorrhage and cystic degeneration [30]. On histologic examination, parathyroid adenomas are well-circumscribed nodules, surrounded by a thin, fibrous capsule. They are mainly composed of chief cells, characterized by round nucleus, scant cytoplasm, and high N/C ratio, arranged within a delicate capillary network. The cells are mainly small, uniform, and with a centrally located hyperchromatic nuclei (Fig. 19.4a-c). Focal mild to marked nuclear atypia is seen with enlarged nuclei, irregular nuclei, and even multi-nucleation [57]. Mitotic activity is not seen or it is less than 1 mitosis per 10 high-power fields [58]. Oncocytic cell change may be focally seen, characterized by large cells with abundant pink cytoplasm and variable granularity. A small subset of parathyroid adenomas is exclusively composed of oxyphilic or oncocytic cells. They may be functional and accounting for less than 6% of parathyroid adenomas [59–63]. Lipoadenoma and water-clear cell adenoma are rare variants of parathyroid adenoma. Lipoadenoma of parathyroid is a benign neoplasm that consists of both parenchymal cells and mature adipose tissue comprising greater than 50% of the tumor. Parenchymal cells of lipoadenoma are predominantly chief cells and scattered oncocytes. There are reported cases of lipoadenoma causing primary hyperparathyroidism [64–67]. Water-clear cell adenomas are extremely rare. They are composed of intermediate to large cells with abundant clear cytoplasm containing small vesicles and glycogen. Clear-cell lipoadenoma is occasionally associated with primary hyperparathyroidism [68–71].

Stromal fat is usually absent or very sparse in parathyroid adenomas. A rim of atrophic or normal parathyroid tissue is seen adjacent to the adenoma in almost half of the cases. Large adenomas may show areas of fibrosis, calcification, hemorrhage, hemosiderin deposition, or cholesterol clefts [30]. GATA-3 and PTH immunostains highlight neoplastic cells [56, 72].

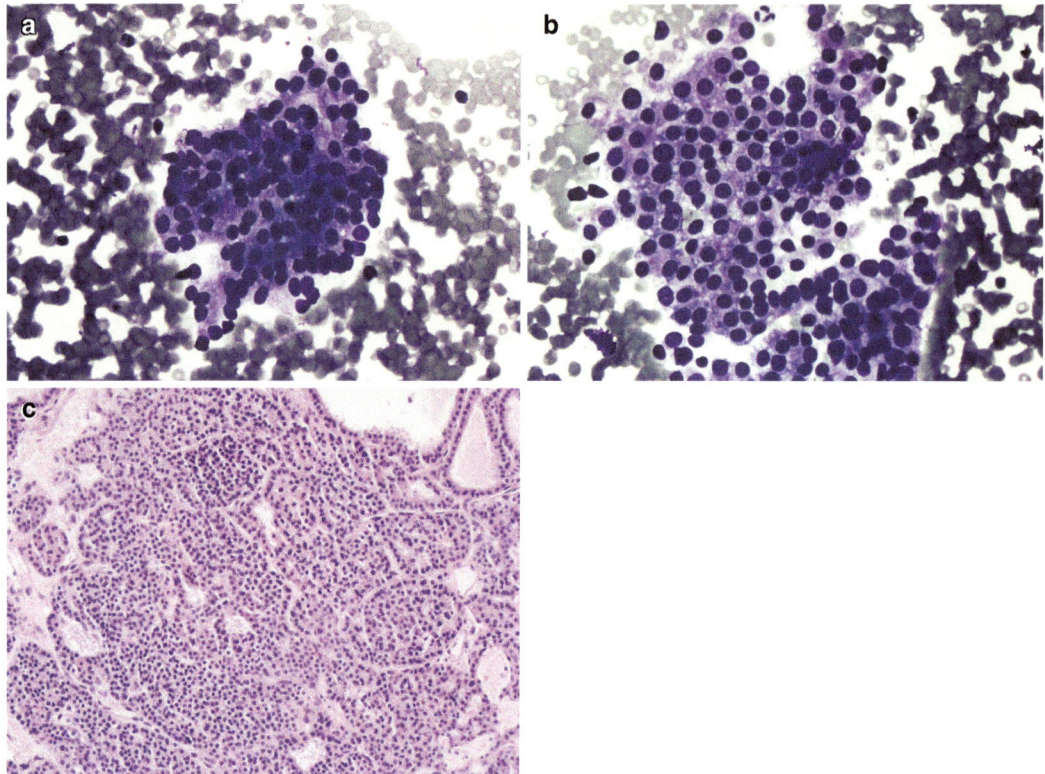

Fig. 19.4 (**a**) **Enlarged parathyroid:** A large fragment of parathyroid cells arranged in follicular pattern simulating the thyroid follicles on a smear (Diff-Quik). (**b**) **Enlarged parathyroid:** Parathyroid cells are characterized by a moderate amount of finely vacuolated cytoplasm and uniform round nuclei arranged in a sheet and small area of follicular pattern at the lower right on a smear (Diff-Quik). (**c**) **Enlarged parathyroid:** Parathyroid cells are arranged in ribbons and sheets with focal cystic areas. The cells are uniform and the nuclei are euchromatin on surgical excision (H&E)

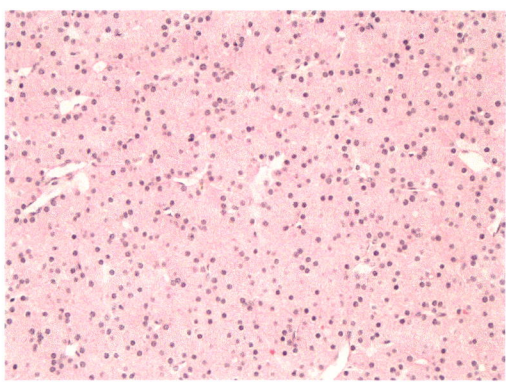

Fig. 19.5 **Parathyroid adenoma:** Parathyroid oxyphilic cells are characterized by abundant eosinophilic cytoplasm, distinct cytoplasmic membrane, and round uniform small nuclei, arranged in sheets (H&E)

19.1.8 Atypical Parathyroid Adenoma

Atypical adenomas are parathyroid adenomas with features concerning for malignancy such as mitotic figures, necrosis, nuclear atypia, broad bands of fibrosis, and a desmoplastic stromal reaction. However, they fail to show definitive features of malignancy including infiltration to the surrounding tissue, vascular invasion, and neural invasion [57]. Atypical parathyroid adenomas are also the underlying cause of primary hyperparathyroidism [73]. They are classified as tumors with uncertain malignant potential [74]. Lack of Parafibromin (CDC73) nuclear expres-

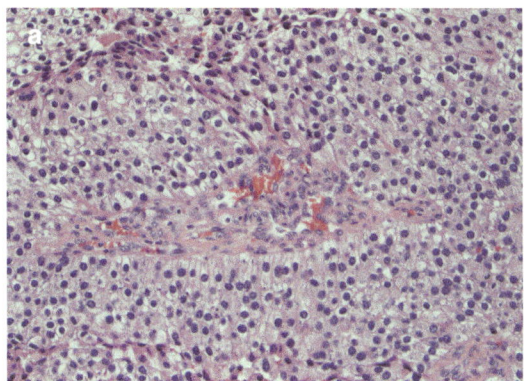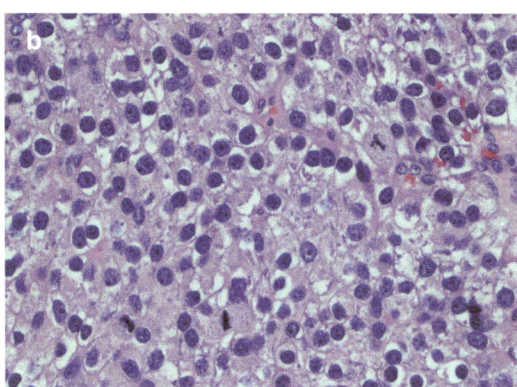

Fig. 19.6 (**a**) **Parathyroid carcinoma:** Malignant parathyroid cells are arranged in solid sheet, characterized by moderate to abundant cytoplasm, round nuclei with coarse chromatin and occasional nucleoli (H&E). (**b**) **Parathyroid carcinoma:** Malignant parathyroid cells contain round nuclei with coarse chromatin and prominent nucleoli. Several atypical mitotic figures and focal necrosis are seen (H&E)

sion is associated with tumor recurrence in 10% of atypical adenomas while no recurrences have been reported in cases positive for Parafibromin (CDC73) [75]. The patients are treated with surgery and clinical follow-up [51]. More studies are needed for better understanding of the biologic behavior of atypical parathyroid adenomas.

19.1.9 Parathyroid Carcinoma

Parathyroid carcinoma was first described by Fritz De Quervain, a Swiss surgeon in 1904 [76] It is a rare endocrine malignancy. It has the same prevalence between women and men. It tends to occur in younger patients by about a decade, mainly between 40 to 50 years [77, 78]. Parathyroid carcinoma account for less than 1% of cases of primary hyperparathyroidism [29, 78]. The etiology of parathyroid carcinoma remains unknown and it occurs as a sporadic or a genetic syndrome including MEN1, MEN2A, isolated familial hyperparathyroidism, and hyperparathyroidism jaw-tumor syndrome [1, 78, 79]. History of head and neck radiation and end-stage renal disease as a result of secondary and tertiary hyperparathyroidism are known risk factors in sporadic cases [77]. In patients with parathyroid carcinoma, clinical symptoms and signs of hypercalcemia are more severe and renal

and skeletal manifestations of the disease are more common [77, 78]. The severe hypercalcemia in parathyroid carcinoma causes extreme weakness, weight loss, psychosis or mental depression, anemia, cardiac arrythmia, thirst, anorexia, constipation, nausea and vomiting, abdominal pain, pancreatitis, and osteoporosis or osteitis fibrosa cystica [80].

Hypercalcemic crisis manifested with neurologic symptoms such as profound weakness and coma and severe hypercalcemia (>16 mg/dl) can be the clinical presentation of parathyroid carcinoma in 7–12% of patients [81]. Parathyroid carcinoma is non functional in up to 10% of the patients and a neck mass and its effects such as hoarseness, dysphagia, and dyspnea can be the initial clinical presentation in this group. Nonfunctional parathyroid carcinoma can be mistaken as a thyroid nodule [82]. Serum calcium level is elevated in most patients (greater than 14 mg/dL) and PTH level is reported to be several times (3–15 times) higher than normal PTH level [77, 78, 83, 84]. In patients with non-functioning parathyroid carcinoma, both serum calcium and PTH levels remain within normal range.

Prior to surgical treatment, imaging studies are done to localize the affected parathyroid gland. Features suggestive of malignancy are the presence of a large, lobulated, hypoechoic, parathyroid gland with ill-defined borders. Local infiltration, increased vascularity, calcifications, and a thick capsule are additional features described in parathyroid carcinoma imaging [85, 86].

Fine-needle aspiration of parathyroid carcinoma shows highly cellular smears comprised of a large number of small and large single cells with scant or no cytoplasm, fragments, tightly cohesive and loose clusters of atypical cells, and papillary-like fragments with vascular cores. Clusters of clear cells with abundant cytoplasm and ill-defined cell borders can be seen mixed with the atypical cells. The clear cells may surround fibrovascular cores, forming papillary structures [87].The nuclei are hyperchromatic and display stippled chromatin, marked anisonucleosis, with occasional nucleoli, nuclear grooving, and intranuclear inclusions [87]. Scattered giant nuclei with multiple enlarged nucleoli can be seen [87–89]. The cytoplasm is mainly granular with less commonly vacuolated. Macrophages and bare nuclei may be seen in the background [50]. The PTH level of aspirates or needle washout from parathyroid carcinoma is markedly elevated [90]. In surgical removal of the tumor, adherence of the gland to adjacent structures may cause difficulty in tumor removal [77]. On gross examination, parathyroid carcinoma is white-gray, spherical shape, and firm. The tumor can be surrounded by thick capsule and its weight ranges between 600 mg to 110 g [83, 91]. The affected gland may show partial cystic changes as high as 22% of the cases [90]. Histologically, frequent mitotic figures, cellular atypia, and invasion of adjacent tissue and blood vessels are features associated with parathyroid carcinoma (Fig. 19.6a, b). Local recurrence and distant metastasis can occur in up to half of patients who underwent surgery [90]. Metastasis to cervical lymph nodes, bones, liver, mediastinum, and lung is reported [90, 92]. Death is usually due to persistent hypercalcemia and its related complications such as renal failure, pancreatitis, and cardiac arrhythmia [90].

19.2 Diagnostic Workflow

A clinical suspicion for parathyroidism warrants measurement of serum calcium and serum PTH. Elevated levels of serum calcium and PTH is followed up by neck imaging studies. Most surgeons recommend ultrasound and sestamibi studies to localize the abnormal parathyroid gland [90]. If FNA of the parathyroid nodule is performed, the diagnosis of parathyroid tissue can be confirmed by assessment of PTH on needle washout or immunohistochemistry on cell block preparation. The parathyroid cells are immunoreactive for PTH and GATA-3 and negative for TTF-1, PAX-8, and calcitonin. Surgical removal of an enlarged parathyroid/parathyroids is considered the standard treatment when hypercalcemia is refractory to medical therapy.

19.3 Framed Text with the Main Massage

Parathyroid glands are two pairs located adjacent to the thyroid gland, producing PTH, which is the main regulator of calcium metabolism. The location of the upper parathyroid glands is more consistent, while the lower parathyroid glands can have variable location from the neck to as far as mediastinum. Primary hyperparathyroidism accounts for majority of cases with hypercalcemia and parathyroid adenomas (85%) are the most common cause of primary hypercalcemia. Symptomatic patients may seek medical advice, while asymptomatic or mildly symptomatic patients with hypercalcemia are discovered during screening tests. Parathyroid FNA specimens have higher sensitivity and specificity when the biopsy is performed under ultrasound guidance and needle washout samples are assessed for the PTH level. Parathyroid imaging is used for localization of the affected parathyroid preoperatively. Surgical removal of the enlarged parathyroid is treatment of choice when hypercalcemia is refractory to medical treatment. Parathyroid hyperplasia, adenoma including atypical adenomas, and carcinoma share morphologic features. However, capsular invasion, vascular invasion, perineural invasion, local recurrence, and distant metastasis (lymph nodes, bone, liver, lung) are features seen in carcinoma.

19.3.1 Take-Home Message

Hypercalcemia can be detected in screening tests in mildly symptomatic or asymptomatic patients or by measurement of serum calcium in symptomatic patients. Primary hyperparathyroidism is the most common cause of hypercalcemia and it is caused by parathyroid adenoma (80% to 85%), primary parathyroid hyperplasia (15%), and rarely parathyroid carcinoma (5%).

Clinical, radiographic, and biochemical testing including intraoperative assessment of PTH level, number, size, and weight of the affected parathyroid glands are of paramount importance for an accurate diagnosis of parathyroid lesion [44].

Minimally invasive surgical removal of the enlarged glands is treatment of choice when hypercalcemia is not responsive to medical treatment.

The surgical specimen should be carefully examined for features associated with carcinoma including capsular invasion, infiltration to the surrounding tissue, and perineural invasion.

References

1. Cummings otolaryngology: head and neck surgery, Seventh Edition, Elsevier, Mosby.
2. Berson SA, Yalow RS, Aurbach GD, Potts JT. Immunoassay of bovine and human parathyroid hormone. Proc Natl Acad Sci USA. 1963;49(5):613–7.
3. Akerstrom G, Malmaeus J, Bergstrom R. Surgical anatomy of human parathyroid glands. Surgery. 1984;95(1):14–21.
4. Som PM, Curtin HD. Head and Neck Imaging, 5th Edition, 2011, Elsevier.
5. Baloch Z, Mete O, Asa SL. Immunohistochemical biomarkers in thyroid pathology. Endocr Pathol. 2018;29(2):91–112.
6. Patel KN, Yip L, Lubitz CC, Grubbs EG, Miller BS, Shen W, Angelos P, Chen H, Doherty GM, Fahey TJ 3rd, Kebebew E, Livolsi VA, Perrier ND, Sipos JA, Sosa JA, Steward D, Tufano RP, McHenry CR, Carty SE. The American Association of Endocrine Surgeons Guidelines for the definitive surgical Management of Thyroid Disease in adults. Ann Surg. 2020;271(3):e21–93.
7. Chang MC, Tsai SC, Lin WY. Dual-phase 99mTc-MIBI parathyroid imaging reveals synchronous parathyroid adenoma and papillary thyroid carcinoma: a case report. Kaohsiung J Med Sci. 2008;24(10):542–7.
8. Sippel RS, Ozgul O, Hartig GK, Mack EA, Chen H. Risks and consequences of incidental parathyroidectomy during thyroid resection. ANZ J Surg. 2007;77(1–2):33–6.
9. Monroe DP, Edeiken-Monroe BS, Lee JE, Evans DB, Perrier ND. Impact of preoperative thyroid ultrasonography on the surgical management of primary hyperparathyroidism. Br J Surg. 2008;95(8):957–60.
10. Abraham D, Duick DS, Baskin HJ. Appropriate administration of fine-needle aspiration (FNA) biopsy on selective parathyroid adenomas is safe. Thyroid. 2008;18(5):581–2. author reply 583-4
11. Elliott DD, Monroe DP, Perrier ND. Parathyroid histopathology: is it of any value today? J Am Coll Surg. 2006;203(5):758–65.
12. Dufour DR, Wilkerson SY. Factors related to parathyroid weight in normal persons. Arch Pathol Lab Med. 1983;107(4):167–72.
13. Dekker A, Dunsford HA, Geyer SJ. The normal parathyroid gland at autopsy: the significance of stromal fat in adult patients. J Pathol. 1979;128(3):127–32.
14. Halsted WS, Evans HM, I. The parathyroid glandules. Their blood supply and their preservation in operation upon the thyroid gland. Ann Surg. 1907;46(4):489–506.
15. Gley ME: Sur les fonctions du corps thyroid. CR Soc Biol. 1891,43.pp. 841–843.
16. Rasmussen H, Craig LC. Purification of parathyroid hormone by use of countercurrent distribution. J Am Chem Soc. 1959;81:5003.
17. Bringhurst DM, Kronenberg HM. Bone and mineral metabolism in health and disease. In: Jameson J, Fauci AS, Kasper DL, Hauser SL, Longo DL, Loscalzo J, editors. Harrison's principles of internal medicine, 20th Edition. Chapter 402. McGraw Hill; 2018.
18. R.F. Recklinghausen FV, Recklinghausen V: Die fibrose oder deformierende Ostitis, die Osteomalacie und die osteoplastische Carcinose in ihren gegenseitigen Beziehungen. 1st Edition. 1891
19. Christensson T, Hellstrom K, Wengle B, Alveryd A, Wikland B. Prevalence of hypercalcaemia in a health screening in Stockholm. Acta Med Scand. 1976;200(1–2):131–7.
20. Bilezikian JP, Silverberg SJ. Normocalcemic primary hyperparathyroidism. Arq Bras Endocrinol Metabol. 2010;54(2):106–9.
21. Silverberg SJ, Lewiecki EM, Mosekilde L, Peacock M, Rubin MR. Presentation of asymptomatic pri-

mary hyperparathyroidism: proceedings of the third international workshop. J Clin Endocrinol Metab. 2009;94(2):351–65.

22. Heath DA. Primary hyperparathyroidism. Clinical presentation and factors influencing clinical management. Endocrinol Metab Clin North Am. 1989;18(3):631–46.

23. Ronni-Sivula H, Sivula A. Long-term effect of surgical treatment on the symptoms of primary hyperparathyroidism. Ann Clin Res. 1985;17(4):141 7.

24. Bilezikian JP, Bandeira L, Khan A, Cusano NE. Hyperparathyroidism. Lancet. 2018;391(10116):168–78.

25. Cope O. The study of hyperparathyroidism at the Massachusetts General Hospital. N Engl J Med. 1966;274(21):1174–82.

26. Silverberg SJ, Clarke BL, Peacock M, Bandeira F, Boutroy S, Cusano NE, Dempster D, Lewiecki EM, Liu JM, Minisola S, Rejnmark L, Silva BC, Walker MD, Bilezikian JP. Current issues in the presentation of asymptomatic primary hyperparathyroidism: proceedings of the fourth international workshop. J Clin Endocrinol Metab. 2014;99(10):3580–94.

27. Nose V, Khan A. Recent developement in the Molecular biology of the parathyroid. Lloyd RV. Endocrine Pathology: Differential Diagnosis and Molecular Advances. 2010. Springer, New York, pp. 173.

28. Brandi ML, Falchetti A. Genetics of primary hyperparathyroidism. Urol Int. 2004;72(Suppl 1):11–6.

29. Ruda JM, Hollenbeak CS, Stack BC Jr. A systematic review of the diagnosis and treatment of primary hyperparathyroidism from 1995 to 2003. Otolaryngol Head Neck Surg. 2005;132(3):359–72.

30. Guilmette J, Sadow PM. Parathyroid pathology. Surg Pathol Clin. 2019;12(4):1007–19.

31. Cunningham J, Locatelli F, Rodriguez M. Secondary hyperparathyroidism: pathogenesis, disease progression, and therapeutic options. Clin J Am Soc Nephrol. 2011;6(4):913–21.

32. Messa P, Alfieri CM. Secondary and tertiary hyperparathyroidism. Front Horm Res. 2019;51:91–108.

33. Obolonczyk L, Karwacka I, Wisniewski P, Sworczak K, Oseka T. The current role of parathyroid fine-needle biopsy (P-FNAB) with iPTH-washout concentration (iPTH-WC) in primary hyperparathyroidism: A single center experience and literature review. Biomedicines. 2022;10(1)

34. Abraham D, Sharma PK, Bentz J, Gault PM, Neumayer L, McClain DA. Utility of ultrasound-guided fine-needle aspiration of parathyroid adenomas for localization before minimally invasive parathyroidectomy. Endocr Pract. 2007;13(4):333–7.

35. Iwen KA, Kussmann J, Fendrich V, Lindner K, Zahn A. Accuracy of parathyroid adenoma localization by preoperative ultrasound and Sestamibi in 1089 patients with primary hyperparathyroidism. World J Surg. 2022;46(9):2197–205.

36. Carral F, Jimenez AI, Tome M, Alvarez J, Diez A, Garcia C, Vega V, Ayala C. Safety and diagnostic performance of parathyroid hormone assay

in fine-needle aspirate in suspicious parathyroid adenomas. Endocrinol Diabetes Nutr (Engl Ed). 2021;68(7):481–8.

37. Bancos I, Grant CS, Nadeem S, Stan MN, Reading CC, Sebo TJ, Algeciras-Schimnich A, Singh RJ, Dean DS. Risks and benefits of parathyroid fine-needle aspiration with parathyroid hormone washout. Endocr Pract. 2012;18(4):441–9.

38. Boerner SL, Asa SL. Biopsy Interpretation of the Thyroid. 2ed Edition. Philadelphia, PA: Wolters Kluwer, 2017.

39. Dahiya N, Patel MD, Young SW. Neck procedures: thyroid and parathyroid. Radiol Clin North Am. 2020;58(6):1085–98.

40. Gokcay Canpolat A, Sahin M, Ediboglu E, Erdogan MF, Gullu S, Demir O, Emral R, Corapcioglu D. Diagnostic accuracy of parathyroid hormone levels in washout samples of suspicious parathyroid adenomas: A single-Centre retrospective cohort study. Clin Endocrinol. 2018;89(4):489–95.

41. Triggiani V, Resta F, Giagulli VA, Iovino M, Licchelli B, De Pergola G, Tafaro A, Benigno M, Sabba C, Guastamacchia E. Parathyroid hormone determination in ultrasound-guided fine needle aspirates allows the differentiation between thyroid and parathyroid lesions: our experience and review of the literature. Endocr Metab Immune Disord Drug Targets. 2013;13(4):351–8.

42. Vignali E, Picone A, Materazzi G, Steffe S, Berti P, Cianferotti L, Cetani F, Ambrogini E, Miccoli P, Pinchera A, Marcocci C. A quick intraoperative parathyroid hormone assay in the surgical management of patients with primary hyperparathyroidism: a study of 206 consecutive cases. Eur J Endocrinol. 2002;146(6):783–8.

43. Uljanovs R, Sinkarevs S, Strumfs B, Vidusa L, Merkurjeva K, Strumfa I. Immunohistochemical profile of parathyroid Tumours: A comprehensive review. Int J Mol Sci. 2022;23(13)

44. Duan K, Gomez Hernandez K, Mete O. Clinicopathological correlates of hyperparathyroidism. J Clin Pathol. 2015;68(10):771–87.

45. Yu Q, Hardin H, Chu YH, Rehrauer W, Lloyd RV. Parathyroid neoplasms: Immunohistochemical characterization and long noncoding RNA (lncRNA) expression. Endocr Pathol. 2019;30(2):96–105.

46. Orell and Sterrett's Fine Needle Aspiration Cytology. Svante R Orell & Gregory F. Sterrett, 5th Edition. Sydney, Australia.

47. Absher KJ, Truong LD, Khurana KK, Ramzy I. Parathyroid cytology: avoiding diagnostic pitfalls. Head Neck. 2002;24(2):157–64.

48. Wani S, Hao Z. Atypical cystic adenoma of the parathyroid gland: case report and review of literature. Endocr Pract. 2005;11(6):389–93.

49. Silva BC, Cusano NE, Bilezikian JP. Primary hyperparathyroidism. Best Pract Res Clin Endocrinol Metab. 2018;32(5):593–607.

50. Ha HJ, Kim EJ, Kim JS, Shin MS, Noh I, Park S, Koh JS, Lee SS. Major clues and pitfalls in the differential diagnosis of parathyroid and thyroid lesions using

fine needle aspiration cytology. Medicina (Kaunas). 2020;56(11)

51. Fernandez-Ranvier GG, Khanafshar E, Jensen K, Zarnegar R, Lee J, Kebebew E, Duh QY, Clark OH. Parathyroid carcinoma, atypical parathyroid adenoma, or parathyromatosis? Cancer. 2007;110(2):255–64.

52. Fraser WD. Hyperparathyroidism. Lancet. 2009;374(9684):145–58.

53. Debruyne F, Ostyn F, Delaere P. Distribution of the solitary adenoma over the parathyroid glands. J Laryngol Otol. 1997;111(5):459–60.

54. Wieneke JA, Smith A. Parathyroid adenoma. Head Neck Pathol. 2008;2(4):305–8.

55. Summers GW. Parathyroid update: a review of 220 cases. Ear Nose Throat J. 1996;75(7):434–9.

56. Suzuki A, Hirokawa M, Kanematsu R, Tanaka A, Yamao N, Higuchi M, Hayashi T, Kuma S, Miya A, Miyauchi A. Fine-needle aspiration of parathyroid adenomas: indications as a diagnostic approach. Diagn Cytopathol. 2021;49(1):70–6.

57. Stojadinovic A, Hoos A, Nissan A, Dudas ME, Cordon-Cardo C, Shaha AR, Brennan MF, Singh B, Ghossein RA. Parathyroid neoplasms: clinical, histopathological, and tissue microarray-based molecular analysis. Hum Pathol. 2003;34(1):54–64.

58. Snover DC, Foucar K. Mitotic activity in benign parathyroid disease. Am J Clin Pathol. 1981;75(3):345–7.

59. Erickson LA, Jin L, Papotti M, Lloyd RV. Oxyphil parathyroid carcinomas: a clinicopathologic and immunohistochemical study of 10 cases. Am J Surg Pathol. 2002;26(3):344–9.

60. Giorgadze T, Stratton B, Baloch ZW, Livolsi VA. Oncocytic parathyroid adenoma: problem in cytological diagnosis. Diagn Cytopathol. 2004;31(4):276–80.

61. Paul A, Villepelet A, Lefevre M, Perie S. Oncocytic parathyroid adenoma. Eur Ann Otorhinolaryngol Head Neck Dis. 2015;132(5):301–3.

62. Paker I, Yilmazer D, Yandakci K, Arikok AT, Alper M. Intrathyroidal oncocytic parathyroid adenoma: a diagnostic pitfall on fine-needle aspiration. Diagn Cytopathol. 2010;38(11):833–6.

63. Howson P, Kruijff S, Aniss A, Pennington T, Gill AJ, Dodds T, Delbridge LW, Sidhu SB, Sywak MS. Oxyphil cell parathyroid adenomas causing primary hyperparathyroidism: a Clinico-pathological correlation. Endocr Pathol. 2015;26(3):250–4.

64. Chow LS, Erickson LA, Abu-Lebdeh HS, Wermers RA. Parathyroid lipoadenomas: a rare cause of primary hyperparathyroidism. Endocr Pract. 2006;12(2):131–6.

65. Cetani F, Torregrossa L, Marcocci C. A large functioning parathyroid lipoadenoma. Endocrine. 2016;53(2):615–6.

66. Johnson N, Serpell JW, Johnson WR, Thomson K. Parathyroid lipoadenoma. ANZ J Surg. 2015;85(6):489–90.

67. Hyrcza MD, Sargin P, Mete O. Parathyroid Lipoadenoma: a Clinicopathological diagnosis and possible trap for the unaware pathologist. Endocr Pathol. 2016;27(1):34–41.

68. Kodama H, Iihara M, Okamoto T, Obara T. Water-clear cell parathyroid adenoma causing primary hyperparathyroidism in a patient with neurofibromatosis type 1: report of a case. Surg Today. 2007;37(10):884–7.

69. Murakami K, Watanabe M, Nakashima N, Fujimori K, Ishida K, Ohuchi N, Sasano H. Water-clear cell adenoma associated with primary hyperparathyroidism: report of a case. Surg Today. 2014;44(4):773–7.

70. Piggott RP, Waters PS, Ashraf J, Colesky F, Kerin MJ. Water-clear cell adenoma: A rare form of hyperparathyroidism. Int J Surg Case Rep. 2013;4(10):911–3.

71. Chou YH, Jhuang JY, Hsieh MS. Water-clear cell parathyroid adenoma in a patient with acute pancreatitis. J Formos Med Assoc. 2014;113(11):872–3.

72. Takada N, Hirokawa M, Suzuki A, Higuchi M, Kuma S, Miyauchi A. Diagnostic value of GATA-3 in cytological identification of parathyroid tissues. Endocr J. 2016;63(7):621–6.

73. Yener S, Saklamaz A, Demir T, Kebapcilar L, Bayraktar F, Canda S, Yesil S. Primary hyperparathyroidism due to atypical parathyroid adenoma presenting with peroneus brevis tendon rupture. J Endocrinol Investig. 2007;30(5):442–4.

74. Guiter GE, DeLellis RA. Risk of recurrence or metastases in atypical parathyroid adenomas (APTAs). Modern Pathol. 2002;15(1):115a–115a.

75. Kruijff S, Sidhu SB, Sywak MS, Gill AJ, Delbridge LW. Negative parafibromin staining predicts malignant behavior in atypical parathyroid adenomas. Ann Surg Oncol. 2014;21(2):426–33.

76. de Quevain F. Parastruma maligna aberrata. Dtsch Z Fuer Chir:334–52.

77. Shane E. Clinical review 122: parathyroid carcinoma. J Clin Endocrinol Metab. 2001;86(2):485–93.

78. Al-Kurd A, Mekel M, Mazeh H. Parathyroid carcinoma. Surg Oncol. 2014;23(2):107–14.

79. Bricaire L, Odou MF, Cardot-Bauters C, Delemer B, North MO, Salenave S, Vezzosi D, Kuhn JM, Murat A, Caron P, Sadoul JL, Silve C, Chanson P, Barlier A, Clauser E, Porchet N, Groussin L, G.T.E. Group. Frequent large germline HRPT2 deletions in a French national cohort of patients with primary hyperparathyroidism. J Clin Endocrinol Metab. 2013;98(2):E403–8.

80. Holmes EC, Morton DL, Ketcham AS. Parathyroid carcinoma: a collective review. Ann Surg. 1969;169(4):631–40.

81. Schoretsanitis G, Daskalakis M, Melissas J, Tsiftsis DD. Parathyroid carcinoma: clinical presentation and management. Am J Otolaryngol. 2009;30(4):277–80.

82. Messerer CL, Bugis SP, Baliski C, Wiseman SM. Normocalcemic parathyroid carcinoma: an unusual clinical presentation. World J Surg Oncol. 2006;4:10.

83. Wynne AG, van Heerden J, Carney JA, Fitzpatrick LA. Parathyroid carcinoma: clinical and patho-

logic features in 43 patients. Medicine (Baltimore). 1992;71(4):197–205.

84. Obara T, Fujimoto Y. Diagnosis and treatment of patients with parathyroid carcinoma: an update and review. World J Surg. 1991;15(6):738–44.

85. Tamler R, Lewis MS, LiVolsi VA, Genden EM. Parathyroid carcinoma: ultrasonographic and histologic features. Thyroid. 2005;15(7):744–5.

86. Mohebati A, Shaha A, Shah J. Parathyroid carcinoma: challenges in diagnosis and treatment. Hematol Oncol Clin North Am. 2012;26(6):1221–38.

87. Koea JB, Shaw JH. Parathyroid cancer: biology and management. Surg Oncol. 1999;8(3):155–65.

88. de la Garza S, Flores de la Garza E, Hernandez Batres F. Functional parathyroid carcinoma. Cytology, histology, and ultrastructure of a case. Diagn Cytopathol. 1985;1(3):232–5.

89. Holmquist N. Fine-needle aspiration and parathyroid carcinoma. Diagn Cytopathol. 1986;2(2):179–80.

90. Harari A, Waring A, Fernandez-Ranvier G, Hwang J, Suh I, Mitmaker E, Shen W, Gosnell J, Duh QY, Clark O. Parathyroid carcinoma: a 43-year outcome and survival analysis. J Clin Endocrinol Metab. 2011;96(12):3679–86.

91. Thompson SD, Prichard AJ. The management of parathyroid carcinoma. Curr Opin Otolaryngol Head Neck Surg. 2004;12(2):93–7.

92. Kassahun WT, Jonas S. Focus on parathyroid carcinoma. Int J Surg. 2011;9(1):13–9.

Zahra Maleki Associate Professor of pathology at the Johns Hopkins University School of Medicine, at the Johns Hopkins Hospital, Division of Cytopathology, Baltimore, MD, USA. Director of the Johns Hopkins Medical School Scientific Foundations of Medicine, Histology and Pathobiology course. Member of Cancer Registry Committee, co-chair of the Membership Committee at the American Society of Cytopathology and an active committee member at the American Society of Cytopathology and the United States and Canadian Academy of Pathology.

Bayan Alzumaili and William C. Faquin

20.1 General Features

Metastatic cancer of unknown primary site including carcinomas (head and neck carcinoma of unknown primary, HNCUP) and other cancer types is a metastatic tumor which at presentation, has no identifiable site of origin clinically and radiologically [1–3]. Metastases to the cervical lymph nodes of the head and neck are of particular importance as many sites of origin and subtypes of cancer are possible. In a majority of cases, the site of origin is identified after tissue biopsy, most often by fine-needle aspiration (FNA); however, a small subset of cases remains of unknown primary despite extensive diagnostic workup (e.g. immunochemical and molecular studies).

20.2 Diagnostic Workflow

Cancers of unknown primary have been reported in up to 5% of head and neck tumors [4, 5]. Patients present with cervical lymph node enlargement which can vary in size, but most palpable lymph nodes will be 1.0 cm or larger.

B. Alzumaili · W. C. Faquin (✉)
Department of Pathology, Massachusetts General Hospital and Harvard Medical School, Boston, MA, USA
e-mail: balzumaili@mgh.harvard.edu; wfaquin@mgh.harvard.edu

The metastatic disease can be unifocal or in some cases it can be multifocal. Information about the location of the involved cervical lymph node (e.g. level I, II, III, etc.) can be very useful in formulating a differential diagnosis and potential site of origin when combined with the cytomorphologic features and results of ancillary studies [6]. As such, radiologic evaluation, usually using CT scan, is a critical component in the diagnostic workflow as well as a focused ear, nose, and throat (ENT) clinical examination. A fine needle aspiration (FNA) should be performed, and in most cases, it will be done under U/S guidance. The workup of head and neck cancers of unknown primary is therefore an integrated, multidisciplinary task shared by the ENT clinician, radiologist, cyto pathologist, and oncologist. It typically will begin with the ENT clinical assessment followed by CT studies, and an FNA coupled with ancillary immunochemical and/or molecular tests for definitive classification of the tumor.

20.3 Differential Diagnosis of the Most Common Head and Neck Cancers of Unknown Primary

A broad range of tumors can metastasize to cervical lymph nodes, but some are much more common than others. Metastatic squamous cell carcinoma is by far the most frequently encountered CUP in the head and neck [7]. Among cervical compartments, those in levels II–III are most often involved by metastatic cancers of unknown primary followed by levels I and IV–V. Table 20.1 shows the most common metastatic cancers involving cervical lymph nodes.

20.3.1 Head and Neck CUP with Squamous Differentiation

HNCUP with squamoid features include a wide range of entities, although a majority will be conventional keratinizing or non-keratinizing squamous cell carcinomas. A significant subset will

Table 20.1 Cervical lymph node metastasis with corresponding differential diagnosis and key immunochemical markers

Cervical lymph node level	Site of origin	Most common metastasis	Immunochemistry
Level I (1A: Submental and 1B: Submandibular) Preauricular/Parotid	Skin (lips, chin, face) Oral cavity (anterior tongue and floor of mouth) Skin (eyelids, scalp, and upper neck)	HPV-independent squamous cell carcinoma (skin)	Keratin 5/6, p63, p40
		Melanoma (skin)	S-100, SOX-10, MART-1, MITF, Melan-A
		Merkel cell carcinoma	CK20, Synaptophysin, Chromogranin, INSM1, MCPyV
Level IIA/B (upper internal jugular) Level III (mid jugular) Level IV (lower internal jugular)	Oropharynx (II) Oral cavity (II) Hypopharynx, Larynx (III and IV) Parotid and Submandibular (III and IV)	HPV-associated squamous cell carcinoma	P16, HPV-high risk
		HPV-independent squamous cell carcinoma (oral cavity)	Keratin 5/6, p63, p40
		Salivary gland tumors	S100, SMA, Calponin, CD117, CAM5.2, PLAG1, HMGA2, Androgen receptor, NR4A3, DOG1, MYB
	Nasopharynx (IV)	EBV-positive nasopharyngeal carcinoma	Keratins, EBER
Level V (spinal accessory, posterior triangle) Level VI (prelaryngeal and paralaryngeal) and Delphian LN (pretracheal)	Posterior scalp (V) Hypopharynx, Larynx, and esophagus (VI)	Squamous cell carcinoma	Keratin, p63, p40
	Thyroid (V and VI)	Papillary thyroid carcinoma Anaplastic thyroid carcinoma	PAX8, TTF1, thyroglobulin, BRAF
Virchow LN (supraclavicular, thoracic duct, and left subclavian vein)	Gastrointestinal, Lung	Adenocarcinoma Squamous cell carcinoma Neuroendocrine carcinoma	CK7, CK20, CDX2, STAB2 TTF1, NapsinA, Keratin, p63, p40, Synaptophysin, Chromogranin, INSM, Ki-67
Level VII (infraclavicular and thymic)	Anterior mediastinum	Thymoma and thymic carcinoma	CD117, CD5, keratin, p63, p40, CD1a, TdT, CD3, CD20

be high-risk human papilloma virus- (HR-HPV) associated squamous cell carcinomas, and a much smaller subset will be Epstein Barr Virus- (EBV) associated nasopharyngeal carcinomas. A very small subset of cases can include *NUT carcinoma* and carcinomas deficient in *SMARCB1 (INI-1)*, *SMARCA4 (BRG1)*, or *SMARCA2 (BRM)*.

A. *Cutaneous keratinizing squamous cell carcinoma* (Fig. 20.1):
   Origin: Skin (lips, chin, face, eyelids, scalp, and upper neck).
   Lymph node levels: Preauricular or parotid lymph nodes.
   Cytology: Keratinizing squamous cells with hyperchromatic, angulated nuclei, and background keratotic debris. In some cases, aspirates may be comprised predominantly of cystic degeneration, necrotic parakeratotic cells, and amorphous debris.
   Ancillary studies: Not necessary in well- and moderately differentiated cases, but for poorly differentiated and spindle cell subtypes: Keratin 5/6, p63, and p40.
   Molecular: Ultraviolet signature, *TP53, KRAS, HRAS, MYC, CDKN2A, EGFR,* and *NOTCH1* [8].

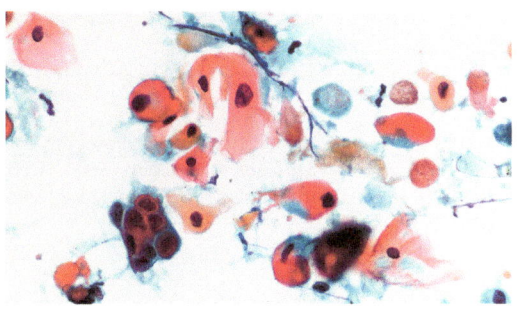

Fig. 20.1 Metastatic keratinizing squamous cell carcinoma. The aspirate demonstrates polygonal cells with moderate amounts of dense cytoplasm and keratinizing features. The follow-up histology identified this as cutaneous squamous cell carcinoma metastasis. (×600, Papanicolaou stain)

B. *Oral cavity keratinizing/non-keratinizing squamous cell carcinoma (HPV-independent):*
   Origin: Tongue, floor of mouth, lip, gingiva, and buccal mucosa.
   Lymph node levels: I, IIA/B, III.
   Cytology: Squamous cells with enlarged nuclei, variable distinct nucleoli, and cytoplasmic keratinization. May present with cystic degeneration, necrotic parakeratotic cells, and amorphous debris.
   Ancillary studies: Pan-Keratin, keratin 5/6, p63, and p40.
   Molecular: CDKN2A, TP53, CCND1, EGFR, PIK3CA, PTEN, and *NOTCH1* [9].

C. *Oropharyngeal HPV-associated non-keratinizing squamous cell carcinoma* (Fig. 20.2):
   Origin: Palatine tonsils, base of tongue, lingual tonsils, soft palate, and posterior pharyngeal wall.
   Lymph node levels: IIA/B and III.
   Cytology: Cohesive groups of non-keratinizing, high nuclear/cytoplasmic ratio squamous cells with basaloid features.
   Ancillary studies: P16+ and positive for HR-HPV-specific markers such as RNA in situ hybridization (ISH) or polymerase chain reaction (PCR).
   Molecular: PIK3CA, 3q copy number alterations, and 16q loss [9].

D. *Nasopharyngeal carcinoma (Epstein-Barr Virus-; EBV-associated)* (Fig. 20.3):
   Origin: Nasopharynx.
   Lymph node levels: II and VII.
   Cytology: Epithelial cells with large vesicular nuclei and prominent nucleoli, syncytial pattern admixed with lymphocytes.
   Ancillary studies: Keratin 5/6, p63, p40 and ISH for Epstein-Barr encoding region (EBER).
   Molecular: Bcl-2, MYC, NF-κB, JNK, JAK/STAT, PI3K/Akt, TP53, PRDM1, DICE1, and *PTEN* [10].

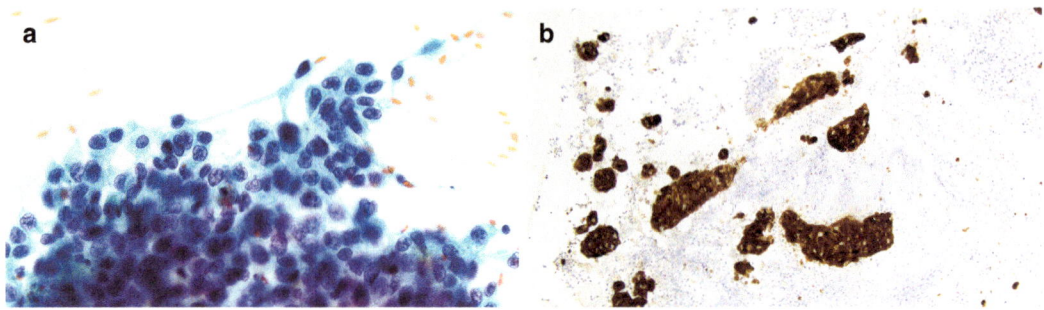

Fig. 20.2 Metastatic HPV-associated non-keratinizing squamous cell carcinoma. (**a**) The aspirate demonstrates a cohesive group of malignant cells with small amounts of dense cytoplasm and pleomorphic oval nuclei. The cells have a basaloid appearance (×400, Papanicolaou stain).

(**b**) The cell block demonstrates groups of malignant cells which are strongly and diffusely positive for p16, a surrogate marker for high-risk HPV. This result should be verified using an HPV-specific test such as RNA in situ hybridization or PCR (×100, Immunohistochemical stain)

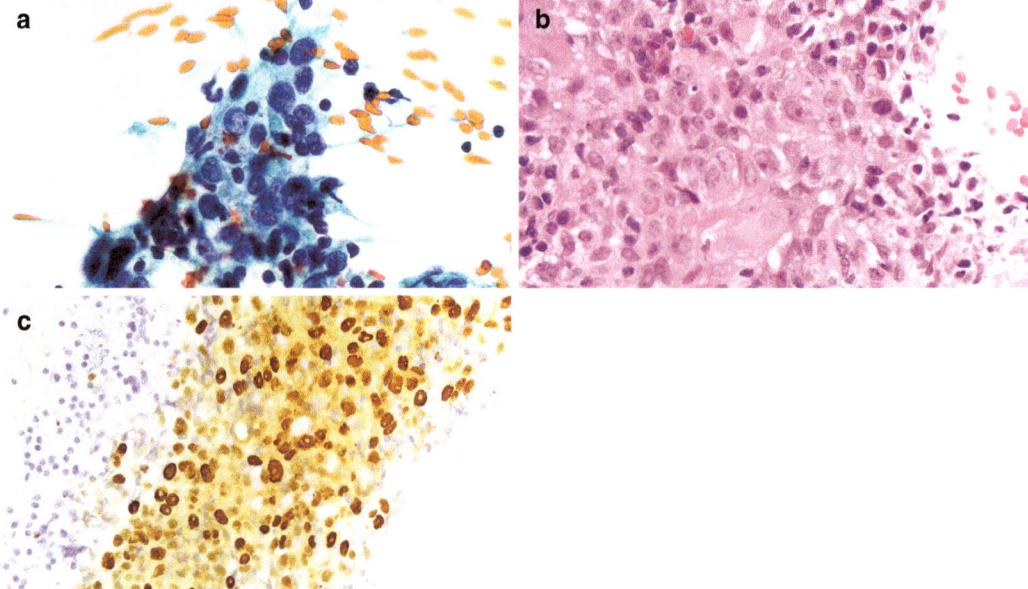

Fig. 20.3 Metastatic nasopharyngeal carcinoma. (**a**) The malignant cells are present in a loosely cohesive arrangement with admixed lymphocytes. The cells have moderate amounts of pale cytoplasm and a large round to oval nucleus with distinct nucleolus (×600, Papanicolaou

stain). (**b**) The corresponding cell block shows the large malignant cells with a prominent nucleolus (×600, H&E), and (**c**) in situ hybridization for EBER is positive (×400, in situ hybridization)

20.3.2 Carcinomas of Thyroid Origin

A. *Classic papillary thyroid carcinoma* (Fig. 20.4):
   Lymph node levels: V, VI, and VII.
   Cytology: Syncytial groups of cells with enlarged, oval, overlapping nuclei with chromatin pallor, nuclear grooves, intra-
   nuclear pseudoinclusions, and papillary architecture.
   Ancillary studies: PAX8, TTF1, BRAF, and thyroglobulin.
   Molecular: BRAF is most common; others may include RET/PTC [11].
B. *Anaplastic thyroid carcinoma* (Fig. 20.5):
   Lymph node levels: V, VI, and VII.

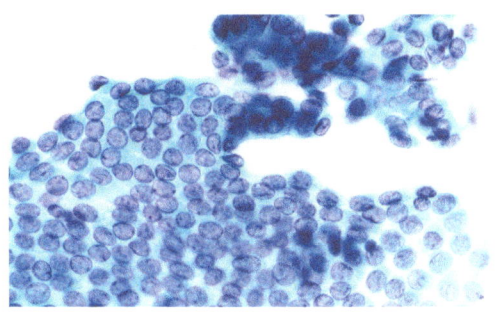

Fig. 20.4 Metastatic classic papillary thyroid carcinoma. The aspirate demonstrates cells in syncytial sheets and papillary arrangements. Nuclei are oval, grooved, overlapping, and have pale chromatin. (×600, Papanicolaou stain)

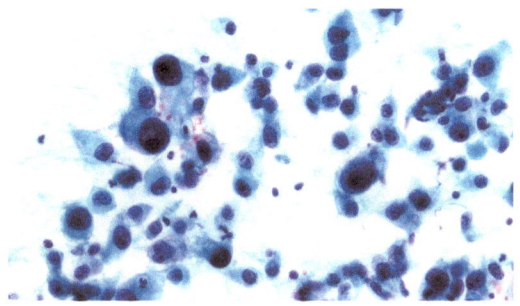

Fig. 20.5 Metastatic anaplastic thyroid carcinoma. The FNA is cellular and comprised of markedly atypical epithelial cells including occasional cells with very large nuclei. The degree of nuclear pleomorphism and overall atypia in the context of a concurrent thyroid mass would identify this as anaplastic thyroid carcinoma. PAX-8 is one of the most useful ancillary markers, and many cases will be positive for BRAF mutation (×400, Papanicolaou stain)

Cytology: Overtly malignant epithelial cells in crowded groups and as single cells. Tumor cells have markedly pleomorphic, hyperchromatic nuclei with mitoses, and background tumor diathesis. Some cases will have tumor giant cells and/or spindled cells.
Ancillary studies: Keratins, PAX8, p53.
Molecular: BRAF, RAS, TERT promoter, *TP53, PIK3CA, E1F1AX, and PTEN* [12].
C. *Medullary thyroid carcinoma* (Fig. 20.6):
 Lymph node levels: V, VI, and VII.
 Cytology: Dispersed population of uniform plasmacytoid cells with round to oval nuclei showing granular "salt and pepper"

chromatin. A variety of cell shapes and patterns can be seen. Background amyloid resembling colloid can be seen.
Ancillary studies: Calcitonin, CEA, PAX8+/−, and Congo red for amyloid.
Molecular: RET [13, 14].

20.3.3 Other Selected Metastatic Cancers of Unknown Primary

A. *Melanoma (cutaneous and mucosal)* (Fig. 20.7):
 Lymph node levels: Any level (regional or distant metastasis).
 Cytology: Enlarged atypical pleomorphic cells, binucleated, with prominent nucleoli, melanin pigment, and cytoplasmic inclusions. Single cells are common; occasional loose clusters.
 Ancillary studies: S-100, SOX-10, MART-1, MITF, and Melan-A.
 Molecular: BRAF, BAP, CDKN2A, GNAQ, GNA11, NRAS, NF1, MAP2K1/MAP2K2, KIT, PTEN, and *TERT* promoter [15].
B. *Merkel cell carcinoma (Skin)* (Fig. 20.8):
 Lymph node levels: Regional lymph nodes (Preauricular/Parotid).
 Cytology: Monotonous small round cells, single cells or loosely cohesive clusters, with round to elongated nuclei, coarsely granular chromatin, nuclear molding, and scant basophilic cytoplasm.
 Ancillary studies: Merkel cell polyomavirus (MCPyV), INSM1, Synaptophysin, Chromogranin, CK20, and TTF-1 negative.
 Molecular: Ultraviolet signature, Human Merkel Cell Polyoma Virus, *TP53,* and *RB* [16].
C. *Small cell carcinoma:*
 Lymph node levels: Any level (distant metastasis: lung).
 Cytology: See above (same as Merkel cell carcinoma).
 Ancillary studies: Keratin, INSM1, Synaptophysin, Chromogranin, and TTF-1.
 Molecular: TP53, RB, and *IKK/NF-κB* [17].

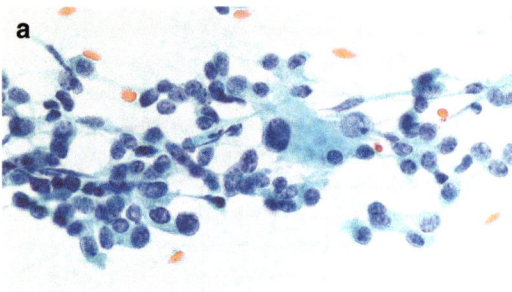 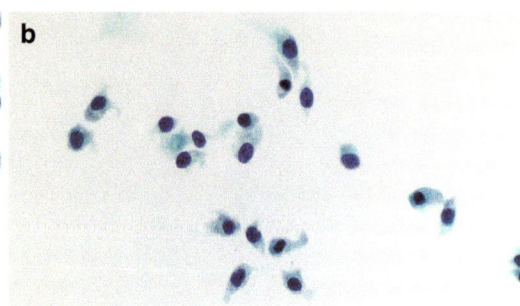

Fig. 20.6 Metastatic medullary thyroid carcinoma. (**a**, **b**) The cells are dispersed, and most nuclei are oval and cytologically bland with a pale granular chromatin pattern. Occasional cells (**a**) have much larger nuclei. Ancillary stains for calcitonin or CEA can be useful (×600, Papanicolaou stain)

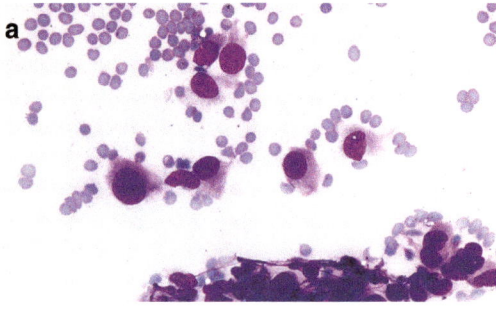 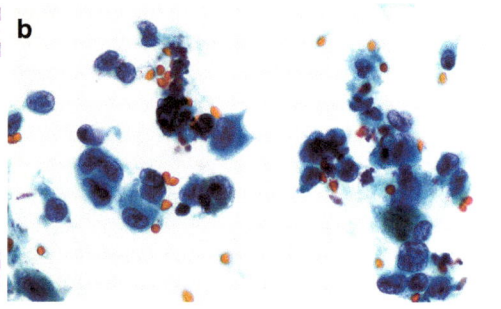

Fig. 20.7 Metastatic Melanoma. (**a**, **b**) The malignant cells are dispersed and present in a loose cluster. Nuclei are large with focal intranuclear inclusion, and there is a moderate amount of cytoplasm. Occasional histiocytes with cytoplasmic pigment are also present (**a**, ×400, Diff-Quik stain; **b**, ×600, Papanicolaou stain)

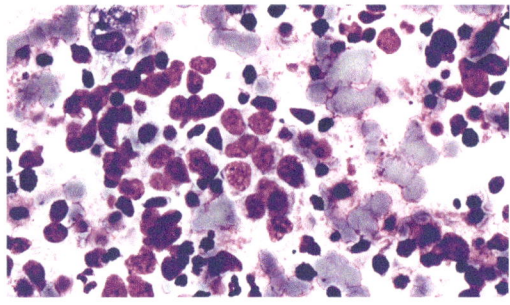

Fig. 20.8 Metastatic Merkel cell carcinoma. The malignant cells have large atypical nuclei and very scant cytoplasm. There are stripped nuclei, necrosis, and some cells demonstrate nuclear molding. Background lymphocytes are present (×600, Diff-Quik stain)

D. *Olfactory neuroblastoma:*
   Lymph node levels: Level II.
   Cytology: Small round blue cell tumor with loosely cohesive clusters. Scant fibrillary cytoplasm, granular chromatin, occasional rosettes, and nuclear molding.
   Ancillary studies: Synaptophysin, Chromogranin, INSM1, NSE, and S100 (sustentacular cells).
   Molecular: GLI1, GLI2, ASH1/ASCL1, and *IDH2 R172* [18].
E. *Distant Metastases* (Fig. 20.9):
   Lymph node levels: Supraclavicular lymph nodes.

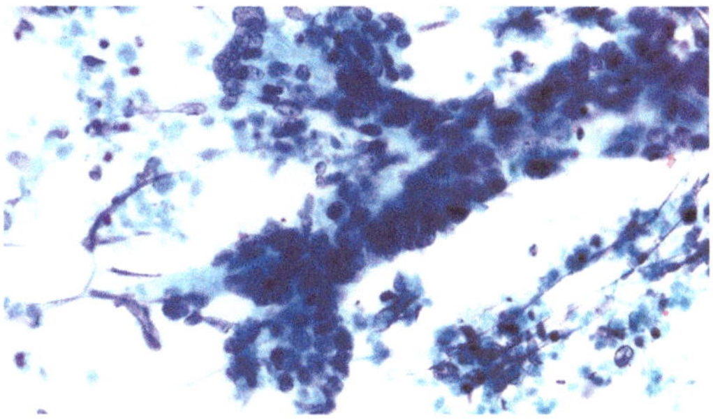

Fig. 20.9 Metastatic colon carcinoma. The aspirate is cellular and shows 3-dimensional glandular groups of high-grade adenocarcinoma. Individual cells have a columnar morphology, pleomorphic nuclei, and background necrosis. These features are characteristic of metastatic colon cancer to any anatomic site (×400, Papanicolaou stain)

Cytology: Adenocarcinoma cytomorphology with variable features depending on specific subtype. Distant metastases are uncommon but include lung, GI, breast, prostate, GYN.

Ancillary studies: Lung (TTF1, CK7, NapsinA); Gastrointestinal tract: CDX2 and CK7: upper GI, CK20: lower GI, CK19: pancreaticobiliary.

References

1. Sinnathamby K, Peters LJ, Laidlaw C, Hughes PG. The occult head and neck primary: to treat or not to treat? Clin Oncol (R Coll Radiol). 1997;9(5):322–9.
2. Friesland S, Lind MG, Lundgren J, Munck-Wikland E, Fernberg JO. Outcome of ipsilateral treatment for patients with metastases to neck nodes of unknown origin. Acta Oncol. 2001;40(1):24–8.
3. Grau C, Johansen LV, Jakobsen J, Geertsen P, Andersen E, Jensen BB. Cervical lymph node metastases from unknown primary tumours. Results from a national survey by the Danish Society for Head and Neck Oncology. Radiother Oncol. 2000;55(2):121–9.
4. Kennel T, Garrel R, Costes V, Boisselier P, Crampette L, Favier V. Head and neck carcinoma of unknown primary. Eur Ann Otorhinolaryngol Head Neck Dis. 2019;136(3):185–92.
5. Barbora U, Marcela N, Vladimir C, Andrej H. Carcinoma of unknown primary in head and neck region. Klin Onkol. 2018;31(4):277–81.
6. Calabrese L, Jereczek-Fossa BA, Jassem J, Rocca A, Bruschini R, Orecchia R, et al. Diagnosis and management of neck metastases from an unknown primary. Acta Otorhinolaryngol Ital. 2005;25(1):2–12.
7. Chernock RD, Lewis JS. Approach to metastatic carcinoma of unknown primary in the head and neck: squamous cell carcinoma and beyond. Head Neck Pathol. 2015;9(1):6–15.
8. Kraft S, Granter SR. Molecular pathology of skin neoplasms of the head and neck. Arch Pathol Lab Med. 2014;138(6):759–87.
9. Leemans CR, Snijders PJF, Brakenhoff RH. The molecular landscape of head and neck cancer. Nat Rev Cancer. 2018;18(5):269–82.
10. Yin H, Qu J, Peng Q, Gan R. Molecular mechanisms of EBV-driven cell cycle progression and oncogenesis. Med Microbiol Immunol. 2019;208(5):573–83.
11. Lee YC, Hsu CY, Lai CR, Hang JF. NTRK-rearranged papillary thyroid carcinoma demonstrates frequent subtle nuclear features and indeterminate cytologic diagnoses. Cancer Cytopathol. 2022;130(2):136–43.
12. Xu B, Fuchs T, Dogan S, Landa I, Katabi N, Fagin JA, et al. Dissecting anaplastic thyroid carcinoma: a comprehensive clinical, histologic, immunophenotypic, and molecular study of 360 cases. Thyroid. 2020;30(10):1505–17.
13. Xu B, Fuchs TL, Ahmadi S, Alghamdi M, Alzumaili B, Bani MA, et al. International medullary thyroid carcinoma grading system: a validated grading system for medullary thyroid carcinoma. J Clin Oncol. 2022;40(1):96–104.
14. Najdawi F, Ahmadi S, Capelletti M, Dong F, Chau NG, Barletta JA. Evaluation of grade in a genotyped cohort of sporadic medullary thyroid carcinomas. Histopathology. 2021;79(3):427–36.
15. Zob DL, Augustin I, Caba L, Panzaru MC, Popa S, Popa AD, et al. Genomics and epigenomics in the molecular biology of melanoma-a prerequisite for biomarkers studies. Int J Mol Sci. 2022;24(1):716.
16. Gauci ML, Aristei C, Becker JC, Blom A, Bataille V, Dreno B, et al. Diagnosis and treatment of Merkel cell carcinoma: European consensus-based interdisciplinary guideline—update 2022. Eur J Cancer. 2022;171:203–31.
17. Koerner L, Schmiel M, Yang TP, Peifer M, Buettner R, Pasparakis M. NEMO- and RelA-dependent NF-kappaB signaling promotes small cell lung cancer. Cell Death Differ. 2023.
18. Bell D, Brandea AI, Hanna EY. Olfactory neuroblastoma: morphological reappraisal and molecular insights with quantum leap in clinical perspectives. Curr Oncol Rep. 2022.

Bayan Alzumaili is an Instructor at Harvard Medical School, Boston, MA, USA, and an Assistant in Head and Neck and Breast Pathology at Massachusetts General Hospital, Boston, MA, USA. His areas of expertise include thyroid, salivary gland, and sinonasal lesions.

William C. Faquin is the Professor of pathology at Harvard Medical School, Boston, MA, USA. He has authored over 400 peer-reviewed publications. He is the Editor-in-Chief for *Cancer Cytopathology*, which is one of the three journals of the American Cancer Society. He is a co-author of *The Bethesda System for Reporting Thyroid Cytopathology*, co-chair of the College of American Pathologists' Evidence-Based Guidelines Committee for the testing of head and neck squamous cell carcinomas for high-risk HPV, and co-chair of *The Milan System for Reporting Salivary Gland Cytopathology*, sponsored by the ASC and IAC.

Dermatopathologic Approach to Diagnostic Challenges in the Head and Neck

21

Raymond L. Barnhill and Jennifer Ko

21.1 Pigmented Lesions

Lesions that may be pigmented and occur on the head and neck include seborrheic keratosis (SK), pigmented actinic keratosis (AK), pigmented basal cell carcinomas (BCC), solar lentigines (SL), melanocytic nevi, pigmented Spitz tumors, and melanoma. Seborrheic keratosis, pigmented AK, and pigmented BCC are relatively easily diagnosed and treated, and this section will focus on the other entities in the differential.

Most biopsies of pigmented head/neck neoplasms are submitted to evaluate for the possibility of melanoma. In the case of relatively thin, flat epidermal lesions, the clinical differential diagnosis is typically lentigo or lentiginous junctional nevus versus lentigo maligna or lentigo maligna melanoma (LMM). In these cases, it is important to obtain a significant proportion of the epidermis and superficial dermis with a biopsy, often more easily accomplished with a deep or "scoop" shave biopsy. This is because tumor spread is irregular, and often shows areas of skip or regression. For particularly large lesions, scouting shave or small punch biopsies may also be helpful, to more thoroughly assess for melanoma arising in a SL or SK and to aid in surgical planning [1, 2].

21.1.1 Lentigo Maligna

Lentigo maligna remains a controversial term since it signifies a melanocytic dysplasia or precursor to melanoma in situ, lentigo maligna type, to some, and simply melanoma in situ to others. This controversy has never been completely resolved. The defining histopathologic features of lentigo maligna as a dysplasia include a broad, disorganized, predominantly single cell, junctional melanocytic proliferation with cytological atypia on significantly sun-damaged skin with conspicuous solar elastotic change in the dermis. Melanocytes typically are arranged in a lentiginous or "lining up" pattern with back to back spread along the basement membrane, and frequent involvement of adnexal structures. Melanocytes can show a variety of cytomorphologic features, but most commonly demonstrate variable nuclear enlargement, hyperchromasia, and variably enlarged nucleoli. Increased retraction artifact from surrounding keratinocytes is often also noted. Confluence of atypical basilar melanocytes, pagetoid spread, junctional nesting, and conspicuous adnexal involvement are criteria

R. L. Barnhill (✉)
Department of Translational Research, Institut Curie and University of Paris, Paris, France
e-mail: raymond.barnhill@curie.fr

J. Ko
Department of Pathology, Cleveland Clinic, Cleveland, OH, USA
e-mail: koj2@ccf.org

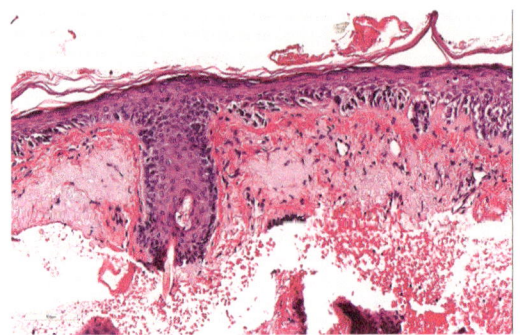

Fig. 21.1 Lentigo maligna. Hyperchromatic single melanocytes and small nests of melanocytes are lined up along the dermoepidermal junction. There is marked solar elastosis (H&E, 200X)

signifying the beginnings of melanoma in situ (Fig. 21.1) [3]. Invasion into the dermis is indicative of lentigo maligna melanoma.

Solar lentigines (SL) and (atypical/dysplastic) junctional lentiginous nevi are the main differential diagnostic considerations. Because melanocytic nevi are known to regress with age, because the degree of sun exposure to the head and neck, and because of the minimal cytologic atypia that can been seen in LM(M), extreme caution is required in considering a diagnosis of atypical or "dysplastic" nevus in this area. From a practical consideration, the diagnosis of a dysplastic nevus in this location should be approached with great caution in anyone older than 40 years. Immunohistochemical (IHC) stains for SOX10 are often helpful in highlighting focal melanocyte nesting and confluence, excluding a SL, which should only show melanocytic hyperplasia [4]. SOX10 stains also make the nuclear enlargement and architectural disarray typical of LM(M) easier to identify. PRAME is another useful IHC stain in this setting; however, positivity should only be interpreted in the setting of strong and diffuse positivity (>75% of cells), because sun-damaged skin can show lower level background staining in melanocytes [5]. In many institutions, a modified variant of Mohs micrographic surgery, known as "slow Mohs" is frequently performed in melanoma in situ or early invasive melanoma involving the face, in order to maximally conserve the surrounding healthy tissue in

this cosmetically sensitive area, while allowing for complete circumferential margin assessment. In this procedure, oriented en face margin specimens are submitted for histopathologic examination. Quick pathologic turnaround (1–2 days) is important in these cases, as wounds are left open until the final report is received.

21.1.2 Spitz Tumors

Spitz tumors, including Spitz nevi and atypical Spitz tumors (AST), commonly occur on the head and neck as pink papules or plaques, and may prove quite difficult to distinguish from Spitz or spitzoid melanoma. In evaluating these lesions, patient age is extremely informative (true Spitz melanoma under the age of 10 years appears almost nonexistent), and complete removal is again optimal, in order to assess the architecture and cytological features of these lesions. Spitz nevi characteristically exhibit diameters <5–6 mm, sharp-circumscription, symmetry, epidermal hyperplasia, and clefting between vertically oriented melanocytic nests and adjacent keratinocytes (Fig. 21.2), dull pink (Kamino) bodies, maturation of the dermal component, and low mitotic rates (usually <2 per mm^2 [6, 7]. Cytomorphologically, uniform epithelioid and spindled melanocytes with abundant cytoplasm, enlarged nuclei, open chromatin, and prominent nucleoli are seen [1–2, 7]. After assessment of the parameters mentioned above, spitzoid neoplasms with one or more atypical features (atypical Spitz tumors), such as diameter >5 mm, **especially >10 mm**, **ulceration**, **involvement of subcutaneous fat**, asymmetry, lack of maturation, dermal nodule formation, **increased mitotic rates >5–6 per mm^2**, deep mitoses, and conspicuous cytological atypia, especially in patients >10 years of age and adult patients, may merit additional ancillary testing with immunohistochemistry such as p16, Ki67, PRAME, BRAFV600E, possibly comprehensive molecular studies, and referral to an expert in order to exclude Spitz or spitzoid melanoma. BRAFV600E positivity excludes a true Spitz lineage and raises the possibility of a spitzoid

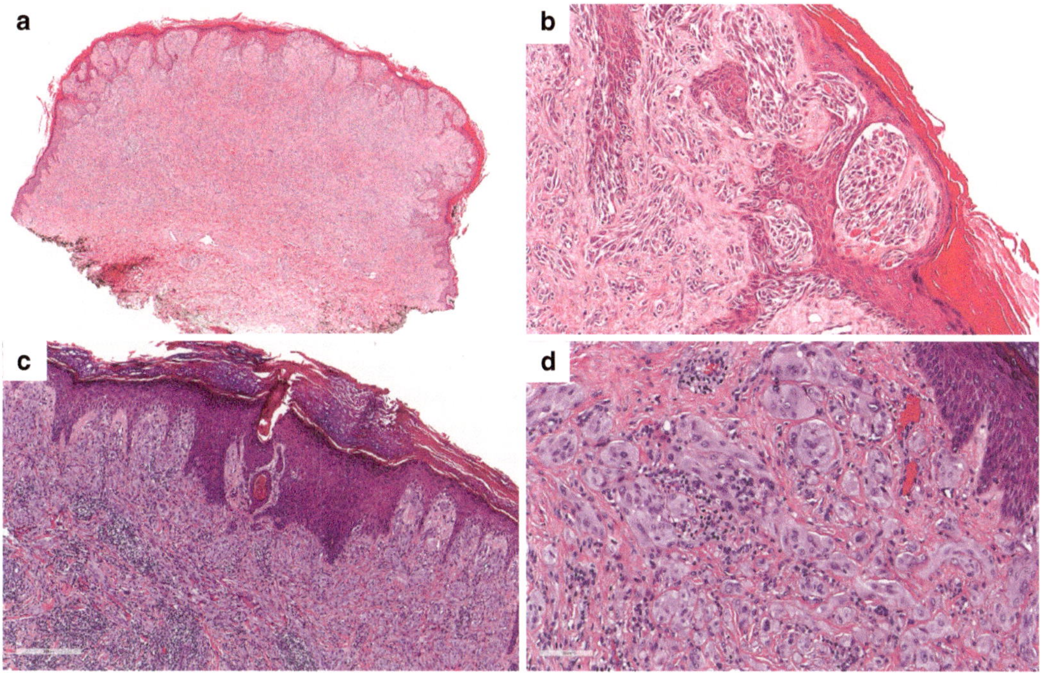

Fig. 21.2 Atypical Spitz Tumor. (**a**) Sections show a large, circumscribed, symmetric compound melanocytic proliferation on non-sun damaged skin with epidermal hyperplasia (H&E, 20X). (**b**) Junctional nests are vertically and horizontally oriented with clefting from kerati-nocytes, and clusters of Kamino bodies (H&E, 200X). (**c**) Another tumor shows a more ill-defined junctional component, and dermal inflammation (H&E, 100X). (**d**) Cells are relatively more epithelioid and less spindled, and are uniformly atypical (H&E, 200X)

tumor, whether non-atypical, atypical, or melanoma [8, 9]. Complete loss of p16 expression suggests homozygous deletion of 9p21, requires molecular confirmation, and raises suspicion for Spitz or spitzoid melanoma [10, 11]. Since true Spitz melanomas and even other melanomas with spitzoid features are rare, such diagnoses should be made only with sufficient evidence (e.g., age >10–20 years, diameter >1 cm, ulceration, subcutaneous fat involvement, mitotic rate >6 per mm^2, p16 loss, three or more genetic alterations (especially TERT promoter mutations)), and consultation with an expert [12].

21.1.3 Desmoplastic Melanoma

Another melanocytic tumor seen in this region that is very difficult to recognize by both clinicians and pathologists is desmoplastic melanoma (DM) (Fig. 21.3). DM presents in older white men > women (mean age: 65 years), involving predominately sun-exposed skin of the head and neck. DM often appears clinically as a nondescript raised, firm amelanotic nodule or depressed indurated plaque. The irregular and variegated features of LM or lentiginous melanoma in situ may be the most notable clinical feature of DM. In approximately 50% of cases, there is no epidermal component. Indeed, tumors often come in labeled "epidermoid cyst," often from the scalp. The essential histopathologic criteria for DM are a predominant spindle cell phenotype and an associated densely collagenized (or "desmoplastic") stroma of the invasive dermal component. Other features including atypical lentiginous melanocytic proliferation and melanoma in situ, neurotropism, and lymphocytic infiltrates within the tumor stroma, aid in diagnosis but may be absent. Cytological atypia and mitotic activity vary from being absent to florid. Tumor cells demonstrate tapered ends

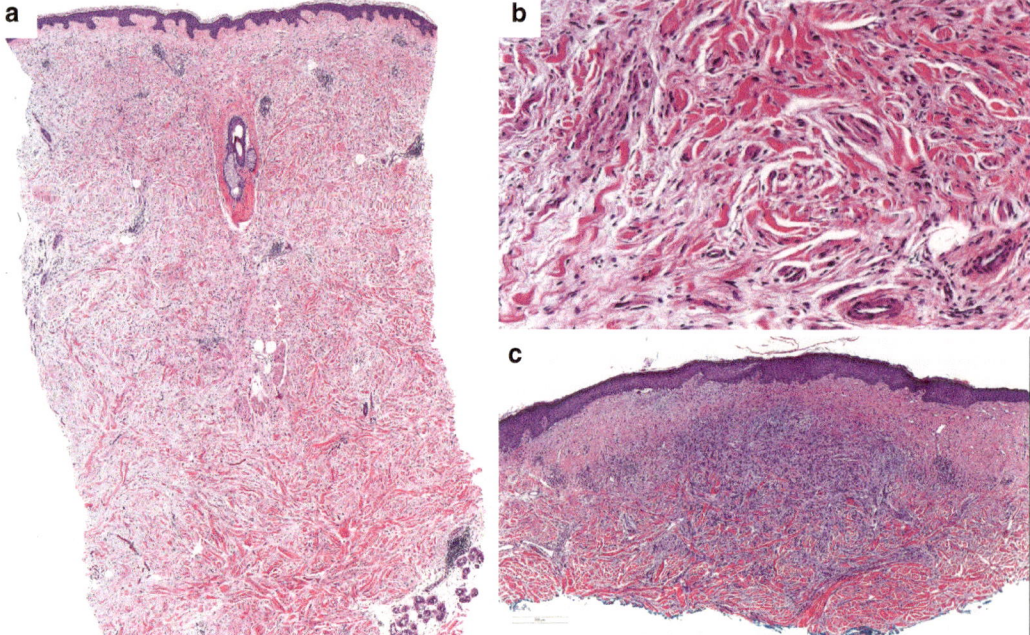

Fig. 21.3 **Desmoplastic Melanoma**. (**a**) At low magnification, there is an ill-defined, dermal spindle cell proliferation on sun-damaged skin with scattered lymphoid aggregates (H&E, 20X). (**b**) At higher magnification, scattered cells show hyperchromatic, mildly enlarged nuclei with wavy contours and tapered ends (H&E 200X). (**c**) Here, the tumor shows areas of increased cellularity centrally, and a focal overlying junctional component (H&E, 20X)

with variable, subtle nuclear atypia. Perineural invasion is common [13–15]. The differential diagnosis is wide and includes scar, various fibromas, dermatofibroma, atypical fibroxanthoma, pleomorphic sarcoma, nerve sheath tumors, especially neurofibroma, benign and malignant, spindle cell and desmoplastic squamous cell carcinoma, angiosarcoma, and leiomyosarcoma. Confirmation of DM by a panel of immunomarkers, both positive and pertinent negatives, in the spindle cell component is usually necessary. These include S100 protein, SOX10, p75NGFR, and MITF (variable); whereas, melan-A/MART-1, HMB45, tyrosinase, cytokeratin, p63, p40, and desmin are usually negative. Wide excision and SLNB is typically performed for "mixed" DMs with conventional melanoma component. There is a rela-tively reduced incidence of lymph node spread, especially with "pure" variants of DM, and outcome is more favorable compared to other melanoma subtypes with similar Breslow thickness [15, 16].

21.2 Non-Pigmented Epidermal Tumors

Non-pigmented epidermal tumors most commonly seen on the head and neck include basal cell carcinoma (BCC), squamous cell carcinoma in situ (SCCIS), and squamous cell carcinoma (SCC), as well as basaloid tumors with relatively more aggressive potential—Merkel cell carcinoma (MCC), sebaceous carcinoma (sebCA), and microcystic adnexal carcinoma (MAC) [17].

21.2.1 Basal Cell Carcinoma

BCC is the most common cancer, and resembles the basal layer of keratinocytes, and is thought to arise from the outer root sheath of the pilosebaceous unit. BCC show a variety of growth patterns, associated with relatively indolent to more aggressive behavior, although nearly all patients have an excellent prognosis following tumor excision. BCC show enlarged ovoid to polygonal tumor nuclei, with minimal amounts of pale cytoplasm, arranged in variably sized nodules in the dermis, often with connection to the epidermis, and at least focal mucinous stroma. Tumor nuclei palisade peripherally, around the outer aspect of tumor nodules, and nodules often retract from adjacent dermal stroma with cleft formation. Several types exist including, and not limited to (in order of most to least indolent), superficial, nodular, micronodular, infiltrative, and morpheaform (Fig. 21.4) [18]. The main alternative diagnostic considerations include trichoblastoma, trichoepithelioma, poorly differentiated SCC, sebCA, and MCC [19]. Basal cell carcinomas have the same IHC staining pattern as other adnexal tumors of follicular origin, including trichoblastoma (TB) and trichoepithelioma (TE) (BerEP4 positive); however, BCC shows loss of benign colonizing CK20+ Merkel cells, whereas the other tumors retain CK20+ Merkel cells. Additionally, TB and TE show more pronounced follicular stroma changes, including fibrotic stroma with delicate spindled cells and papillary mesenchymal bodies, and less cytologic atypia, no necrosis, and no stromal mucin with peripheral clefting (Fig. 21.5) [20].

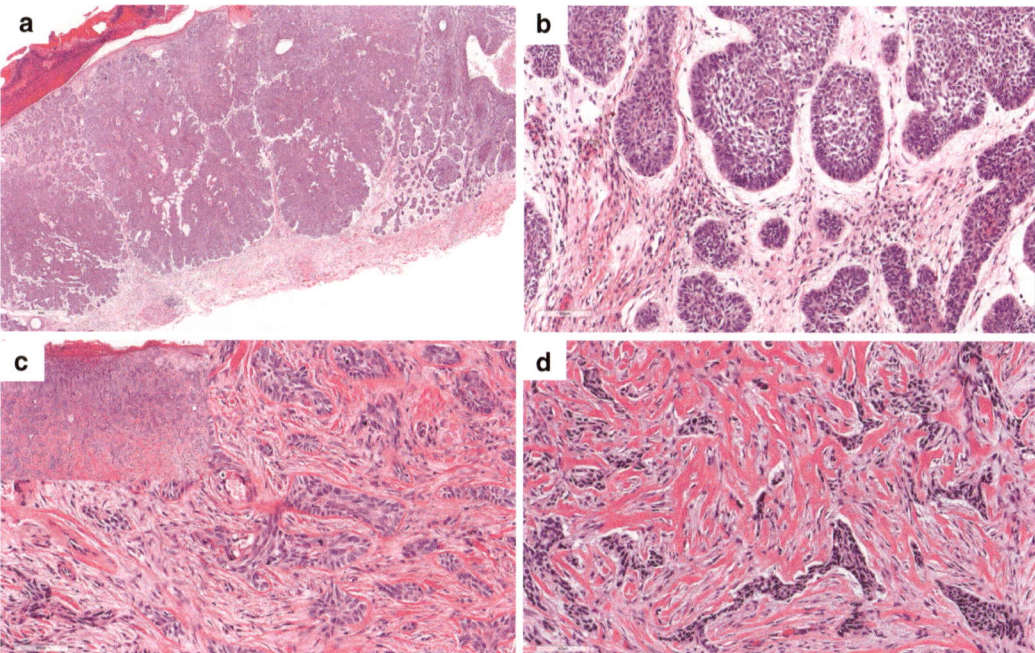

Fig. 21.4 Basal Cell Carcinoma. (**a**) Sections show an ulcerated dermal tumor arranged in large nodules with a pushing border (H&E, 10X, nodular type). (**b**) Cells show peripheral nuclear palisading and clefting from surrounding stroma with slight mucin (H&E, 200X, nodular and micronodular types). (**c**) Cells are arranged in infiltrative cords with surrounding stromal desmoplasia (H&E, 200X, infiltrative type). (**d**) Infiltrative tumor cords are compressing and stroma shows dense collagen (H&E, 200x, morpheaform type)

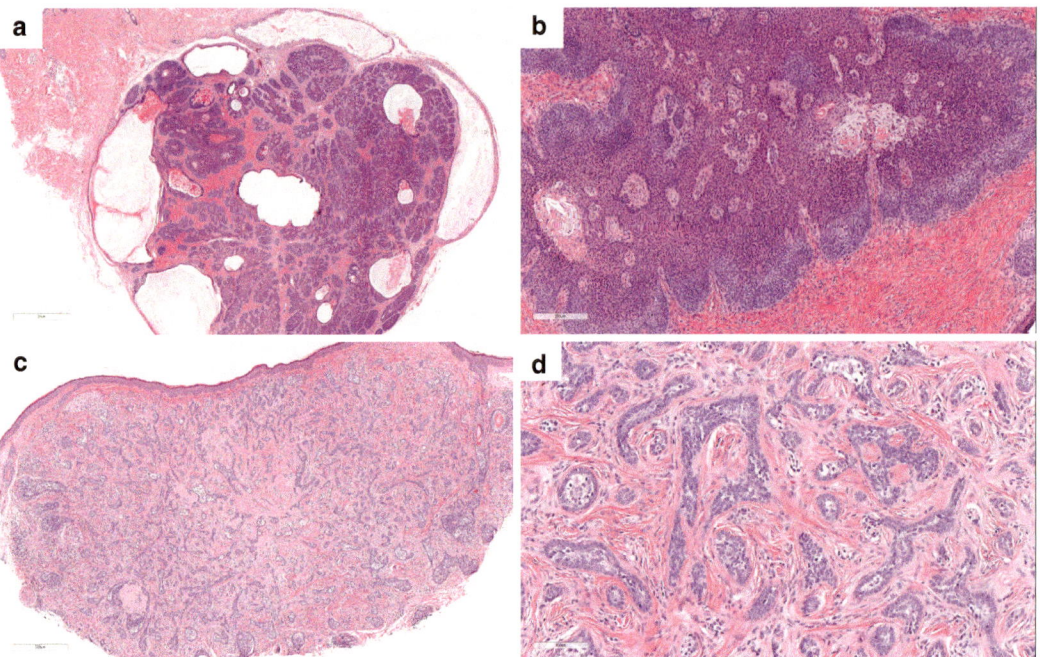

Fig. 21.5 **Trichoblastoma**. (**a**) The tumor is circumscribed, nodular, and dermal based, comprised of basaloid cells with palisading, keratin microcysts, and a cellular stroma (H&E, 20x). (**b**) Subtle areas of pilomatrical differentiation are noted on closer inspection (H&E, 100X). **Trichoepithelioma**. (**c**) Basaloid tumor cells are arranged in islands and cords in a cellular, fibrotic stroma (H&E, 20X). (**d**) There is no stromal retraction, and no significant cytologic atypia (H&E, 200X)

21.2.2 Squamous Cell Carcinoma

SCC is the second most common skin cancer. It arises from the keratinizing cells of the epidermis (Fig. 21.6). Well-differentiated SCC closely resembles normal epidermis, but shows an endophytic growth pattern, with irregularly shaped infiltrative islands and a desmoplastic stromal response. Paradoxical maturation, with deep parakeratosis and keratin formation is typical, along with subtle cytologic atypia characterized by increased watery, pale pink cytoplasm, irregular nuclear membranes and prominent nucleoli. Moderately and poorly differentiated SCC show increased nuclear to cytoplasmic ratios and less to no keratin. They can be confirmed by cytokeratins, and, if available, p63, and p40 IHC staining

positivity with an absence of BerEP4 positivity. Risk factors for SCC recurrence/spread include immune compromise, poor differentiation, perineural invasion, and/or incomplete initial excision [21].

21.2.3 Merkel Cell Carcinoma

MCC is a somewhat rare, but extremely aggressive and potentially lethal, cutaneous malignancy of increasing incidence, comprised of malignant Merkel cells—neuroendocrine cells involved in light touch. Approximately 80% of cases in the US are initiated by the Merkel cell polyoma virus (MPV), and the remaining are caused by UV exposure [22]. Tumors are treated

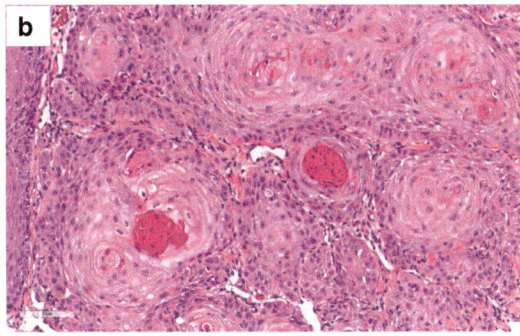

Fig. 21.6 Invasive Squamous Cell Carcinoma. (**a**) Sections show an endophytic tumor comprised of irregular squamoid islands with deep, paradoxical keratinization and a desmoplastic stroma interface (H&E, 20x). (**b**) Cells show watery pale pink cytoplasm and abrupt parakeratin, with subtle nuclear atypia (H&E, 200)

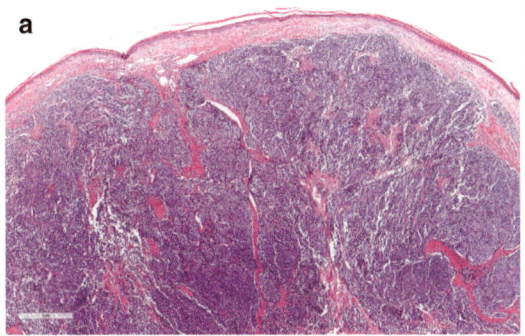
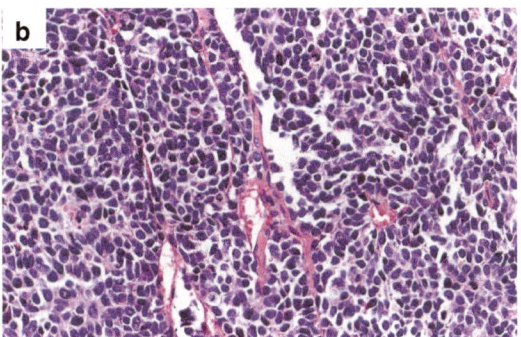

Fig. 21.7 Merkel Cell Carcinoma. (**a**) There is a basaloid tumor arranged in sheets with intervening fibrous stroma and absence of stromal retraction or palisading (H&E, 20X). (**b**) Tumor cells have scant cytoplasm, and polygonal nuclei with molding and fine, neuroendocrine chromatin, and no nucleoli. There are scattered mitotic and necrotic tumor cells (H&E, 200X)

with wide excision in addition to sentinel lymph node biopsy (SLNB). And SLN status, along with age, and immune status have prognostic significance [23, 24]. Tumors can mimic BCC at low magnification, as a dermal based, variably nodular to infiltrative tumor of small to medium-sized blue cells with scant cytoplasm. On closer inspection, MCC lack peripheral nuclear palisading, and show fine, salt and pepper chromatin with nuclear molding, crush artifact, increased mitoses, and single cell necrosis (Fig. 21.7). MCC is positive for CK20, although rare cases of CK20-negative tumors are seen, typically unassociated with the MPV [22, 25]. MCC is positive for neuroendocrine markers INSM1, synaptophysin, and chromogranin. As a caveat, it should be pointed out that BCC may be positive for synaptophysin or chromogranin (but not INSM1), and MCC may be positive for Ber-EP4 [26, 27].

21.2.4 Sebaceous Carcinoma

Sebaceous carcinoma is another potentially aggressive tumor that commonly occurs on the head, specifically the periorbital region of middle-aged to elderly patients. A subset of sebCA occurs in association with Muir-Torre syndrome; however, most arise sporadically [28, 29]. SebCA can recur locally, spread to the draining lymph node, and/or metastasize, resulting in death. For this reason, SLNB is often performed with excision [30]. Histologically, tumors resemble BCC at low magnification, with large, relatively more lobulated nodules of basaloid cells in the dermis. Pagetoid spread can be seen in the overlying epidermis, unlike BCC. Typically, at least a small subset of cells show histopathologically evident sebaceous differentiation, with ample, clear, microvacuolated cytoplasm and small, indented nuclei. That said, this can be absent in high-grade tumors. In this setting, there is typically more pleomorphism and greater mitotic activity than that seen in BCC. In contrast to BCC, there is strong expression of EMA in SebCA, negative staining for Ber-EP4, and often diffuse staining with androgen receptor, adipophilin, and PRAME [31].

21.2.5 Microcystic Adnexal Carcinoma

Microcystic adnexal carcinoma (MAC) is another rare, aggressive malignancy which commonly occurs on the head and neck, typically the central face, of patients of all ages. MAC has both follicular and eccrine differentiation, showing (typically more superficial) squamoid islands with keratinous microcysts, which become small, bland but infiltrative basaloid islands, cords, and tubules, some of which contain eccrine duct lumens (Fig. 21.8). Subcutaneous and perineural invasion are common. Syringomas and trichoepitheliomas are benign eccrine and follicular tumors, respectively, that also show strands of basaloid tumor cells in a fibrotic stroma, with micro- (sweat or keratin) cysts, and thus require differentiation from MAC and BCC. Table 21.1 demonstrates the most useful differentiating immunohistochemical features of these entities [32].

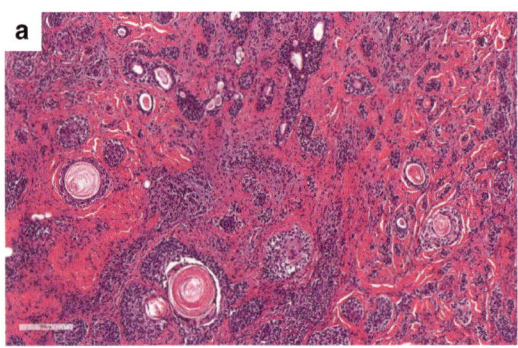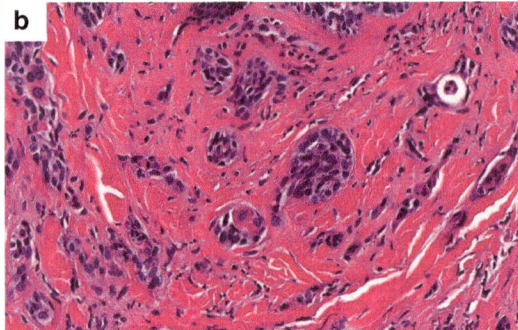

Fig. 21.8 Microcystic Adnexal Carcinoma. (**a**) Tumor cells are arranged in infiltrative irregular islands, cords, and tadpole shapes with keratin microcysts and ductular structures (H&E 100X). (**b**) Cells do not show significant cytologic atypia or pleomorphism (H&E, 300X)

Table 21.1 Immunohistochemical staining pattern of basal cell carcinoma and mimics

	Basal Cell Carcinoma	Trichoblastoma	Sebaceous Carcinoma	Merkel Cell Carcinoma	Microcystic Adnexal Carcinoma	Trichoepithelioma	Syringoma
BerEP4	+	+	–	+/–	–	+/–	–
CK20	–	–	–	+	–	–	–
CK20+ Merkel cells	–	+	–	+	–	+	+
Androgen receptor	Patchy +	–	+	–	–	–	
EMA	–	–	+	–	Focal ducts	–	+
Adipophilin	–	–	+	–	–	–	–
Bcl2	Diffuse + epithelium	Peripheral	–	+	Focal	Peripheral	Focal
CD10	Diffuse + epithelium; negative stroma	–/weak epithelium; positive stroma	+/–	–	–	–/weak epithelium; positive stroma	–

21.3   Dermal and Subcutaneous Tumors

Dermal and subcutaneous-based tumors on the head and neck have a somewhat limited differential, and most tumors are relatively rare compared to epidermal tumors. A relatively deep scoop shave, or an incisional or large (6 mm) punch biopsy is most useful for sampling dermal-based tumors, and excision may be necessary if a subcutaneous process is suspected. Desmoplastic melanoma is arguably the most important malignant dermal tumor in this location (see above). Other spindled and epithelioid tumors to consider in the differential diagnosis mainly consist of atypical fibroxanthoma (AFX), pleomorphic dermal sarcoma (PDS), and angiosarcoma (AS).

21.3.1   Atypical Fibroxanthoma and Pleomorphic Dermal Sarcoma

Atypical fibroxanthoma is an undifferentiated dermal neoplasm which typically occurs on sun-damaged skin of older patients. By definition, the tumor is limited to the dermis, and does not involve the subcutis or deep soft tissue. When this strict definition is applied, outcome following wide excision is excellent. Overall, tumor cells are round to spindled and arranged in fascicles, sheets, or rarely a storiform pattern. There is

often multinucleation, pleomorphism, and conspicuous mitotic activity (Fig. 21.9). There is negative staining with any lineage-defining markers, including SOX10, S100, cytokeratins, desmin, CD31, or ERG. Smooth muscle actin can show patchy positivity and CD10 is diffusely positive, but this is not a specific finding [33]. Pleomorphic dermal sarcomas represent the deeper, more aggressive counterpart of AFX, and are diagnosed when a similar tumor to AFX shows tumor necrosis or extends into the subcutis or deeper. PDS has a worse prognosis, with risk of recurrence and distant spread [34, 35].

21.3.2 Epithelioid Hemangioma

Of particular note, epithelioid hemangiomas are known to arise in the head and neck, particularly in a periauricular location, in middle aged adults, with female predominance. They present as erythematous nodules and can have multiple coalescing lesions. Microscopically, tumors are circumscribed and dermal or subcutaneous, typically with a dense inflammatory infiltrate, imparting a low-power appearance resembling a lymph node. Tumoral endothelial cells are arranged in well-formed capillaries in a lobular distribution around a larger central vessel. They are epithelioid and protrude into vascular lumina with "hobnail" appearance, but lack pleomorphism (Fig. 21.10) [36].

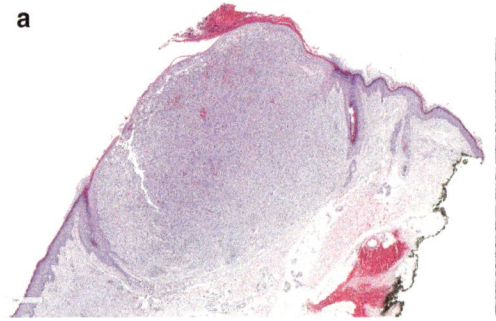
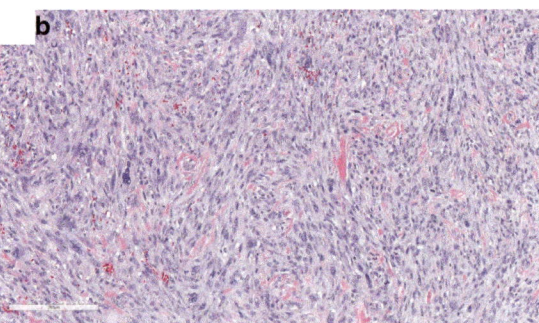

Fig. 21.9 Atypical Fibroxanthoma. (**a**) There is a dermal-based tumor on sun-damaged skin with overlying epidermal ulceration (H&E, 20X). (**b**) Pleomorphic spindled and epithelioid cells are arranged in short and long fascicles and sheets (H&E, 200X)

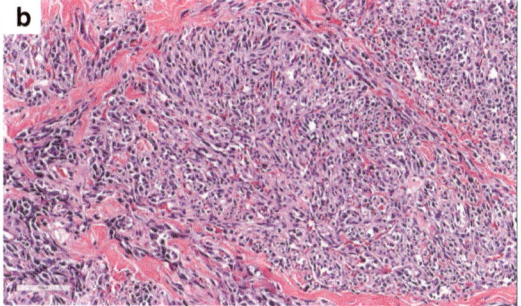

Fig. 21.10 Epithelioid Hemangioma. (**a**) Sections show an ill-defined tumor nodule with scattered lymphoid aggregates (H&E, 20X). (**b**) Closer inspection reveals a lobular proliferation of capillaries with plump endothelial cells and surrounding inflammation and fibrosis (H&E, 100X)

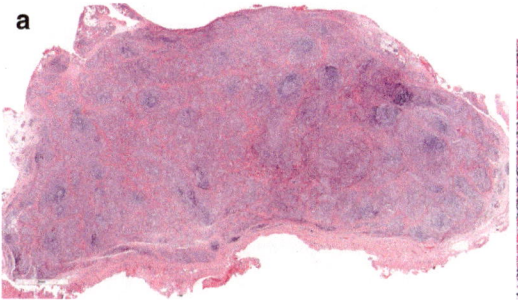
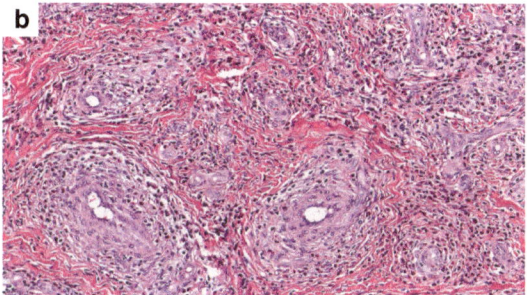

Fig. 21.11 Angiosarcoma. (**a**) Sections show a vague increase in dermal cellularity with dilated, thin-walled, irregular vascular channels, hemorrhage, and inflammation. Scattered hyperchromatic spindled cells are noted (H&E, 100X). (**b**) Tumor nodules are comprised of sheets of hyperchromatic spindled to epithelioid cells with occasional small lumens and extravasated erythrocytes (H&E, 100X)

21.3.3 Angiosarcoma

Angiosarcoma also commonly occurs on the head and neck of elderly patients as a result of chronic sun exposure. Additionally, radiation to the head and neck could increase the risk for post-radiation angiosarcoma [37]. Angiosarcoma typically appears clinically as a purpuric patch or plaque. Histologically, well-differentiated tumors show infiltrative, vasoformative channels and ectatic to compressed vascular spaces with scattered extravasated red blood cells and subtle atypia, including nuclear hob nailing into vascular lumens, multi-layering, hyperchromasia, enlargement, and mitoses (Fig. 21.11). Other, less-differentiated tumors can show nodules, sheets, or fascicles of atypical epithelioid or spindled cells with frank hemorrhage. Tumors stain positively with ERG (nuclear) and CD34. CD31 is also typically expressed, but can be lost in more poorly differentiated cases [38].

21.4 Palpable Lymph Nodes

Palpable lymph nodes are commonly encountered clinically in the head and neck region. On the head, they most commonly occur in the lateral jaw area, in association with the parotid. In general, sustained, non-mobile, firm, asymmetric, and painless growth is more indicative of tumor, versus that of a reactive process such as infection. In these cases, a fine-needle aspiration biopsy (FNA) is often obtained, rather than excision, for diagnosis. Lymph nodes are typically palpable, and samples can be obtained without the need for ultrasound or CT-scan. The most commonly encountered tumors include metastatic squamous cell carcinoma and metastatic melanoma [39]. In the case of squamous cell carcinoma, tumors can either arise from the oropharynx/tonsillar region or from the skin. Often times, if tumors arise from the skin, there is a clinical history of multiple lesions on the face and scalp, treated with freezing and multiple surgeries. Immunosuppression, such as from organ transplantation, is also a frequent precipitating factor. Squamous tumors can grow under epidermal scars, and spread to lymph nodes with delayed clinical detection. Nodal involvement by melanoma almost always results from loco-regional cutaneous spread. However, not uncommonly, melanoma can arise in a lymph node with no identifiable primary tumor [40].

References

1. Barnhill RL. Editor in Chief. Piepkorn M, Busam KJ, Co-Editors. Pathology of melanocytic nevi and melanoma. 3rd. New York: Springer; 2014.
2. Massi G, LeBoit PE. Histological diagnosis of nevi and melanoma. 2nd ed. Springer: New York; 2014.
3. Clark WH Jr, Mihm MC Jr. Lentigo maligna and lentigo-maligna melanoma. Am J Pathol. 1969;55(1):39–67. PMID: 5776171; PMCID: PMC2013384.
4. Star P, Rawson RV, Drummond M, Lo S, Scolyer RA, Guitera P. Lentigo maligna: defining margins and predictors of recurrence utilizing clinical, dermoscopic, confocal microscopy and histopathology features. J Eur Acad Dermatol Venereol. 2021. https://doi.org/10.1111/jdv.17349. Epub ahead of print. PMID: 33998703.
5. Lezcano C, Jungbluth AA, Nehal KS, Hollmann TJ, Busam KJ. PRAME expression in melanocytic tumors. Am J Surg Pathol. 2018;42(11):1456–65. https://doi.org/10.1097/PAS.0000000000001134. PMID: 30045064; PMCID: PMC6631376.
6. Gerami P, Busam K, Cochran A, Cook MG, Duncan LM, Elder DE, Fullen DR, Guitart J, LeBoit PE, Mihm MC Jr, Prieto VG, Rabkin MS, Scolyer RA, Xu X, Yun SJ, Obregon R, Yazdan P, Cooper C, Weitner BB, Rademaker A, Barnhill RL. Histomorphologic assessment and interobserver diagnostic reproducibility of atypical spitzoid melanocytic neoplasms with long-term follow-up. Am J Surg Pathol. 2014;38(7):934–40.

7. Spatz A, Calonje E, Handfield-Jones S, Barnhill RL. Spitz tumors in children: a grading system for risk stratification. Arch Dermatol. 1999;135(3):282–5. https://doi.org/10.1001/archderm.135.3.282. PMID: 10086449.
8. Zarabi SK, Azzato EM, Tu ZJ, Ni Y, Billings SD, Arbesman J, Funchain P, Gastman B, Farkas DH, Ko JS. Targeted next generation sequencing (NGS) to classify melanocytic neoplasms. J Cutan Pathol. 2020;47(8):691–704. https://doi.org/10.1111/cup.13695. Epub 2020 Jun 2. PMID: 32291779.
9. Quan VL, Zhang B, Zhang Y, Mohan LS, Shi K, Wagner A, Kruse L, Taxter T, Beaubier N, White K, Zou L, Gerami P. Integrating next-generation sequencing with morphology improves prognostic and biologic classification of Spitz neoplasms. J Invest Dermatol. 2020;140(8):1599–608. https://doi.org/10.1016/j.jid.2019.12.031. Epub 2020 Jan 29. PMID: 32004563.
10. Gerami P, Scolyer RA, Xu X, Elder DE, Abraham RM, Fullen D, Prieto VG, Leboit PE, Barnhill RL, Cooper C, Yazdan P, Guitart J, Liu P, Pestova E, Busam K. Risk assessment for atypical spitzoid melanocytic neoplasms using FISH to identify chromosomal copy number aberrations. Am J Surg Pathol. 2013;37(5):676–84. https://doi.org/10.1097/PAS.0b013e3182753de6. PMID: 23388126.
11. Gerami P, Cooper C, Bajaj S, Wagner A, Fullen D, Busam K, Scolyer RA, Xu X, Elder DE, Abraham RM, Prieto VG, Guitart J, Liu P, Pestova E, Barnhill RL. Outcomes of atypical Spitz tumors with chromosomal copy number aberrations and conventional melanomas in children. Am J Surg Pathol. 2013;37(9):1387–94. https://doi.org/10.1097/PAS.0b013e31828fc283. PMID: 23797719.
12. Lee S, Barnhill RL, Dummer R, Dalton J, Wu J, Pappo A, Bahrami A. TERT promoter mutations are predictive of aggressive clinical behavior in patients with spitzoid melanocytic neoplasms. Sci Rep. 2015;5:11200. https://doi.org/10.1038/srep11200. PMID: 26061100; PMCID: PMC4462090.
13. Carlson JA, Dickersin GR, Sober AJ, Barnhill RL. Desmoplastic neurotropic melanoma. A clinicopathologic analysis of 28 cases. Cancer. 1995;75(2):478–94. https://doi.org/10.1002/1097-0142(19950115)75:2<478::aid-cncr2820750211>3.0.co;2-o. PMID: 7812919.
14. Busam KJ, Mujumdar U, Hummer AJ, et al. Cutaneous desmoplastic melanoma: reappraisal of morphologic heterogeneity and prognostic factors. Am J Surg Pathol. 2004;28:1518–25.
15. Hughes TM, Williams GJ, Gyorki DE, Kelly JW, Stretch JR, Varey AHR, Hong AM, Scolyer RA, Thompson JF. Desmoplastic melanoma: a review of its pathology and clinical behaviour, and of management recommendations in published guidelines. J Eur Acad Dermatol Venereol. 2021;35(6):1290–8.

16. Howard MD, Wee E, Wolfe R, McLean CA, Kelly JW, Pan Y. Differences between pure desmoplastic melanoma and superficial spreading melanoma in terms of survival, distribution and other clinicopathologic features. J Eur Acad Dermatol Venereol. 2019;33(10):1899–906. https://doi.org/10.1111/jdv.15759. Epub 2019 Jul 22. PMID: 31237040.

17. Preston DS, Stern RS. Nonmelanoma cancers of the skin. N Engl J Med. 1992;327:1649–62.

18. Sexton M, Jones DB, Maloney ME. Histologic patterns analysis of basal cell carcinoma: a study of a series of 1039 consecutive neoplasms. J Am Acad Dermatol. 1990;23:1118–26.

19. Alsaazd KO, Obaidat NA, Ghazarian D. Skin adnexal neoplasms—part 1: an approach to tumors of the pilosebaceous unit. J Clin Pathol. 2007;60:129–44.

20. Stanoszek LM, Wang GY, Harms PW. Histologic mimics of basal cell carcinoma. Arch Pathol Lab Med. 2017;141(11):1490–502. https://doi.org/10.5858/arpa.2017-0222-RA. PMID: 29072946.

21. Schmitt AR, Brewer JD, Bordeaux JS, Baum CL. Staging for cutaneous squamous cell carcinoma as a predictor of sentinel lymph node biopsy results: meta-analysis of American Joint Committee on Cancer criteria and a proposed alternative system. JAMA Dermatol. 2014;150:19–24.

22. Miner AG, Patel RM, Wilson DA, Procop GW, Minca EC, Fullen DR, Harms PW, Billings SD. Cytokeratin 20-negative Merkel cell carcinoma is infrequently associated with the Merkel cell polyomavirus. Mod Pathol. 2015;28(4):498–504. https://doi.org/10.1038/modpathol.2014.148. Epub 2014 Nov 14. PMID: 25394777.

23. Ko JS, Prieto VG, Elson PJ, Vilain RE, Pulitzer MP, Scolyer RA, Reynolds JP, Piliang MP, Ernstoff MS, Gastman BR, Billings SD. Histological pattern of Merkel cell carcinoma sentinel lymph node metastasis improves stratification of Stage III patients. Mod Pathol. 2016;29(2):122–30. https://doi.org/10.1038/modpathol.2015.109. Epub 2015 Nov 6. PMID: 26541273; PMCID: PMC5063050.

24. Erstine EM, Tetzlaff MT, Jia X, Aung PP, Prieto VG, Funchain P, Gastman BR, Billings SD, Ko JS. Prognostic significance of "nonsolid" microscopic metastasis in Merkel cell carcinoma sentinel lymph nodes. Am J Surg Pathol. 2019;43(7):907–19. https://doi.org/10.1097/PAS.0000000000001277. PMID: 31094923.

25. Harms PW, Collie AM, Hovelson DH, Cani AK, Verhaegen ME, Patel RM, Fullen DR, Omata K, Dlugosz AA, Tomlins SA, Billings SD. Next generation sequencing of Cytokeratin 20-negative Merkel cell carcinoma reveals ultraviolet-signature mutations and recurrent TP53 and RB1 inactivation. Mod Pathol. 2016;29(3):240–8. https://doi.org/10.1038/modpathol.2015.154. Epub 2016 Jan 8. PMID: 26743471; PMCID: PMC4769666.

26. Gill P, Naugler C, Abi Daoud MS. Utility of Ber-EP4 and MOC-31 in basaloid skin tumor detection. Appl Immunohistochem Mol Morphol. 2019;27(8):584–8. https://doi.org/10.1097/PAI.0000000000000664.

27. Lilo MT, Chen Y, LeBlanc RE. INSM1 is more sensitive and interpretable than conventional immunohistochemical stains used to diagnose Merkel cell carcinoma. Am J Surg Pathol. 2018;42(11):1541–8. https://doi.org/10.1097/PAS.0000000000001136. PMID: 30080705.

28. North JP. Molecular genetics of sebaceous neoplasia. Surg Pathol Clin. 2021;14(2):273–84. https://doi.org/10.1016/j.path.2021.03.005. PMID: 34023105.

29. Plotzke JM, Adams DJ, Harms PW. Molecular pathology of skin adnexal tumors. Histopathology. 2021. https://doi.org/10.1111/his.14441. Epub ahead of print. PMID: 34197659.

30. Sethi R, Emerick K. Sentinel node biopsy for nonmelanoma skin cancer of the head and neck. Otolaryngol Clin N Am. 2021;54(2):295–305. https://doi.org/10.1016/j.otc.2020.11.005. PMID: 33743888.

31. Donnell SA, LeBlanc RE, Yan S, Parra O, Momtahen S, Sriharan A, Linos K. Comparison of adipophilin and recently introduced PReferentially expressed Antigen in MElanoma immunohistochemistry in the assessment of sebaceous neoplasms: a pilot study. J Cutan Pathol. 2021. https://doi.org/10.1111/cup.14043. Epub ahead of print. PMID: 33949693.

32. Danialan R, Mutyambizi K, Aung P, Prieto VG, Ivan D. Challenges in the diagnosis of cutaneous adnexal tumours. J Clin Pathol. 2015;68(12):992–1002. https://doi.org/10.1136/jclinpath-2015-203228. PMID: 26602416.

33. Mentzel T, Requena L, Brenn T. Atypical fibroxanthoma revisited. Surg Pathol Clin. 2017;10(2):319–35.

34. Miller K, Goodlad JR, Brenn T. Pleomorphic dermal sarcoma: adverse histologic features predict aggressive behavior and allow distinction from atypical fibroxanthoma. Am J Surg Pathol. 2012;36(9):1317–26. https://doi.org/10.1097/PAS.0b013e31825359e1. PMID: 22510760.

35. Griewank KG, Wiesner T, Murali R, et al. Atypical fibroxanthoma and pleomorphic dermal sarcoma harbor frequent NOTCH1/2 and FAT1 mutations and similar DNA copy number alteration profiles. Mod Pathol. 2018;31(3):418–28.

36. Ko JS, Billings SD. Diagnostically challenging epithelioid vascular tumors. Surg Pathol Clin. 2015;8(3):331–51. https://doi.org/10.1016/j.path.2015.05.001. PMID: 26297060.

37. Mentzel T, Schildhaus HU, Palmedo G, Büttner R, Kutzner H. Postradiation cutaneous angiosarcoma after treatment of breast carcinoma is characterized by MYC amplification in contrast to atypical vascular lesions after radiotherapy and control cases: clinicopathological, immunohistochemical and molecular

analysis of 66 cases. Mod Pathol. 2012;25(1):75–85. https://doi.org/10.1038/modpathol.2011.134.   Epub 2011 Sep 9. PMID: 21909081.

38. Ronchi A, Cozzolino I, Zito Marino F, De Chiara A, Argenziano G, Moscarella E, Pagliuca F, Franco R. Primary and secondary cutaneous angiosarcoma: distinctive clinical, pathological and molecular features. Ann Diagn Pathol. 2020;48:151597. https://doi.org/10.1016/j.anndiagpath.2020.151597. Epub 2020 Aug 15. PMID: 32829071.

39. O'Brien CJ, McNeil EB, McMahon JD, Pathak I, Lauer CS. Incidence of cervical node involvement in metastatic cutaneous malignancy involving the parotid gland. Head Neck. 2001;23(9):744–8. https://doi.org/10.1002/hed.1106. PMID: 11505484.

40. Chernock RD, Lewis JS. Approach to metastatic carcinoma of unknown primary in the head and neck: squamous cell carcinoma and beyond. Head Neck Pathol.   2015;9(1):6–15.   https://doi.org/10.1007/s12105-015-0616-2. Epub 2015 Mar 25. PMID: 25804376; PMCID: PMC4382479.

Raymond L. Barnhill is a Professor at the University of Paris Cité and anatomic pathologist, dermatopathologist, and researcher at Institut Curie, Paris, France. He is the Founder of the North American Melanoma Pathology Study Group and the International Melanoma Pathology Study Group (current president). He is a current or past member of professional societies, including the WHO Melanoma Programme (now defunct), EORTC, ECOG, USCAP/IAP, Cancer and Blood Vessels Research Group, Liver Metastasis Research Network, and the International Melanoma Working Group. He is the author of more than 300 articles, over 40 chapters, and 5 books.

Jennifer Ko is a dermatopathologist at Cleveland Clinic since 2015, Cleveland, OH, USA. She is also Medical Director of the Cleveland Clinic Central Biorepositories, and of the Immune Monitoring Lab in the CITI. She is a member of the International Melanoma Pathology Study Group, and current or past member of numerous professional societies including the ASDP, USCAP, and the SITC. She is author of more than 80 articles and book chapters.

Soft Tissue and Bone Tumors of the Head and Neck

Henryk A. Domanski and Pawel Gajdzis

Soft tissue tumors are relatively uncommon in the head and neck region and count approximately 5–10% of all soft tissue sarcomas. With the exceptions of nasopharyngeal angiofibroma and biphenotypic sinonasal sarcoma, all other mesenchymal neoplasms have a predilection to other parts of the body and only occasionally present in the head and neck area. Tumors that are relatively frequent arising in this site include benign fibroblastic/myofibroblastic lesions, nerve sheath, vascular and fatty tumors, and small round cell tumors, commonly rhabdomyosarcoma in young individuals. Table 22.1 shows the most common soft tissue malignancy in children and adults in the head and neck.

Some of the soft tissue tumors have recurrent genetic abnormalities, which in many cases help to provide a final diagnosis (Table 22.2).

Table 22.1 Most common head and neck sarcomas in children and adults

Children	Adults
Rhabdomyosarcoma (40–50%)	Undifferentiated sarcoma (30–40%)
Undifferentiated sarcoma (up to 10%)	Kaposi sarcoma (20–25%)
Osteosarcoma (up to 10%)	Angiosarcoma (10%)
Ewing sarcoma (5–10%)	Leiomyosarcoma (5–10%)
Malignant peripheral nerve sheath tumor (up to 5%)	Chondrosarcoma (5–10%)
Chondrosarcoma (up to 5%)	Osteosarcoma (up to 5%)
Synovial sarcoma (up to 5%)	Chordoma (up to 5%)
	Malignant peripheral nerve sheath tumor (up to 5%)
	Rhabdomyosarcoma (<5%)

H. A. Domanski (✉)
Department of Clinical Sciences, Lund University, Lund, Sweden

Department of Clinical Genetics, Pathology and Molecular Diagnostics, Division of Laboratory Medicine, Lund, Sweden
e-mail: henryk.domanski@med.lu.se

P. Gajdzis
Department of Clinical and Experimental Pathology, Wroclaw Medical University, Wroclaw, Poland

Department of Pathomorphology, 4th Military Clinical Hospital, Wroclaw, Poland

© The Author(s), under exclusive license to Springer Nature Switzerland AG 2024
J. Klijanienko et al. (eds.), *Diagnostic Procedures in Patients with Neck Masses*,
https://doi.org/10.1007/978-3-031-67675-8_22

Table 22.2 Genetic alterations in the most common soft tissue tumors of the head and neck

Neoplasms	Genetic alteration
Fibroblastic/ myofibroblastic tumors	
Nodular fasciitis	*USP6* gene
Desmoid fibromatosis	rearrangement
Dermatofibrosarcoma protuberans	*CTNNB1* or *APC* mutation
Solitary fibrous tumor	*COL1A1-PDGFB* gene fusion
Inflammatory myofibroblastic tumor	*NAB2-STAT6* gene fusion
	ALK gene rearrangement (in up to 60% of cases)
Skeletal muscle tumors	
Embryonal rhabdomyosarcoma	*PAX3-FOXO1* or *PAX7-FOXO1* gene fusion
Spindle cell/sclerosing rhabdomyosarcoma	*VGLL2* or *NCOA2* rearrangement (in congenital or infant cases) and *MyoD1* mutation (in adolescence or young adult cases)
Vascular tumors	
Epithelioid hemangioendothelioma	*WWTR1-CAMTA1* or rarely *YAP1-TFE3* rearrangement
Radiation-associated angiosarcoma	Amplification of *MYC*
Undifferentiated small round cell sarcomas	
Ewing sarcoma	*EWSR1* or *FUS* genes fusion
Adipocytic tumors	
Atypical lipomatous tumor/well-differentiated liposarcoma	Amplification of *MDM2* or/and *CDK4*
Myxoid liposarcoma	*DDIT3* gene rearrangement
Distinctive tumors of the nasal cavity	
Sinonasal tract angiofibroma	*CTNNB1* mutation
Biphenotypic sinonasal sarcoma	*PAX3* gene rearrangement

22.1 Adipocytic Tumors

Adipocytic tumors represent a broad variety of benign and low-grade/high-grade malignant neoplasms with variable clinical presentations and a spectrum of morphologic findings overlapping other soft tissue lesions such as spindle cells, floret cells, lipoblasts, collagenous tissue, prominent vas-

culature, and myxoid changes. The head and neck is an infrequent localization for lipomatous tumors. However, benign lipoma is the most common soft tissue tumor of adults and is not uncommon in the subcutaneous tissue of the head and neck, and spindle cell/pleomorphic lipoma has a predisposition to this anatomical localization. Other subtypes of benign, locally aggressive, and malignant adipose tissue tumors such as lipoblastoma, hibernoma, chondroid lipoma, atypic lipomatous tumor (ALT)/ well-differentiated liposarcoma (WDLPS), dedifferentiated liposarcoma (DDLPS), myxoid liposarcoma (MLPS), pleomorphic liposarcoma, and myxoid pleomorphic liposarcoma rarely arise in this location.

22.1.1 Benign Adipocytic Tumors

22.1.1.1 Lipoma

Lipoma is the most common soft tissue tumor in adults, rarely presented before the third decade of life.

Most lipomas in the head and neck arise in the buccal mucosa, lower lip, and tongue. Intraoral, hypopharyngeal, and laryngeal sites are rarely involved [1, 2]. Lipomas usually appear as slowly growing, solitary, or less common multiple, subcutaneous masses and can be occasionally deeply seated (intramuscular or intermuscular lipoma). They are usually well-circumscribed lesions, although intramuscular lipomas may show infiltration into surrounding muscle.

Histologically, lipomas are composed of mature adipose tissue, small blood vessels, and occasionally presented paucicellular, thin fibrous septa. Occasional multivacuolated histiocytes (lipophages) may be seen in areas with trauma or fat necrosis. Rarely lipomas may contain other connective tissue elements such as metaplastic bone and cartilage, fibrotic tissue (fibrolipoma), or degenerative/myxoid areas (myxolipoma).

Fine needle aspiration (FNA) smears from lipoma are identical to those from normal adipose tissue containing clusters of uniform adipocytes with a single fat vacuole, small peripheral nucleus, and variable number of capillaries within the fatty tissue fragments. Fragments of striated muscle or regenerating muscle may be visible in smears from inter/intramuscular lipomas. The uncommon presence of other connective tissue elements may cause difficulties in FNA examination.

Lipomas are a heterogenous group of tumors from a genetic perspective with three major subgroups of genetic changes. The most common involves chromosome 12q13–15 and the pathogenetic important *HMGA2* gene. This aberration is present in 65% of lipoma cases. The other two subgroups involve loss of material from chromosome 13q and changes in 6p21–23 and are present in 10 and 5% of lipomas, respectively [3, 4]. Lipomas are cured by simple excision, and local recurrence is rare.

22.1.1.2 Spindle Cell Lipoma and Pleomorphic Lipoma

Spindle cell lipoma (SCL) and pleomorphic lipoma (PL) represent morphological variants of benign neoplasm that share clinical, immunohistochemical, cytogenetic, and prognostic features.

SCL and PL have a predilection to subcutaneous tissues of the head and neck region, back, and shoulders of middle-aged to elderly individuals, particularly men [5–8]. The face (Fig. 22.1a), scalp, oral cavity, tongue, orbit, limbs, and trunk are less common sites [5–10].

Histologically, both neoplasms are composed of variable amounts of bland spindle cells, fat tissue, and ropy collagen bundles in a fibromyx-

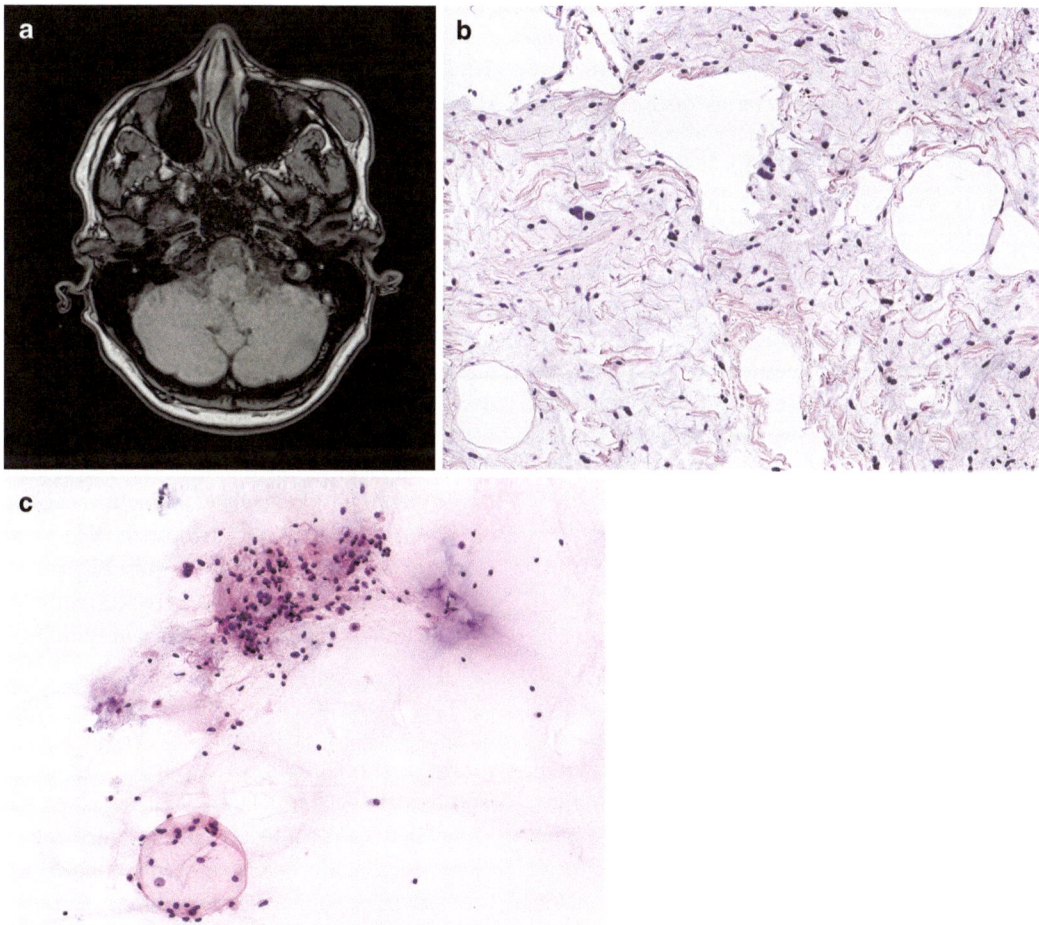

Fig. 22.1 (**a**) Pleomorphic lipoma. MRI discloses well-circumscribed subcutaneous mass in the cheek. (**b**) Pleomorphic lipoma. CNB. Spindle cells, few floret cells in the myxoid stroma (H&E). (**c**) Pleomorphic lipoma. FNAB. Mature fat, variable pleomorphic spindle cells, floret cells, and mast cells (H&E)

oid stroma [5–8]. Additional components of PLs are multinucleated floret-like cells and pleomorphic spindle cells (Fig. 22.1b) [8]. Mast cells are common findings, while lipoblasts or mitoses may be rarely seen in a subset of cases. There are some different histologic patterns of SCL such as fat-poor [11, 12], myxoid [13–15], (pseudo) angiomatous [13, 15], and plexiform [16] subtypes.

The cytomorphology of SCL is often distinct although the proportions of different elements vary from case to case. FNA smears contain clusters of mature adipose tissue mixed with fascicles of uniform, bland spindle cells with elongated nuclei and collagen fibers, often in a myxoid background matrix [17]. Cytomorphologic findings of pleomorphic lipoma (Fig. 22.1c) include the presence of floret cells and pleomorphic spindle cells in addition to adipose tissue [18, 19]. Collagen fibers may not be as distinctive as in smears of SCLs.

Both SCL and PL show more complex karyotypes compared to ordinary lipomas, and complete or partial loss of chromosomes 13 and/or 16 has been reported [20, 21]. By immunohistochemistry, spindle cells are positive for CD34 [13]. Demonstration of loss of the *RB1* locus or/and RB1 protein expression can support diagnosis in selected cases [22]. SCL/PL are cured by simple excision, and local recurrence is rare [5, 6, 8].

22.1.1.3 Lipoblastoma/ Lipoblastomatosis

Lipoblastoma is a benign neoplasm of embryonal white fat, which may be a localized or diffuse tumor. This tumor of infancy most commonly involves the extremities and rarely the head and neck region including retropharynx, oral mucosa, and salivary gland. Lipoblastoma presents either as a well-circumscribed subcutaneous tumor (lipoblastoma) or a deep-seated, diffusely infiltrative, and ill-defined mass (lipoblastomatosis). Histologically, lipoblastoma is composed of lobules of immature fat with mesenchymal and myxoid areas containing primitive spindle or stellate cells, separated by fibrovascular septa and with plexiform vasculature [23, 24].

The typical cytopathological features include small uniform adipocytes with vacuolated cytoplasm and round uniform nuclei in a myxoid background matrix, admixed with uniform spindle cells and branching strands of capillaries [25–27]. Smears may also be dominated by large ordinary univacuolated adipocytes.

By immunohistochemistry, spindle cells show cytoplasmic staining for desmin [28]. Approximately 70% of lipoblastomas harbor genetic rearrangement of the chromosome region 8q11–13 involving the *PLAG1* gene which is detectable by Fluorescence in situ hybridization (FISH) [29, 30] or nuclear staining for PLAG1 [31].

Lipoblastoma is benign neoplasm. The recurrence occurs usually due to incomplete excision [32, 33].

22.1.1.4 Hibernoma

Hibernoma is a benign lipomatous tumor of brown fat derivation.

Hibernomas account for 1% of all adipocytic tumors and typically occur in young adults. Most cases are presented as a slow-growing, well-defined, painless subcutaneous mass, and are most often located in the interscapular region, on the back or chest wall, the extremities, and head and neck. Fewer than 15% of cases occur in the deep intramuscular, intra-abdominal, retroperitoneal, and intrathoracic locations [34–36].

Histologically, hibernomas are composed of large (brown fat-like) cells with finely vacuolated or granular, eosinophilic cytoplasm, and small, bland centrally situated nuclei. Most hibernomas have a prominent capillary network. Subtypes include lipoma-like, rare myxoid, and spindle cell variants [35, 36]. Hibernomas mimicking atypical lipomatous tumor have been reported although nuclear atypia and mitoses are absent [37]. In FNA smears, clusters or fragments of round to oval and polygonal cells of variable sizes, with vacuolated or granular cytoplasm and centrally placed small uniform nuclei are intermingled with ordinary large adipocytes. The clusters and tissue fragments often contain numerous capillary vessels. Ordinary lipoma-like fat cells may dominate the smears, and the typical hibernoma cells may be in minority, thus posing challenges to diagnose

[38–40]. Most hibernomas are characterized by recurrent genetic changes involving structural rearrangements of 11q13 [41].

Hibernoma is a benign neoplasm and does not recur after complete local excision [35].

22.1.1.5 Chondroid Lipoma

Chondroid lipoma is a rare, benign lipomatous tumor that primarily affects adult women.

Most arise in the deep soft tissue or deep subcutaneous fat of the proximal extremities, limb girdles, and less often in the trunk, head, and neck [42–45].

Histologically, chondroid lipoma is composed of lipoblasts that intermingle with mature adipocytes and small chondroblast-like cells in a myxohyaline chondroid matrix.

By immunohistochemistry, fatty and lipoblastic components display positivity for S100 and rarely and only focally for keratins and negative results for smooth muscle actin (SMA) and epithelial membrane antigen (EMA) [42–44].

FNA smears show clusters of mature adipocytes with an admixture of uni- or multivacuolated lipoblasts and small strands and clusters of chondroblast-like cells in a background of abundant myxochondroid matrix. Despite variation in size and shape, the nuclei of small chondroid cells are bland appearing. Chondroid lipomas lack a plexiform capillary network of lipoblastoma or myxoid liposarcoma [46–48].

Surgical excision is curative and local recurrences are rare.

22.1.2 Locally Aggressive and Malignant Adipocytic Tumors

This category includes clinically, morphologically, and cytogenetically distinct entities: atypical lipomatous tumor/well-differentiated ALT/WDLS/dedifferentiated liposarcoma (DDLPS), low- and high-grade myxoid liposarcoma (MLPS), and pleomorphic liposarcoma. Liposarcomas comprise 2–9% of sarcomas in the head and neck. The most common subtype in this location is ALT/WDLS, followed by MLPS, pleomorphic, and DDLPS [49].

22.1.2.1 Atypical Lipomatous Tumor/Well-Differentiated Liposarcoma and Dedifferentiated Liposarcoma

Atypical lipomatous tumor (ALT)/well-differentiated liposarcoma (WDLPS) is a locally aggressive, non-metastasizing adipocytic neoplasm showing nuclear atypia and characterized by a ring or giant marker chromosomes derived from 12q13–15, which are present in most cases. They contain an amplification of 12q13-15 involving *MDM2* and *CDK4* genes [50, 51].

Dedifferentiated liposarcoma is diagnosed when a well-differentiated liposarcoma also displays non-lipogenic sarcomatous areas.

The presence of heterologous osteosarcomatous or rhabdomyosarcomatous differentiation in dedifferentiated liposarcoma is not uncommon. ALT/WDLPS accounting for approximately 40–45% of all liposarcomas occurs in adults with a peak incidence between the fourth and fifth decades of life. Head and neck location is uncommon and includes scalp and face, pharynx, mouth, larynx, and neck. The tongue is a common location for intraoral cases. Most cases occur as deeply located, slowly growing masses on proximal extremities, trunk, and the retroperitoneum/paratesticular region, less commonly in the mediastinum [52–54]. When the same tumor arises at surgically curable sites such as the lower extremities, the term "atypical lipomatous tumor" (ALT) is preferred [55]. Variants of ALT/WDLPS include lipoma-like, sclerotic, and inflammatory liposarcomas [55].

Histologically, ALT/WDLPS is composed of solid sheaths and strands of adipocytes showing variability of the cell size and variable nuclear atypia (Fig. 22.2a). Variable fibrotic septation and enlarged, hyperchromatic, and pleomorphic nuclei of both adipocytes and stromal cells are common findings. Multinucleated "floret" cells, atypical lipoblasts, and rarely hibernoma-like cells may be encountered. Occasionally, areas with myxoid matrix may be present. The occur-

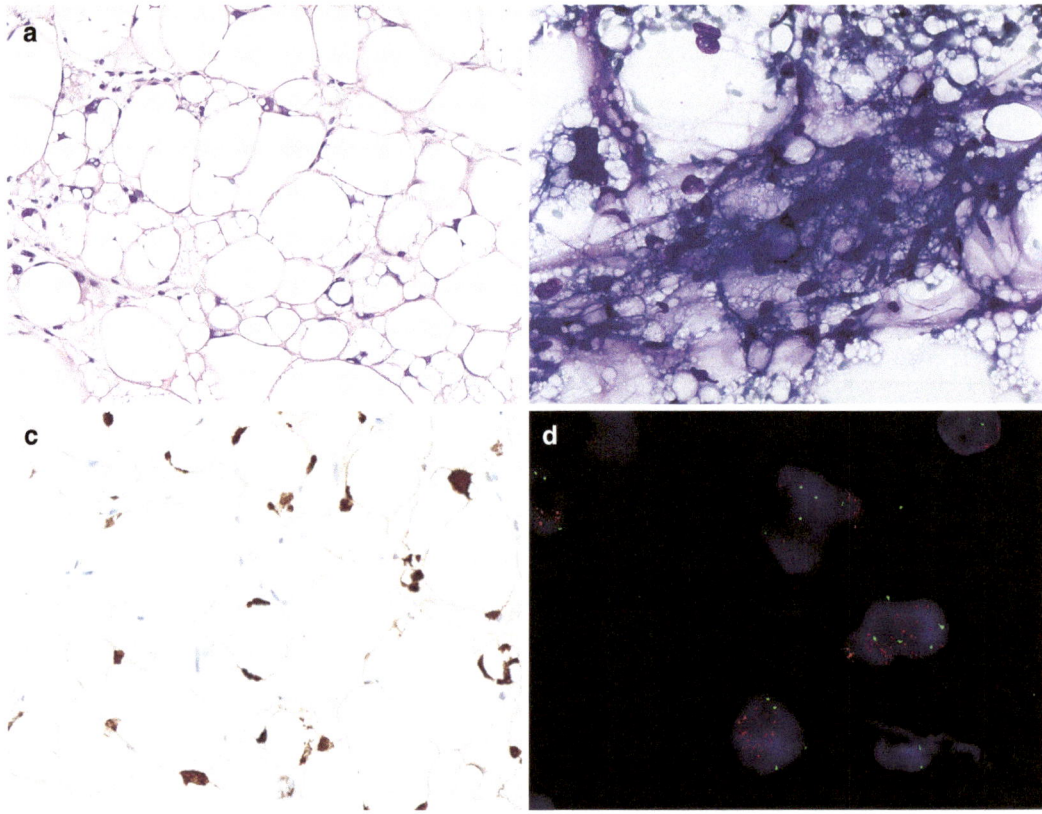

Fig. 22.2 (**a**) Atypical lipomatous tumor/well-differentiated liposarcoma. The presence of variation in adipocytic size and atypical hyperchromatic stroma cells is a diagnostic feature. Lipoblasts are variably presented (H&E). (**b**) Atypical lipomatous tumor/well-differentiated liposarcoma. FNAB. Fat cells and atypical stromal cells with enlarged, irregular, hyperchromatic nuclei (MGG). (**c**) Atypical lipomatous tumor/well-differentiated liposarcoma. The presence of MDM2 positivity in the tumor cells. (**d**) Atypical lipomatous tumor/well-differentiated liposarcoma. FISH showing high-level amplification of *MDM2*

rence of nonlipogenic spindle cells or pleomorphic areas lacking lipomatous components and with abrupt transition signifies the progression to the DDLPS.

Cytologic findings in these tumors include the mixture of clusters of adipocytes showing the variability of the cell size, variable nuclear atypia with ordinary lipoma-like fragments, and atypical stromal cells with enlarged, irregular hyperchromatic nuclei (Fig. 22.2b). Atypical lipoblasts with cytoplasmic vacuoles and scalloped nuclei as well as multinucleated "floret" cells may be present but are not necessary for the diagnosis.

ALT/WDLPS/DDLPS is characterized by supernumerary ring and giant marker chromosomes, resulting in MDM2 and CDK4 amplification. These genetic abnormalities can be detected by FISH showing MDM2 amplification (Fig. 22.2c), by immunohistochemistry showing MDM2 (Fig. 22.2d), and/or CDK4 nuclear reactivities [50, 56–59].

ALT/WDLPS shows no potential for metastasis unless it undergoes dedifferentiation. The risk of dedifferentiation varies according to site and lesional duration [60, 61]. Surgically amenable tumors do not recur after complete excision. Local recurrence of DDLPS occurs in at least 40% of cases and distant metastases in 15–20% of cases [61–63].

22.1.2.2 Myxoid Liposarcoma

Myxoid liposarcoma (MLS) is a malignant tumor composed of small ovoid to round cells with a myxoid stroma, a branching capillary vasculature, variable numbers of lipoblasts, and characterized by translocation producing *FUS::DDIT3* or rarely *EWSR1::DDIT3* fusion transcripts.

MLS is graded as low or high grade based on the degree of cellularity. Low-grade MLS shows abundant myxoid matrix and low cellularity, while high-grade MLS often demonstrates dense cellularity with a round cell appearance.

MLS accounts for 20–30% of liposarcomas [64] and is the most common liposarcoma subtype in children, adolescents, and young adults although peak incidence is at 45 years of age [65, 66]. The most common site of involvement is in the deep soft tissue, preferably the thigh. Rarely, MLS arises in the soft tissues of the head and neck and in this site involves connective tissue of the neck, face, and scalp [49]. Most cases occurring in the head and neck location are metastatic in nature [67].

Histologically, low-grade MLS is composed of small cells varying in shape from round, spindled, primitive cells to lipoblasts and a variable number of branching, capillary-sized vessels often arranged in a plexiform pattern, both components embedded in an abundant extracellular myxoid matrix. Cellular and nuclear atypia are usually minimal or absent, and mitoses are seldom seen. Nuclear atypia is usually minimal, and mitoses are seldom seen [68]. High-grade MLS shows hypercellular areas that may exhibit an undifferentiated round cell morphology with elevated nuclear grade, less apparent myxoid matrix, capillary vasculature, and increased mitotic activity [64, 68].

The cytological features at the FNA smears include abundant myxoid background matrix, fragments of tumor tissue with a branching network of thin capillaries, and slightly atypical lipoblasts as well as round to ovoid primitive cells, often associated with the capillaries in tissue fragments.

The high-grade MLS shows increased cellularity and scant myxoid matrix. Tumor cells display rather prominent round cell morphology, increased nuclear/cytoplasmic ratio, and increased mitotic activity. Neoplastic cells may be adherent around thin capillaries. In hypercellular areas, however, the capillary network is often less prominent, obscured by tight clusters of tumor cells [69–71].

In 95% of MLS, a balanced translocation involving the *DDIT3* gene on chromosome 12 with either *FUS* on chromosome 16 or, less frequently, *EWSR1* on chromosome 22 is present. FISH for DDIT3 rearrangement is very helpful in difficult cases, especially the high-grade variant [72]. By immunocytochemistry, variable positivity for S100 and positivity for an immunohistochemical marker of DDIT3 (nuclear localization) occur in both the low- and high-grade forms of MLS [73, 74].

Recurrence and metastatic disease of MLS depends on the grade. Most tumors behave as low-grade sarcomas. When metastasized, the outcome is worse [75].

22.1.2.3 Pleomorphic Liposarcoma

Pleomorphic liposarcoma is a rare, high-grade liposarcoma containing markedly atypical, bizarre, and giant multinucleated tumor cells with adipocytic differentiation. Pleomorphic liposarcoma is a rare subtype of liposarcoma, accounting for <5% of all liposarcomas [76, 77]. Pleomorphic liposarcoma is infrequently seen in the head and neck region with reported cases in the scalp and orbit [55, 78]. Most cases arise in the extremities in elderly patients, with a peak incidence in the seventh decade of life and a slightly higher incidence in males than females. Pediatric cases are very rare [66].

Histologically, all tumors contain a varying proportion of areas of the nonlipogenic component that resembles undifferentiated pleomorphic sarcoma with spindle and multinucleated giant cells often showing clear or vacuolated cytoplasm and areas of myxofibrosarcoma-like morphology. The number of pleomorphic lipoblasts varies between cases and between areas within the same tumor. Some pleomorphic liposarcomas may consist only of pleomorphic lipoblasts. Many cases show at least focal areas of necrosis and increased mitotic activity [79–81].

The most important clue to the cytological diagnosis is the presence of highly atypical uni- or multinucleated lipoblasts in FNA samples. FNA smears of pleomorphic liposarcoma most frequently yield smears representative of pleomorphic sarcoma with markedly pleomorphic spindle, polygonal, and epithelioid cells with an admixture of anaplastic multinucleated tumor cells without evidence of atypical lipoblasts. Mitoses and necrosis are common [82, 83].

Pleomorphic liposarcomas are aggressive sarcomas exhibiting local recurrence and metastatic rates of 30–50%, with an overall 5-year survival rate of about 60%. Metastases occur mostly in the lungs and pleura. Central location, increased tumor depth, greater size, and higher mitotic count have been associated with a worse prognosis [78, 81].

22.1.2.4 Myxoid Pleomorphic Liposarcoma

Myxoid pleomorphic liposarcoma is a rare, malignant adipocytic neoplasm, typically occurring in children and adolescents. Many cases are associated with Li–Fraumeni syndrome [84, 85].

Myxoid pleomorphic liposarcoma may arise in the head and neck [66, 85], but has a predilection for the mediastinum [66, 86].

Histologically, the tumors show variable proportions of liposarcoma-like areas including prominent myxoid matrix, curvilinear to plexiform capillary network, and hypercellular atypical areas resembling pleomorphic liposarcoma [66, 86, 87].

Myxoid pleomorphic liposarcoma is an extremely aggressive tumor type with a high recurrence/metastasis rate and poor overall survival [66, 88].

22.2 Fibroblastic/Myofibroblastic Tumors

22.2.1 Nodular Fasciitis

Nodular fasciitis (NOF) is a self-limiting, benign, and myofibroblastic neoplasm characterized by recurrent *USP6* gene rearrangements (most commonly *MYH9-USP6*). Up to 25% of NOF cases are located in the head and neck region, and the most common sites are the face (most commonly cheeks), neck, and parotid glands. Typically, it

presents a subcutaneous and painful mass measuring less than 3 cm. Due to its rapid growth and worrisome histopathological features (high cellularity and mitotic activity), it can mimic malignancy. Subset of NOF called cranial fasciitis, commonly found in infants and children, can affect deep layers of the scalp and underlying bones [89–91].

NOF is usually suitable for FNA in the head and neck region and is most often needled in the early phase of tumor growth. At this stage, aspirates are usually hypercellular and contain spindle cells with bland-looking spindle or ovoid nuclei, which are dispersed or present within tissue fragments. Loose tissue fragments consisting of haphazardly arranged tumor cells may produce a tissue culture appearance. The older lesion shows less myxoid stroma and a collagenous matrix may be present [91–93].

Histologically, the tumor is composed of plump spindle cells without any significant atypia, but usually with a high mitotic rate, especially in its early phase. The lesion usually may have highly cellular areas, where cells grow in fascicles, in storiform pattern, or in myxoid areas with a tissue culture appearance. In older lesions, stroma can be very collagenous. Despite the benign nature of the tumor, its border is typically infiltrative [89, 90, 94].

Immunohistochemical studies show a tramtrack pattern of SMA expression typical for myofibroblasts, and desmin is usually negative. To confirm the diagnosis, molecular studies should be performed to find *USP6* gene rearrangement [89, 91].

22.2.2 Desmoid Fibromatosis

Desmoid fibromatosis (DF) is a rare, locally aggressive myofibroblastic neoplasm without a metastatic ability [89]. There is up to a 30% recurrent rate after surgical treatment, but modern guidelines opt for a less aggressive approach if possible, including active surveillance [95, 96]. In the head and neck region, it is usually diagnosed in children and young adults and most often affects the neck. The etiology factors of DF can be variable, from genetic factors (like *CTNNB1* and *APC* gene mutations) to external factors (like trauma or surgery) [89, 97, 98].

FNA is a useful procedure to recognize a non-malignant behavior of the tumor [99]. Cytological specimens contain bland spindle cells with elongated, fusiform nuclei. Cells can be dispersed or seen within the collagenous stroma. In some cases, degenerating skeletal muscle cells and inflammatory cells can be observed [100, 101].

In histopathological specimens, a characteristic feature of DF is an infiltration into surrounding tissues. DF may have variable morphological patterns, but some number of long fascicles composed of bland fibroblasts or myofibroblasts are visible in all cases. Neoplastic cells are characterized by slender nuclei with inconspicuous nucleoli and without hyperchromasia or other features of atypia. Other most commonly encountered morphological patterns are hyalinized areas, myxoid changes, keloidal changes, or prominent staghorn vessels [102, 103].

Ancillary studies show nuclear expression of β-catenin in the majority of cases, but in equivocal cases, *CTNNB1* mutation analysis may be needed [104].

22.2.3 Fibromatosis Colli

Fibromatosis colli (FC) is an uncommon, usually self-limited, and benign fibroblastic proliferation affecting sternocleidomastoid muscle in infants and may lead to torticollis in some cases [105, 106].

Besides cervical ultrasonography, FNA is one of the most important diagnostic procedures, especially to exclude neoplastic or inflammatory lesions, which allows for the elimination of surgical procedures [106–108]. Smears are composed of bland, spindle-shaped, and plump fibroblasts which are dispersed or form loose clusters within collagen fibers. Atrophic or degenerated skeletal muscles are also usually found [107–109].

Surgical specimens are rarely obtained, and surgical procedures are a treatment in selected cases, not a diagnostic approach. Histologically, there is a bland, paucicellular fibroblastic pro-liferation that entraps skeletal muscle fibers [110].

22.2.4 Dermatofibrosarcoma Protuberans

Dermatofibrosarcoma protuberans (DFSP) is a dermal-based sarcoma, and up to 15% of cases occur in the head and neck (mostly on the forehead and cheeks). It is a locally aggressive fibroblastic neoplasm characterized by *COL1A1-PDGFB* fusion genes and has a low metastatic potential, but a high local recurrence rate [111–113]. Most commonly, it is diagnosed in young or middle-aged adults but can be found in any age [112].

DFSP is rarely diagnosed by FNA. Smears show neoplastic spindle cells which are dissociated or arranged in three-dimensional clusters or fascicles within fibrillary stromal fragments. The storiform pattern can be observed in most cases. Slight to moderate atypia may be visible in some cases, especially with sarcomatous transformation. Apart from the recurrences, a confident diagnosis of DFSP is usually not possible based on cytomorphological features alone [114–116].

In histological slides, DFSP is an ill-defined tumor located in the dermis and infiltrating subcutaneous tissue with a honeycomb pattern (infiltrating and expanding fibrous connective tissue septae). The classic variant of DFSP is composed of uniform spindle cells arranged in storiform or cartwheel patterns [112, 113]. Multiple morphological variants of DFSP exist, which can be characterized by features such as myxoid areas, the presence of pigmented cells, myoid differentiation, or fibrosarcomatous changes. This latter variant is distinguished by higher metastatic potential [89, 112].

Diagnosis of DFSP can be supported by strong and diffuse expression of CD34. In areas of fibrosarcomatous changes, CD34 expression can be diminished or even absent [111, 112]. In problematic cases, the detection of *COL1A1-PDGFB* fusion can be helpful to confirm the diagnosis [112].

22.2.5 Solitary Fibrous Tumor

Solitary fibrous tumor (SFT) is a fibroblastic neoplasm that is found in the head and neck in up to 15% of cases (most commonly in the oral cavity, orbits, sinonasal tract, and neck) and is often smaller in other locations [117, 118]. It is most often diagnosed in middle-aged adults and is one of the most common mesenchymal neoplasms diagnosed in the head and neck in adults [119]. SFT harbors pathognomonic *NAB2-STAT6* gene fusion. The majority of the cases behave like benign tumors. While more than a quarter of the cases bear recurrence or distant metastasis potential, it seems that metastatic risk in the head and neck SFT is lower in other locations [117, 120]. The risk of malignancy assessment using clinical and histological features, such as size of the tumor, mitotic index, or tumor necrosis, is crucial for proper management [117, 121, 122].

In smears, bland spindle cells are observed as dispersed cells or tight clusters. Neoplastic cells have spindle or rounded nuclei and indistinct nucleoli (Fig. 22.3a). There is a variable amount of dense, collagenous stroma. In malignant cases, nuclear pleomorphism, mitotic activity, or necrotic background may be seen. Cytomorphological features alone are usually nonspecific, and in most cases, it is impossible to provide a proper diagnosis without ancillary studies [123–125].

Histologically, conventional SFT is composed of spindle or ovoid cells randomly arranged ("patternless" growth). A stroma is made of fibrous tissue, frequently with dense hyalinization or sometimes with myxoid changes. Prominent vas-

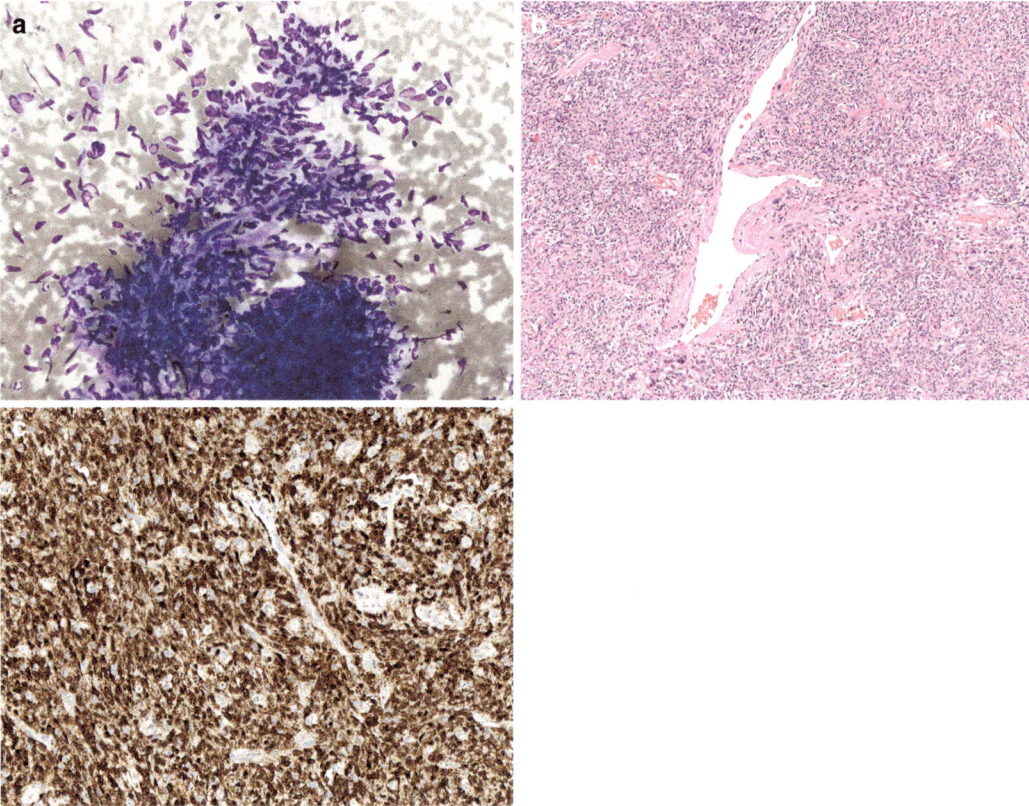

Fig. 22.3 (**a**) Solitary fibrous tumor. FNAB. Loosely clusters and dispersed spindle cells with poorly preserved cytoplasm and uniform or slightly pleomorphic nuclei (MGG). (**b**) Solitary fibrous tumor. Patternless architecture of spindled and ovoid tumor cells and prominent vasculature (H&E). (**c**) Solitary fibrous tumor. Tumor cells show immunoreactivity for STAT6

culature is characterized by staghorn-shaped (hemangiopericytoma-like) vessels with perivascular hyalinization (Fig. 22.3b) [126–128].

STAT6 positivity in immunohistochemical studies is a very sensitive and specific surrogate marker for *NAB2-STAT6* gene fusion (Fig. 22.3c). Another helpful immunohistochemical staining is CD34 positivity [129, 130].

22.2.6 Low-Grade Fibromyxoid Sarcoma

Low-grade fibromyxoid sarcoma (LGFMS) is a fibroblastic malignancy that is very rarely found in the head and neck region, most commonly in the neck. It usually affects young adults [131, 132]. LGFMS has up to 50% metastatic rate and a slightly higher recurrence rate in the long-term follow-up (more than 10 years) [133].

FNA specimens show a monomorphic population of spindle cells with elongated or oval nuclei, and only a minor subset of cases presents mildly atypical nuclei. In the background, there is a variable myxoid and collagenous stroma. Due to its bland appearance, it may be misdiagnosed as a benign spindle cell tumor [134, 135].

Histological finding is bland spindle cell neoplasm arranged in short fascicles or in a whorled pattern within the collagenous or more cellular myxoid stroma (Fig. 22.4). In myxoid areas, blood vessels are typically seen as arcades with perivascular sclerosis [133, 136].

Diffuse strong MUC4 immunoexpression is a very specific feature which can support the diagnosis. Molecular studies, including identification of the most common *FUS-CREB3L2* gene fusion, are helpful in problematic cases [137].

22.2.7 Low-Grade Myofibroblastic Sarcoma

Low-grade myofibroblastic sarcoma (LGMS) is a neoplasm with myofibroblastic differentiation and predilection to the deep layers of the head and neck region, particularly in the oral cavity (usually in the tongue) or larynx. It occurs mainly in

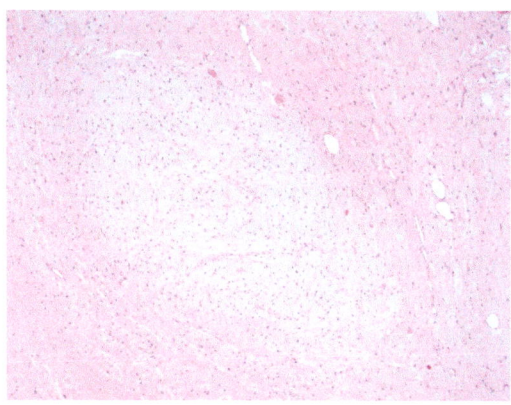

Fig. 22.4 Low-grade fibromyxoid sarcoma. The tumor consists of myxoid areas (in the center of the photo) surrounded by less cellular collagenous bands (H&E)

adults and has a high risk of recurrence. Distant metastasis is rarely found [138, 139].

Cytological features have not been well established. Histologically, it contains atypical spindle cells arranged in fibromatosis-like fascicles with a typical diffusely infiltrative growth pattern, the so-called checkerboard pattern (infiltration between individual skeletal muscle fibers) [139, 140].

Myofibroblastic differentiation can be shown by immunohistochemistry. Tumor cells can present variable SMA, desmin, and calponin positivity [139].

22.2.8 Inflammatory Myofibroblastic Tumor

Inflammatory myofibroblastic tumor (IMT) is a myofibroblastic neoplasm mixed with chronic inflammatory cells. Up to 15% of cases arise in the head and neck region (mainly in the sinonasal tract and larynx). Head and neck IMT has a predilection to young adults. IMT is a very rare metastatic disease, and the course is most often benign. Recurrences happen in a minority of cases [89, 141], [142].

FNAs of IMT consist of a mixture of plump, usually bland spindle myofibroblastic cells, chronic inflammatory cells, and ganglion-like cells in some cases. These cytomorphological features may lead to reactive myofibroblastic proliferation misdiagnosis [143, 144].

In surgical specimens, myofibroblastic cells may be seen in different patterns: with prominent myxoid stroma, in tight fascicles, or in hypocellular fibrous stroma. Predominant populations of chronic inflammatory cells in the background are lymphocytes and plasma cells [142, 145].

In about half of the cases, Anaplastic lymphoma kinase (ALK) immunohistochemical positivity or *ALK* rearrangement can be found [141, 145, 146].

22.3 Smooth Muscle Tumors

22.3.1 Leiomyoma

Leiomyoma is a benign tumor presenting smooth muscle differentiation, and primary head and neck leiomyomas account for less than 1% of all leiomyomas. In this region, it is most commonly diagnosed within the oral cavity, sinonasal tract, and skin of the face. Leiomyoma occurs mainly in middle-aged adults [147–149].

The cytomorphological features of leiomyoma are similar to normal smooth muscle tissue. In smears, it is composed of bland spindle cells with cigar-shaped nuclei which are in clusters or are dispersed. At low magnification, it may look like desmoid fibromatosis, but without collagenous stromal fragments [150, 151].

In histological sections, bland spindle cells without atypia form intersecting fascicles. In the head and neck region, some of the benign smooth muscle tumors are presented as angioleiomyomas—characterized by prominent vessels with thick muscular walls [148, 149, 152, 153].

22.3.2 Leiomyosarcoma

Leiomyosarcoma (LMS) is a smooth muscle malignancy. The head and neck region is very rarely involved by the LMS, and patients are typically older adults. The most common sites of the primary lesions are deep soft tissues and skin, followed by the oral cavity and sinonasal tract [154, 155]. Radiation exposure and immunosuppression are important risk factors [156, 157]. The overall prognosis of the head and neck LMS is poor, but it is slightly better in retroperitoneal or vascular tumors, especially in patients with superficial LMS who are eligible for complete surgical excision [158]. Distant metastasis, larger size of the primary tumor, and higher grade are the most important adverse prognostic factors [158, 159].

FNA is a highly sensitive method for diagnosing LMS as a malignancy. In smears, there are typically spindle cells with cigar-shaped nuclei and some number of pleomorphic cells or epithelioid cells (Fig. 22.5a–b). The degree of atypia depends on the tumor grade. In high-grade LMS markedly atypical cells, mitotic activity and necrotic background may be visible [151, 160].

The main histological differences that can differentiate between LMS and leiomyoma are pleomorphism (Fig. 22.5c), mitotic activity, and tumor cell necrosis [161].

By immunohistochemistry, neoplastic cells show positivity for at least one myogenic marker (Fig. 22.3d). Also, in many cases, epithelial markers are at least focally positive [161, 162].

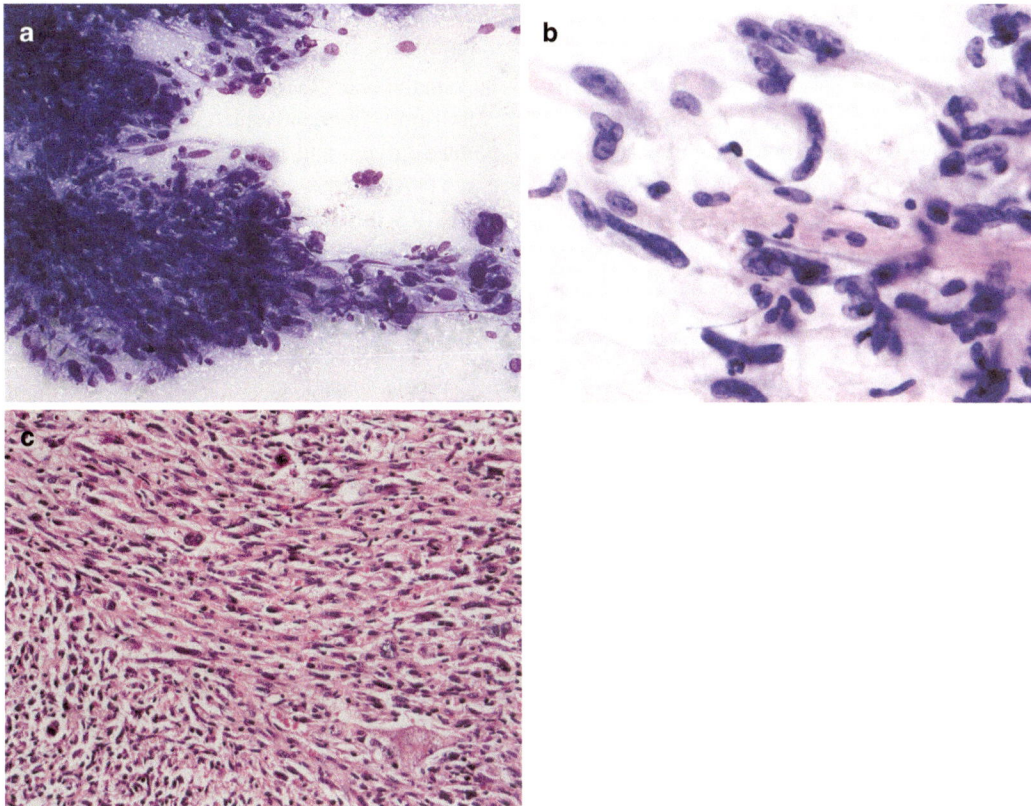

Fig. 22.5 (**a–b**) Leiomyosarcoma. FNAB. Clusters and dispersed, pleomorphic tumor cells with elongated, cigar-shaped nuclei mixed with epithelioid and multinucleated tumor cells (MGG and H&E). (**c**) Leiomyosarcoma. High-grade leiomyosarcoma is composed of fascicles of spindle cells with hyperchromatic nuclei, eosinophilic cytoplasm, and scattered pleomorphic cells (H&E)

22.4 Skeletal Muscle Tumors

22.4.1 Rhabdomyoma

Rhabdomyoma is an uncommon benign neoplasm presenting skeletal muscle differentiation. According to WHO classification, it is divided into adult rhabdomyoma (ARM) and fetal rhabdomyoma (FRM). Both variants arise predominantly within the head and neck area. ARM usually affects older adults, while FRM affects infants and children. Male predominance is seen in both variants [163].

Cytologically and histopathologically, ARM contains large polygonal neoplastic cells with abundant, eosinophilic cytoplasm with fine granules and small, located peripherally nucleoli [163, 164]. FRM is characterized by a predominant nonatypical spindle cell population with dispersed larger cells with abundant, eosinophilic cytoplasm. Myxoid material can be found in the background [163, 165].

22.4.2 Rhabdomyosarcoma

Rhabdomyosarcoma (RMS) is a malignant neoplasm presenting skeletal muscle differentiation and is the most common soft tissue sarcoma in children. They can arise in different locations in the body, but about 35% are located within the head and neck region, where they can be divided into (in order of decreasing frequency): nonparameningeal/nonorbital (superficial sites of the head and neck, oral cavity, oropharynx, or hypopharynx), parameningeal (middle ear, infratemporal fossa, paranasal sinuses, and nasopharynx), and orbital. Pathological features of RMS allowed us to distinguish four subtypes of RMS: embryonal rhabdomyosarcoma (ERMS), alveolar rhabdomyosarcoma (ARMS), spindle cell/sclerosing rhabdomyosarcoma (SRMS), and pleomorphic rhabdomyosarcoma (PRMS). In the head and neck, ERMS is the most common subtype, followed by ARMS, SRMS is rare, and PRMS is exceedingly rare. RMS is usually diagnosed in children or young adults (generally, EMRS is diagnosed in younger children; ARMS in older children, adolescents, and adults; SRMS in children, adolescents, and adults; and PRMS in adults >50 y.o.) [166–169]. Generally, RMS has a poor prognosis. The lower stage at presentation, younger age, orbital location of the tumor, and embryonal subtype are the most important prognostic factors correlated with more favorable outcomes [163, 168]. Clinicopathological differences among RMS subtypes are presented in Table 22.3.

FNA is a very sensitive method for diagnosing RMS. Smears from all subtypes of RMS usually show round neoplastic cells, very often with rhabdomyoblastic morphology (Fig. 22.6a–b). In some cases, spindle-shaped cells (more frequently in nonalveolar RMS) or multinucleated giant cells (more frequently in ARMS) are observed. Nuclear atypia and mitoses are evident in most cases [170, 171].

AMRS in histopathology presents itself as a primitive round cell tumor with small cells containing scant cytoplasm. Tumor cells form nests separated by fibrovascular septa. In ERMS, besides primitive round cells, there is a population of spindle-shaped cells. Neoplastic cells are located within a myxoid matrix, and, in some cases, there is a linear arrangement of tumor cells below the mucosal surface (the so-called cambium layer). In SRMS, spindle cells are the predominant population of neoplastic cells, sometimes within sclerotic stroma. PRMS is characterized by the presence of large, pleomorphic tumor cells [163].

Immunohistochemical positivity of myogenic regulatory proteins, MyoD1 and Myogenin, confirms the diagnosis of RMS (Fig. 22.6c). AMRS and SRMS usually harbor specific molecular alterations (AMRS *PAX3-FOXO1* or *PAX7-FOXO1* fusion, while SRMS *VGLL2* and *NCOA2* rearrangements or *MyoD1* mutations) [163, 169].

Table 22.3 Clinicopathological features of different subtypes of the head and neck rhabdomyosarcoma

	Embryonal RMS	Alveolar RMS	Spindle cell/sclerosing RMS	Pleomorphic RMS
Frequency	The most common	Common	Rare	Exceedingly rare
Age group	<5 y.o.	10–25 y.o.	Children and adults	>50 y.o.
Molecular alterations	Gains of chromosomes 2, 8, 12, 13, and/or 20 LOH at 11p15.5	*PAX3-FOXO1* and *PAX7-FOXO1* gene fusions	*VGLL2, NCOA2* gene rearrangements in infantile RMS *MyoD1* mutations in adolescents and adults	Not specific
Immunohistochemistry	Desmin positivity Focal myogenin and MyoD1 staining Occasional keratin staining	Desmin positivity Myogenin strong and diffuse positivity Focal MyoD1 staining Occasional keratin staining	Desmin positivity Myogenin focal staining MyoD1 usually diffuse staining (most commonly in sclerosing variant) Occasional keratin staining	Desmin positivity Focal Myogenin and MyoD1 staining Occasional keratin staining
Prognosis	Better prognosis (5-year OS: about 80%)	Good prognosis (5-year OS: 60–70%)	Infantile RMS—better prognosis (5-year OS: about 90%) RMS with *MyoD1* mutation—Worse prognosis	Highly aggressive behavior

RMS rhabdomyosarcoma, *LOH* loss of heterozygosity, *OS* overall survival

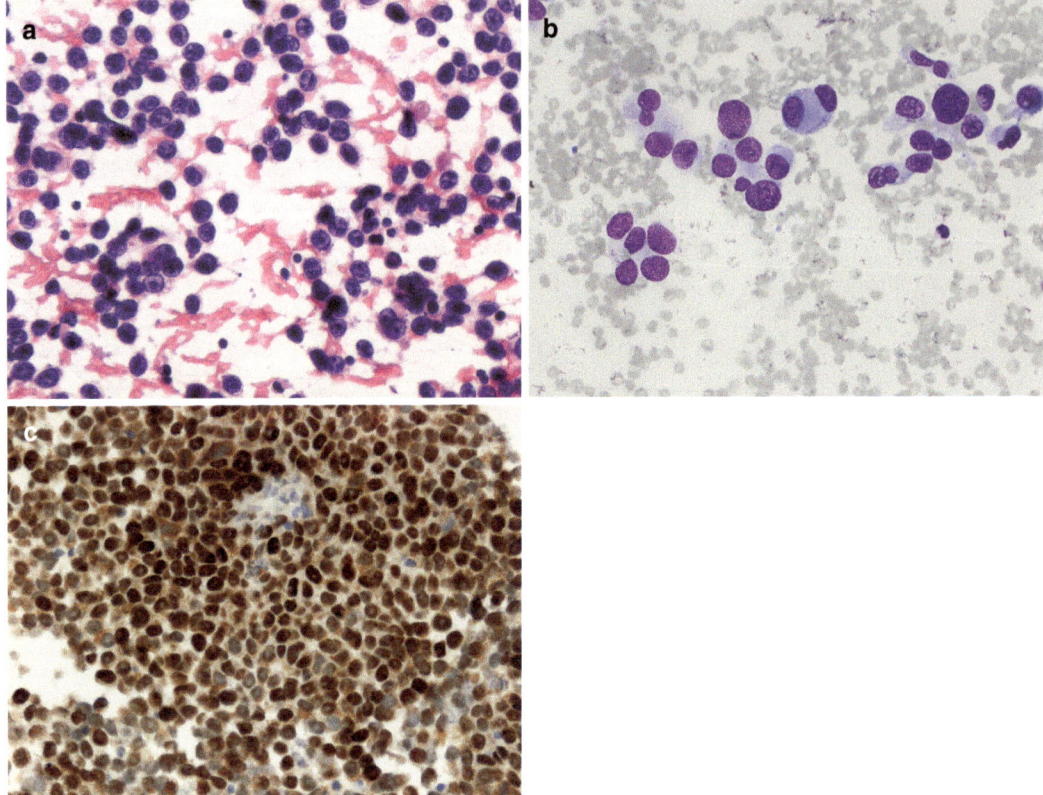

Fig. 22.6 (a–b) Alveolar rhabdomyosarcoma. FNAB. Dispersed, single, small- and medium-sized round cells with hyperchromatic nuclei and prominent nucleoli (H&E), and occasional rhabdomyoblastic morphology (MGG). (c) Rhabdomyosarcoma, positivity for MyoD1, confirms the diagnosis of RMS (MyoD1-Cell block section)

22.5 Vascular Tumors

22.5.1 Hemangioma

Hemangioma is a group of benign vascular neoplastic lesions. There are many different morphological variants, but the most common are as follows: capillary hemangioma, cavernous hemangioma, and lobular capillary hemangioma (previously called pyogenic granuloma). It is most commonly found in the skin or subcutaneous tissue, followed by the oral cavity or sinonasal tract. Clinically, it presents as a solitary tumor, but some patients, especially in the pediatric population, may have multiple lesions. The median age of patients is 40, but a subset of hemangiomas occurs in infants (several days or weeks after birth). Lobular capillary hemangioma mostly presents itself in children and young adults (women are affected two times more than men). An involution or even spontaneous regression is seen in many cases in infants and children [172–175]. Infantile hemangiomas should be differentiated from vascular malformations which persist throughout life.

FNAB of hemangiomas is rarely performed. Due to poor cellularity (usually small groups of poorly preserved spindle cells without atypia) and abundant hemorrhagic background, the diagnosis should be supplemented by clinical and radiological data [176].

Histopathological slides show the proliferation of blood vessels of different sizes lined by nonatypical endothelial cells (Fig. 22.7). Lobular capillary hemangioma is characterized by lobular architecture in which each lobule has a bigger central vein surrounded by capillary type of vessels [177].

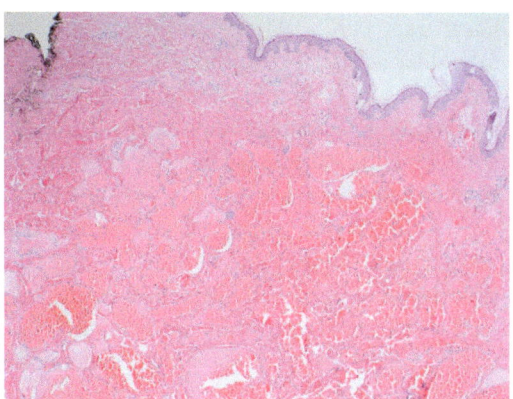

Fig. 22.7 Cavernous hemangioma. The tumor is composed of cystically dilated, blood-filled vascular channels (H&E)

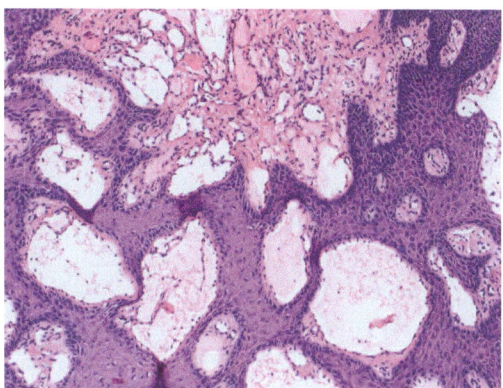

Fig. 22.8 Lymphangioma. Variably sized lymphatic channels located directly under the oral mucosal epithelium (H&E)

In most cases, ancillary studies are not required for diagnosing hemangiomas. In more problematic cases, usually in rarer subtypes, immunohistochemical positivity of endothelial markers (like CD34, CD31, or ERG) may be helpful. GLUT1 positivity in infantile hemangiomas can be used to differentiate it from vascular malformations. Some rare variants of hemangioma may present recurrent genetic alterations, like in epithelioid hemangioma, *FOS* and *FOSB* fusions may be observed in up to 50% of cases (less often in superficial head and neck tumors) [177, 178].

22.5.2 Lymphangioma

Lymphangioma is a benign tumor showing proliferation of dilated lymphatic vessels and having a predilection for the head and neck region. Most often, it is localized in the skin or subcutaneous tissue, but the oral cavity can also be affected. Lymphangioma is an uncommon tumor, and typically, it is diagnosed in infancy and early childhood. These lesions do not regress like hemangiomas but rather grow up with the patient's age [179–181].

FNAB can be contributive when there is a clinical suspicion of other tumors [181]. In aspired fluid, there are a lot of lymphocytes and macrophages.

Histopathology shows the proliferation of dilated lymphatic channels (Fig. 22.8). The lym-

phatic endothelial lining shows no atypia [177, 180].

D2-40 is positive in lymphatic endothelial cells, and staining can be used to discriminate lymphangiomas from hemangiomas, which are D2-40 negative [177, 182].

22.5.3 Kaposi Sarcoma

Kaposi sarcoma (KS) is defined as a locally aggressive neoplasm presenting vascular endothelial differentiation and is induced by human herpesvirus 8 (HHV8). Most cases of head and neck KS are AIDS-related subtypes and are located within the oral cavity (with the hard palate being the most often affected site) [169, 183]. The KS incidence is increasing with more pronounced immunodeficiency. The prognosis depends on the immune status. In most cases, KS behaves as a locally aggressive tumor, but in very immunocompromised patients, it can rarely develop distant metastasis in visceral organs [169, 184, 185].

As it is mainly an oral cavity tumor, cytological examination is carried out extremely rarely. Smears typically show bland or mildly atypical spindle cells with crushed nuclear artifacts, which form small groups or they are dispersed [176, 186].

In the early stages of the disease, histopathology reveals only subtle proliferation of small vascular spaces surrounded by extravasated erythrocytes and chronic inflammatory cells. In the advanced stages, proliferation of fascicles composed of mildly atypical spindle cells with increased mitotic activity is observed.

HHV8 immunohistochemical staining can be performed to confirm the diagnosis [187].

22.5.4 Epithelioid Hemangioendothelioma

Epithelioid hemangioendothelioma (EHE) is considered to be a malignant vascular neoplasm harboring *WWTR1-CAMTA1* or rarely *YAP1-TFE3* gene fusion. It is a very rare tumor that can be diagnosed at any age, but the incidence peak is between the fourth and fifth decades [188]. Up to 20% of cases are found in the head and neck, most commonly in the neck soft tissue, oral cavity, or bones. The clinical course of the majority of cases is indolent, but 20-25% of the patients develop distant metastasis. A 5-year overall survival rate is about 80% [169, 177, 189, 190].

In cytological specimens, epithelioid or rarely spindle cells with low-grade atypia can be seen. Infrequently, cells may contain a small lumen containing erythrocytes [191–193].

Histopathology reveals cords of epithelioid or spindle-shaped neoplastic cells embedded in myxohyaline stroma. The characteristic feature is the presence of the cells with a single cytoplasmic vacuole. Significant atypia may be observed in some cases [178, 190].

Besides vascular markers (like CD31 and ERG), CAMTA1 and TFE3 immunohistochemical positivity are highly sensitive to EHE [178].

22.5.5 Angiosarcoma

Angiosarcoma is a malignancy showing endothelial differentiation. The head and neck region is the most common location of this tumor. UV-exposed skin of the head and neck is most commonly affected, but angiosarcoma can also be found in the oral cavity and sino-

nasal tract [177, 194, 195]. Patients are usually older adults. The etiology in most cases is unknown, but previous radiation therapy, trauma, or UV damage may be risk factors in some patients. Angiosarcoma is a very aggressive disease with a high rate of local recurrences, and 5-year overall survival is less than 30%. Primary tumor site in the head and neck is believed to be an independent factor associated with improved overall survival, other than younger age, lower tumor grade, and smaller tumor size [196].

Most of the head and neck angiosarcomas are easily accessible for FNA, and cytological features of angiosarcoma are well described. Neoplastic cells show a wide variety of shapes; they can be epithelioid, spindle, polymorphous, or multinucleated (Fig. 22.9a–b). Vasoformative features, like hemophagocytosis or the presence of cells with vacuoles containing erythrocytes, can be seen in most cases [197–199].

In histopathological specimens, angiosarcoma may present very diverse features. In low-grade tumors, the formation of vascular channels lined by mildly atypical neoplastic cells may be easily found (Fig. 22.9c), while high-grade tumors are typically composed of undifferentiated cells, which can be difficult to discern from other high-grade sarcomas. Epithelioid angiosarcoma usually appears as a tumor with a diffuse, solid growth pattern and comprises large, atypical epithelioid cells with prominent nucleoli. This subtype is characterized by more aggressive behavior [177, 200].

Immunohistochemically, neoplastic cells present vascular markers positivity (mainly CD31 and ERG). A potential diagnostic pitfall, especially in epithelioid angiosarcoma, is an expression of cytokeratins, which can cause a misdiagnosis as carcinoma [201, 202].

Genetically, angiosarcoma is a very heterogenous tumor. Various molecular abnormalities have been described, but in radiation-associated angiosarcoma, the characteristic feature is the presence of *MYC* amplification, which corresponds with immunohistochemical strong positivity for MYC protein [203, 204].

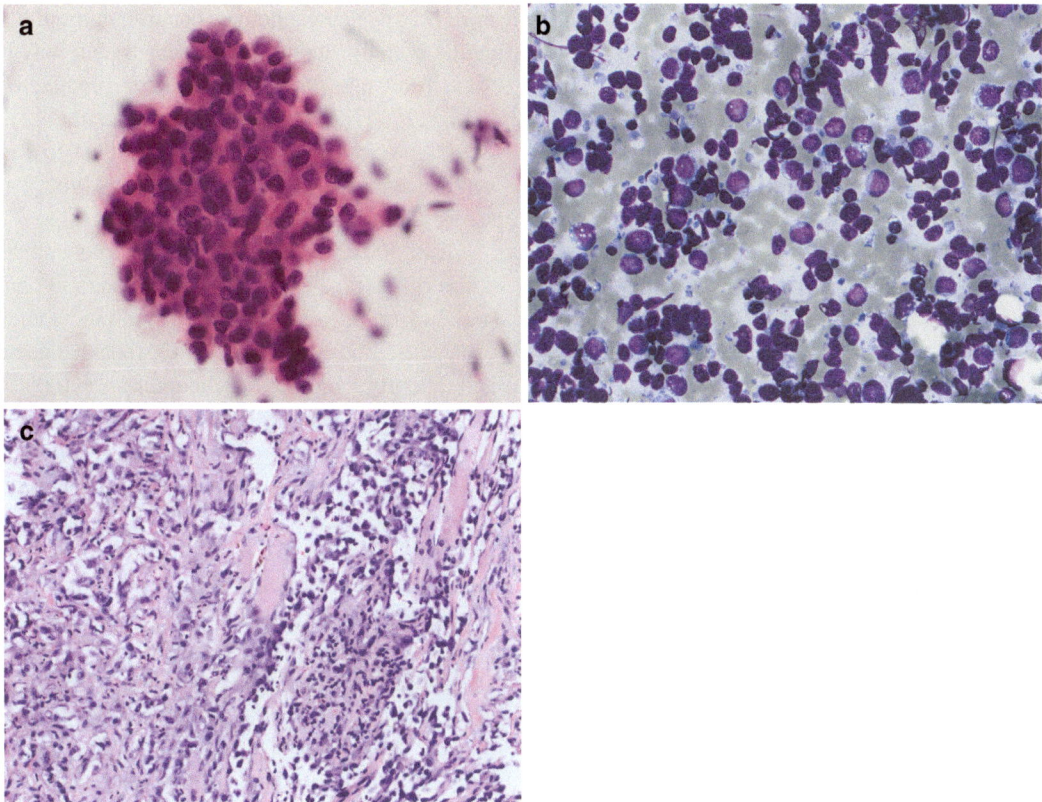

Fig. 22.9 (**a**–**b**) Angiosarcoma. FNAB. Dispersed single cells and cohesive three-dimensional clusters of neoplastic cells showing a wide variety of shapes; they can be epithelioid, spindle, polymorphous, or multinucleated. (**c**) Angiosarcoma. Poorly formed vascular channels lined by atypical neoplastic cells (H&E)

22.6   Nerve Sheath Tumors

Nerve sheath tumors arise relatively often in the head and neck area. Among benign nerve sheath neoplasms, approximately 40% of cases of schwannoma occur in this location, while MPNST accounts for 5-10% of all soft tissue sarcomas occurring in the head and neck. This region is a rare site of hybrid peripheral nerve sheath tumors and is a newly recognized subtype of peripheral nerve sheath tumors.

22.6.1 Neurofibroma

Neurofibroma is a nerve sheath tumor composed of Schwann cells, fibroblasts, and perineurial cells with an admixture of residual axons and mast cells within a fibromyxoid matrix. Four subtypes of neurofibroma are ancient neurofibroma, cellular neurofibroma, atypical neurofibroma, and plexiform neurofibroma.

Neurofibroma is the most common peripheral nerve sheath tumor affecting individuals of all ages with a peak incidence occurring between the second and fourth decades of life. About 15% of neurofibromas arise in the head and neck region [205–207]. Most neurofibromas are sporadic, while approximately 10% are associated with neurofibromatosis type 1. Most arise in the skin, but deep lesions associated with medium-sized nerves, a major nerve trunk, or a nerve plexus are seen. Any head and neck site may be affected [208–212]. Intraorally, the tongue is the most common location [213–216]. Multiple and plexiform neurofibromas are frequently associated with neurofibromatosis type 1 [206, 217, 218]. Plexiform neurofibroma may arise in superficial or deep soft tissue and occasionally in the large nerve trunks in the head and neck area, with the orbitotemporal region commonly affected [205].

Histologically, neurofibromas show commonly nodular and less often diffuse or plexiform growth patterns [219] Lesions are composed of randomly distributed spindle cells with inconspicuous cytoplasm and wavy and tapered nuclei in the background of fibromyxoid stroma. The collagen bundles resemble shredded carrots, and mast cells are often presented [207, 220, 221].

In the majority of neurofibromas, the tumor matrix is typically fibromyxoid, collagenous, or hyalinized, and FNA smears are hypocellular with small fragments of cohesive spindle cells in a myxoid, fibromyxoid, or collagenous matrix. Spindle cells show comma-shaped, bent, or wavy nuclei [222, 223].

By immunohistochemistry, stromal cells display positivity for S100 and CD34, scattered perineurial cells show variable positivity for claudin-1, GLUT1, and EMA, and scattered axons show positivity for neurofilament.

Localized cutaneous neurofibromas are benign neoplasms. Subtypes of neurofibroma associated with neurofibromatosis type 1 may undergo malignant transformation with a lifetime risk for MPNST estimated at 9-13% [224].

22.6.2 Schwannoma

Schwannoma is a benign nerve sheath tumor composed of neoplastic Schwann cells. Subtypes include ancient schwannoma, cellular schwannoma, plexiform schwannoma, epithelioid schwannoma, and microcystic/reticular schwannoma.

Schwannomas are typically encapsulated and arise sporadically in the superficial or, less often, the deep soft tissues of the head and neck and limbs. Up to 40% of schwannomas occur in the head and neck [217, 221]. Any head and neck site may be affected by schwannoma [217, 225]. Intraorally, the tongue is the most common location [226]. Spinal intradural extramedullary and cranial nerve schwannomas are commonly associated with neurofibromatosis type 2 [227]. Rare sites include spinal intramedullary and CNS loca-

tion [228]. Schwannomas occur commonly in adults in their second to fifth decades but may be seen in all age groups with no sex predilection [218, 225–228]. Most cases are sporadic [217, 218], but approximately 10% are associated with syndromes such as neurofibromatosis type 2 or schwannomatosis [221].

Histologically, most schwannomas are well circumscribed (Fig. 22.10a), encapsulated, and composed of uniform or slightly pleomorphic spindle cells with spindled, oval, tapered, or buckled nuclei and poorly defined eosinophilic cytoplasm (Fig. 22.10b). Tumor cells are arranged in variable proportions of compact hypercellular Antoni A areas with common nuclear palisading occasionally creating Verocay bodies (Fig. 22.10c), alternating with hypocellular, loosely arranged myxoid Antoni B areas. Thick-walled, hyalinized blood vessels, foamy macrophages, and peripheral lymphoid aggregates are common [218, 229]. Microcystic/reticular changes, intranuclear cytoplasmic inclusions, nuclear pleomorphism, and mitoses may exist. The ancient subtype shows marked degenerative nuclear atypia and often presents ischemic and cystic changes, hemorrhage, and hyalinization. The cellular variant of schwannoma shows a predominantly hypercellular Antoni A pattern. Necrosis and mitotic activity may be present [218]. The cell morphology of plexiform schwannoma commonly arising in the head and neck region resembles that of classical schwannoma with the exception of an intraneural multinodular/plexiform architecture [221]. Rare epithelioid schwannomas show multilobular architecture and tumor cells with predominantly epithelioid morphology in nests or linear arrays within a myxoid or hyalinized stroma [229]. Microcystic/reticular schwannomas are extremely rare with only two cases reported at the head and neck location [230, 231].

Schwannomas are common targets for fine needle aspiration. Smears may vary with respect to cellularity but are often hypercellular, containing irregular tissue fragments of spindle cells embedded in a fibrillary stroma and occasionally or rarely presented single cells in the background (Fig. 22.10d) [223, 234–236]. Most of the spindle cells exhibit neurogenic differentiation, including

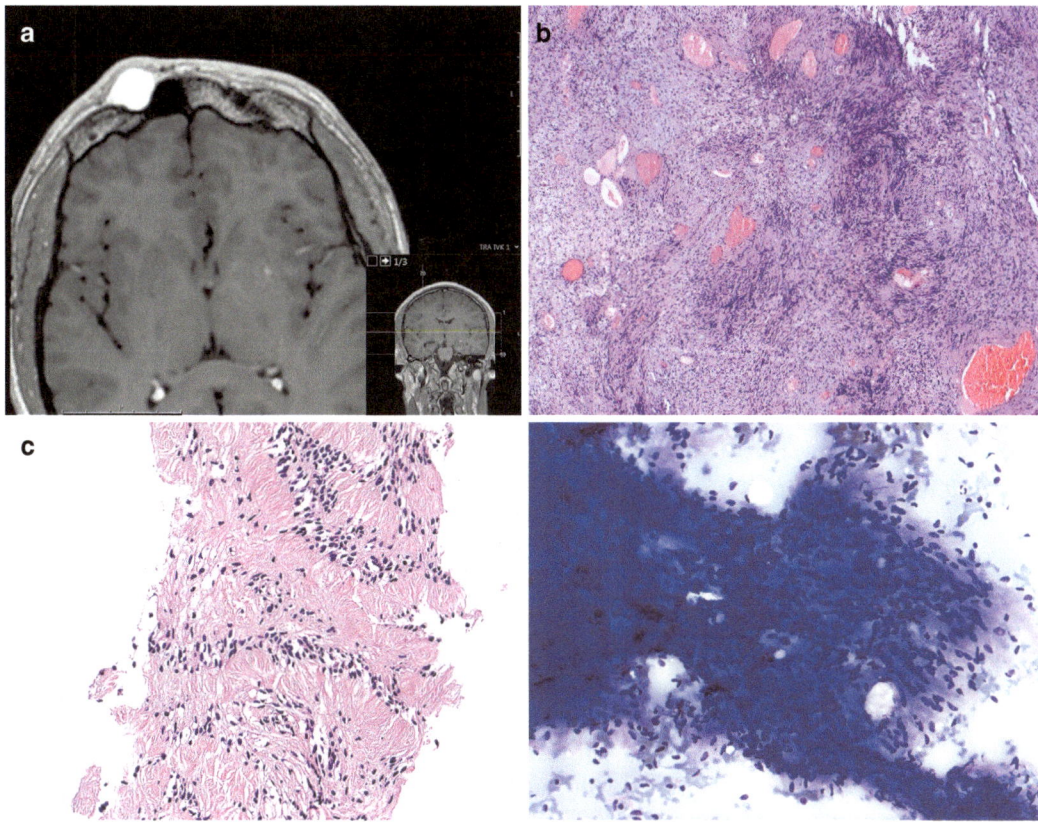

Fig. 22.10 (**a**) Schwannoma. MRI showing well-circumscribed subcutaneous tumor in the forehead. (**b**) Schwannoma. Spindle cell neoplasm with typical nuclear palisading and hyalinized blood vessels (H&E). (**c**) Schwannoma. CNB. Nuclear palisades, known as Verocay bodies, are presented (H&E). (**d**) Schwannoma. FNAB. Typically, cohesive clusters of spindle cells embedded in a fibrillary stroma and some dispersed single cells (MGG)

elongated, wavy nuclei that are often pointed or folded and sometimes show a fishhook-like appearance. Many aspirates also contain variable amounts of small- or medium-sized cells with round, bland-looking nuclei. It may be possible occasionally to identify both the highly cellular Antoni A and the poorly cellular myxoid Antoni B components corresponding to histopathologic patterns of tissue sections [235, 236]. Intranuclear inclusions are common. A subset of ancient schwannoma may cause problems in the cytologic diagnosis as FNA smears from these contain atypical cells with marked anisonucleosis and hyperchromasia [237]. FNA smears of schwannomas with cystic degeneration may be pluricellular and nondiagnostic [235, 238].

By immunohistochemistry, tumor cells display strong and diffuse positivity for S100 and SOX10 [232, 233]. The perineurial cells in the capsule are positive for EMA.

Schwannomas are benign neoplasms, and malignant transformation of conventional schwannoma is exceptionally rare [239, 240].

22.6.3 Perineurioma

Soft tissue perineurioma is a rare benign peripheral nerve sheath neoplasm composed of cells resembling normal perineural cells.

Head and neck location is uncommon and soft tissue perineuriomas commonly arise on the limbs and trunk. Perineuriomas occur over a wide age range with a peak incidence between the fourth and fifth decades of life [241]. Children are rarely affected.

Histologically, most tumors show variable cellularity and are composed of spindle cells with wavy or tapering nuclei, indistinct nucleoli, and delicate bipolar cytoplasmic extensions. Tumor cells are arranged in a storiform, whorled, or fascicular growth pattern within collagenous and myxoid stroma [241–243].

FNAB features are not specific with variable cellularity and the presence of elongated spindle cells with bland oval nuclei and characteristic long, thin, bipolar cytoplasmic processes in a collagenous to myxoid background [244–246].

By immunohistochemistry, perineuriomas express EMA, Claudin-1, GLUT1, and CD34 in about 60% of cases [241, 247].

22.6.4 Granular Cell Tumor

Granular cell tumor (GCT) is a benign neoplasm of neuroectodermal origin that occurs in a wide anatomic distribution but commonly arises in the skin and subcutaneous tissue of the head and neck region, particularly oral cavity with the tongue, representing approximately 25% of cases [248–250]. Other locations include the breast, trunk, limbs, aerodigestive tract, and genital region. Multicentric GCT occurs in approximately 10% of cases [251–253]. GCT most commonly occurs in adults and rarely in children and adolescents [254, 255]. Malignant GCTs are rare, usually arising in adults in deep soft tissues and metastasizing early in up to 50% of cases [256–259].

Histologically, GCT is an ill-defined, nonencapsulated, and infiltrating tumor characterized by large epithelial and polygonal cells with an abundant, eosinophilic faintly granular cytoplasm, and a central dark nucleus. Infiltrative cords or nests of tumor cells can cause stromal fibrosis and can be associated with epithelial hyperplasia.

FNA smears of GCT are often moderately to richly cellular showing small clusters, sheets, and singly dispersed, uniform or slightly atypical tumor cells with round to oval nuclei, inconspicuous nucleoli, and abundant granular cytoplasm. Because of the fragility of the tumor cells, FNA smears from granular cell tumors are often dominated by naked, bland nuclei in a background of finely granular material [259–263].

By immunohistochemistry, GCT expresses S100, and many cases are also immunoreactive for SOX10, inhibin, nestin, NSE, CD68, and calretinin [264–266].

GCTs are benign neoplasms, and local recurrence can be seen after incomplete excision. Malignant GCTs metastasize early and are aggressive neoplasms with poor prognosis [256].

22.6.5 Malignant Peripheral Nerve Sheath Tumor (MPNST)

Malignant peripheral nerve sheath tumor (MPNST) is a malignant spindle cell neoplasm that usually arises from a peripheral nerve and shows variable Schwannian differentiation.

MPNST, accounting for 5-10% of all soft tissue sarcomas occurring in the head and neck, is the second most common location after limbs and trunk [267–270]. Approximately 50% of cases arise in patients with neurofibromatosis type 1 (NF1) [268, 271, 272], and ~10% is associated with radiation therapy [270, 272]. MPNST occurs in adults between 20 and 50 years of age, but younger patients and children with NF1 may be affected.

Histologically, MPNST shows alternating hypercellular and hypocellular areas with often presented geographical necrosis, mitotic activity, and a haemangiopericytoma-like vascular pattern. It is composed of fascicles of spindle cells with hyperchromatic nuclei, pale, and eosinophilic cytoplasm with occasional prominent cell and nuclear pleomorphism and heterologous components [267–270]. Epithelioid subtype of MPNST is not associated with NF1 and is composed of epithelioid cells with eosinophilic cytoplasm within a hyalinizing and myxoid matrix [273, 274].

The cytomorphologic features, reflecting very diverse histologic appearances, are variable and nonspecific. FNA smears are often hypercellular with clusters of spindle cells showing vague fascicular growth and an admixture of singly dispersed cells. The tumor cells may be uniform in size and shape, elongated with fusiform, often comma-shaped, wavy, or buckled nuclei, but other forms of neoplastic cells are also present. The nuclei are hyperchromatic with evenly dispersed chromatin and small or inconspicuous nucleoli, and the cytoplasm varies from sparse to moderate. Pleomorphic and multinucleated tumor cells and background necrosis are seen in high-grade tumors. Polygonal or rounded cells may predominate smears of epithelioid MPNST. Heterologous components (cartilage, bone, epithelial glands, or rhabdoid cells) that are present focally in approximately 10–15% of MPNST are rarely sampled by FNA [275–280].

By immunohistochemistry, MPNST displays variable positivity for S-100, SOX10, or GFAP and loss of H3K27me3. Loss of SMARCB1 expression is a common finding in epithelioid MPNST [281, 282].

MPNST often displays complex karyotypes with both structural and numerical changes [283]. Common aberrations are gains of chromosome arms 7p, 8q, and 17q, and loss of 9p, 11q, 13q, and 17p [284]. Mutations of both copies of the tumor suppressor gene NF1 at 17q11.2 are found in many MPNSTs [285]. Deletion and inactivation of another known tumor suppressor gene, CDKN2A, at 9p21 is also common [286].

Overall, MPNST is an aggressive neoplasm with a poor prognosis.

22.7 Tumors of Uncertain Differentiation

22.7.1 Ossifying Fibromyxoid Tumor

Ossifying fibromyxoid tumor (OFMT) is a rare mesenchymal neoplasm of uncertain lineage, commonly arising in the subcutis/superficial soft tissues in adults, with a 2:1 male predominance.

The common primary sites are the extremities, followed by the trunk and the head and neck region [287–289].

Histologically, OFMT shows variable cellularity and is composed of lobules of uniform, round to oval, or spindled cells arranged in cords or trabeculae in variable amounts of a fibromyxoid stroma. The tumor is usually well circumscribed, and, in most cases, encapsulated and surrounded by a complete or incomplete shell of mature metaplastic bone [287, 290]. Most OFMTs are multinodular due to fibrous septa and metaplastic bone extending into the tumor. Most tumors have low mitotic activity and behave in a benign fashion. OFMTs can rarely show atypical or malignant features, having the potential for local recurrence and metastasis [287, 291–294].

The cytology of OFMT in FNA has not been sufficiently investigated, except for a few case reports. FNA smears show variable cellularity and present single cells, clusters of cells, and/or acinar-like structures of uniform or slightly pleomorphic cells with round to ovoid nuclei with inconspicuous nucleoli and moderate to abundant cytoplasm [295–298].

By immunohistochemistry, about two-thirds of OFMTs are positive for S100, 50% of tumors express desmin, and may also express EMA, MUC4, keratins, and SMA [294, 299]. INI1 expression is lost in a mosaic pattern in approximately 75% of cases, and 80% of tumors display gen fusion, commonly involving rearrangements *PHF1* gene [294, 299–302].

OFMTs have unpredictable biological potential. Both benign, atypical and malignant tumors may recur or metastasize. For the malignant subtype of OFMT, the metastasis rate is reported as 20-60% [287, 291, 293, 294].

22.7.2 Angiomatoid Fibrous Histiocytoma

Angiomatoid fibrous histiocytoma (AFH) is a rare neoplasm of intermediate malignant potential and uncertain differentiation, commonly occurring in the subcutis and characterized by sheets of spindled to ovoid histiocytoid cells, pseudoangiomatoid spaces, intralesional hemorrhage, and lymphoplasmocytoid infiltrate.

Most cases occur in the extremities, trunk, and head and neck region in children and young adults, although the age distribution is wide, and AFH can occur at unusual sites [303–308].

Histologically, most tumors display characteristic microscopic features of circumscribed and lobulated or multinodular growth of ovoid, epithelioid, or spindle cells with bland, vesicular nuclei, eosinophilic cytoplasm, and a fibroblastic or "histiocytoid" appearance. The tumor cells are often arranged in syncytial-like sheets and short fascicles with variably sized blood-filled pseudoangiomatous spaces lined by neoplastic cells and intralesional hemorrhage. Most tumors are surrounded by a dense lymphoplasmacytic infiltrate and a thick, often incomplete fibrous pseudocapsule. Mitotic figures are usually infrequent [303, 304, 309]. AFH may show a spectrum of microscopic features, and smaller numbers of myxoid, reticular, small round cell, or pleomorphic variants have been described [310–312].

FNA cytomorphology is nonspecific. Clinical correlation and ancillary studies are necessary to render the diagnosis. FNA smears show variable cellularity with small and large cellular clusters, containing ovoid to spindled histiocytoid cells with a moderate amount of vacuolated cytoplasm and an ovoid or folded nucleus with vesicular chromatin and a small inconspicuous nucleolus. Large cellular clusters with a capillary structure and a whorled arrangement of tumor cells can be appreciated in some cases. Other cytological features include occasional nuclear atypia and pleomorphism and variable amounts of single histiocytoid cells, hemosiderin-laden cells, lymphocytes, and plasma cells [313–315].

By immunohistochemistry, most cases express TLE1 [316], ALK and in approximately 50% of cases, desmin and EMA. Many cases show variable nonspecific staining for CD99 and CD68 [317–319]. Most tumors show *EWSR1::CREB1*, *EWSR1::ATF1*, and *FUS::ATF1* gen fusions which can be detected by FISH studies [320, 321].

Most AFHs behave indolently, with local recurrence in up to 15% of cases and metastasis in less than 5% of cases [304, 317].

22.7.3 Synovial Sarcoma

Synovial sarcoma (SS) is a spindle cell sarcoma showing variable epithelial differentiation and characterized by a specific *SS18::SSX1, SSX2,* or *SSX4* fusion gene. Based on their morphology, SS are divided into monophasic, biphasic, or poorly differentiated subtypes.

Most SS arises in the deep soft tissue of the extremities, followed by the trunk/abdomen, head and neck (7% of cases), mediastinum, retroperitoneum, and visceral organs [322, 323]. SS may occur at any age, with 70% affecting patients less than 50 years [322–326].

Histopathologic patterns include monophasic (Fig. 22.11a) or biphasic morphologies with cellular sheets and/or vague fascicles of uniform spindle cells with dark chromatin, sparse cytoplasm, and admixture of epithelial structures in biphasic tumors. Many SSs display areas with calcification and/or ossification, a staghorn-shaped vascular pattern, and prominent fascicular growth with occasional nuclear palisading or a herringbone pattern. Hypercellular areas with high-grade nuclear features, round cell patterns resembling Ewing sarcoma, increased mitotic activity, and necrosis may be seen in the poorly differentiated subset of SS. Rare findings include rosette-like structures, clear cell changes, and rhabdoid cells [327, 328].

FNA smears of SS are usually hypercellular, and, in low magnification, show a distinctive pattern of tight clusters of bland spindle cells mixed with dispersed cells or bare nuclei in almost equal proportions (Fig. 22.11b). Fragments of fibromyxoid or fibrous matrix, capillaries bordered by tumor cells, and scattered mast cells are other frequent findings in smears. Smears occasionally contain delicate capillaries within cell clusters. Aspirates of biphasic SS contain clusters and dispersed spindle cells mixed with acinar-like and alveolar structures [329–336].

By immunohistochemistry, SS typically expresses nuclear TLE1 (Fig. 22.11c), and at least focally EMA and keratins. They may also express S100, CD99, and BCL-2 [337–340]. A translocation t(X;18)(p11;q11) is present in most SSs, resulting in *SS18::SSX1, SS18::SSX2,* and *SS18::SSX4* gene fusions, which can be detected by FISH, PCR, and NGS [324, 341, 342].

SS may metastasize to lungs, bone, and regional lymph nodes. The prognosis depends mainly on staging, grading, resectability, use of radiation therapy, site of primary tumor, and presence of metastases [343, 344].

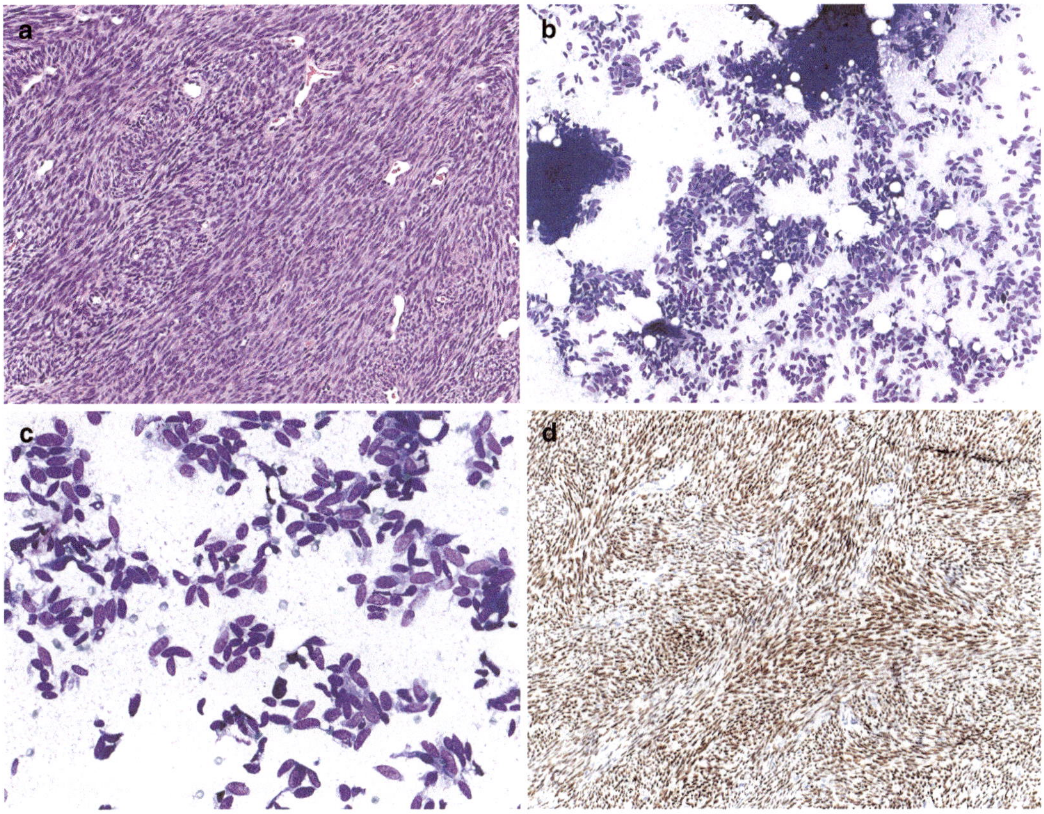

Fig. 22.11 (**a**) Synovial sarcoma. Tumor cells arranged in cellular sheets, with occasional herringbone architectural pattern (H&E). (**b**) Synovial sarcoma. FNAB. Hypercellular smears showing cohesive clusters mixed with dispersed uniform spindle cells (MGG). (**c**) Synovial sarcoma. FNAB. Single-cell population of uniform spindle cells with scant cytoplasm (MGG). (**d**) Synovial sarcoma. Tumor cells show immunoreactivity for TLE1

22.7.4 Alveolar Soft Part Sarcoma

Alveolar soft part sarcoma (ASPS) is a rare malignant mesenchymal neoplasm of uncertain histogenesis with a characteristic *ASPSCR1::TFE*3 gene fusion.

Common sites are deep soft tissue of the lower limbs or limb girdles, trunk, and head and neck region (9%) [345–347]. ASPS accounting for less than 1% of all sarcomas mainly occurs in adolescents and young adults with a slight female predominance [345].

ASPS is composed of large, polygonal-shaped cells arranged in an organoid and a uniform nesting and/or alveolar growth pattern with the tumor nests surrounded by a capillary vasculature. Tumor cells show central to eccentric nuclei with prominent nucleoli. Variable microscopic features of tumor cells include multinucleation, rhabdold-like cells, pleomorphic and xanthomatous cells, cytoplasmic vacuolization, and mitotic figures. Cystic change, myxoid stroma, and dystrophic calcification may be seen [348–350].

The cytomorphologic features of ASPS include cohesive clusters, alveolar aggregates, and scattered dyshesive tumor cells with round nuclei and prominent centrally situated nucleoli. Tumor cells have abundant granular to finely vacuolated, fragile cytoplasm. The presence of bare nuclei in a cytoplasmic granular background is a useful clue to the diagnosis. Binucleate to multinucleate giant cells, intracytoplasmic rod-like crystals, and a thin fibrillary stroma may be seen in the FNA smears [351–356].

ASPS is characterized by an *ASPSCR1::TFE3* gene fusion and nuclear overexpression of TFE3 protein [357–359]. The tumor cells contain PAS-positive/diastase-resistant rhomboid or rod-shaped intracytoplasmic crystals and granules that might be focally or diffusely present [348].

ASPS is regarded as high-grade sarcoma metastasizing to the lungs, liver, bone, brain, and rarely to lymph nodes. Local recurrence occurs in up to 50% of cases [348, 360–362].

22.7.5 Clear Cell Sarcoma of Soft Tissue

Clear cell sarcoma (CCS) of soft tissue is a rare, aggressive sarcoma with melanocytic differentiation of unknown etiology, characterized by recurrent *EWS::ATF1* fusion gene in most cases.

CCS typically occurs in young adults with a peak of incidence in the third decade of life and is slightly more common in females. Most cases arise in the lower extremities, especially the foot and ankle, while the head and neck region is rarely affected [363–369].

CCS exhibits a characteristic pattern of infiltrative growth of uniform epithelioid to fusiform and plump spindled cells divided into nests and fascicles by dense fibrous septa. Tumor cells have pale eosinophilic cytoplasm and vesicular nuclei with macronucleoli. Scattered wreath-like giant cells and melanin pigment are common findings. Necrosis is found in one-third of the cases [363, 364, 366, 369].

FNA smears are moderately to highly cellular, containing mostly dispersed cells and loose or cohesive clusters of rounded, polygonal, or spindly shaped cells. Tumor cells have rather abundant clear or pale cytoplasm and large round to ovoid, hyperchromatic nuclei with prominent nucleoli, and occasionally presented intranuclear cytoplasmic pseudoinclusions. Binucleated or wreath-like multinucleated cells, cytoplasmic melanin, and tigroid background may be present [370–375].

By immunohistochemistry, tumor cells express S100, HBM45, Melan-A, and SOX10 and typically express the MITF-M [376]. Most cases display a specific translocation, t(12; 22)(q13;q12), resulting in an *EWSR1::ATF1* gene fusion, detectable by conventional cytogenetics, FISH, PCR, or NGS [377, 378].

Overall CCSs are aggressive neoplasms with recurrence rates of 40% and pulmonary or lymph node metastasis in up to 50% of patients [366, 368, 379, 380].

22.7.6 Extraskeletal Myxoid Chondrosarcoma

Extraskeletal myxoid chondrosarcoma (EMC) is a myxoid sarcoma of uncertain differentiation characterized by *NR4A3* gene rearrangement.

Most EMCs arise in the deep soft tissues of the proximal extremities and limb girdles, followed by the trunk, head and neck, and other rare locations in middle-aged adults with a mean age of 50 years (range 4-92 years) [381, 382]. Head and neck sites include orbit, intracranial and sinonasal tract, parapharyngeal space, parotid gland, eyelid, and bucca [383–387].

EMC exhibits a multinodular or lobular architecture and characteristic reticular arrangement of uniform tumor cells with round to oval and/or spindled nuclei, often with a small, inconspicuous nucleolus, and eosinophilic cytoplasm, with delicate cytoplasmic processes (Fig. 22.12a). Common histopathologic features of EMC include cords, small clusters, and complex trabecular or cribriform arrays of tumor cells in a chondromyxoid stroma. A subset of high-grade tumors shows hypercellular areas with epithelioid to rhabdoid morphology [381, 382, 388].

FNA smears show moderately cellular to hypercellular smears of uniform tumor cells arranged as cords, strands, or balls in a myxoid and fibrillary matrix (Fig. 22.12b–c). Cell shapes are variable, including polygonal/epithelioid to rhabdoid and spindled cells with oval to spindled nuclei with small nucleoli, frequent intranuclear inclusions, and grooves. Tumor cells contain moderate to abundant, eosinophilic to vacuolated cytoplasm and occasional unipolar or bipolar cytoplasmic processes of variable length [389–393].

The immunophenotype is not specific, up to 20% stain for S-100 protein and about 30% for CD117 (KIT), and occasionally for neuroendocrine markers [393–396]. INI1 loss has been

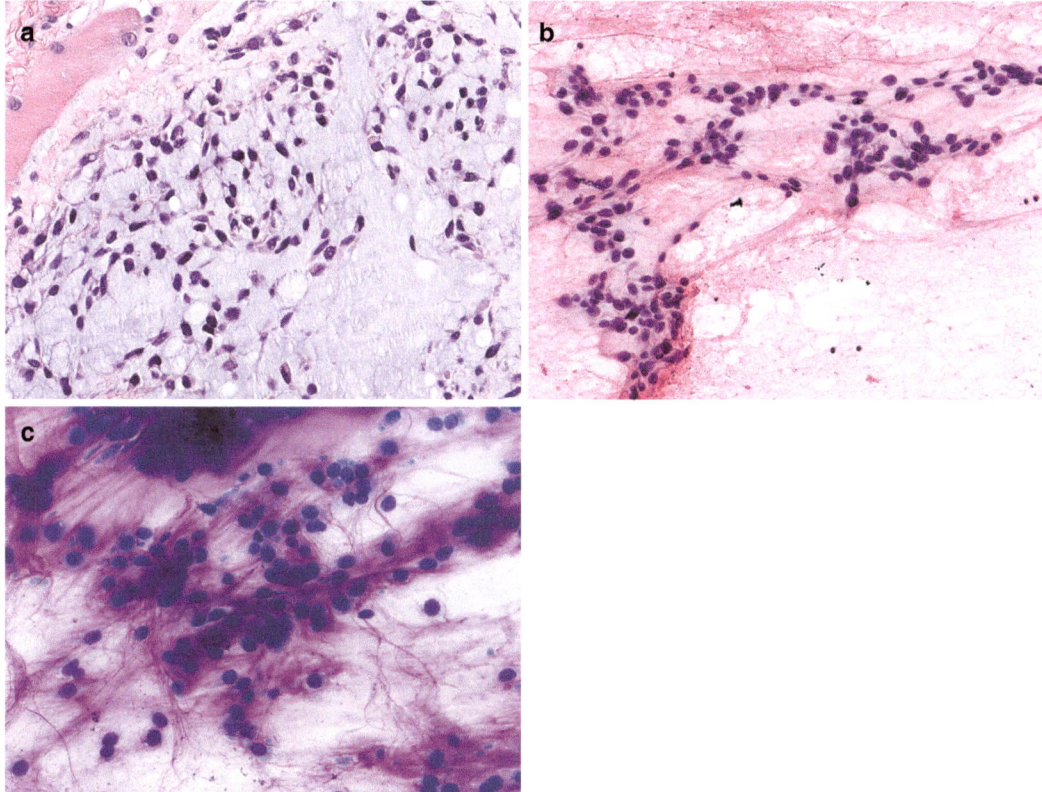

Fig. 22.12 (**a**) Extraskeletal myxoid chondrosarcoma. The tumor is composed of interconnecting cords and strands of uniform spindled and epithelioid cells with cytoplasmic processes, embedded in a myxoid matrix (H&E). (**b**) Extraskeletal myxoid chondrosarcoma. FNAB. Dispersed single cells and poorly cohesive cords of fusiform and round cells in the myxoid background matrix (MGG). (**c**) Extraskeletal myxoid chondrosarcoma. FNAB. Dispersed single cells and cords of ovoid and round cells within the myxoid matrix. Occasional nuclei show nuclear grooves (H&E)

reported in tumors with rhabdoid morphology. A characteristic translocation t(9;22)(q22/q3;q12), resulting in *EWSR1::NR4A3* fusion gene, is present in most cases. In about 25% of cases, a translocation t(9;17)(q22;q11) is identified, which is probably connected with neuroendocrine differentiation [393, 396–398].

EMC is associated with prolonged survival despite high rates of recurrences, distant metastases, and death from the disease [382, 399, 400].

22.8   Undifferentiated Sarcoma

Undifferentiated sarcoma (US) of the soft tissue, previously called malignant fibrous histiocytoma, is a malignant tumor that shows no identifiable differentiation. This tumor cannot be classified by available diagnostic methods as any other known sarcoma, so it is treated as a diagnosis of exclusion. It can be found in any age, but mainly in adults. It accounts for about 20% of all soft tissue sarcomas and is one of the most commonly diagnosed sarcomas in the head and neck region in adults and in children [401–403]. Head and neck US is most often localized in the soft tissue of the scalp, face, and neck, but also in the sinonasal or upper aerodigestive tract [404, 405]. Due to the heterogeneity of this group of tumors, the prognosis can be variable.

US is a very heterogenous group of tumors that is characterized by an extremely high burden of genomic alterations. Morphologically, most of the US are high-grade tumors and can be divided into

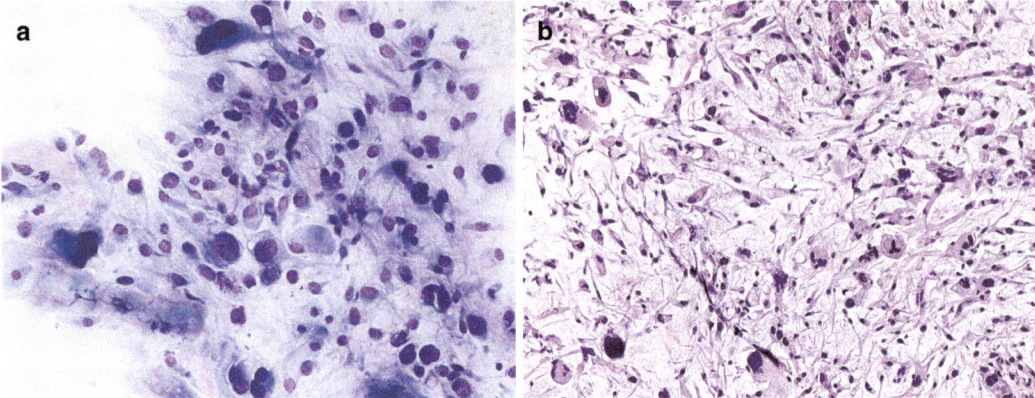

Fig. 22.13 (**a**) Undifferentiated sarcoma. FNAB. Polygonal and epithelioid cells with marked cellular and nuclear pleomorphism (MGG). (**b**) Undifferentiated sarcoma. Variable cellular morphology, spindle, polygonal, and epithelioid cells with marked cellular and nuclear pleomorphism, coarse chromatin, and scattered mitotic figs. (H&E)

spindle cell, pleomorphic, round cell, or epithelioid neoplasms depending on dominant cell types [401, 402]. FNA is a very sensitive method to diagnose US as a malignancy, and cytological features can show a lot of diversity (Fig. 22.13a) [406]. In histopathological specimens, high-grade atypia, tumor giant cells, areas of necrosis, and mitotic figures including atypical ones are seen in many cases (Fig. 22.13b). There are no specific morphological features of any other known neoplasms. All potential mimics should be ruled out microscopically or molecularly before diagnosing the US [401, 402].

22.9 Undifferentiated Small Round Cell Sarcomas

22.9.1 Ewing Sarcoma

Ewing sarcoma (ES) is an aggressive small round cell sarcoma characterized by recurrent gene fusions including *EWSR1* or *FUS* and ETS transcription factors family. It arises in children and young adults [407, 408]. Up to 9% of all ES are diagnosed in the head and neck, and in this region, it is one of the most common sarcomas in children. Unlike other body sites, in the head and neck, ES is almost equally located in the bones (mainly the cervical spine, skull, and mandible) and in the soft tissue (mainly the neck, scalp, and

face) [409, 410]. Adamantinoma-like ES (ALES), a rare subtype of ES, occurs in older age than conventional ES and shows predilection to the head and neck, mainly salivary glands, thyroid gland, and sinonasal tract [411, 412]. Head and neck ES is associated with improved prognosis compared to tumors located in other sites, but it seems that it is due to a less advanced stage at presentation [410, 413].

In most cases, ES is eligible for FNA. Smears are composed of small round cells with scant cytoplasm, and, in many cases, there are two populations of neoplastic cells: (1) smaller and darker and (2) larger and paler. Rosette formation may be seen in some cases, and mitotic activity is present in all cases. FNA assisted by molecular studies can be helpful to provide accurate diagnosis [414].

Histopathology shows hypercellular tumor compromising quite uniform small round cells with indistinct nucleoli, or sometimes cells are larger and more polymorphic with prominent nuclei (so-called atypical ES) [407]. In ALES cases, there are nests and sheets of basaloid neoplastic cells within fibromyxoid or hyalinized stroma and sometimes focal keratin pearl formation can be observed [412].

Diagnosis of ES has to be confirmed by ancillary techniques. Immunohistochemical studies show strong and diffuse CD99 expression. Other useful markers are NKX2.2 and FLI1. ALES cases are consistently keratin and p63/p40 positive. The most common genetic alteration is translocation involving *EWSR1* gene and, in a minority of cases, translocation involves *FUS* gene [407, 412].

22.9.2 Other Undifferentiated Small Round Cell Sarcomas with Recurring Genetic Alterations

A subset of undifferentiated small round cell sarcomas is characterized by different recurrent genetic abnormalities than gene fusions found in ES such as *CIC* rearrangement (CIC-rearranged sarcoma), *BCOR* abnormalities (sarcoma with BCOR genetic alterations), and *EWSR1* or *FUS* fusions involving genes other than ETS transcription factors family (round cell sarcoma with EWSR1-non-ETS fusions). These sarcomas are very rare, and only up to 10% of cases are located in the head and neck. While CIC-rearranged sarcoma has a predilection to deep soft tissue, sarcoma with BCOR genetic alterations and round cell sarcoma with EWSR1-non-ETS fusions are more commonly found in bones [408, 415, 416]. CIC-rearranged sarcoma is significantly more aggressive than ES, while the clinical course of sarcoma with BCOR genetic alterations is similar to ES [415–417]. Round cell sarcoma with EWSR1-non-ETS fusions is a very heterogenous group of neoplasms and outcome data are limited.

Cytologically and histopathologically, these tumors have subtle differences from classic ES, like the population of ovoid or spindle cells or myxoid stroma [417, 418].

Immunohistochemical and molecular studies are crucial to make a proper diagnosis.

22.10 Distinctive Soft Tissue Neoplasms of the Sinonasal Tract

Sinonasal tract angiofibroma and biphenotypic sinonasal sarcoma are very rare, site-specific soft tissue tumors that exclusively involve the sinonasal tract.

22.10.1 Sinonasal Tract Angiofibroma

Sinonasal tract angiofibroma is defined as a locally aggressive, fibrovascular tumor. It is most commonly located in the nasopharynx followed by the nasal cavity and is almost exclusively found in young males (mean age is about 17 years) [419, 420]. The APC/β-catenin pathway aberrations (mainly *CTNNB1* mutations) seem to play a major role in the pathogenesis of sinonasal tract angiofibroma, which explains >25 times the likelihood of developing tumor in patients with familial adenomatous polyposis than population without germline *APC* mutations. Recurrences after resection are reported in up to a quarter of cases, but distant metastases are not observed [420–422].

Histopathology shows the proliferation of fibrous stroma with variably sized blood vessels lined by one layer of nonatypical endothelial cells. By immunohistochemistry, stromal cells present androgen receptor and β-catenin positivity, and endothelial cells show CD31, CD34, and ERG positivity, while characteristic for hemangiomas GLUT-1 expression is lacking [421, 422].

22.10.2 Biphenotypic Sinonasal Sarcoma

Biphenotypic sinonasal sarcoma is a low-grade malignant tumor showing neural and myogenic differentiation. The tumor commonly invades multiple subsites of the sinonasal tract; the nasal cavity and ethmoid sinuses are the most commonly affected. Biphenotypic sinonasal sarcoma is found in adults with women predominance. The recurrences are seen in almost half of the patients, but metastases are not reported. The prognosis is very good with an almost 100% of 5-year survival rate [423–426].

In histological sections, biphenotypic sinonasal sarcoma is an infiltrative cellular tumor composed of monotonous spindle cells that form fascicles, sometimes with herringbone patterns. Mitotic activity is low, and necrosis is not present. By immunohistochemistry, S100 as a neural marker and SMA as a myogenic marker are consistently positive, at least focally [423, 425]. Molecularly, biphenotypic sinonasal sarcoma is characterized by recurrent *PAX3* rearrangement (most commonly with *MAML3* as a fusion partner), and the presence of immunohistochemical expression of PAX3 protein seems to be highly sensitive and specific for this entity [427].

22.11 Bone Neoplasms

Primary bone tumors arise relatively often in the head and neck area. In many cases of benign bone lesions, radiography may be diagnostic, obviating the need for any biopsy. In the majority of benign and malignant bone neoplasms, radiography may exclude or establish malignancy and limit the diagnostic options to one diagnosis or a few differential diagnoses. Morphologic examinations, however, are considered to be a necessary part of the diagnostic workup of malignant and some benign bone neoplasms since therapeutic regiments may differ significantly for both malignant and benign/locally aggressive neoplasms.

22.11.1 Osteosarcoma

Osteosarcoma is a primary malignant bone tumor composed of cells producing osteoid and tumoral bone. Osteosarcoma is the most frequent primary nonhematopoietic malignant bone tumor and accounts for approximately 20% of all primary bone sarcomas. Conventional osteosarcoma is the most common and aggressive subtype, whereas periosteal osteosarcoma is of intermediate grade, and low-grade central and parosteal osteosarcomas are low-grade subtypes. Most patients are children, adolescents, and young adults, but up to 30% of osteosarcomas occur in patients older than 40 years, with a second peak at the age of 60 years. Most osteosarcomas arise in the metaphysis of long bones but the jawbones, particularly the mandible, account for about 6% of cases. Any other craniofacial bone can be involved [428–431].

Conventional osteosarcomas are composed of highly atypical and pleomorphic tumor cells that produce immature osteoid and show osteode-structive and aggressive growth, permeating morrow spaces. The tumor cells may have densely eosinophilic cytoplasm resembling osteoblasts but often display prominent nuclear atypia. The osteoid may be variable in amount and may consist of broad, irregular, or thin lace-like trabeculae. Mitotic activity is usually brisk, including atypical mitotic figures. Osteosarcomas may have different histopathological patterns, and depending on the predominant matrix, they are subdivided into osteoblastic, chondroblastic, and fibroblastic subtypes. In osteoblastic osteosarcoma, neoplastic bone is the principal matrix; in the chondroblastic subtype, the predominant component is neoplastic hyaline cartilage; and fibroblastic osteosarcoma is composed of predominantly spindled, highly atypical tumor cells.

Periosteal subtypes generally demonstrate a predominant chondroblastic differentiation, with intermediate-grade atypia, but are exceedingly rare in the head and neck region. Low-grade medullary and parosteal osteosarcomas generally demonstrate more subtle atypia and scarce mitotic activity. Giant cell-rich osteosarcoma is a morphologic subtype that should be distinguished from other giant cell-rich lesions affecting the jaws [432–434].

FNA cytology is an efficient technique in the diagnosis of high-grade osteosarcoma in conjunction with imaging and appropriate clinical data [435–445]. The high-grade conventional type is also the most common target for FNA examination. FNAB is less useful in the evaluation of low-grade osteosarcoma, often providing nonspecific or aspiration smears insufficient for a diagnosis. FNA smears display variable cellularity but are often hypercellular. A mixture of single cells and loosely or somewhat cohesive clusters of moderately to highly pleomorphic rounded, ovoid, and polygonal tumor cells in a hemorrhagic background is a common pattern in smears. Most tumor cells have a moderate or abundant amount of well-demarcated cytoplasm, often containing small vacuoles. The nuclei have coarse chromatin and one or more, often prominent macronucleoli. The nuclei may be eccentrically placed, and such tumor cells resemble atypical osteoblasts. A background matrix is present in most of the smears, and strands of tumor matrix stained pinkish-violet-grey and red-violet-grey in DiffQuick and May-Grünwald-Giemsa (MGG) stains are considered to represent osteoid. Cartilaginous matrix and chondroid tissue fragments with atypical cells lying within lacunae may be identified in the FNA smears of chondroblastic osteosarcoma. It can be difficult to distinguish chondroid matrix material from osteoid or fragments of normal bone presented in aspirate. A variable number of pleomorphic often multinucleated tumor cells is almost always visible in smears irrespective of subtype. Osteoclast-like cells and mitoses are also frequent findings, while necrosis and calcifications are occasional findings in smears of high-grade osteosarcomas [435–445].

By immunohistochemistry, positivity for SATB2 may be useful to detect osteoblastic differentiation. Positive staining with antibodies against MDM2 and CDK4 might help in distinguishing low-grade osteosarcoma from benign fibro-osseous mimics [446–449].

Aggressive local growth and rapid systemic dissemination characterize the clinical course of conventional high-grade osteosarcoma. Osteosarcomas of the jaws metastasize far less frequently (in 6–21% of cases) than their peripheral counterparts [450–453].

22.11.2 Chondrosarcoma

Chondrosarcoma is a malignant bone neoplasm that produces a cartilaginous matrix.

Subtypes of chondrosarcoma include conventional grade 1-3 chondrosarcoma, periosteal, dedifferentiated, and clear cell chondrosarcomas. Conventional chondrosarcoma is a malignant bone neoplasm that arises in the medullary cavity and produces a cartilaginous matrix. Periosteal chondrosarcoma develops on the surface of bone. Dedifferentiated chondrosarcoma shows an abrupt transition into a high-grade, noncartilaginous sarcoma. Clear-cell chondrosarcoma is a low-grade neoplasm composed of lobules of cells with abundant clear cytoplasm.

Chondrosarcomas occur in adults, predominantly in the fourth to seventh decades of life but all age groups can be affected [454].

Conventional chondrosarcoma affects all parts of the skeleton arising from endochondral ossification, the long tubular bones, the flat bones, and occasionally the spine or base of the skull. Maxillo-facial chondrosarcoma commonly arises in the maxilla, nasal septum, and mandible. Other specific sites include the larynx, trachea, skull base, cervical spine, clivus, and orbit, but any maxillofacial bone may be affected [454–459].

Chondrosarcomas generally have a lobular morphology. Well-differentiated tumors resemble hyaline cartilage with uniform oval to polygonal cells in lacunar spaces. The nuclei are small and uniform, with round to oval outlines and evenly distributed dense chromatin. Nuclear atypia, increased cellularity with an irregular distribution, decreased volume of cytoplasm, myxoid background, and mitoses are associated with higher tumor grade {890,662}. High-grade chondrosarcomas may be highly cellular and are composed of nests of atypical, less differentiated, and occasionally spindled cells within the myxoid matrix. The tumors may destroy and grow through the cortex and necrosis may be present [460, 461].

The cytologic features of chondrosarcomas are closely related to the grade of malignancy. Low-grade chondrosarcomas yield tumor cells in fragments of variable size, and dispersed cell pattern is an infrequent finding. Variable cellularity occurs in the fragments of cartilaginous tissue, with some cells lying in lacunar spaces. Individual tumor cells display a slight to moderate atypia and occasional binucleation. Smears from high-grade (grades 2 and 3) chondrosarcoma are generally hypercellular with cellular tissue fragments and often prominent myxoid background matrix. The cellular and nuclear pleomorphism is marked, and occasional mitoses may be seen in smears, especially in grade 3 tumors [462–467].

By immunohistochemistry, the tumor cells usually stain for S-100 protein, SOX9, ERG, and podoplanin [468]. Detection of *IDH1/2* mutations can be helpful in distinguishing conventional, periosteal, and dedifferentiated chondrosarcoma from chondroblastic osteosarcoma in selected cases [469, 470].

Histologic grade and complete resection are the most important prognostic factors. The prognosis of dedifferentiated chondrosarcoma is usually poor.

22.11.3 Mesenchymal Chondrosarcoma

Mesenchymal chondrosarcomas (MCS) are high-grade, biphasic malignant cartilaginous neoplasm characterized by sheets of small blue round to spindle-shaped cells interspersed with lobules of hyaline cartilage.

MCSs have widespread anatomical distribution in bone, soft tissue, and intracranial sites [471]. The most common sites in the head and neck are the jaws (50% of cases) and mandible followed by the skull [472–479]. The most common sites within the sinonasal tract are the maxillary sinus, followed by the ethmoid and nasal cavities [480].

The peak incidence is in the second and third decades of life (age range 7 to 80 years) [471, 480].

MCS is composed of areas of small, uniform, and round to spindle-shaped cells, which resemble those of Ewing sarcoma admixed with islands of well-differentiated cartilage that can exhibit calcification and immature ossification. Many tumors show a perivascular arrangement of tumor cells and hemangiopericytoma-like vascular pattern, necrosis, and mitoses [481–484].

The cytologic features of mesenchymal chondrosarcoma include small, round monomorphic (Ewing sarcoma-like) tumor cells in cohesive clusters, some embedded in a fibrillar matrix. Fragments of cartilaginous matrix may be observed, as well as osteoclast-like giant cells. The main differential diagnoses include Ewing sarcoma and small-cell osteosarcoma [485–487].

By immunohistochemistry, tumor cells express S100, CD99, and nuclear SOX9 [480]. NKX3-1 has been suggested to be highly specific [488]. Aberrant expression of EMA, desmin, myogenin, and MYOD1 may be identified, whereas INI1 is retained [471, 489]. *HEY1::NCOA2* recurrent fusion is present in almost all MCS [490, 491] and more rarely *IRF2BP2::CDX1* [492].

MCS is an aggressive neoplasm with a high local recurrence rate and with estimated overall 5-year and 10-year survival rates of 51 and 43%, respectively [481, 492]. Jaw tumors generally have a better prognosis [473, 476].

22.11.4 Chordoma

Chordoma is a primary malignant bone tumor that shows notochordal differentiation and arises in the axial skeleton.

Subtypes include conventional chordoma, chondroid chordoma, poorly differentiated chordoma, and dedifferentiated chordoma.

The majority of chordomas arise in the axial skeleton with approximately 30% present in the base of skull (32%), sacrum/coccyx (29.2%), and mobile spine (32.8%) [493, 494]. Chordoma most commonly occurs in the sixth to seventh decades. However, all ages are affected, and most poorly differentiated chordomas arise in the base of the skull in pediatric patients [495].

Histologically, conventional chordoma exhibits a characteristic pattern of lobules separated by fibrous septa and composed of middle-sized and large epithelioid cells with bubbly cytoplasm (physaliphorous cells) embedded in a myxoid or chondroid matrix (Fig. 22.14a). Chondroid chordoma represents a subtype composed predominantly of hyaline cartilage-like extracellular matrix [496–498]. Poorly differentiated chordoma is composed of solid epithelioid cells with areas of rhabdoid morphology and loss of SMARCB1 immunoreactivity. Dedifferentiated chordoma is a biphasic tumor characterized by conventional chordoma and high-grade sarcoma.

FNA smears are usually cellular with round, cuboidal, and epithelioid cells arranged in clusters and cords. The cytoplasm of tumor cells can be granular or show varying vacuolization, ranging from signet ring-like to abundantly vacuolated physaliphorous cells. The characteristic features in smears are the abundant, myxoid, often fibrillar background substance, which encircles groups of cells and/or single tumor cells and the presence of the physaliferous cells with their abundant, bubbly cytoplasm, and round nuclei with inconspicu-

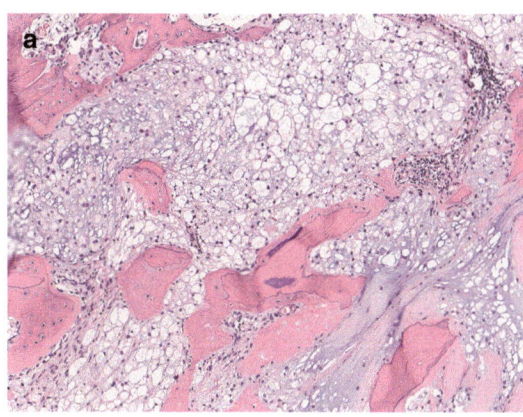
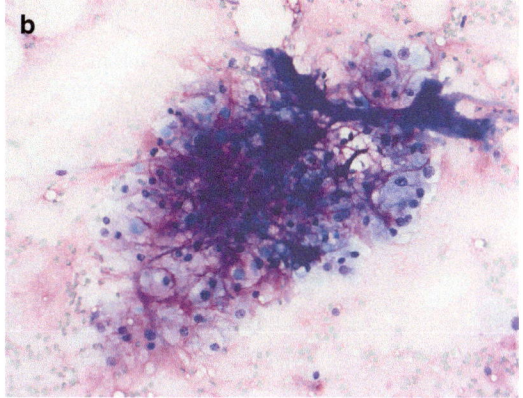

Fig. 22.14 (**a**) Chordoma. Tumor cells with abundant clear, vacuolated cytoplasm mimicking renal clear cell carcinoma (H&E). (**b**) Chordoma. FNAB. Loosely clusters of tumor cells embedded in a fibrillary blue–violet myxoid matrix. Large cells corresponding to physaliferous cells, with abundant, multivacuolated cytoplasm, and uniform, round nuclei with small nucleoli (MGG)

ous nucleoli (Fig. 22.14b). The myxoid matrix stains red, blue, or violet in MGG and Diff-Quik, pale pink in H&E, and pale green, gray in Papanicolaou. Bi- and multinucleated cells and occasional mitoses may be seen [499–503].

By immunohistochemistry, neoplastic cells are strongly immunoreactive with cytokeratin, EMA, and brachyury (TBXT), with variable S100 protein, CEA, and GFAP [504–506].

The median overall survival is 7 years for conventional chordoma. Poorly differentiated chordoma and dedifferentiated chordoma are associated with poor prognosis [495, 506–509].

References

1. Pires FR, Souza L, Arruda R, Cantisano MH, Picciani BL, Dos Santos TC. Intraoral soft tissue lipomas: clinicopathological features from 91 cases diagnosed in a single Oral Pathology service. Med Oral Patol Oral Cir Bucal. 2021;26(1):e90–6.
2. Linares MF, Leonel AC, Carvalho EJ, de Castro JF, de Almeida OP, Perez DE. Intraoral lipomas: a clinicopathological study of 43 cases, including four cases of spindle cell/pleomorphic subtype. Med Oral Patol Oral Cir Bucal. 2019;24(3):e373–8.
3. Bartuma H, Hallor KH, Panagopoulos I, Collin A, Rydholm A, Gustafson P, Bauer HC, Brosjo O, Domanski HA, Mandahl N, Mertens F. Assessment of the clinical and molecular impact of different cytogenetic subgroups in a series of 272 lipomas with abnormal karyotype. Genes Chromosomes Cancer. 2007;46:594–606.
4. Ashar HR, Fejzo MS, Tkachenko A, Zhou X, Fletcher JA, Weremowicz S, Morton CC, Chada K. Disruption of the architectural factor HMGI-C: DNA-binding AT hook motifs fused in lipomas to distinct transcriptional regulatory domains. Cell. 1995;82:57–65.
5. Enzinger FM, Harvey DA. Spindle cell lipoma. Cancer. 1975;36(5):1852–9.
6. Angervall L, Dahl I, Kindblom LG, Säve-Söderbergh. Spindle cell lipoma. Acta Pathol Microbiol Scand A. 1976;84(6):477–87.
7. Fletcher CD, Martin-Bates E. Spindle cell lipoma: a clinicopathological study with some original observations. Histopathology. 1987;11(8):803–17.
8. Shmookler BM, Enzinger FM. Pleomorphic lipoma: a benign tumor simulating liposarcoma. A clinicopathologic analysis of 48 cases. Cancer. 1981;47(1):126–33.
9. Ud Din N, Zhang P, Sukov WR, Sattler CA, Jenkins SM, Doyle LA, Folpe AL, Fritchie KJ. Spindle cell lipomas arising at atypical locations. Am J Clin Pathol. 2016;146(4):487–95.
10. Cheah A, Billings S, Goldblum J, Hornick J, Uddin N, Rubin B. Spindle cell/pleomorphic lipomas of the face: an under-recognized diagnosis. Histopathology. 2015;66(3):430–7.
11. Sachdeva MP, Goldblum JR, Rubin BP, Billings SD. Low-fat and fat-free pleomorphic lipomas: a diagnostic challenge. Am J Dermatopathol. 2009;31(5):423–6.
12. Billings SD, Folpe AL. Diagnostically challenging spindle cell lipomas: a report of 34 "low-fat" and "fat-free" variants. Am J Dermatopathol. 2007;29(5):437–42.
13. Chen S, Huang H, He S, Wang W, Zhao R, Li L, Cui Z, Zhang R. Spindle cell lipoma: clinicopathologic

characterization of 40 cases. Int J Clin Exp Pathol. 2019;12(7):2613–21.

14. Wong YP, Chia WK, Low SF, Mohamed-Haflah NH, Sharifah NA. Dendritic fibromyxolipoma: a variant of spindle cell lipoma with extensive myxoid change, with cytogenetic evidence. Pathol Int. 2014;64(7):346–51.

15. Hawley IC, Krausz T, Evans DJ, Fletcher CD. Spindle cell lipoma--a pseudoangiomatous variant. Histopathology. 1994;24(6):565–9.

16. Zelger BW, Zelger BG, Plörer A, Steiner H, Fritsch PO. Dermal spindle cell lipoma: plexiform and nodular variants. Histopathology. 1995;27(6):533–40.

17. Domanski HA, Carlen B, Jonsson K, Mertens F, Akerman M. Distinct cytologic features of spindle cell lipoma. A cytologic-histologic study with clinical, radiologic, electron microscopic, and cytogenetic correlations. Cancer. 2001;93:381–9.

18. Yong M, Raza AS, Greaves TS, Cobb CJ. Fine-needle aspiration of a pleomorphic lipoma of the head and neck: a case report. Diagn Cytopathol. 2005;32(2):110–3.

19. Chen X, Yu K, Tong GX, Hood M, Storper I, Hamele-Bena D. Fine needle aspiration of pleomorphic lipoma of the neck: report of two cases. Diagn Cytopathol. 2010;38(3):184–7.

20. Dahlén A, Debiec-Rychter M, Pedeutour F, Domanski HA, Höglund M, Bauer HC, Ryd holm A, Sciot R, Mandahl N, Mertens F. Clustering of deletions on chromosome 13 in benign and low-malignant lipomatous tumors. Int J Cancer. 2003;103(5):616–23.

21. Bartuma H, Nord KH, Macchia G, Isaksson M, Nilsson J, Domanski HA, Mandahl N, Mertens F. Gene expression and single nucleotide polymorphism array analyses of spindle cell lipomas and conventional lipomas with 13q14 deletion. Genes Chromosomes Cancer. 2011;50(8):619–32.

22. Libbrecht S, Van Dorpe J, Creytens D. The rapidly expanding group of *RB1*-deleted soft tissue tumors: an updated review. Diagnostics (Basel). 2021;11(3):430.

23. Coffin CM, Lowichik A, Putnam A. Lipoblastoma (LPB): a clinicopathologic and immunohistochemical analysis of 59 cases. Am J Surg Pathol. 2009;33(11):1705–12.

24. Hicks J, Dilley A, Patel D, Barrish J, Zhu SH, Brandt M. Lipoblastoma and lipoblastomatosis in infancy and childhood: histopathologic, ultrastructural, and cytogenetic features. Ultrastruct Pathol. 2001;25(4):321–33.

25. Ferreira J, Esteves G, Fonseca R, Martins C, André S, Lemos MM. Fine-needle aspiration of lipoblastoma: cytological, molecular, and clinical features. Cancer Cytopathol. 2017;125(12):934–9.

26. Agrawal P, Srinivasan R, Rajwanshi A, Gupta N, Dey P, Kakkar N, Samujh R. Fine needle aspiration cytology of paediatric soft tissue tumours highlighting challenges in diagnosis of benign lesions and unusual malignant tumours. Cytopathology. 2019;30(3):301–8.

27. Kloboves-Prevodnik VV, Us-Krasovec M, Gale N, Lamovec J. Cytological features of lipoblastoma: a report of three cases. Diagn Cytopathol. 2005;33(3):195–200.

28. Kubota F, Matsuyama A, Shibuya R, Nakamoto M, Hisaoka M. Desmin-positivity in spindle cells: under-recognized immunophenotype of lipoblastoma. Pathol Int. 2013;63(7):353–7.

29. Dadone B, Refae S, Lemarié-Delaunay C, Bianchini L, Pedeutour F. Molecular cytogenetics of pediatric adipocytic tumors. Cancer Genet. 2015;208(10):469–81.

30. Gisselsson D, Hibbard MK, Dal Cin P, Sciot R, Hsi BL, Kozakewich HP, Fletcher JA. PLAG1 alterations in lipoblastoma: involvement in varied mesenchymal cell types and evidence for alternative oncogenic mechanisms. Am J Pathol. 2001;159(3):955–62.

31. Matsuyama A, Hisaoka M, Hashimoto H. PLAG1 expression in mesenchymal tumors: an immunohistochemical study with special emphasis on the pathogenetical distinction between soft tissue myoepithelioma and pleomorphic adenoma of the salivary gland. Pathol Int. 2012;62(1):1–7.

32. Han JW, Kim H, Youn JK, Oh C, Jung SE, Park KW, Lee SC, Kim HY. Analysis of clinical features of lipoblastoma in children. Pediatr Hematol Oncol. 2017;34(4):212–20.

33. Speer AL, Schofield DE, Wang KS, Shin CE, Stein JE, Shaul DB, Mahour GH, Ford HR. Contemporary management of lipoblastoma. J Pediatr Surg. 2008;43(7):1295–300.

34. Beals C, Rogers A, Wakely P, Mayerson JL, Scharschmidt TJ. Hibernomas: a single-institution experience and review of literature. Med Oncol. 2014;31(1):769.

35. Furlong MA, Fanburg-Smith JC, Miettinen M. The morphologic spectrum of hibernoma: a clinicopathologic study of 170 cases. Am J Surg Pathol. 2001;25(6):809–14.

36. Mavrogenis AF, Coll-Mesa L, Drago G, Gambarotti M, Ruggieri P. Hibernomas: clinicopathological features, diagnosis, and treatment of 17 cases. Orthopedics. 2011;34(11):e755–9.

37. Al Hmada Y, Schaefer IM, Fletcher CDM. Hibernoma mimicking atypical lipomatous tumor: 64 cases of a morphologically distinct subset. Am J Surg Pathol. 2018;42(7):951–7.

38. Lemos MM, Kindblom LG, Meis-Kindblom JM, Remotti F, Ryd W, Gunterberg B, et al. Fine-needle aspiration characteristics of hibernoma. Cancer. 2001;93:206–10.

39. Walaas L, Kindblom LG. Lipomatous tumors: a correlative cytologic and histologic study of 27 tumors examined by fine needle aspiration cytology. Hum Pathol. 1985;16(1):6–18.

40. Saqi A, Yu GH, Marshall MB. Fine needle aspiration of hibernoma. Diagn Cytopathol. 2003;29(1):44–5.

41. Maire G, Forus A, Foa C, Bjerkehagen B, Mainguené C, Kresse SH, Myklebost O, Pedeutour F. 11q13 alterations in two cases of hibernoma: large heterozygous deletions and rearrangement breakpoints near GARP in 11q13.5. Genes Chromosomes Cancer. 2003;37(4):389–95.

42. Meis JM, Enzinger FM, Chondroid lipoma. A unique tumor simulating liposarcoma and myxoid chondrosarcoma. Am J Surg Pathol. 1993;17(11):1103–12.

43. Kindblom LG, Meis-Kindblom JM. Chondroid lipoma: an ultrastructural and immunohistochemical analysis with further observations regarding its differentiation. Hum Pathol. 1995;26(7):706–15.

44. Nielsen GP, O'Connell JX, Dickersin GR, Rosenberg AE. Chondroid lipoma, a tumor of white fat cells. A brief report of two cases with ultrastructural analysis. Am J Surg Pathol. 1995;19(11):1272–6.

45. Furlong MA, Fanburg-Smith JC, Childers EL. Lipoma of the oral and maxillofacial region: site and subclassification of 125 cases. Oral Surg Oral Med Oral Pathol Oral Radiol Endod. 2004;98(4):441–50.

46. Gisselsson D, Domanski HA, Höglund M, Carlén B, Mertens F, Willén H, Mandahl N. Unique cytological features and chromosome aberrations in chondroid lipoma: a case report based on fine-needle aspiration cytology, histopathology, electron microscopy, chromosome banding, and molecular cytogenetics. Am J Surg Pathol. 1999;23(10):1300–4.

47. Thomson TA, Horsman D, Bainbridge TC. Cytogenetic and cytologic features of chondroid lipoma of soft tissue. Mod Pathol. 1999;12(1):88–91.

48. Yang YJ, Damron TA, Ambrose JL. Diagnosis of chondroid lipoma by fine-needle aspiration biopsy. Arch Pathol Lab Med. 2001;125(9):1224–6.

49. Gerry D, Fox NF, Spruill LS, Lentsch EJ. Liposarcoma of the head and neck: analysis of 318 cases with comparison to non-head and neck sites. Head Neck. 2014;36(3):393–400.

50. Wong DD, Low IC, Peverall J, Robbins PD, Spagnolo DV, Nairn R, Carey-Smith RL, Wood D. MDM2/CDK4 gene amplification in large/deep-seated 'lipomas': incidence, predictors and clinical significance. Pathology. 2016;48(3):203–9.

51. Sandberg AA. Updates on the cytogenetics and molecular genetics of bone and soft tissue tumors: liposarcoma. Cancer Genet Cytogenet. 2004;155(1):1–24.

52. Enzinger FM, Winslow DJ. Liposarcoma. A study of 103 cases. Virchows Arch Pathol Anat Physiol Klin Med. 1962;335:367–88.

53. Hahn HP, Fletcher CD. Primary mediastinal liposarcoma: clinicopathologic analysis of 24 cases. Am J Surg Pathol. 2007;31(12):1868–74.

54. Nascimento AF, McMenamin ME, Fletcher CD. Liposarcomas/atypical lipomatous tumors of the oral cavity: a clinicopathologic study of 23 cases. Ann Diagn Pathol. 2002;6(2):83–93.

55. Cai YC, McMenamin ME, Rose G, Sandy CJ, Cree IA, Fletcher CD. Primary liposarcoma of the orbit: a clinicopathologic study of seven cases. Ann Diagn Pathol. 2001;5(5):255–66.

56. Evans HL. Atypical lipomatous tumor, its variants, and its combined forms: a study of 61 cases, with a minimum follow-up of 10 years. Am J Surg Pathol. 2007;31(1):1–14.

57. Demicco EG. Molecular updates in adipocytic neoplasms*. Semin Diagn Pathol. 2019;36(2):85–94.

58. Mariño-Enríquez A, Hornick JL, Dal Cin P, Cibas ES, Qian X. Dedifferentiated liposarcoma and pleomorphic liposarcoma: a comparative study of cytomorphology and MDM2/CDK4 expression on fine-needle aspiration. Cancer Cytopathol. 2014;122(2):128–37.

59. Binh MB, Sastre-Garau X, Guillou L, de Pinieux G, Terrier P, Lagacé R, Aurias A, Hostein I, Coindre JM. MDM2 and CDK4 immunostainings are useful adjuncts in diagnosing well-differentiated and dedifferentiated liposarcoma subtypes: a comparative analysis of 559 soft tissue neoplasms with genetic data. Am J Surg Pathol. 2005;29(10):1340–7.

60. Lucas DR, Nascimento AG, Sanjay BK, Rock MG. Well-differentiated liposarcoma. The Mayo Clinic experience with 58 cases. Am J Clin Pathol. 1994;102(5):677–83.

61. Weiss SW, Rao VK. Well-differentiated liposarcoma (atypical lipoma) of deep soft tissue of the extremities, retroperitoneum, and miscellaneous sites. A follow-up study of 92 cases with analysis of the incidence of "dedifferentiation". Am J Surg Pathol. 1992;16(11):1051–8.

62. Henricks WH, Chu YC, Goldblum JR, Weiss SW. Dedifferentiated liposarcoma: a clinicopathological analysis of 155 cases with a proposal for an expanded definition of dedifferentiation. Am J Surg Pathol. 1997;21(3):271–81.

63. McCormick D, Mentzel T, Beham A, Fletcher CD. Dedifferentiated liposarcoma. Clinicopathologic analysis of 32 cases suggesting a better prognostic subgroup among pleomorphic sarcomas. Am J Surg Pathol. 1994;18(12):1213–23.

64. Orvieto E, Furlanetto A, Laurino L, Dei Tos AP. Myxoid and round cell liposarcoma: a spectrum of myxoid adipocytic neoplasia. Semin Diagn Pathol. 2001;18(4):267–73.

65. Huh WW, Yuen C, Munsell M, Hayes-Jordan A, Lazar AJ, Patel S, Wang WL, Barahmani N, Okcu MF, Hicks J, Debelenko L, Spunt SL. Liposarcoma in children and young adults: a multi-institutional experience. Pediatr Blood Cancer. 2011;57(7):1142–6.

66. Alaggio R, Coffin CM, Weiss SW, Bridge JA, Issakov J, Oliveira AM, Folpe AL. Liposarcomas in young patients: a study of 82 cases occurring in patients younger than 22 years of age. Am J Surg Pathol. 2009;33(5):645–58.

67. Been L, Olar A, Powers MP, López-Terrada D, Lauriria R. Myxoid liposarcoma: a case report of a sentinel metastasis to the parotid gland with molecular confirmation. Diagn Cytopathol. 2011;39(10):780–3.

68. Fritchie KJ, Goldblum JR, Tubbs RR, Sun Y, Carver P, Billings SD, Rubin BP. The expanded histologic spectrum of myxoid liposarcoma with an emphasis on newly described patterns: implications for diagnosis on small biopsy specimens. Am J Clin Pathol. 2012;137(2):229–39.

69. Kilpatrick SE, Ward WG, Bos GD. The value of fine-needle aspiration biopsy in the differential diagnosis of adult myxoid sarcoma. Cancer. 2000;90(3):167–77.

70. Layfield LJ, Dodd L, Klijanienko J. Myxoid neoplasms of bone and soft tissue: a pattern-based approach. J Am Soc Cytopathol. 2021;10(3):278–92.

71. Chufal SS, Chufal KS, Pant P, Rizvi G, Pandey HS, Shahi KS. Hypercellular round cell liposarcoma: a comprehensive cytomorphologic study and review of 8 cases. J Cytol. 2017;34(2):78–83.

72. Narendra S, Valente A, Tull J, Zhang S. DDIT3 gene break-apart as a molecular marker for diagnosis of myxoid liposarcoma--assay validation and clinical experience. Diagn Mol Pathol. 2011;20(4):218–24.

73. Baranov E, Black MA, Fletcher CDM, Charville GW, Hornick JL. Nuclear expression of DDIT3 distinguishes high-grade myxoid liposarcoma from other round cell sarcomas. Mod Pathol. 2021;34(7):1367–72.

74. Scapa JV, Cloutier JM, Raghavan SS, Peters-Schulze G, Varma S, Charville GW. DDIT3 immunohistochemistry is a useful tool for the diagnosis of myxoid liposarcoma. Am J Surg Pathol. 2021;45(2):230–9.

75. Haniball J, Sumathi VP, Kindblom LG, Abudu A, Carter SR, Tillman RM, Jeys L, Spooner D, Peake D, Grimer RJ. Prognostic factors and metastatic patterns in primary myxoid/round-cell liposarcoma. Sarcoma. 2011;2011:538085.

76. Anderson WJ, Jo VY. Pleomorphic liposarcoma: updates and current differential diagnosis. Semin Diagn Pathol. 2019;36(2):122–8.

77. Hornick JL. Subclassification of pleomorphic sarcomas: how and why should we care? Ann Diagn Pathol. 2018;37:118–24.

78. Hornick JL, Bosenberg MW, Mentzel T, McMenamin ME, Oliveira AM, Fletcher CD. Pleomorphic liposarcoma: clinicopathologic analysis of 57 cases. Am J Surg Pathol. 2004;28(10):1257–67.

79. Carvalho SD, Pissaloux D, Crombé A, Coindre JM, Le Loarer F. Pleomorphic sarcomas: the state of the art. Surg Pathol Clin. 2019;12(1):63–105.

80. Dei Tos AP. Liposarcomas: diagnostic pitfalls and new insights. Histopathology. 2014;64(1):38–52.

81. Gebhard S, Coindre JM, Michels JJ, Terrier P, Bertrand G, Trassard M, Taylor S, Château MC, Marquès B, Picot V, Guillou L. Pleomorphic liposarcoma: clinicopathologic, immunohistochemical, and follow-up analysis of 63 cases: a study from the French Federation of Cancer Centers Sarcoma Group. Am J Surg Pathol. 2002;26(5):601–16.

82. Klijanienko J, Caillaud JM, Lagacé R. Fine-needle aspiration in liposarcoma: cytohistologic correlative study including well-differentiated, myxoid, and pleomorphic variants. Diagn Cytopathol. 2004;30(5):307–12.

83. Dodd LG, Sara Jiang X, Rao K, Bui MM. Pleomorphic liposarcoma: a cytologic study of five cases. Diagn Cytopathol. 2015;43(2):138–43.

84. Sinclair TJ, Thorson CM, Alvarez E, Tan S, Spunt SL, Chao SD. Pleomorphic myxoid liposarcoma in an adolescent with Li-Fraumeni syndrome. Pediatr Surg Int. 2017;33(5):631–5.

85. Francom CR, Leoniak SM, Lovell MA, Herrmann BW. Head and neck pleomorphic myxoid liposarcoma in a child with Li-Fraumeni syndrome. Int J Pediatr Otorhinolaryngol. 2019;123:191–4.

86. Boland JM, Colby TV, Folpe AL. Liposarcomas of the mediastinum and thorax: a clinicopathologic and molecular cytogenetic study of 24 cases, emphasizing unusual and diverse histologic features. Am J Surg Pathol. 2012;36(9):1395–403.

87. Creytens D, van Gorp J, Ferdinande L, Van Roy N, Libbrecht L. Array-based comparative genomic hybridization analysis of a pleomorphic myxoid liposarcoma. J Clin Pathol. 2014;67(9):834–5.

88. Coffin CM, Alaggio R. Adipose and myxoid tumors of childhood and adolescence. Pediatr Dev Pathol. 2012;15(1 Suppl):239–54.

89. Baranov E, Hornick JL. Soft tissue special issue: fibroblastic and myofibroblastic neoplasms of the head and neck. Head Neck Pathol. 2020;14(1):43–58. https://doi.org/10.1007/S12105-019-01104-3.

90. Shimizu S, Hashimoto H, Enjoji M. Nodular fasciitis: an analysis of 250 patients. Pathology. 1984;16(2):161–6. https://doi.org/10.3109/00313028409059097.

91. Allison DB, Wakely PE, Siddiqui MT, Ali SZ. Nodular fasciitis: a frequent diagnostic pitfall on fine-needle aspiration. Cancer Cytopathol. 2017;125(1):20–9. https://doi.org/10.1002/CNCY.21768.

92. Matusik J, Wiberg A, Sloboda J, Andersson O. Fine needle aspiration in nodular fasciitis of the face. Cytopathology. 2002;13(2):128–32. https://doi.org/10.1046/J.1365-2303.2002.00385.X.

93. Peng WX, et al. Nodular fasciitis in the parotid gland: a case report and review of the literature. Diagn Cytopathol. 2013;41(9):829–33. https://doi.org/10.1002/DC.22983.

94. Sápi Z, et al. Nodular fasciitis: a comprehensive, time-correlated investigation of 17 cases. Mod Pathol. 2021;34(12):2192–9. https://doi.org/10.1038/S41379-021-00883-X.

95. Penel N, Kasper B, Van Der Graaf WTA. Desmoid-type fibromatosis: toward a holistic management. Curr Opin Oncol. 2021;33(4):309–14. https://doi.org/10.1097/CCO.0000000000000743.

96. Alman B, et al. The management of desmoid tumours: a joint global consensus-based guideline approach for adult and paediatric patients. Eur J

Cancer. 2020;127:96–107. https://doi.org/10.1016/J.
EJCA.2019.11.013.

97. Kasper B, et al. An update on the management of sporadic desmoid-type fibromatosis: a European consensus initiative between Sarcoma PAtients EuroNet (SPAEN) and European Organization for Research and Treatment of Cancer (EORTC)/Soft Tissue and Bone Sarcoma Group (STBSG). Ann Oncol. 2017;28(10):2399–408. https://doi.org/10.1093/ANNONC/MDX323.

98. Ferenc T, et al. Aggressive fibromatosis (desmoid tumors): definition, occurrence, pathology, diagnostic problems, clinical behavior, genetic background. Pol J Pathol. 2006;57(1):5–15. [Online]. Available: https://europepmc.org/article/med/16739877. Accessed 30 Apr 2023

99. Dalén BPM, Meis-Kindblom JM, Sumathi VP, Ryd W, Kindblom LG. Fine-needle aspiration cytology and core needle biopsy in the preoperative diagnosis of desmoid tumors. Acta Orthop. 2006;77(6):926–31. https://doi.org/10.1080/17453670610013240.

100. Raab SS, Silverman JF, McLeod DL, Benning TL, Geisinger KR. Fine needle aspiration biopsy of fibromatoses. Acta Cytol. 1993;37(3):323–8. [Online]. Available: https://europepmc.org/article/med/8498134. Accessed 30 Apr 2023.

101. Owens CL, Sharma R, Ali SZ. Deep fibromatosis (desmoid tumor): cytopathologic characteristics, clinicoradiologic features, and immunohistochemical findings on fine-needle aspiration. Cancer. 2007;111(3):166–72. https://doi.org/10.1002/CNCR.22689.

102. Zreik RT, Fritchie KJ. Morphologic spectrum of desmoid-type fibromatosis. Am J Clin Pathol. 2016;145(3):332–40. https://doi.org/10.1093/AJCP/AQV094.

103. Burke AP, Sobin LH, Shekitka KM, Federspiel BII, Helwig EB. Intra abdominal fibromatosis. A pathologic analysis of 130 tumors with comparison of clinical subgroups. Am J Surg Pathol. 1990;14(4):335–41. https://doi.org/10.1097/00000478-199004000-00004.

104. Carlson JW, Fletcher CDM. Immunohistochemistry for β-catenin in the differential diagnosis of spindle cell lesions: analysis of a series and review of the literature. Histopathology. 2007;51(4):509–14. https://doi.org/10.1111/J.1365-2559.2007.02794.X.

105. Cheng JCY, Tang SP, Chen TMK. Sternocleidomastoid pseudotumor and congenital muscular torticollis in infants: a prospective study of 510 cases. J Pediatr. 1999;134(6):712–6. https://doi.org/10.1016/S0022-3476(99)70286-6.

106. Porter SB, Blount BW. Pseudotumor of infancy and congenital muscular torticollis. Am Fam Physician. 1995;52(6):1731–6. [Online]. Available: https://europepmc.org/article/med/7484683. Accessed 30 Apr 2023.

107. Rajalakshmi V, Selvambigai G, Jaiganesh. Cytomorphology of fibromatosis colli.

J Cytol. 2009;26(1):41–2. https://doi.org/10.4103/0970-9371.54869.

108. Sharma S, Mishra K, Khanna G. Fibromatosis colli in infants. A cytologic study of eight cases. Acta Cytol. 2003;47(3):359–62. https://doi.org/10.1159/000326533.

109. Kurtycz DF, Logroo R, Hoerl HD, Heatley DG. Diagnosis of fibromatosis colli by fine-needle aspiration. Diagn Cytopathol. 2000;23(5):338–42. https://doi.org/10.1002/1097-0339(200011)23:5<338::aid-dc11>3.0.co;2-9.

110. The WHO Classification of Tumours Editorial Board. WHO classification of tumours soft tissue and bone tumours. 5th ed. Lyon: IARC Press; 2020.

111. Mentzel T, Beham A, Katenkamp D, Dei Tos AP, Fletcher CDM. Fibrosarcomatous ('high-grade') dermatofibrosarcoma protuberans: clinicopathologic and immunohistochemical study of a series of 41 cases with emphasis on prognostic significance. Am J Surg Pathol. 1998;22(5):576–87. https://doi.org/10.1097/00000478-199805000-00009.

112. Thway K, Noujaim J, Jones RL, Fisher C. Dermatofibrosarcoma protuberans: pathology, genetics, and potential therapeutic strategies. Ann Diagn Pathol. 2016;25:64–71. https://doi.org/10.1016/J.ANNDIAGPATH.2016.09.013.

113. Mark RJ, Bailet JW, Tran LM, Poen J, Yao YS, Calcaterra TC. Dermatofibrosarcoma protuberans of the head and neck. A report of 16 cases. Arch Otolaryngol Head Neck Surg. 1993;119(8):891–6. https://doi.org/10.1001/ARCHOTOL.1993.01880200097014.

114. Domanski HA, Gustafson P. Cytologic features of primary, recurrent, and metastatic dermatofibrosarcoma protuberans. Cancer. 2002;96(6):351–61. https://doi.org/10.1002/CNCR.10760.

115. Klijanienko J, Caillaud JM, Lagacé R. Fine-needle aspiration of primary and recurrent dermatofibrosarcoma protuberans. Diagn Cytopathol. 2004;30(4):261–5. https://doi.org/10.1002/DC.20024.

116. Domanski HA. FNA diagnosis of dermatofibrosarcoma protuberans. Diagn Cytopathol. 2005;32(5):299–302. https://doi.org/10.1002/DC.20238.

117. Smith SC, et al. Solitary fibrous tumors of the head and neck: a multi-institutional clinicopathologic study. Am J Surg Pathol. 2017;41(12):1642–56. https://doi.org/10.1097/PAS.0000000000000940.

118. Stanisce L, et al. Solitary fibrous tumors in the head and neck: comprehensive review and analysis. Head Neck Pathol. 2020;14(2):516–24. https://doi.org/10.1007/S12105-019-01058-6.

119. Harrison L, McCulloch T, Beasley N. Soft tissue head and neck sarcoma: experience of a tertiary referral Centre over a 15-year period. J Laryngol Otol. 2019;133(12):1053–8. https://doi.org/10.1017/S0022215119002299.

120. Bowe SN, Wakely PE, Ozer E. Head and neck solitary fibrous tumors: diagnostic and therapeutic chal-

lenges. Laryngoscope. 2012;122(8):1748–55. https://doi.org/10.1002/LARY.23350.

121. Van Houdt WJ, et al. Prognosis of solitary fibrous tumors: a multicenter study. Ann Surg Oncol. 2013;20(13):4090–5. https://doi.org/10.1245/S10434-013-3242-9.

122. Demicco EG, et al. Solitary fibrous tumor: a clinicopathological study of 110 cases and proposed risk assessment model. Mod Pathol. 2012;25(9):1298–306. https://doi.org/10.1038/MODPATHOL.2012.83.

123. Wakely PE, Rekhi B. Cytopathology of solitary fibrous tumor: a series of 34 cases. J Am Soc Cytopathol. 2021;10(4):382–90. https://doi.org/10.1016/J.JASC.2021.03.005.

124. Tani E, Wejde J, Åström K, Wingmo IL, Larsson O, Haglund F. FNA cytology of solitary fibrous tumors and the diagnostic value of STAT6 immunocytochemistry. Cancer Cytopathol. 2018;126(1):36–43. https://doi.org/10.1002/CNCY.21923.

125. Bishop JA, Rekhtman N, Chun J, Wakely PE, Ali SZ. Malignant solitary fibrous tumor: cytopathologic findings and differential diagnosis. Cancer Cytopathol. 2010;118(2):83–9. https://doi.org/10.1002/CNCY.20069.

126. O'Regan EM, Vanguri V, Allen CM, Eversole LR, Wright JM, Bin Woo S. Solitary fibrous tumor of the oral cavity: clinicopathologic and immunohistochemical study of 21 cases. Head Neck Pathol. 2009;3(2):106. https://doi.org/10.1007/S12105-009-0111-8.

127. Tariq MU, Din NU, Abdul-Ghafar J, Park YK. The many faces of solitary fibrous tumor; diversity of histological features, differential diagnosis and role of molecular studies and surrogate markers in avoiding misdiagnosis and predicting the behavior. Diagn Pathol. 2021;16(1) https://doi.org/10.1186/S13000-021-01095-2.

128. Chan JK. Solitary fibrous tumour--everywhere, and a diagnosis in vogue. Histopathology. 1997;31(6):568–76. https://doi.org/10.1046/J.1365-2559.1997.2400897.X.

129. Smrke A, Thway K, Huang PH, Jones RL, Hayes AJ. Solitary fibrous tumor: molecular hallmarks and treatment for a rare sarcoma. Future Oncol. 2021;17(27):3627–36. https://doi.org/10.2217/FON-2021-0030/ASSET/IMAGES/LARGE/FIGURE2.JPEG.

130. Karpathiou G, Papoudou-Bai A, Ferrand E, Dumollard JM, Peoc'h M. STAT6: a review of a signaling pathway implicated in various diseases with a special emphasis in its usefulness in pathology. Pathol Res Pract. 2021;223:153477. https://doi.org/10.1016/J.PRP.2021.153477.

131. Gjorgova Gjeorgjievski S, Fritchie K, Thangaiah JJ, Folpe AL, Din NU. Head and neck Low-grade fibromyxoid sarcoma: a clinicopathologic study of 15 cases. Head Neck Pathol. 2022;16(2):434–43. https://doi.org/10.1007/S12105-021-01380-Y.

132. Cowan ML, Thompson LD, Leon ME, Bishop JA. Low-grade fibromyxoid sarcoma of the head and neck: a clinicopathologic series and review of the literature. Head Neck Pathol. 2016;10(2):161–6. https://doi.org/10.1007/S12105-015-0647-8.

133. Evans HL. Low-grade fibromyxoid sarcoma: a clinicopathologic study of 33 cases with long-term follow-up. Am J Surg Pathol. 2011;35(10):1450 62. https://doi.org/10.1097/PAS.0B013E31822B3687.

134. Mustafa S, VandenBussche CJ, Ali SZ, Siddiqui MT, Wakely PE. Cytomorphologic findings of low-grade fibromyxoid sarcoma. J Am Soc Cytopathol. 2020;9(3):191–201. https://doi.org/10.1016/J.JASC.2020.01.006.

135. Domanski HA, Mertens F, Panagopoulos I, Åkerman M. Low-grade fibromyxoid sarcoma is difficult to diagnose by fine needle aspiration cytology: a cytomorphological study of eight cases. Cytopathology. 2009;20(5):304–14. https://doi.org/10.1111/J.1365-2303.2008.00587.X.

136. Mertens F, et al. Clinicopathologic and molecular genetic characterization of low-grade fibromyxoid sarcoma, and cloning of a novel FUS/CREB3L1 fusion gene. Lab Invest. 2005;85(3):408–15. https://doi.org/10.1038/LABINVEST.3700230.

137. Doyle LA, et al. MUC4 is a sensitive and extremely useful marker for sclerosing epithelioid fibrosarcoma: association with FUS gene rearrangement. Am J Surg Pathol. 2012;36(10):1444–51. https://doi.org/10.1097/PAS.0B013E3182562BF8.

138. Yonezawa H, et al. Low-grade myofibroblastic sarcoma of the levator scapulae muscle: a case report and literature review. BMC Musculoskelet Disord. 2020;21(1):836. https://doi.org/10.1186/S12891-020-03857-3.

139. Mentzel T, Dry S, Katenkamp D, Fletcher CDM. Low-grade myofibroblastic sarcoma: analysis of 18 cases in the spectrum of myofibroblastic tumors. Am J Surg Pathol. 1998;22(10):1228–38. https://doi.org/10.1097/00000478-199810000-00008.

140. Cai C, Dehner LP, El-Mofty SK. In myofibroblastic sarcomas of the head and neck, mitotic activity and necrosis define grade: a case study and literature review. Virchows Arch. 2013;463(6):827–36. https://doi.org/10.1007/S00428-013-1494-1.

141. Pierry C, et al. Polypoid laryngeal inflammatory myofibroblastic tumors: misleading lesions: description of six cases showing ALK overexpression. Am J Clin Pathol. 2015;144(3):511–6. https://doi.org/10.1309/AJCPCG8D6JAQBVLG.

142. He CY, Dong GH, Yang DM, Liu HG. Inflammatory myofibroblastic tumors of the nasal cavity and paranasal sinus: a clinicopathologic study of 25 cases and review of the literature. Eur Arch Otorrinolaringol. 2015;272(4):789–97. https://doi.org/10.1007/S00405-014-3026-2.

143. Sastre-Garau X, Couturier J, Derré J, Aurias A, Klijanienko J, Lagacé R. Inflammatory myofibroblastic tumour (inflammatory pseudotumour) of

the breast. Clinicopathological and genetic analysis of a case with evidence for clonality. J Pathol. 2002;196(1):97–102. https://doi.org/10.1002/PATH.1004.

144. Stoll LM, Li QK. Cytology of fine-needle aspiration of inflammatory myofibroblastic tumor. Diagn Cytopathol. 2011;39(9):663–72. https://doi.org/10.1002/DC.21444.

145. Coffin CM, Watterson J, Priest JR, Dehner LP. Extrapulmonary inflammatory myofibroblastic tumor (inflammatory pseudotumor). A clinicopathologic and immunohistochemical study of 84 cases. Am J Surg Pathol. 1995;19(8):859–72. https://doi.org/10.1097/00000478-199508000-00001.

146. Coffin CM, Patel A, Perkins S, Elenitoba-Johnson KSJ, Perlman E, Griffin CA. ALK1 and p80 expression and chromosomal rearrangements involving 2p23 in inflammatory myofibroblastic tumor. Mod Pathol. 2001;14(6):569–76. https://doi.org/10.1038/MODPATHOL.3880352.

147. Veeresh M, Sudhakara M, Girish G, Naik C. Leiomyoma: a rare tumor in the head and neck and oral cavity: report of 3 cases with review. J Oral Maxillofac Pathol. 2013;17(2):281–7. https://doi.org/10.4103/0973-029X.119770.

148. Yoon TM, Yang HC, Choi YD, Lee DH, Lee JK, Lim SC. Vascular leiomyoma in the head and neck region: 11 years experience in one institution. Clin Exp Otorhinolaryngol. 2013;6(3):171–5. https://doi.org/10.3342/CEO.2013.6.3.171.

149. Kilpatrick SE, Mentzel T, Fletcher CDM. Leiomyoma of deep soft tissue. Clinicopathologic analysis of a series. Am J Surg Pathol. 1994;18(6):576–82. https://doi.org/10.1097/00000478-199406000-00003.

150. Val-Bernal JF, Martino M, Terán A, Yllera E, Castro-Senosiain B. Endoscopic ultrasound-guided fine-needle aspiration cytology in the diagnosis of leiomyomas of the gastrointestinal tract. Rev Esp Patol. 2019;52(3):154–62. https://doi.org/10.1016/J.PATOL.2018.09.003.

151. Domanski HA, Åkerman M, Rissler P, Gustafson P. Fine-needle aspiration of soft tissue leiomyosarcoma: an analysis of the most common cytologic findings and the value of ancillary techniques. Diagn Cytopathol. 2006;34(9):597–604. https://doi.org/10.1002/DC.20499.

152. Liu Y, Li B, Li L, Liu Y, Wang C, Zha L. Angioleiomyomas in the head and neck: a retrospective clinical and immunohistochemical analysis. Oncol Lett. 2014;8(1):241–7. https://doi.org/10.3892/OL.2014.2124.

153. Agaimy A, Michal M, Thompson LDR, Michal M. Angioleiomyoma of the sinonasal tract: analysis of 16 cases and review of the literature. Head Neck Pathol. 2015;9(4):463–73. https://doi.org/10.1007/S12105-015-0636-Y.

154. Workman AD, et al. Leiomyosarcoma of the head and neck: a 17-year single institution experience and review of the National Cancer Data Base. Head Neck. 2018;40(4):756–62. https://doi.org/10.1002/HED.25054.

155. Eppsteiner RW, DeYoung BR, Milhem MM, Pagedar NA. Leiomyosarcoma of the head and neck: a population-based analysis. Arch Otolaryngol Head Neck Surg. 2011;137(9):921–4. https://doi.org/10.1001/ARCHOTO.2011.147.

156. MacCarthy A, et al. Second and subsequent tumours among 1927 retinoblastoma patients diagnosed in Britain 1951-2004. Br J Cancer. 2013;108(12):2455–63. https://doi.org/10.1038/BJC.2013.228.

157. Agaimy A, Semrau S, Koch M, Thompson LDR. Sinonasal leiomyosarcoma: clinicopathological analysis of nine cases with emphasis on common association with other malignancies and late distant metastasis. Head Neck Pathol. 2018;12(4):463–70. https://doi.org/10.1007/S12105-017-0876-0.

158. Bathan AJ, Constantinidou A, Pollack SM, Jones RL. Diagnosis, prognosis, and management of leiomyosarcoma: recognition of anatomic variants. Curr Opin Oncol. 2013;25(4):384–9. https://doi.org/10.1097/CCO.0B013E3283622C77.

159. Saluja TS, Iyer J, Singh SK. Leiomyosarcoma: prognostic outline of a rare head and neck malignancy. Oral Oncol. 2019;95:100–5. https://doi.org/10.1016/J.ORALONCOLOGY.2019.06.010.

160. Klijanienko J, Caillaud JM, Lagacé R, Vielh P. Fine-needle aspiration of leiomyosarcoma: a correlative cytohistopathological study of 96 tumors in 68 patients. Diagn Cytopathol. 2003;28(3):119–25. https://doi.org/10.1002/DC.10249.

161. George S, Serrano C, Hensley ML, Ray-Coquard I. Soft tissue and uterine leiomyosarcoma. J Clin Oncol. 2018;36(2):144–50. https://doi.org/10.1200/JCO.2017.75.9845.

162. Oda Y, et al. Pleomorphic leiomyosarcoma: clinicopathologic and immunohistochemical study with special emphasis on its distinction from ordinary leiomyosarcoma and malignant fibrous histiocytoma. Am J Surg Pathol. 2001;25(8):1030–8. https://doi.org/10.1097/00000478-200108000-00007.

163. Kohashi K, Kinoshita I, Oda Y. Soft tissue special issue: skeletal muscle tumors: a clinicopathological review. Head Neck Pathol. 2020;14(1):12–20. https://doi.org/10.1007/S12105-019-01113-2.

164. Domanski HA, Dawiskiba S. Adult rhabdomyoma in fine needle aspirates. A report of two cases. Acta Cytol. 2000;44(2):223–6. https://doi.org/10.1159/000326364.

165. Al Rikabi AC, Al Kharfy T, Al Sohaibani MO, Al Samarrai AI. Fetal rhabdomyoma. A case report with the diagnosis suggested by intraoperative cytology. Acta Cytol. 1996;40(4):786–8. https://doi.org/10.1159/000333959.

166. Häußler SM, Stromberger C, Olze H, Seifert G, Knopke S, Böttcher A. Head and neck rhabdomyosarcoma in children: a 20-year retrospective study at a tertiary referral center. J Cancer Res Clin

Oncol. 2018;144(2):371–9. https://doi.org/10.1007/S00432-017-2544-X.

167. Wu Y, Li C, Zhong Y, Guo W, Ren G. Head and neck rhabdomyosarcoma in adults. J Craniofac Surg. 2014;25(3):922–5. https://doi.org/10.1097/SCS.0000000000000704.

168. Darwish C, et al. Pediatric head and neck rhabdomyosarcoma: an analysis of treatment and survival in the United States (1975–2016). Int J Pediatr Otorhinolaryngol. 2020;139:110403. https://doi.org/10.1016/J.IJPORL.2020.110403.

169. Jo VY, Demicco EG. Update from the 5th edition of the World Health Organization classification of head and neck Tumors: soft tissue Tumors. Head Neck Pathol. 2022;16(1):87–100. https://doi.org/10.1007/S12105-022-01425-W.

170. Klijanienko J, et al. Cyto-histological correlations in primary, recurrent and metastatic rhabdomyosarcoma: the institut Curie's experience. Diagn Cytopathol. 2007;35(8):482–7. https://doi.org/10.1002/DC.20662.

171. Pohar-Marinsek Z, Bracko M. Rhabdomyosarcoma. Cytomorphology, subtyping and differential diagnostic dilemmas. Acta Cytol. 2000;44(4):524–32. https://doi.org/10.1159/000328524.

172. WHO Classification of Tumours Editorial Board. Head and neck tumours [Internet; beta version ahead of print]. Lyon: International Agency for Research on Cancer; 2022.

173. Thompson LD. Lobular capillary hemangioma (pyogenic granuloma) of the oral cavity. Ear Nose Throat J. 2017;96(7):240. https://doi.org/10.1177/014556131709600716.

174. Sachin K, Rashmi S, Manish S, Siddhartha W, Uday L. Haemangiomas and venous malformations of the head and neck: a retrospective analysis of endovascular management in 358 patients. Indian J Plast Surg. 2013;46(1):109. https://doi.org/10.4103/0970-0358.113727.

175. Putra J, Al-Ibraheemi A. Vascular anomalies of the head and neck: a pediatric overview. Head Neck Pathol. 2021;15(1):59–70. https://doi.org/10.1007/S12105-020-01236-X.

176. Domanski HA, Stanley DE. Skin and subcutis. In: Atlas of fine needle aspiration cytology. Cham: Springer; 2019. p. 553–98. https://doi.org/10.1007/978-3-319-76980-6_15.

177. Flucke U, Karanian M, ten Broek RW, Thway K. Soft tissue special issue: perivascular and vascular tumors of the head and neck. Head Neck Pathol. 2020;14(1):21. https://doi.org/10.1007/S12105-020-01129-Z.

178. Papke DJ, Hornick JL. What is new in endothelial neoplasia? Virchows Arch. 2020;476(1):17–28. https://doi.org/10.1007/S00428-019-02651-4.

179. Damaskos EAAC, Garmpis N, Manousi M, Garmpi A, Margonis G-A, Spartalis E, Doula C, Michail-Strantzia C, Patelis N, Schizas D, Arkoumanis P-T, Andreatos N, Tsourouflis G, Zavras N, Markatos K, Kontzoglou K. Cystic hygroma of the neck: single

center experience and literature review. Eur Rev Med Pharmacol Sci. 2017;21(21):4918–23.

180. Nelson BL, Bischoff EL, Nathan A, Ma L. Lymphangioma of the dorsal tongue. Head Neck Pathol. 2020;14(2):512–5. https://doi.org/10.1007/S12105-019-01108-Z.

181. Lerat J, et al. Guidelines (short version) of the French Society of Otorhinolaryngology (SFORL) on cervical lymphatic malformation in adults and children: diagnosis. Eur Ann Otorhinolaryngol Head Neck Dis. 2019;136(2):109–12. https://doi.org/10.1016/J.ANORL.2019.02.005.

182. Arai E, et al. Usefulness of D2-40 immunohistochemistry for differentiation between kaposiform hemangioendothelioma and tufted angioma. J Cutan Pathol. 2006;33(7):492–7. https://doi.org/10.1111/J.1600-0560.2006.00461.X.

183. Ramírez-Amador V, Anaya-Saavedra G, Martínez-Mata G. Kaposi's sarcoma of the head and neck: a review. Oral Oncol. 2010;46(3):135–45. https://doi.org/10.1016/J.ORALONCOLOGY.2009.12.006.

184. Berberi A, Aoun G. Oral lesions associated with human immunodeficiency virus in 75 adult patients: a clinical study. J Korean Assoc Oral Maxillofac Surg. 2017;43(6):388–94. https://doi.org/10.5125/jkaoms.2017.43.6.388.

185. Levine AM, Tulpule A. Clinical aspects and management of AIDS-related Kaposi's sarcoma. Eur J Cancer. 2001;37(10):1288–95. https://doi.org/10.1016/S0959-8049(01)00109-5.

186. Hales M, Bottles K, Miller T, Donegan E, Ljung BM. Diagnosis of Kaposi's sarcoma by fine-needle aspiration biopsy. Am J Clin Pathol. 1987;88(1):20–5. https://doi.org/10.1093/AJCP/88.1.20.

187. Patel RM, Goldblum JR, Hsi ED. Immunohistochemical detection of human herpes virus-8 latent nuclear antigen-1 is useful in the diagnosis of Kaposi sarcoma. Mod Pathol. 2004;17(4):456–60. https://doi.org/10.1038/MODPATHOL.3800061.

188. Stacchiotti S, et al. Epithelioid hemangioendothelioma, an ultra-rare cancer: a consensus paper from the community of experts. ESMO Open. 2021;6(3):100170. https://doi.org/10.1016/J.ESMOOP.2021.100170.

189. Deyrup AT, Tighiouart M, Montag AG, Weiss SW. Epithelioid hemangioendothelioma of soft tissue: a proposal for risk stratification based on 49 cases. Am J Surg Pathol. 2008;32(6):924–7. https://doi.org/10.1097/PAS.0B013E31815BF8E6.

190. Flucke U, et al. Epithelioid Hemangioendothelioma: clinicopathologic, immunhistochemical, and molecular genetic analysis of 39 cases. Diagn Pathol. 2014;9(1):131. https://doi.org/10.1186/1746-1596-9-131.

191. Tong GX, Hamele-Bena D, Borczuk A, Monaco S, Khosh MM, Greenebaum E. Fine needle aspiration biopsy of epithelioid hemangioendothelioma of the oral cavity: report of one case and review of litera-

ture. Diagn Cytopathol. 2006;34(3):218–23. https://doi.org/10.1002/DC.20397.

192. Jurczyk M, Zhu B, Laskin W, Lin X. Pitfalls in the diagnosis of hepatic epithelioid hemangioendothelioma by FNA and needle core biopsy. Diagn Cytopathol. 2014;42(6):516–20. https://doi.org/10.1002/DC.22943.

193. Jebastin Thangaiah J, Hanley K, Nomani L, Policarpio-Nicolas ML. Cytologic features and immunohistochemical findings of epithelioid hemangioendothelioma (EHE) in effusion: a case series. Diagn Cytopathol. 2021;49(1):E24–30. https://doi.org/10.1002/DC.24565.

194. Mark RJ, Tran LM, Sercarz J, Yao YS, Calcaterra TC, Juillard GF. Angiosarcoma of the head and neck. The UCLA experience 1955 through 1990. Arch Otolaryngol Head Neck Surg. 1993;119(9):973–8. https://doi.org/10.1001/ARCHOTOL.1993.01880210061009.

195. Ramakrishnan N, Mokhtari R, Charville GW, Bui N, Ganjoo K. Cutaneous angiosarcoma of the head and neck-A retrospective analysis of 47 patients. Cancers (Basel). 2022;14(15):3841. https://doi.org/10.3390/CANCERS14153841.

196. Yan Q, Fernandez RA, Elmi M, Gelfond J, Davies MG. Outcomes of interventions for angiosarcoma. Front Surg. 2022;9:819099. https://doi.org/10.3389/FSURG.2022.819099.

197. Klijanienko J, Caillaud JM, Lagacé R, Vielh P. Cytohistologic correlations in angiosarcoma including classic and epithelioid variants: Institut Curie's experience. Diagn Cytopathol. 2003;29(3):140–5. https://doi.org/10.1002/DC.10335.

198. Pohar-Marinšek Ž, Lamovec J. Angiosarcoma in FNA smears: diagnostic accuracy, morphology, immunocytochemistry and differential diagnoses. Cytopathology 2010;21(5):311–9. https://doi.org/10.1111/J.1365-2303.2009.00726.X.

199. Geller RL, Hookim K, Sullivan HC, Stuart LN, Edgar MA, Reid MD. Cytologic features of angiosarcoma: a review of 26 cases diagnosed on FNA. Cancer Cytopathol. 2016;124(9):659–68. https://doi.org/10.1002/CNCY.21726.

200. Koch M, Nielsen GP, Yoon SS. Malignant tumors of blood vessels: angiosarcomas, hemangioendotheliomas, and hemangiopericytomas. J Surg Oncol. 2008;97(4):321–9. https://doi.org/10.1002/JSO.20973.

201. Miettinen M, et al. ERG transcription factor as an immunohistochemical marker for vascular endothelial tumors and prostatic carcinoma. Am J Surg Pathol. 2011;35(3):432–41. https://doi.org/10.1097/PAS.0B013E318206B67B.

202. Thum C, Husain EA, Mulholland K, Hornick JL, Brenn T. Atypical fibroxanthoma with pseudoangiomatous features: a histological and immunohistochemical mimic of cutaneous angiosarcoma. Ann Diagn Pathol. 2013;17(6):502–7. https://doi.org/10.1016/J.ANNDIAGPATH.2013.08.004.

203. Shon W, Sukov WR, Jenkins SM, Folpe AL. MYC amplification and overexpression in primary cutaneous angiosarcoma: a fluorescence in-situ hybridization and immunohistochemical study. Mod Pathol. 2014;27(4):509–15. https://doi.org/10.1038/MODPATHOL.2013.163.

204. Flucke U, Requena L, Mentzel T. Radiation-induced vascular lesions of the skin: an overview. Adv Anat Pathol. 2013;20(6):407–15. https://doi.org/10.1097/PAP.0B013E3182A92E19.

205. Abdel Razek AAK, Gamaleldin OA, Elsebaie NA. Peripheral nerve sheath tumors of head and neck: imaging-based review of World Health Organization classification. J Comput Assist Tomogr. 2020;44(6):928–40.

206. Cates JM, Coffin CM. Neurogenic tumors of soft tissue. Pediatr Dev Pathol. 2012;15(1 Suppl):62–107.

207. Rodriguez FJ, Folpe AL, Giannini C, Perry A. Pathology of peripheral nerve sheath tumors: diagnostic overview and update on selected diagnostic problems. Acta Neuropathol. 2012;123(3):295–319.

208. Sakata A, Hirokawa Y, Kuwahara R, Hamada A, Kuroda M, Araki N, Ito T. Solitary oropharyngeal neurofibroma: MR appearance with pathologic correlation and review of the literature. Clin Imaging. 2013;37(3):554–7.

209. Chinn SB, Collar RM, McHugh JB, Hogikyan ND, Thorne MC. Pediatric laryngeal neurofibroma: case report and review of the literature. Int J Pediatr Otorhinolaryngol. 2014;78(1):142–7. https://doi.org/10.1016/j.ijporl.2013.10.047.

210. Guraya SS, Prayson RA. Peripheral nerve sheath tumors arising in salivary glands: a clinicopathologic study. Ann Diagn Pathol. 2016;23:38–42.

211. Azani AB, Bishop JA, Thompson LD. Sinonasal tract Neurofibroma: a clinicopathologic series of 12 cases with a review of the literature. Head Neck Pathol. 2015;9(3):323–33.

212. Perzin KH, Panyu H, Wechter S. Nonepithelial tumors of the nasal cavity, paranasal sinuses and nasopharynx. A clinicopathologic study. XII: schwann cell tumors (neurilemoma, neurofibroma, malignant schwannoma). Cancer. 1982;50(10):2193–202.

213. de Pontes Santos HB, de Morais EF, Moreira DGL, Marinho LCN, Galvão HC, de Almeida FR. Neurofibromas of the oral and maxillofacial complex: a 48-year retrospective study. J Cutan Pathol. 2020;47(3):202–6.

214. Alotaiby FM, Fitzpatrick S, Upadhyaya J, Islam MN, Cohen D, Bhattacharyya I. Demographic, clinical and histopathological features of Oral neural neoplasms: a retrospective study. Head Neck Pathol. 2019;13(2):208–14.

215. Thompson LDR, Koh SS, Lau SK. Sporadic neurofibroma of the tongue unassociated with neurofibromatosis type I: a clinicopathologic study of ten cases. Head Neck Pathol. 2020;14(2):374–80.

216. Tamiolakis P, Chrysomali E, Sklavounou-Andrikopoulou A, Nikitakis NG. Oral neural tumors: clinicopathologic analysis of 157 cases

and review of the literature. J Clin Exp Dent. 2019;11(8):e721–31.

217. Handschel J, Heikaus S, Depprich R, Kübler NR, Yekta SS, Smeets R, Ommerborn M, Naujoks C. Intraoral schwannoma: review of the literature and presentation of a rare case. Cranio. 2012;30(2):150–3.

218. Hasegawa SL, Mentzel T, Fletcher CD. Schwannomas of the sinonasal tract and nasopharynx. Mod Pathol. 1997;10(8):777–84. PMID: 9267819.

219. Megahed M. Histopathological variants of neurofibroma. A study of 114 lesions. Am J Dermatopathol. 1994;16(5):486–95.

220. Belakhoua SM, Rodriguez FJ. Diagnostic pathology of tumors of peripheral nerve. Neurosurgery. 2021;88(3):443–56.

221. Cortes-Santiago N, Patel K. Review of pediatric head and neck neoplasms that raise the possibility of a cancer predisposition syndrome. Head Neck Pathol. 2021;15(1):16–24.

222. Wakely PE Jr. Myxomatous soft tissue tumors: correlation of cytopathology and histopathology. Ann Diagn Pathol. 1999;3(4):227–42.

223. Resnick JM, Fanning CV, Caraway NP, Varma DG, Johnson M. Percutaneous needle biopsy diagnosis of benign neurogenic neoplasms. Diagn Cytopathol. 1997;16(1):17–25.

224. Evans DG, Huson SM, Birch JM. Malignant peripheral nerve sheath tumours in inherited disease. Clin Sarcoma Res. 2012;2(1):17.

225. Sinkkonen ST, Hildén O, Hagström J, Leivo I, Bäck LJ, Mäkitie AA. Experience of head and neck extracranial schwannomas in a whole population-based single-center patient series. Eur Arch Otorrinolaringol. 2014;271(11):3027–34.

226. Thompson LDR, Koh SS, Lau SK. Tongue schwannoma: a clinicopathologic study of 19 cases. Head Neck Pathol. 2020;14(3):571–6.

227. Evans DG. Neurofibromatosis type 2 (NF2): a clinical and molecular review. Orphanet J Rare Dis. 2009;4:16.

228. Casadei GP, Komori T, Scheithauer BW, Miller GM, Parisi JE, Kelly PJ. Intracranial parenchymal schwannoma. A clinicopathological and neuroimaging study of nine cases. J Neurosurg. 1993;79(2):217–22.

229. Hart J, Gardner JM, Edgar M, Weiss SW. Epithelioid schwannomas: an analysis of 58 cases including atypical variants. Am J Surg Pathol. 2016;40(5):704–13.

230. Zhao X, Zhou X, Chen X, Pan J, Li B. Primary microcystic/reticular schwannoma of the frontal bone: illustrative case. J Neurosurg Case Lessons. 2021;1(25):CASE21175.

231. Yin Y, Wang T, Cai YP, Huang XJ, Li YJ, Chen SH, Qin R, Wang CF, Wu Q. Microcystic/reticular schwannoma of the mandible first case report and review of the literature. Medicine (Baltimore). 2015;94(45):e1974.

232. Nonaka D, Chiriboga L, Rubin BP. Sox10: a pan-schwannian and melanocytic marker. Am J Surg Pathol. 2008;32(9):1291–8.

233. Karamchandani JR, Nielsen TO, van de Rijn M, West RB. Sox10 and S100 in the diagnosis of soft-tissue neoplasms. Appl Immunohistochem Mol Morphol. 2012;20(5):445–50.

234. Chebib I, Hornicek FJ, Nielsen GP, Deshpande V. Cytomorphologic features that distinguish schwannoma from other low-grade spindle cell lesions. Cancer Cytopathol. 2015;123(3):171–9.

235. Domanski HA, Akerman M, Engellau J, Gustafson P, Mertens F, Rydholm A. Fine-needle aspiration of neurilemoma (schwannoma). A clinicocytopathologic study of 116 patients. Diagn Cytopathol. 2006;34(6):403–12.

236. Dahl I, Hagmar B, Idvall I. Benign solitary neurilemoma (Schwannoma). A correlative cytological and histological study of 28 cases. Acta Pathol Microbiol Immunol Scand A. 1984;92(2):91–101.

237. Dodd LG, Marom EM, Dash RC, Matthews MR, McLendon RE. Fine-needle aspiration cytology of "ancient" schwannoma. Diagn Cytopathol. 1999;20(5):307–11.

238. Satarkar RN, Kolte SS, Vujhini SK. Cystic schwannoma in neck: fallacious diagnosis arrived on fine needle aspiration cytology. Diagn Cytopathol. 2011;39(11):866–7.

239. Woodruff JM, Selig AM, Crowley K, Allen PW. Schwannoma (neurilemoma) with malignant transformation. A rare, distinctive peripheral nerve tumor. Am J Surg Pathol. 1994;18(9):882–95.

240. McMenamin ME, Fletcher CD. Expanding the spectrum of malignant change in schwannomas: epithelioid malignant change, epithelioid malignant peripheral nerve sheath tumor, and epithelioid angiosarcoma: a study of 17 cases. Am J Surg Pathol. 2001;25(1):13–25.

241. Hornick JL, Fletcher CD. Soft tissue perineurioma: clinicopathologic analysis of 81 cases including those with atypical histologic features. Am J Surg Pathol. 2005;29(7):845–58.

242. Rankine AJ, Filion PR, Platten MA, Spagnolo DV. Perineurioma: a clinicopathological study of eight cases. Pathology. 2004;36(4):309–15.

243. Zelger B, Weinlich G, Zelger B. Perineuroma. A frequently unrecognized entity with emphasis on a plexiform variant. Adv Clin Pathol. 2000;4(1):25–33.

244. Yang EJ, Hornick JL, Qian X. Fine-needle aspiration of soft tissue perineurioma: a comparative analysis of cytomorphology and immunohistochemistry with benign and malignant mimics. Cancer Cytopathol. 2016;124(9):651–8.

245. Housini I, Dabbs DJ. Fine needle aspiration cytology of perineurioma. Report of a case with histologic, immunohistochemical and ultrastructural studies. Acta Cytol. 1990;34(3):420–4.

246. Domanski HA, Walther ChS. pp. 96–7. https://doi.org/10.1159/000475092.

247. Folpe AL, Billings SD, McKenney JK, Walsh SV, Nusrat A, Weiss SW. Expression of claudin-1, a recently described tight junction-associated protein,

distinguishes soft tissue perineurioma from potential mimics. Am J Surg Pathol. 2002;26(12):1620–6.

248. Andrade ES, Filho JR, Rocha NS, Neto IC, Camargo IB. Isolated intra-oral granular cell tumor: report of two cases and review of the literature. Acta Odontol Latinoam. 2010;23(2):99–104.

249. Giuliani M, Lajolo C, Pagnoni M, Boari A, Zannoni GF. Granular cell tumor of the tongue (Abrikossoff's tumor). A case report and review of the literature. Minerva Stomatol. 2004;53(7-8):465–9.

250. Dias Ferraz PN, Danu V, Almeida R, Figueiredo J. Granular cell tumour (Abrikossoff's tumour) of the tongue. BMJ Case Rep. 2020;13(7):e235637.

251. Serpa MS, Costa-Neto H, de Oliveira PT, da Silveira ÉJ, de Medeiros AM. Granular cell tumor in two oral anatomic sites. Eur Arch Otorrinolaringol. 2016;273(10):3439–41. https://doi.org/10.1007/s00405-016-4006-5. Epub 2016 Mar 23. PMID: 27007285.

252. Billeret LV. La tumeur à cellules granuleuses. Epidémiologie de 263 cas [Granular cell tumor. Epidemiology of 263 cases]. Arch Anat Cytol Pathol. 1999;47(1):26–30.

253. Lack EE, Worsham GF, Callihan MD, Crawford BE, Klappenbach S, Rowden G, Chun B. Granular cell tumor: a clinicopathologic study of 110 patients. J Surg Oncol. 1980;13(4):301–16.

254. Ashbrook C, Batie SF, Sengupta A, Peters CA. Granular cell tumor in the scrotum of a pediatric patient: a case report of a rare clinical entity. Urol Case Rep. 2023;47:102327.

255. Kitahara Y, Hook CE, Miyagi K, Burrows NP. Atypical granular cell tumour in a child: a rare case report. Skin Health Dis. 2023;3(3):e218.

256. Fanburg-Smith JC, Meis-Kindblom JM, Fante R, Kindblom LG. Malignant granular cell tumor of soft tissue: diagnostic criteria and clinicopathologic correlation. Am J Surg Pathol. 1998;22(7):779–94. Erratum in: Am J Surg Pathol 1999 Jan;23(1):136.

257. Mobarki M, Dumollard JM, Dal Col P, Camy F, Peoc'h M, Karpathiou G. Granular cell tumor a study of 42 cases and systemic review of the literature. Pathol Res Pract. 2020;216(4):152865.

258. Moten AS, Zhao H, Wu H, Farma JM. Malignant granular cell tumor: clinical features and long-term survival. J Surg Oncol. 2018;118(6):891–7.

259. Wieczorek TJ, Krane JF, Domanski HA, Akerman M, Carlén B, Misdraji J, Granter SR. Cytologic findings in granular cell tumors, with emphasis on the diagnosis of malignant granular cell tumor by fine-needle aspiration biopsy. Cancer. 2001;93(6):398–408.

260. Gibbons D, Leitch M, Coscia J, Lindberg G, Molberg K, Ashfaq R, Saboorian MH. Fine needle aspiration cytology and histologic findings of granular cell tumor of the breast: review of 19 cases with clinical/radiologic correlation. Breast J. 2000;6(1):27–30.

261. Pal S, Nautiyal N, Kaira K, Bharosay V. Cytological features of cutaneous granular cell tumor: a brief report. J Cytol. 2019;36(4):217–8.

262. Das S, Das RN, Sen A, Chatterjee U, Datta C, Choudhuri M. Cytological and histological correlation of granular cell tumor in a series of three cases. J Cancer Res Ther. 2018;14(2):459–61.

263. Toi PC, Siddaraju N, Basu D. Fine-needle aspiration cytology of granular cell tumor: a report of two cases. J Cytol. 2013;30(3):195–7.

264. Parfitt JR, McLean CA, Joseph MG, Streutker CJ, Al-Haddad S, Driman DK. Granular cell tumours of the gastrointestinal tract: expression of nestin and clinicopathological evaluation of 11 patients. Histopathology. 2006;48(4):424–30.

265. Chamberlain BK, McClain CM, Gonzalez RS, Coffin CM, Cates JM. Alveolar soft part sarcoma and granular cell tumor: an immunohistochemical comparison study. Hum Pathol. 2014;45(5):1039–44.

266. Filie AC, Lage JM, Azumi N. Immunoreactivity of S100 protein, alpha-1-antitrypsin, and CD68 in adult and congenital granular cell tumors. Mod Pathol. 1996;9(9):888–92.

267. Ducatman BS, Scheithauer BW, Piepgras DG, Reiman HM, Ilstrup DM. Malignant peripheral nerve sheath tumors. A clinicopathologic study of 120 cases. Cancer. 1986;57(10):2006–21.

268. Ma C, Ow A, Shan OH, Wu Y, Zhang C, Sun J, Ji T, Pingarron Martin L, Wang L. Malignant peripheral nerve sheath tumours in the head and neck region: retrospective analysis of clinicopathological features and treatment outcomes. Int J Oral Maxillofac Surg. 2014;43(8):924–32.

269. Owosho AA, Estilo CL, Huryn JM, Chi P, Antonescu CR. A clinicopathologic study of head and neck malignant peripheral nerve sheath tumors. Head Neck Pathol. 2018;12(2):151–9.

270. Le Guellec S, Decouvelaere AV, Filleron T, Valo I, Charon-Barra C, Robin YM, Terrier P, Chevreau C, Coindre JM. Malignant peripheral nerve sheath tumor is a challenging diagnosis: a systematic pathology review, immunohistochemistry, and molecular analysis in 160 patients from the French Sarcoma Group Database. Am J Surg Pathol. 2016;40(7):896–908.

271. Ferner RE, Gutmann DH. International consensus statement on malignant peripheral nerve sheath tumors in neurofibromatosis. Cancer Res. 2002;62(5):1573–7.

272. Watson KL, Al Sannaa GA, Kivlin CM, Ingram DR, Landers SM, Roland CL, Cormier JN, Hunt KK, Feig BW, Ashleigh Guadagnolo B, Bishop AJ, Wang WL, Slopis JM, McCutcheon IE, Lazar AJ, Torres KE. Patterns of recurrence and survival in sporadic, neurofibromatosis type 1-associated, and radiation-associated malignant peripheral nerve sheath tumors. J Neurosurg. 2017;126(1):319–29.

273. Laskin WB, Weiss SW, Bratthauer GL. Epithelioid variant of malignant peripheral nerve sheath tumor (malignant epithelioid schwannoma). Am J Surg Pathol. 1991;15(12):1136–45.

274. Jo VY, Fletcher CD. Epithelioid malignant peripheral nerve sheath tumor: clinicopathologic analysis of 63 cases. Am J Surg Pathol. 2015;39(5):673–82.

275. Schaefer IM, Al-Ibraheemi A, Qian X. Cytomorphologic spectrum of SMARCB1-deficient soft tissue neoplasms. Am J Clin Pathol. 2021;156(2):229–45.

276. Jiwani S, Gokden M, Lindberg M, Ali S, Jeffus S. Fine-needle aspiration cytology of epithelioid malignant peripheral nerve sheath tumor; a case report and review of the literature. Diagn Cytopathol. 2016;44(3):226–31.

277. Gupta K, Dey P, Vashisht R. Fine-needle aspiration cytology of malignant peripheral nerve sheath tumors. Diagn Cytopathol. 2004;31(1):1–4.

278. Jiménez-Heffernan JA, López-Ferrer P, Vicandi B, Hardisson D, Gamallo C, Viguer JM. Cytologic features of malignant peripheral nerve sheath tumor. Acta Cytol. 1999;43(2):175–83.

279. Klijanienko J, Caillaud JM, Lagacé R, Vielh P. Cytohistologic correlations of 24 malignant peripheral nerve sheath tumor (MPNST) in 17 patients: the Institut Curie experience. Diagn Cytopathol. 2002;27(2):103–8.

280. Dodd LG, Scully S, Layfield LJ. Fine-needle aspiration of epithelioid malignant peripheral nerve sheath tumor (epithelioid malignant schwannoma). Diagn Cytopathol. 1997;17(3):200–4.

281. Kang Y, Pekmezci M, Folpe AL, Ersen A, Horvai AE. Diagnostic utility of SOX10 to distinguish malignant peripheral nerve sheath tumor from synovial sarcoma, including intraneural synovial sarcoma. Mod Pathol. 2014;27(1):55–61.

282. Schaefer IM, Dong F, Garcia EP, Fletcher CDM, Jo VY. Recurrent SMARCB1 inactivation in epithelioid malignant peripheral nerve sheath tumors. Am J Surg Pathol. 2019;43(6):835–43.

283. Lothe RA, Karhu R, Mandahl N, Mertens F, Saeter G, Heim S, Borresen-Dale AL, Kallioniemi OP. Gain of 17q24-qter detected by comparative genomic hybridization in malignant tumors from patients with von Recklinghausen's neurofibromatosis. Cancer Res. 1996;56(20):4778–81.

284. Brekke HR, Ribeiro FR, Kolberg M, Agesen TH, Lind GE, Eknaes M, Hall KS, Bjerkehagen B, van den Berg E, Teixeira MR, Mandahl N, Smeland S, Mertens F, Skotheim RI, Lothe RA. Genomic changes in chromosomes 10, 16, and X in malignant peripheral nerve sheath tumors identify a high-risk patient group. J Clin Oncol. 2010;28(9):1573–82.

285. Bottillo I, Ahlquist T, Brekke H, Danielsen SA, van den Berg E, Mertens F, Lothe RA, Dallapiccola B. Germline and somatic NF1 mutations in sporadic and NF1-associated malignant peripheral nerve sheath tumours. J Pathol. 2009;217:693–701.

286. Agesen TH, Florenes VA, Molenaar WM, Lind GE, Berner JM, Plaat BE, Komdeur R, Myklebost O, van den Berg E, Lothe RA. Expression patterns of cell cycle components in sporadic and neurofibromatosis type 1-related malignant peripheral nerve sheath tumors. J Neuropathol Exp Neurol. 2005;64:74–81.

287. Folpe AL, Weiss SW. Ossifying fibromyxoid tumor of soft parts: a clinicopathologic study of 70 cases with emphasis on atypical and malignant variants. Am J Surg Pathol. 2003;27(4):421–31.

288. Enzinger FM, Weiss SW, Liang CY. Ossifying fibromyxoid tumor of soft parts. A clinicopathological analysis of 59 cases. Am J Surg Pathol. 1989;13(10):817–27.

289. Micttinen M, Finnell V, Fetsch JF. Ossifying fibromyxoid tumor of soft parts--a clinicopathologic and immunohistochemical study of 104 cases with long-term follow-up and a critical review of the literature. Am J Surg Pathol. 2008;32(7):996–1005.

290. Schneider N, Fisher C, Thway K. Ossifying fibromyxoid tumor: morphology, genetics, and differential diagnosis. Ann Diagn Pathol. 2016;20:52–8.

291. Dantey K, Schoedel K, Yergiyev O, McGough R, Palekar A, Rao UNM. Ossifying fibromyxoid tumor: a study of 6 cases of atypical and malignant variants. Hum Pathol. 2017;60:174–9.

292. Kilpatrick SE, Ward WG, Mozes M, Miettinen M, Fukunaga M, Fletcher CD. Atypical and malignant variants of ossifying fibromyxoid tumor. Clinicopathologic analysis of six cases. Am J Surg Pathol. 1995;19:1039–46.

293. Atanaskova Mesinkovska N, Buehler D, McClain CM, Rubin BP, Goldblum JR, Billings SD. Ossifying fibromyxoid tumor: a clinicopathologic analysis of 26 subcutaneous tumors with emphasis on differential diagnosis and prognostic factors. J Cutan Pathol. 2015;42(9):622–31.

294. Graham RP, Dry S, Li X, Binder S, Bahrami A, Raimondi SC, Dogan A, Chakraborty S, Souchek JJ, Folpe AL. Ossifying fibromyxoid tumor of soft parts: a clinicopathologic, proteomic, and genomic study. Am J Surg Pathol. 2011;35(11):1615–25.

295. Mohanty SK, Srinivasan R, Rajwanshi A, Vasishta RK, Vignesh PS. Cytologic diagnosis of ossifying fibromyxoid tumor of soft tissue: a case report. Diagn Cytopathol. 2004;30:41–5.

296. Ahmed OI, Qasem SA, Salih ZT. Ossifying fibromyxoid tumor: report of a case with cytomorphologic description. Diagn Cytopathol. 2015;43(8):646–9.

297. Gupta S, Gupta R, Singh S, Pant L. Ossifying fibromyxoid tumour of soft parts: report of a case diagnosed on fine needle aspiration cytology. Cytopathology. 2012;23:126–8.

298. Minami R, Yamamoto T, Tsukamoto R, Maeda S. Fine needle aspiration cytology of the malignant variant of ossifying fibromyxoid tumor of soft parts: a case report. Acta Cytol. 2001;45:745–55.

299. Graham RP, Weiss SW, Sukov WR, Goldblum JR, Billings SD, Dotlic S, Folpe AL. PHF1 rearrangements in ossifying fibromyxoid tumors of soft parts: a fluorescence in situ hybridization study of 41 cases with emphasis on the malignant variant. Am J Surg Pathol. 2013;37(11):1751–5.

300. Endo M, Kohashi K, Yamamoto H, Ishii T, Yoshida T, Matsunobu T, Iwamoto Y, Oda Y. Ossifying fibromyxoid tumor presenting EP400-PHF1 fusion gene. Hum Pathol. 2013;44(11):2603–8.

301. Gebre-Medhin S, Nord KH, Möller E, Mandahl N, Magnusson L, Nilsson J, Jo VY, Vult von Steyern F, Brosjö O, Larsson O, Domanski HA, Sciot R, Debiec-Rychter M, Fletcher CD, Mertens F. Recurrent rearrangement of the PHF1 gene in ossifying fibromyxoid tumors. Am J Pathol. 2012;181(3):1069–77.

302. Suurmeijer AJH, Song W, Sung YS, Zhang L, Swanson D, Fletcher CDM, Dickson BC, Antonescu CR. Novel recurrent PHF1-TFE3 fusions in ossifying fibromyxoid tumors. Genes Chromosomes Cancer. 2019;58(9):643–9.

303. Enzinger FM. Angiomatoid malignant fibrous histiocytoma: a distinct fibrohistiocytic tumor of children and young adults simulating a vascular neoplasm. Cancer. 1979;44(6):2147–57.

304. Costa MJ, Weiss SW. Angiomatoid malignant fibrous histiocytoma. A follow-up study of 108 cases with evaluation of possible histologic predictors of outcome. Am J Surg Pathol. 1990;14(12):1126–32.

305. Argenyi ZB, Van Rybroek JJ, Kemp JD, Soper RT. Congenital angiomatoid malignant fibrous histiocytoma. A light-microscopic, immunopathologic, and electron-microscopic study. Am J Dermatopathol. 1988;10(1):59–67.

306. Chen G, Folpe AL, Colby TV, Sittampalam K, Patey M, Chen MG, Chan JK. Angiomatoid fibrous histiocytoma: unusual sites and unusual morphology. Mod Pathol. 2011;24(12):1560–70.

307. Bohelay G, Kluger N, Battistella M, Biaggi-Frassati A, Plantier F, Harraudeau A, Avril MF, Pedeutour F, Fraitag S. Histiocytome fibreux angiomatoïde de l'enfant: 6 cas [Angiomatoid fibrous histiocytoma in children: 6 cases]. Ann Dermatol Venereol. 2015;142(10):541–8.

308. Saito K, Kobayashi E, Yoshida A, Araki Y, Kubota D, Tanzawa Y, Kawai A, Yanagawa T, Takagishi K, Chuman H. Angiomatoid fibrous histiocytoma: a series of seven cases including genetically confirmed aggressive cases and a literature review. BMC Musculoskelet Disord. 2017;18(1):31.

309. Thway K, Fisher C. Angiomatoid fibrous histiocytoma: the current status of pathology and genetics. Arch Pathol Lab Med. 2015;139(5):674–82.

310. Schaefer IM, Fletcher CD. Myxoid variant of so-called angiomatoid "malignant fibrous histiocytoma": clinicopathologic characterization in a series of 21 cases. Am J Surg Pathol. 2014;38(6):816–23.

311. Weinreb I, Rubin BP, Goldblum JR. Pleomorphic angiomatoid fibrous histiocytoma: a case confirmed by fluorescence in situ hybridization analysis for EWSR1 rearrangement. J Cutan Pathol. 2008;35(9):855–60.

312. Moura RD, Wang X, Lonzo ML, Erickson-Johnson MR, García JJ, Oliveira AM. Reticular angiomatoid "malignant" fibrous histiocytoma--a case report with cytogenetics and molecular genetic analyses. Hum Pathol. 2011;42(9):1359–63.

313. Pettinato G, Manivel JC, De Rosa G, Petrella G, Jaszcz W. Angiomatoid malignant fibrous histiocytoma: cytologic, immunohistochemical, ultrastructural, and flow cytometric study of 20 cases. Mod Pathol. 1990;3(4):479–87.

314. Lemos MM, Karlen J, Tani E. Fine-needle aspiration cytology of angiomatoid malignant fibrous histiocytoma. Diagn Cytopathol. 2005;33(2):116–21.

315. Qian X, Hornick JL, Cibas ES, Dal Cin P, Domanski HA. Angiomatoid fibrous histiocytoma a series of five cytologic cases with literature review and emphasis on diagnostic pitfalls. Diagn Cytopathol. 2012;40(Suppl 2):E86–93.

316. Pan H, Byers J, Yin H, Rytting H, Logan S, He M, Yu Z, Wang D, Mangray S, Zhou S. The utility of TLE1 and BCOR as immunohistochemical markers for angiomatoid fibrous histiocytoma. Int J Clin Exp Pathol. 2023;16(2):32–9.

317. Fanburg-Smith JC, Miettinen M. Angiomatoid "malignant" fibrous histiocytoma: a clinicopathologic study of 158 cases and further exploration of the myoid phenotype. Hum Pathol. 1999;30(11):1336–43.

318. Rekhi B, Adamane S, Ghodke K, Desai S, Jambhekar NA. Angiomatoid fibrous histiocytoma: clinicopathological spectrum of five cases, including EWSR1-CREB1 positive result in a single case. Indian J Pathol Microbiol. 2016;59(2):148–52.

319. Cheah AL, Zou Y, Lanigan C, Billings SD, Rubin BP, Hornick JL, Goldblum JR. ALK expression in angiomatoid fibrous histiocytoma: a potential diagnostic pitfall. Am J Surg Pathol. 2019;43(1):93–101.

320. Tanas MR, Rubin BP, Montgomery EA, Turner SL, Cook JR, Tubbs RR, Billings SD, Goldblum JR. Utility of FISH in the diagnosis of angiomatoid fibrous histiocytoma: a series of 18 cases. Mod Pathol. 2010;23(1):93–7.

321. Rossi S, Szuhai K, Ijszenga M, Tanke HJ, Zanatta L, Sciot R, Fletcher CD, Dei Tos AP, Hogendoorn PC. EWSR1-CREB1 and EWSR1-ATF1 fusion genes in angiomatoid fibrous histiocytoma. Clin Cancer Res. 2007;13(24):7322–8.

322. Sultan I, Rodriguez-Galindo C, Saab R, Yasir S, Casanova M, Ferrari A. Comparing children and adults with synovial sarcoma in the Surveillance, Epidemiology, and End Results program, 1983 to 2005: an analysis of 1268 patients. Cancer. 2009;115(15):3537–47.

323. Fukushima T, Ogura K, Akiyama T, Takeshita K, Kawai A. Soft tissue sarcoma in adolescent and young adult patients: a retrospective study using a nationwide bone and soft tissue tumor registry in Japan. Jpn J Clin Oncol. 2021;51(7):1080–7.

324. Ladanyi M, Antonescu CR, Leung DH, Woodruff JM, Kawai A, Healey JH, Brennan MF, Bridge JA, Neff JR, Barr FG, Goldsmith JD, Brooks JS, Goldblum JR, Ali SZ, Shipley J, Cooper CS, Fisher C, Skytting B, Larsson O. Impact of SYT-SSX fusion type on the clinical behavior of synovial sarcoma: a multi-institutional retrospective study of 243 patients. Cancer Res. 2002;62(1):135–40.

325. Kerouanton A, Jimenez I, Cellier C, Laurence V, Helfre S, Pannier S, Mary P, Freneaux P, Orbach D. Synovial sarcoma in children and adolescents. J Pediatr Hematol Oncol. 2014;36(4):257–62.

326. Stanbouly D, Litman E, Lee KC, Philipone E. Synovial sarcoma of the head & neck: a review of reported cases in the literature. J Stomatol Oral Maxillofac Surg. 2021;122(5):505–10.

327. Thway K, Fisher C. Synovial sarcoma: defining features and diagnostic evolution. Ann Diagn Pathol. 2014;18(6):369–80.

328. Soule EH. Synovial sarcoma. Am J Surg Pathol. 1986;10(Suppl 1):78–82.

329. Ewing CA, Zakowski MF, Lin O. Monophasic synovial sarcoma: a cytologic spectrum. Diagn Cytopathol. 2004;30(1):19–23.

330. Srinivasan R, Gautam U, Gupta R, Rajwanshi A, Vasistha RK. Synovial sarcoma: diagnosis on fine-needle aspiration by morphology and molecular analysis. Cancer. 2009;117(2):128–36.

331. Kottu R, Prayaga AK. Synovial sarcoma with relevant immunocytochemistry and special emphasis on the monophasic fibrous variant. J Cytol. 2010;27(2):47–50.

332. Klijanienko J, Caillaud JM, Lagacé R, Vielh P. Cytohistologic correlations in 56 synovial sarcomas in 36 patients: the Institut Curie experience. Diagn Cytopathol. 2002;27(2):96–102.

333. Kilpatrick SE, Teot LA, Stanley MW, Ward WG, Savage PD, Geisinger KR. Fine-needle aspiration biopsy of synovial sarcoma. A cytomorphologic analysis of primary, recurrent, and metastatic tumors. Am J Clin Pathol. 1996;106(6):769–75.

334. Rekhi B, Shetty O, Ramadwar M, Rangarajan V, Bajpai J. Role of fine needle aspiration cytology in the diagnosis of a rare case of a poorly differentiated synovial sarcoma with "Rhabdoid" features, including treatment implications. Diagn Cytopathol. 2017;45(7):662–7.

335. Akerman M, Ryd W, Skytting B, Scandinavian Sarcoma Group. Fine-needle aspiration of synovial sarcoma: criteria for diagnosis: retrospective reexamination of 37 cases, including ancillary diagnostics. A Scandinavian Sarcoma Group study. Diagn Cytopathol. 2003;28(5):232–8.

336. Akerman M, Domanski HA. The complex cytological features of synovial sarcoma in fine needle aspirates, an analysis of four illustrative cases. Cytopathology. 2007;18(4):234–40.

337. Viguer JM, Jiménez-Heffernan JA, Vicandi B, López-Ferrer P, Gamallo C. Cytologic features of synovial sarcoma with emphasis on the monophasic fibrous variant: a morphologic and immunocytochemical analysis of bcl-2 protein expression. Cancer. 1998;84(1):50–6.

338. Foo WC, Cruise MW, Wick MR, Hornick JL. Immunohistochemical staining for TLE1 distinguishes synovial sarcoma from histologic mimics. Am J Clin Pathol. 2011;135(6):839–44.

339. Terry J, Saito T, Subramanian S, Ruttan C, Antonescu CR, Goldblum JR, Downs-Kelly E, Corless CL, Rubin BP, van de Rijn M, Ladanyi M, Nielsen TO. TLE1 as a diagnostic immunohistochemical marker for synovial sarcoma emerging from gene expression profiling studies. Am J Surg Pathol. 2007;31(2):240–6.

340. Kosemehmetoglu K, Vrana JA, Folpe AL. TLE1 expression is not specific for synovial sarcoma: a whole section study of 163 soft tissue and bone neoplasms. Mod Pathol. 2009;22(7):872–8.

341. Amary MF, Berisha F, Bernardi Fdel C, Herbert A, James M, Reis-Filho JS, Fisher C, Nicholson AG, Tirabosco R, Diss TC, Flanagan AM. Detection of SS18-SSX fusion transcripts in formalin-fixed paraffin-embedded neoplasms: analysis of conventional RT-PCR, qRT-PCR and dual color FISH as diagnostic tools for synovial sarcoma. Mod Pathol. 2007;20(4):482–96.

342. Choi JH, Ro JY. The recent advances in molecular diagnosis of soft tissue tumors. Int J Mol Sci. 2023;24(6):5934.

343. Krieg AH, Hefti F, Speth BM, Jundt G, Guillou L, Exner UG, von Hochstetter AR, Cserhati MD, Fuchs B, Mouhsine E, Kaelin A, Klenke FM, Siebenrock KA. Synovial sarcomas usually metastasize after >5 years: a multicenter retrospective analysis with minimum follow-up of 10 years for survivors. Ann Oncol. 2011;22(2):458–67.

344. ten Heuvel SE, Hoekstra HJ, Bastiaannet E, Suurmeijer AJ. The classic prognostic factors tumor stage, tumor size, and tumor grade are the strongest predictors of outcome in synovial sarcoma: no role for SSX fusion type or ezrin expression. Appl Immunohistochem Mol Morphol. 2009;17(3):189–95.

345. Wang H, Jacobson A, Harmon DC, Choy E, Hornicek FJ, Raskin KA, Chebib IA, DeLaney TF, Chen YL. Prognostic factors in alveolar soft part sarcoma: a SEER analysis. J Surg Oncol. 2016;113(5):581–6.

346. Fanburg-Smith JC, Miettinen M, Folpe AL, Weiss SW, Childers EL. Lingual alveolar soft part sarcoma; 14 cases: novel clinical and morphological observations. Histopathology. 2004;45(5):526–37.

347. Font RL, Jurco S 3rd, Zimmerman LE. Alveolar soft-part sarcoma of the orbit: a clinicopathologic analysis of seventeen cases and a review of the literature. Hum Pathol. 1982;13(6):569–79.

348. Rekhi B, Ingle A, Agarwal M, Puri A, Laskar S, Jambhekar NA. Alveolar soft part sarcoma 'revisited': clinicopathological review of 47 cases from a tertiary cancer referral Centre, including immunohistochemical expression of TFE3 in 22 cases and 21 other tumours. Pathology. 2012;44(1):11–7.

349. Jong R, Kandel R, Fornasier V, Bell R, Bedard Y. Alveolar soft part sarcoma: review of nine cases including two cases with unusual histology. Histopathology. 1998;32(1):63–8.

350. Folpe AL, Deyrup AT. Alveolar soft-part sarcoma: a review and update. J Clin Pathol. 2006;59(11):1127–32.
351. Xu Y, Zhou T, Yu W, Zarrin-Khameh N. Fine-needle aspiration of alveolar soft part sarcoma: histologic correlation and aberrant CD68 expression. Diagn Cytopathol. 2019;47(2):114–20.
352. Rekhi B, Rao V, Ramadwar M. Revisiting cytomorphology, including unusual features and clinical scenarios of 8 cases of alveolar soft part sarcoma with TFE3 immunohistochemical staining in 7 cases. Cytopathology. 2021;32(1):20–8.
353. Wakely PE Jr, McDermott JE, Ali SZ. Cytopathology of alveolar soft part sarcoma: a report of 10 cases. Cancer. 2009;117(6):500–7.
354. López-Ferrer P, Jiménez-Heffernan JA, Vicandi B, González-Peramato P, Viguer JM. Cytologic features of alveolar soft part sarcoma: report of three cases. Diagn Cytopathol. 2002;27(2):115–9.
355. Shabb N, Sneige N, Fanning CV, Dekmezian R. Fine-needle aspiration cytology of alveolar soft-part sarcoma. Diagn Cytopathol. 1991;7(3):293–8.
356. Drachenberg CB, Papadimitriou JC. Alveolar soft part sarcoma. A case report with correlation of fine needle aspiration and ultrastructural cytologic features. Acta Cytol. 1991;35(6):746–52.
357. Argani P, Antonescu CR, Illei PB, Lui MY, Timmons CF, Newbury R, Reuter VE, Garvin AJ, Perez-Atayde AR, Fletcher JA, Beckwith JB, Bridge JA, Ladanyi M. Primary renal neoplasms with the ASPL-TFE3 gene fusion of alveolar soft part sarcoma: a distinctive tumor entity previously included among renal cell carcinomas of children and adolescents. Am J Pathol. 2001;159(1):179–92.
358. Pang LJ, Chang B, Zou H, Qi Y, Jiang JF, Li HA, Hu WH, Chen YZ, Liu CX, Zhang WJ, Li F. Alveolar soft part sarcoma: a bimarker diagnostic strategy using TFE3 immunoassay and ASPL-TFE3 fusion transcripts in paraffin-embedded tumor tissues. Diagn Mol Pathol. 2008;17(4):245–52.
359. Vistica DT, Krosky PM, Kenney S, Raffeld M, Shoemaker RH. Immunohistochemical discrimination between the ASPL-TFE3 fusion proteins of alveolar soft part sarcoma. J Pediatr Hematol Oncol. 2008;30(1):46–52.
360. Lieberman PH, Brennan MF, Kimmel M, Erlandson RA, Garin-Chesa P, Flehinger BY. Alveolar soft-part sarcoma. A clinico-pathologic study of half a century. Cancer. 1989;63(1):1–13.
361. Pennacchioli E, Fiore M, Collini P, Radaelli S, Dileo P, Stacchiotti S, Casali PG, Gronchi A. Alveolar soft part sarcoma: clinical presentation, treatment, and outcome in a series of 33 patients at a single institution. Ann Surg Oncol. 2010;17(12):3229–33.
362. Portera CA Jr, Ho V, Patel SR, Hunt KK, Feig BW, Respondek PM, Yasko AW, Benjamin RS, Pollock RE, Pisters PW. Alveolar soft part sarcoma: clinical course and patterns of metastasis in 70 patients treated at a single institution. Cancer. 2001;91(3):585–91.
363. Dim DC, Cooley LD, Miranda RN. Clear cell sarcoma of tendons and aponeuroses: a review. Arch Pathol Lab Med. 2007;131(1):152–6.
364. Ibrahim RM, Steenstrup Jensen S, Juel J. Clear cell sarcoma-a review. J Orthop. 2018;15(4):963–6. Erratum in: J Orthop. 2020 Dec 15;24:291.
365. Bianchi G, Charoenlap C, Cocchi S, Rani N, Campagnoni S, Righi A, Frisoni T, Donati DM. Clear cell sarcoma of soft tissue: a retrospective review and analysis of 31 cases treated at Istituto Ortopedico Rizzoli. Eur J Surg Oncol. 2014;40(5):505–10.
366. Lucas DR, Nascimento AG, Sim FH. Clear cell sarcoma of soft tissues. Mayo Clinic experience with 35 cases. Am J Surg Pathol. 1992;16(12):1197–204.
367. Chung EB, Enzinger FM. Malignant melanoma of soft parts. A reassessment of clear cell sarcoma. Am J Surg Pathol. 1983;7(5):405–13.
368. Deenik W, Mooi WJ, Rutgers EJ, Peterse JL, Hart AA, Kroon BB. Clear cell sarcoma (malignant melanoma) of soft parts: a clinicopathologic study of 30 cases. Cancer. 1999;86(6):969–75.
369. Eckardt JJ, Pritchard DJ, Soule EH. Clear cell sarcoma. A clinicopathologic study of 27 cases. Cancer. 1983;52(8):1482–8.
370. Rao V, Rekhi B. Cytomorphological spectrum, including immunohistochemical results of 16 cases of clear cell sarcoma of soft tissue, along with positive EWSR1 gene rearrangement result in two cases. Cytopathology. 2020;31(4):280–7.
371. Caraway NP, Fanning CV, Wojcik EM, Staerkel GA, Benjamin RS, Ordóñez NG. Cytology of malignant melanoma of soft parts: fine-needle aspirates and exfoliative specimens. Diagn Cytopathol. 1993;9(6):632–8.
372. Tong TR, Chow TC, Chan OW, Lee KC, Yeung SH, Lam A, Yu CK. Clear-cell sarcoma diagnosis by fine-needle aspiration: cytologic, histologic, and ultrastructural features; potential pitfalls; and literature review. Diagn Cytopathol. 2002;26(3):174–80.
373. Kumar N, Das PM, Jain S, Sodhani P, Gupta S. Melanoma of the soft parts: diagnosis of metastatic and recurrent tumors by aspiration cytology. Diagn Cytopathol. 2003;28(6):295–300.
374. Rau AR, Kini H, Verghese R. Tigroid background in fine-needle aspiration cytology of clear cell sarcoma. Diagn Cytopathol. 2006;34(5):355–7.
375. Creager AJ, Pitman MB, Geisinger KR. Cytologic features of clear cell sarcoma (malignant melanoma) of soft parts: a study of fine-needle aspirates and exfoliative specimens. Am J Clin Pathol. 2002;117(2):217–24.
376. Granter SR, Weilbaecher KN, Quigley C, Fletcher CD, Fisher DE. Clear cell sarcoma shows immunoreactivity for microphthalmia transcription factor: further evidence for melanocytic differentiation. Mod Pathol. 2001;14(1):6–9.
377. Reeves BR, Fletcher CD, Gusterson BA. Translocation t(12;22)(q13;q13) is a nonrandom rearrangement in clear cell sarcoma. Cancer Genet Cytogenet. 1992;64(2):101–3.

378. Panagopoulos I, Mertens F, Débiec-Rychter M, Isaksson M, Limon J, Kardas I, Domanski HA, Sciot R, Perek D, Crnalic S, Larsson O, Mandahl N. Molecular genetic characterization of the EWS/ATF1 fusion gene in clear cell sarcoma of tendons and aponeuroses. Int J Cancer. 2002;99(4):560–7.

379. Gonzaga MI, Grant L, Curtin C, Gootee J, Silberstein P, Voth E. The epidemiology and survivorship of clear cell sarcoma: a National Cancer Database (NCDB) review. J Cancer Res Clin Oncol. 2018;144(9):1711–6.

380. Hocar O, Le Cesne A, Berissi S, Terrier P, Bonvalot S, Vanel D, Auperin A, Le Pechoux C, Bui B, Coindre JM, Robert C. Clear cell sarcoma (malignant melanoma) of soft parts: a clinicopathologic study of 52 cases. Dermatol Res Pract. 2012;2012:984096.

381. Enzinger FM, Shiraki M. Extraskeletal myxoid chondrosarcoma. An analysis of 34 cases. Hum Pathol. 1972;3(3):421–35.

382. Meis-Kindblom JM, Bergh P, Gunterberg B, Kindblom LG. Extraskeletal myxoid chondrosarcoma: a reappraisal of its morphologic spectrum and prognostic factors based on 117 cases. Am J Surg Pathol. 1999;23(6):636–50.

383. Fidele NB, Tianfu W, Liu B, Sun Y, Yifang Z. Extraskeletal Myxoid chondrosarcoma of the parotid gland. Ann Maxillofac Surg. 2019;9(2):439–43.

384. Qin Y, Zhang HB, Ke CS, Huang J, Wu B, Wan C, Yang CS, Yang KY. Primary extraskeletal myxoid chondrosarcoma in cerebellum: a case report with literature review. Medicine (Baltimore). 2017;96(47):e8684.

385. Ceylan K, Kizilkaya Z, Yavanoglu A. Extraskeletal myxoid chondrosarcoma of the nasal cavity. Eur Arch Otorrinolaringol. 2006;263(11):1044–7.

386. Purkayastha A, Sharma N, Dutta V. Extraskeletal myxoid chondrosarcoma of nasopharynx: an oncologic entity rarely reported. Oman Med J. 2018;33(2):159–62.

387. Romañach MJ, Carlos R, Nuyens M, de Andrade BA, de Almeida OP. Extraskeletal myxoid chondrosarcoma of the masticator space in a pediatric patient. J Clin Exp Dent. 2017;9(6):e825–31.

388. Lucas DR, Fletcher CD, Adsay NV, Zalupski MM. High-grade extraskeletal myxoid chondrosarcoma: a high-grade epithelioid malignancy. Histopathology. 1999;35(3):201–8.

389. Kumar R, Rekhi B, Shirazi N, Pais A, Amare P, Gawde D, Jambhekar N. Spectrum of cytomorphological features, including literature review, of an extraskeletal myxoid chondrosarcoma with t(9;22)(q22;q12) (TEC/EWS) results in one case. Diagn Cytopathol. 2008;36(12):868–75.

390. Wakely PE Jr. Extraskeletal myxoid chondrosarcoma: combining cytopathology with molecular testing to achieve diagnostic accuracy. J Am Soc Cytopathol. 2021;10(3):293–9.

391. Santos F, Martins C, Lemos MM. Fine-needle aspiration features of extraskeletal myxoid chondrosar-

coma: a study of cytological and molecular features. Diagn Cytopathol. 2018;46(11):950–7.

392. Jakowski JD, Wakely PE Jr. Cytopathology of extraskeletal myxoid chondrosarcoma: report of 8 cases. Cancer. 2007;111(5):298–305.

393. Domanski HA, Carlen B, Mertens F, Akerman M. Extraskeletal myxoid chondrosarcoma with neuroendocrine differentiation: a case report with fine-needle aspiration biopsy, histopathology, electron microscopy, and cytogenetics. Ultrastruct Pathol. 2003;27:363–8.

394. Okamoto S, Hisaoka M, Ishida T, Imamura T, Kanda H, Shimajiri S, Hashimoto H. Extraskeletal myxoid chondrosarcoma: a clinicopathologic, immunohistochemical, and molecular analysis of 18 cases. Hum Pathol. 2001;32(10):1116–24.

395. Oliveira AM, Sebo TJ, McGrory JE, Gaffey TA, Rock MG, Nascimento AG. Extraskeletal myxoid chondrosarcoma: a clinicopathologic, immunohistochemical, and ploidy analysis of 23 cases. Mod Pathol. 2000;13(8):900–8.

396. Harris M, Coyne J, Tariq M, Eyden BP, Atkinson M, Freemont AJ, Varley J, Attwooll C, Telford N. Extraskeletal myxoid chondrosarcoma with neuroendocrine differentiation: a pathologic, cytogenetic, and molecular study of a case with a novel translocation t(9;17)(q22;q11.2). Am J Surg Pathol. 2000;24(7):1020–6.

397. Schaefer IM, Hornick JL. SWI/SNF complex-deficient soft tissue neoplasms: an update. Semin Diagn Pathol. 2021;38(3):222–31.

398. Flucke U, Tops BB, Verdijk MA, van Cleef PJ, van Zwam PH, Slootweg PJ, Bovée JV, Riedl RG, Creytens DH, Suurmeijer AJ, Mentzel T. NR4A3 rearrangement reliably distinguishes between the clinicopathologically overlapping entities myoepithelial carcinoma of soft tissue and cellular extraskeletal myxoid chondrosarcoma. Virchows Arch. 2012;460(6):621–8.

399. Drilon AD, Popat S, Bhuchar G, D'Adamo DR, Keohan ML, Fisher C, Antonescu CR, Singer S, Brennan MF, Judson I, Maki RG. Extraskeletal myxoid chondrosarcoma: a retrospective review from 2 referral centers emphasizing long-term outcomes with surgery and chemotherapy. Cancer. 2008;113(12):3364–71.

400. Saleh G, Evans HL, Ro JY, Ayala AG. Extraskeletal myxoid chondrosarcoma. A clinicopathologic study of ten patients with long-term follow-up. Cancer. 1992;70(12):2827–30.

401. Steele CD, et al. Undifferentiated sarcomas develop through distinct evolutionary pathways. Cancer Cell. 2019;35(3):441–456.e8. https://doi.org/10.1016/J.CCELL.2019.02.002.

402. Fletcher CDM. Undifferentiated sarcomas: what to do? And does it matter? A surgical pathology perspective. Ultrastruct Pathol. 2008;32(2):31–6. https://doi.org/10.1080/01913120801896945.

403. Peng KA, Grogan T, Wang MB. Head and neck sarcomas: analysis of the SEER database. Otolaryngol

Head Neck Surg. 2014;151(4):627. https://doi.org/10.1177/0194599814545747.

404. Wang CP, Chang YL, Ting LL, Yang TL, Ko JY, Lou PJ. Malignant fibrous histiocytoma of the sinonasal tract. Head Neck. 2009;31(1):85–93. https://doi.org/10.1002/HED.20936.

405. Sturgis EM, Potter BO. Sarcomas of the head and neck region. Curr Opin Oncol. 2003;15(3):239–52. https://doi.org/10.1097/00001622-200305000-00011.

406. Klijanienko J, Caillaud JM, Lagacé R, Vielh P. Comparative fine-needle aspiration and pathologic study of malignant fibrous histiocytoma: cytodiagnostic features of 95 tumors in 71 patients. Diagn Cytopathol. 2003;29(6):320–6. https://doi.org/10.1002/DC.10363.

407. Kilpatrick SE, Reith JD, Rubin B. Ewing sarcoma and the history of similar and possibly related small round cell tumors: from whence have we come and where are we going? Adv Anat Pathol. 2018;25(5):314–26. https://doi.org/10.1097/PAP.0000000000000203. Lippincott Williams and Wilkins.

408. Gajdzis P, Pierron G, Klijanienko J. Cytology of undifferentiated round-cell sarcomas of bone and soft tissue: Ewing sarcoma or not Ewing sarcoma, that is the question. Acta Cytol. 2022;66(4):295–306. https://doi.org/10.1159/000518146.

409. Olson MD, Van Abel KM, Wehrs RN, Garcia JJ, Moore EJ. Ewing sarcoma of the head and neck: the Mayo Clinic experience. Head Neck. 2018;40(9):1999–2006. https://doi.org/10.1002/HED.25191.

410. Ellis MA, Gerry DR, Neskey DM, Lentsch EJ. Ewing sarcoma of the head and neck. Ann Otol Rhinol Laryngol. 2017;126(3):179–84. https://doi.org/10.1177/0003489416681322.

411. Bal M, et al. Adamantinoma-like Ewing sarcoma of the head and neck: a case-series of a rare and challenging diagnosis. Head Neck Pathol. 2022;16(3):679–94. https://doi.org/10.1007/S12105-022-01412-1.

412. Rooper LM, Bishop JA. Soft tissue special issue: adamantinoma-like Ewing sarcoma of the head and neck: a practical review of a challenging emerging entity. Head Neck Pathol. 2020;14(1):59–69. https://doi.org/10.1007/S12105-019-01098-Y.

413. Martin E, Radomski S, Harley EH. Pediatric Ewing sarcoma of the head and neck: a retrospective survival analysis. Int J Pediatr Otorhinolaryngol. 2019;117:138–42. https://doi.org/10.1016/J.IJPORL.2018.11.026.

414. Klijanienko J, et al. Fine-needle aspiration as a diagnostic technique in 50 cases of primary Ewing sarcoma/peripheral neuroectodermal tumor. Institut Curie's experience. Diagn Cytopathol. 2012;40(1):19–25. https://doi.org/10.1002/dc.21491.

415. Kao YC, et al. BCOR-CCNB3 fusion positive sarcomas: a clinicopathologic and molecular analysis of 36 cases with comparison to morphologic spectrum and clinical behavior of other round cell sarcomas. Am J Surg Pathol. 2018;42(5):604–15. https://doi.org/10.1097/PAS.0000000000000965.

416. Antonescu CR, et al. Sarcomas with CIC-rearrangements are a distinct pathologic entity with aggressive outcome: a clinicopathologic and molecular study of 115 cases. Am J Surg Pathol. 2017;41(7):941–9. https://doi.org/10.1097/PAS.0000000000000846.

417. Antonescu C. Round cell sarcomas beyond Ewing: emerging entities. Histopathology. 2014;64(1):26–37. https://doi.org/10.1111/HIS.12281.

418. Gajdzis P, et al. Fine-needle aspiration features of BCOR-CCNB3 sarcoma. Am J Clin Pathol. 2020;153(3):315–21. https://doi.org/10.1093/ajcp/aqz159.

419. Neel HB, Whicker JH, Devine KD, Weiland LH. Juvenile angiofibroma. Review of 120 cases. Am J Surg. 1973;126(4):547–56. https://doi.org/10.1016/S0002-9610(73)80048-0.

420. Boghani Z, et al. Juvenile nasopharyngeal angiofibroma: a systematic review and comparison of endoscopic, endoscopic-assisted, and open resection in 1047 cases. Laryngoscope. 2013;123(4):859–69. https://doi.org/10.1002/LARY.23843.

421. Abraham SC, Montgomery EA, Giardiello FM, Wu TT. Frequent beta-catenin mutations in juvenile nasopharyngeal angiofibromas. Am J Pathol. 2001;158(3):1073–8. https://doi.org/10.1016/S0002-9440(10)64054-0.

422. Agaimy A, Haller F. CTNNB1 (β-catenin)-altered neoplasia: a review focusing on soft tissue neoplasms and parenchymal lesions of uncertain histogenesis. Adv Anat Pathol. 2016;23(1):1–12. https://doi.org/10.1097/PAP.0000000000000104.

423. Rooper LM, Huang SC, Antonescu CR, Westra WH, Bishop JA. Biphenotypic sinonasal sarcoma: an expanded immunoprofile including consistent nuclear β-catenin positivity and absence of SOX10 expression. Hum Pathol. 2016;55:44–50. https://doi.org/10.1016/J.HUMPATH.2016.04.009.

424. Lewis JT, et al. Low-grade sinonasal sarcoma with neural and myogenic features: a clinicopathologic analysis of 28 cases. Am J Surg Pathol. 2012;36(4):517–25. https://doi.org/10.1097/PAS.0B013E3182426886.

425. Carter CS, East EG, McHugh JB. Biphenotypic sinonasal sarcoma: a review and update. Arch Pathol Lab Med. 2018;142(10):1196–201. https://doi.org/10.5858/ARPA.2018-0207-RA.

426. Bishop JA. Newly described tumor entities in Sinonasal tract pathology. Head Neck Pathol. 2016;10(1):23–31. https://doi.org/10.1007/S12105-016-0688-7.

427. Jo VY, Mariño-Enríquez A, Fletcher CDM, Hornick JL. Expression of PAX3 distinguishes biphenotypic sinonasal sarcoma from histologic mimics. Am J Surg Pathol. 2018;42(10):1275–85. https://doi.org/10.1097/PAS.0000000000001092.

428. Savage SA, Mirabello L. Using epidemiology and genomics to understand osteosarcoma etiology. Sarcoma. 2011;2011:548151.

429. Mirabello L, Troisi RJ, Savage SA. Osteosarcoma incidence and survival rates from 1973 to 2004: data from the Surveillance, Epidemiology, and End Results Program. Cancer. 2009;115(7):1531–43. https://doi.org/10.1002/cncr.24121. PMID: 19197972; PMCID: PMC2813207.

430. Baumhoer D, Brunner P, Eppenberger-Castori S, Smida J, Nathrath M, Jundt G. Osteosarcomas of the jaws differ from their peripheral counterparts and require a distinct treatment approach. Experiences from the DOESAK Registry. Oral Oncol. 2014;50(2):147–53.

431. van den Berg H, Merks JH. Incidence and grading of cranio-facial osteosarcomas. Int J Oral Maxillofac Surg. 2014;43(1):7–12.

432. Klein MJ, Siegal GP. Osteosarcoma: anatomic and histologic variants. Am J Clin Pathol. 2006;125(4):555–81.

433. Bacci G, Longhi A, Versari M, Mercuri M, Briccoli A, Picci P. Prognostic factors for osteosarcoma of the extremity treated with neoadjuvant chemotherapy: 15-year experience in 789 patients treated at a single institution. Cancer. 2006;106(5):1154–61.

434. Hauben EI, Weeden S, Pringle J, Van Marck EA, Hogendoorn PC. Does the histological subtype of high-grade central osteosarcoma influence the response to treatment with chemotherapy and does it affect overall survival? A study on 570 patients of two consecutive trials of the European Osteosarcoma Intergroup. Eur J Cancer. 2002;38(9):1218–25.

435. VandenBussche CJ, Sathiyamoorthy S, Wakely PE Jr, Ali SZ. Chondroblastic osteosarcoma: cytomorphologic characteristics and differential diagnosis on FNA. Cancer Cytopathol. 2016;124(7):493–500.

436. Söderlund V, Skoog L, Unni KK, Bertoni F, Brosjö O, Kreicbergs A. Diagnosis of high-grade osteosarcoma by radiology and cytology: a retrospective study of 52 cases. Sarcoma. 2004;8:31–6.

437. Sathiyamoorthy S, Ali SZ. Osteoblastic osteosarcoma: cytomorphologic characteristics and differential diagnosis on fine-needle aspiration. Acta Cytol. 2012;56(5):481–6.

438. Klijanienko J, Caillaud JM, Orbach D, Brisse H, Lagacé R, Sastre-Gareau X. Cyto-histological correlations in primary, recurrent, and metastatic bone and soft tissue osteosarcoma. Institut Curie's experience. Diagn Cytopathol. 2007;35(5):270–5.

439. Domanski HA, Akerman M. Fine-needle aspiration of primary osteosarcoma: a cytological-histological study. Diagn Cytopathol. 2005;32(5):269–75.

440. Dodd LG, Scully SP, Cothran RL, Harrelson JM. Utility of fine-needle aspiration in the diagnosis of primary osteosarcoma. Diagn Cytopathol. 2002;27(6):350–3. https://doi.org/10.1002/dc.10196. PMID: 12451565.

441. White VA, Fanning CV, Ayala AG, Raymond AK, Carrasco CH, Murray JA. Osteosarcoma and the role of fine-needle aspiration. A study of 51 cases. Cancer. 1988;62:1238–46.

442. Walaas L, Kindblom LG. Light and electron microscopic examination of fine-needle aspirates in the preoperative diagnosis of osteogenic tumors: a study of 21 osteosarcomas and two osteoblastomas. Diagn Cytopathol. 1990;6:27–38.

443. Gupta N, Rajwanshi A, Gupta P, Vaiphei K, Gupta AK. Chondroblastic osteosarcoma of the temporal region: a diagnostic dilemma. Diagn Cytopathol. 2011;39:377–9.

444. Kilpatrick SE, Ward WG, Bos GD, Chauvenet AR, Gold SH. The role of fine needle aspiration biopsy in the diagnosis and management of osteosarcoma. Pediatr Pathol Mol Med. 2001;20:175–87.

445. Bhatia A, Ashokraj G. Cytological diversity of osteosarcoma. Indian J Cancer. 1992;29:56–60.

446. Machado I, Navarro S, Picci P, Llombart-Bosch A. The utility of SATB2 immunohistochemical expression in distinguishing between osteosarcomas and their malignant bone tumor mimickers, such as Ewing sarcomas and chondrosarcomas. Pathol Res Pract. 2016;212(9):811–6.

447. Davis JL, Horvai AE. Special AT-rich sequence-binding protein 2 (SATB2) expression is sensitive but may not be specific for osteosarcoma as compared with other high-grade primary bone sarcomas. Histopathology. 2016;69(1):84–90. https://doi.org/10.1111/his.12911. Epub 2016

448. Dujardin F, Binh MB, Bouvier C, Gomez-Brouchet A, Larousserie F, Muret A, Louis-Brennetot C, Aurias A, Coindre JM, Guillou L, Pedeutour F, Duval H, Collin C, de Pinieux G. MDM2 and CDK4 immunohistochemistry is a valuable tool in the differential diagnosis of low-grade osteosarcomas and other primary fibro-osseous lesions of the bone. Mod Pathol. 2011;24(5):624–37.

449. Yoshida A, Ushiku T, Motoi T, Shibata T, Beppu Y, Fukayama M, Tsuda H. Immunohistochemical analysis of MDM2 and CDK4 distinguishes low-grade osteosarcoma from benign mimics. Mod Pathol. 2010;23(9):1279–88.

450. Smeland S, Bielack SS, Whelan J, Bernstein M, Hogendoorn P, Krailo MD, Gorlick R, Janeway KA, Ingleby FC, Anninga J, Antal I, Arndt C, Brown KLB, Butterfass-Bahloul T, Calaminus G, Capra M, Dhooge C, Eriksson M, Flanagan AM, Friedel G, Gebhardt MC, Gelderblom H, Goldsby R, Grier HE, Grimer R, Hawkins DS, Hecker-Nolting S, Sundby Hall K, Isakoff MS, Jovic G, Kühne T, Kager L, von Kalle T, Kabickova E, Lang S, Lau CC, Leavey PJ, Lessnick SL, Mascarenhas L, Mayer-Steinacker R, Meyers PA, Nagarajan R, Randall RL, Reichardt P, Renard M, Rechnitzer C, Schwartz CL, Strauss S, Teot L, Timmermann B, Sydes MR, Marina N. Survival and prognosis with osteosarcoma: outcomes in more than 2000 patients in the EURAMOS-1 (European and American Osteosarcoma Study) cohort. Eur J Cancer. 2019;109:36–50.

451. Patel SG, Meyers P, Huvos AG, Wolden S, Singh B, Shaha AR, Boyle JO, Pfister D, Shah JP, Kraus DH. Improved outcomes in patients with osteo-

genic sarcoma of the head and neck. Cancer. 2002;95(7):1495–503.

452. Guadagnolo BA, Zagars GK, Raymond AK, Benjamin RS, Sturgis EM. Osteosarcoma of the jaw/craniofacial region: outcomes after multimodality treatment. Cancer. 2009;115(14):3262–70.

453. Seng D, Wu J, Fang Q, Liu F. Prognosis of osteosarcomas in the mandible: 15-year experience of 55 patients. Medicine (Baltimore). 2019;98(1):e13875.

454. Koch BB, Karnell LH, Hoffman HT, Apostolakis LW, Robinson RA, Zhen W, Menck HR. National cancer database report on chondrosarcoma of the head and neck. Head Neck. 2000;22(4):408–25.

455. Saito K, Unni KK, Wollan PC, Lund BA. Chondrosarcoma of the jaw and facial bones. Cancer. 1995;76(9):1550–8.

456. Hong P, Taylor SM, Trites JR, Bullock M, Nasser JG, Hart RD. Chondrosarcoma of the head and neck: report of 11 cases and literature review. J Otolaryngol Head Neck Surg. 2009;38(2):279–85.

457. Pontes HA, Pontes FS, de Abreu MC, de Carvalho PL, de Brito Kato AM, Fonseca FP, de Freitas Silva BS, Neto NC. Clinicopathological analysis of head and neck chondrosarcoma: three case reports and literature review. Int J Oral Maxillofac Surg. 2012;41(2):203–10.

458. Gadwal SR, Fanburg-Smith JC, Gannon FH, Thompson LD. Primary chondrosarcoma of the head and neck in pediatric patients: a clinicopathologic study of 14 cases with a review of the literature. Cancer. 2000;88(9):2181–8.

459. Lee SY, Lim YC, Song MH, Seok JY, Lee WS, Choi EC. Chondrosarcoma of the head and neck. Yonsei Med J. 2005;46(2):228–32.

460. Hameed M. Malignant cartilage-forming tumors. Surg Pathol Clin. 2021;14(4):605–17.

461. Rozeman LB, Hogendoorn PC, Bovée JV. Diagnosis and prognosis of chondrosarcoma of bone. Expert Rev Mol Diagn. 2002;2(5):461–72.

462. Akerman M, Domanski HA. Fine needle aspiration (FNA) of bone tumours. With special emphasis on definitive treatment of primary malignant bone tumours based on FNA. Curr. Diagn Pathol. 1998;5:82–92.

463. Handa U, Bal A, Mohan H, Bhardwaj S. Fine needle aspiration cytology in the diagnosis of bone lesions. Cytopathology. 2005;16:59–64.

464. Abdul-Karim FW, Wasman JK, Pitlik D. Needle aspiration cytology of chondrosarcomas. Acta Cytol. 1993;37:655–60.

465. Dodd LG. Fine-needle aspiration of chondrosarcoma. Diagn Cytopathol. 2006;34:413–8.

466. Lerma E, Tani E, Brosjö O, Bauer H, Söderlund V, Skoog L. Diagnosis and grading of chondrosarcomas on FNA biopsy material. Diagn Cytopathol. 2003;28:13–7.

467. Skoog L, Pereira ST, Tani E. Fine-needle aspiration cytology and immunocytochemistry of soft-tissue tumors and osteo/chondrosarcomas of the head and neck. Diagn Cytopathol. 1999;20:131–6.

468. Oakley GJ, Fuhrer K, Seethala RR. Brachyury, SOX-9, and podoplanin, new markers in the skull base chordoma vs chondrosarcoma differential: a tissue microarray-based comparative analysis. Mod Pathol. 2008;21(12):1461–9.

469. Amary MF, Bacsi K, Maggiani F, Damato S, Halai D, Berisha F, Pollock R, O'Donnell P, Grigoriadis A, Diss T, Eskandarpour M, Presneau N, Hogendoorn PC, Futreal A, Tirabosco R, Flanagan AM. IDH1 and IDH2 mutations are frequent events in central chondrosarcoma and central and periosteal chondromas but not in other mesenchymal tumours. J Pathol. 2011;224(3):334–43.

470. Kerr DA, Lopez HU, Deshpande V, Hornicek FJ, Duan Z, Zhang Y, Rosenberg AE, Borger DR, Nielsen GP. Molecular distinction of chondrosarcoma from chondroblastic osteosarcoma through IDH1/2 mutations. Am J Surg Pathol. 2013;37(6):787–95.

471. Fanburg-Smith JC, Auerbach A, Marwaha JS, Wang Z, Santi M, Judkins AR, Rushing EJ. Immunoprofile of mesenchymal chondrosarcoma: aberrant desmin and EMA expression, retention of INI1, and negative estrogen receptor in 22 female-predominant central nervous system and musculoskeletal cases. Ann Diagn Pathol. 2010;14(1):8–14.

472. Cesari M, Bertoni F, Bacchini P, Mercuri M, Palmerini E, Ferrari S, Mesenchymal chondrosarcoma. An analysis of patients treated at a single institution. Tumori. 2007;93(5):423–7.

473. Vencio EF, Reeve CM, Unni KK, Nascimento AG. Mesenchymal chondrosarcoma of the jaw bones: clinicopathologic study of 19 cases. Cancer. 1998;82(12):2350–5.

474. Pellitteri PK, Ferlito A, Fagan JJ, Suárez C, Devaney KO, Rinaldo A. Mesenchymal chondrosarcoma of the head and neck. Oral Oncol. 2007;43(10):970–5.

475. Chen JY, Hsu SS, Ho JT. Extraskeletal intracranial mesenchymal chondrosarcoma: case report and literature review. Kaohsiung J Med Sci. 2004;20(5):240–6.

476. Huvos AG, Rosen G, Dabska M, Marcove RC, Mesenchymal chondrosarcoma. A clinicopathologic analysis of 35 patients with emphasis on treatment. Cancer. 1983;51(7):1230–7.

477. Bertoni F, Picci P, Bacchini P, Capanna R, Innao V, Bacci G, Campanacci M. Mesenchymal chondrosarcoma of bone and soft tissues. Cancer. 1983;52(3):533–41.

478. Nakashima Y, Unni KK, Shives TC, Swee RG, Dahlin DC. Mesenchymal chondrosarcoma of bone and soft tissue. A review of 111 cases. Cancer. 1986;57(12):2444–53.

479. Knott PD, Gannon FH, Thompson LD. Mesenchymal chondrosarcoma of the sinonasal tract: a clinicopathological study of 13 cases with a review of the literature. Laryngoscope. 2003;113(5):783–90.

480. Fanburg-Smith JC, Auerbach A, Marwaha JS, Wang Z, Rushing EJ. Reappraisal of mesenchymal chondrosarcoma: novel morphologic observations of the hyaline cartilage and endochondral ossification and

beta-catenin, Sox9, and osteocalcin immunostaining of 22 cases. Hum Pathol. 2010;41(5):653–62.

481. Schneiderman BA, Kliethermes SA, Nystrom LM. Survival in mesenchymal chondrosarcoma varies based on age and tumor location: a survival analysis of the SEER database. Clin Orthop Relat Res. 2017;475(3):799–805.

482. Frezza AM, Cesari M, Baumhoer D, Biau D, Bielack S, Campanacci DA, Casanova J, Esler C, Ferrari S, Funovics PT, Gerrand C, Grimer R, Gronchi A, Haffner N, Hecker-Nolting S, Höller S, Jeys L, Jutte P, Leithner A, San-Julian M, Thorkildsen J, Vincenzi B, Windhager R, Whelan J. Mesenchymal chondrosarcoma: prognostic factors and outcome in 113 patients. A European Musculoskeletal Oncology Society study. Eur J Cancer. 2015;51(3):374–81.

483. Arora K, Riddle ND. Extraskeletal mesenchymal chondrosarcoma. Arch Pathol Lab Med. 2018;142(11):1421–4.

484. Shakked RJ, Geller DS, Gorlick R, Dorfman HD. Mesenchymal chondrosarcoma: clinicopathologic study of 20 cases. Arch Pathol Lab Med. 2012;136(1):61–75.

485. Trembath DG, Dash R, Major NM, Dodd LG. Cytopathology of mesenchymal chondrosarcomas: a report and comparison of four patients. Cancer. 2003;99(4):211–6.

486. Cheim AP Jr, Queiroz TL, Alencar WM, Rezende RM, Vencio EF. Mesenchymal chondrosarcoma in the mandible: report of a case with cytological findings. J Oral Sci. 2011;53:245–7.

487. Handa U, Singhal N, Punia RS, Garg S, Mohan H. Cytologic features and differential diagnosis in a case of extraskeletal mesenchymal chondrosarcoma: a case report. Acta Cytol. 2009;53:704–6.

488. Yoshida KI, Machado I, Motoi T, Parafioriti A, Lacambra M, Ichikawa H, Kawai A, Antonescu CR, Yoshida A. NKX3-1 is a useful immunohistochemical marker of EWSR1-NFATC2 sarcoma and mesenchymal chondrosarcoma. Am J Surg Pathol. 2020;44(6):719–28.

489. Folpe AL, Graham RP, Martinez A, Schembri-Wismayer D, Boland J, Fritchie KJ. Mesenchymal chondrosarcomas showing immunohistochemical evidence of rhabdomyoblastic differentiation: a potential diagnostic pitfall. Hum Pathol. 2018;77:28–34.

490. Nakayama R, Miura Y, Ogino J, Susa M, Watanabe I, Horiuchi K, Anazawa U, Toyama Y, Morioka H, Mukai M, Hasegawa T. Detection of HEY1-NCOA2 fusion by fluorescence in-situ hybridization in formalin-fixed paraffin-embedded tissues as a possible diagnostic tool for mesenchymal chondrosarcoma. Pathol Int. 2012;62(12):823–6.

491. Wang L, Motoi T, Khanin R, Olshen A, Mertens F, Bridge J, Dal Cin P, Antonescu CR, Singer S, Hameed M, Bovee JV, Hogendoorn PC, Socci N, Ladanyi M. Identification of a novel, recurrent HEY1-NCOA2 fusion in mesenchymal chondrosarcoma based on a genome-wide screen of exon-level expression data. Genes Chromosomes Cancer. 2012;51(2):127–39.

492. El Beaino M, Roszik J, Livingston JA, Wang WL, Lazar AJ, Amini B, Subbiah V, Lewis V, Conley AP. Mesenchymal chondrosarcoma: a review with emphasis on its fusion-driven biology. Curr Oncol Rep. 2018;20(5):37.

493. Mukherjee D, Chaichana KL, Gokaslan ZL, Aaronson O, Cheng JS, McGirt MJ. Survival of patients with malignant primary osseous spinal neoplasms: results from the Surveillance, Epidemiology, and End Results (SEER) database from 1973 to 2003. J Neurosurg Spine. 2011;14(2):143–50.

494. McMaster ML, Goldstein AM, Bromley CM, Ishibe N, Parry DM. Chordoma: incidence and survival patterns in the United States, 1973–1995. Cancer Causes Control. 2001;12(1):1–11.

495. Shih AR, Cote GM, Chebib I, Choy E, DeLaney T, Deshpande V, Hornicek FJ, Miao R, Schwab JH, Nielsen GP, Chen YL. Clinicopathologic characteristics of poorly differentiated chordoma. Mod Pathol. 2018;31(8):1237–45.

496. Rosenberg AE, Brown GA, Bhan AK, Lee JM. Chondroid chordoma--a variant of chordoma. A morphologic and immunohistochemical study. Am J Clin Pathol. 1994;101(1):36–41.

497. Jeffrey PB, Biava CG, Davis RL, Chondroid chordoma. A hyalinized chordoma without cartilaginous differentiation. Am J Clin Pathol. 1995;103(3):271–9.

498. Hoch BL, Nielsen GP, Liebsch NJ, Rosenberg AE. Base of skull chordomas in children and adolescents: a clinicopathologic study of 73 cases. Am J Surg Pathol. 2006;30(7):811–8.

499. Plaza JA, Ballestín C, Pérez-Barrios A, Martínez MA, de Agustín P. Cytologic, cytochemical, immunocytochemical and ultrastructural diagnosis of a sacrococcygeal chordoma in a fine needle aspiration biopsy specimen. Acta Cytol. 1989;33(1):89–92.

500. Walaas L, Kindblom LG. Fine-needle aspiration biopsy in the preoperative diagnosis of chordoma: a study of 17 cases with application of electron microscopic, histochemical, and immunocytochemical examination. Hum Pathol. 1991;22(1):22–8.

501. Finley JL, Silverman JF, Dabbs DJ, West RL, Dickens A, Feldman PS, Frable WJ. Chordoma: diagnosis by fine-needle aspiration biopsy with histologic, immunocytochemical, and ultrastructural confirmation. Diagn Cytopathol. 1986;2(4):330–7.

502. Rekhi B, Karmarkar S. Clinicocytopathological spectrum, including uncommon forms, of nine cases of chordomas with immunohistochemical results, including brachyury immunostaining: a single institutional experience. Cytopathology. 2019;30(2):229–35.

503. Kay PA, Nascimento AG, Unni KK, Salomão DR. Chordoma. Cytomorphologic findings in 14 cases diagnosed by fine needle aspiration. Acta Cytol. 2003;47(2):202–8.

504. Lauer SR, Edgar MA, Gardner JM, Sebastian A, Weiss SW. Soft tissue chordomas: a clinico-pathologic analysis of 11 cases. Am J Surg Pathol. 2013;37(5):719–26.

505. Jo VY, Hornick JL, Qian X. Utility of brachyury in distinction of chordoma from cytomorphologic mimics in fine-needle aspiration and core needle biopsy. Diagn Cytopathol. 2014;42(8):647–52.

506. O'Connell JX, Renard LG, Liebsch NJ, Efird JT, Munzenrider JE, Rosenberg AE. Base of skull chordoma. A correlative study of histologic and clinical features of 62 cases. Cancer. 1994;74(8):2261–7.

507. Hasselblatt M, Thomas C, Hovestadt V, Schrimpf D, Johann P, Bens S, Oyen F, Peetz-Dienhart S, Crede Y, Wefers A, Vogel H, Riemenschneider MJ, Antonelli M, Giangaspero F, Bernardo MC, Giannini C, Ud Din N, Perry A, Keyvani K, van Landeghem F, Sumerauer D, Hauser P, Capper D, Korshunov A, Jones DT, Pfister SM, Schneppenheim R, Siebert R, Frühwald MC, Kool M. Poorly differentiated chordoma with SMARCB1/INI1 loss: a distinct molecular entity with dismal prognosis. Acta Neuropathol. 2016;132(1):149–51.

508. Zheng W, Huang Y, Guan T, Lu S, Yao L, Wu S, Chen H, Wang N, Liang Y, Xiao W, Jiang X, Wen S. Application of nomograms to predict overall and cancer-specific survival in patients with chordoma. J Bone Oncol. 2019;18:100247.

509. Beccaria K, Tauziède-Espariat A, Monnien F, Adle-Biassette H, Masliah-Planchon J, Pierron G, Maillot L, Polivka M, Laquerrière A, Bouillot-Eimer S, Gimbert E, Gauchotte G, Coffinet L, Sevestre H, Alapetite C, Bolle S, Thompson D, Bouazza S, George B, Zérah M, Sainte-Rose C, Puget S, Varlet P. Pediatric chordomas: results of a multicentric study of 40 children and proposal for a histopathological prognostic grading system and new therapeutic strategies. J Neuropathol Exp Neurol. 2018;77(3):207–15. Erratum in: J Neuropathol Exp Neurol. 2018 Aug 1;77(8):747.

Henryk A. Domanski Professor of pathology at Skåne University Hospital, Lund, Sweden. First/second author or editor in five monographs and atlases, five book chapters and 100 papers published in international journals. Vice-president of the Swedish Society of Clinical Cytology and a member of the European Society of Pathology, the International Academy of Cytology and the Scandinavian Sarcoma Group. President of 42nd European Congress of Cytology 2019 in Malmö, Sweden and a president of European Federation of Cytology Societies 2018–2019.

Pawel Gajdzis, Pathologist at the Wroclaw Medical University, Poland and 4th Military Clinical Hospital in Wroclaw, Poland. Active member in European Federation of Cytology Societies. Author of publications concerning mainly soft tissue and head and neck tumors.

Damjana Verša Ostojić
and Danijela Vrdoljak-Mozetič

23.1   General

Eye diseases are frequent in the general population and are a common reason for visiting an ophthalmologist. A clinical examination in most cases is sufficient to make a diagnosis, but certain cases require additional diagnostic procedures. The eye is specific because in a small space we find different types of tissues and a wide range of pathological processes that include inflammatory, infectious, benign, and malignant neoplastic disorders. In diagnosis and treatment, it is important to preserve the functionality of all parts of the eye as much as possible. Pathological processes can take place on the eye surface, in the anterior aqueous chamber, or in the posterior segment of the eye. The other parts of the ocular region include the eyelid skin, lid margin, palpebral conjunctiva, glandular adnexa, soft tissues, and orbital space. Ocular cytology is relatively a simple, noninvasive, safe, and accurate technique that helps establish a working diagnosis in case of neoplastic lesion, reduces the number of unnecessary biopsies in case of non-neoplastic findings, and is suitable for monitoring the treatment success. Before taking a sample, it is important that the ophthalmologist and cytologist analyze the lesion and clinical data together and discuss the differential diagnosis. They then determine which material retrieval method to apply.

The obtained sample is usually scanty, and the repetition of sampling is often difficult. For this reason, it is important to properly assess the clinical picture, and choose the optimal sampling method as well as appropriate specimen handling with the selection of the necessary additional analysis of a small cell sample (Table 23.1).

D. Verša Ostojić (✉)
Department of Pathology and Cytology, Clinical
Hospital Centre Rijeka, Rijeka, Croatia

D. Vrdoljak-Mozetič
Department of Pathology and Cytology, Clinical
Hospital Centre Rijeka, Rijeka, Croatia

Department of Pathology, Medical Faculty,
University of Rijeka, Rijeka, Croatia
e-mail: danijela.vrdoljak.mozetic@kbc-rijeka.hr

Table 23.1 Ocular cytology specimens and cytopreparatory techniques

Specimen site	Cytopreparatory techniques
Eyelid samples	Direct smears
Corneal and conjunctival samples	Liquid-based cytology
Aqueous and vitrectomy fluid samples	Cytospin preparation
Fine needle aspiration samples of ocular and intraorbital lesions	Cell block preparation
	Sample for molecular testing

23.2 Diagnostic Workflow

The *scraping technique* is simple to perform, relatively noninvasive, rapid, and particularly suitable for small and flat lesions [1, 2]. Primarily, it is used for external eye surfaces including eyelid skin, lid margin, conjunctiva, and cornea. Ulcerated lesions are easily scraped and more cellular compared to fine needle aspiration cytology. These two methods can be combined. Corneal and conjunctival surface lesions must be scrapped under local topical anesthesia under slit-lamp control. It is necessary to make several passes to obtain adequate cellularity from deeper layers as well. Scraping can be done with a small spatula, a brush with short bristles, or with a spherical tip. The scraping technique using the corneal dissector instrument gives very good results due to simple handling and easy transfer of the cellular sample to the slides. The collected material must be evenly smeared on slides and immediately alcohol-fixed for Papanicolaou stain or air-dried for May-Grunwald-Giemsa (MGG) stain or other stains. In addition to conventional smears, the sample can be processed utilizing liquid-based cytology (LBC) placing the material in an appropriate alcohol-based fixative so the sample is suitable for additional testing. Since very scarce materials are usually handled, there is an additional possibility of making immunocytochemistry (ICC) on alcohol-fixed smears.

Impression cytology is performed using a cellulose acetate filter placed on the ocular surface after the application of topical anesthetic drops using gentle pressure and carefully peeled off. The filter removes the two to three epithelial superficial layers of the ocular surface. The strip must then be fixed in alcohol, stained with Papanicolaou stain, and mounted on a glass slide [3].

A *fine needle aspiration cytology* (FNAC) was first applied to orbital tumors in 1975 and published by Schyberg [4]. FNAC plays an important role in deeper orbital lesions, intraocular lesions, or cystic lesions. FNAC can be used for more superficial nonulcerating lesions of the eyelids and conjunctiva using a 23–24 gauge needle. For deeper intraorbital and intraocular lesions, it is necessary to use imaging techniques such as ultrasonography or computed tomography. Cytopathology assistance in performing FNAC is very important due to the usually small samples and the necessity of optimal handling of the precious sample. The material is applied to slides for standard cytology staining. If there is enough material, cytospin smears, LBC, and cell block can be done and used for histochemical and ICC as well as for molecular testing. The material obtained from FNAC is also sent for microbiological analysis if necessary.

Intraoperative cytology diagnosis can be used when there is no preoperative diagnosis of an ocular lesion or there is disagreement with clinical findings [5]. An imprint of the cutting surface of unfixed tissue can be used. The squash technique can also be used, in which a piece of tissue is placed between two slides, pressed lightly, and drawn apart [6].

Intraocular fluids cytology has an important place in the diagnosis of eye diseases. Two chambers divide the interior of the eye. The anterior aqueous chamber is located between the cornea and lens and contains approximately 0.3 ml of aqueous fluid. The posterior chamber is located between the lens and retina and filled with transparent viscous vitreous fluid. Vitrectomy is a type of intervention performed to remove some or all vitreous humor from the posterior segment. Vitectomy specimens contain approximately

1 ml of the sample obtained in both diagnostic and therapeutic vitectomies depending on the clinical diagnosis. Proper handling of the small volume of intraocular fluid is essential to perform the necessary ancillary tests according to the presumed diagnosis. Few drops of fluid can be used to prepare direct smears. The fluids may be diluted with saline and processed in cytospin or LBC or sent for microbiology or molecular testing [2]. The most common questions of differential diagnosis in these samples include infections, noninfectious inflammatory processes, and neoplastic lesions. A typical cytomorphologic picture of a specific infection is usually absent. In chronic uveitis, cytology smears from ocular fluids contain chronic inflammatory cells, including lymphocytes, plasma cells, and macrophages [7].

The front parts of the eye, which include the conjunctiva and cornea as well as the eyelids, are suitable for easy and quick collection of cytological samples. The structure of the *eyelid* is complex with different tissue types in a small space. They are composed of several layers including skin (keratinized stratified squamous epithelium) with subcutaneous tissue, striated muscle, tarsus, and conjunctiva. The eyelids are rich with glandular tissue: sebaceous and apocrine glands and sweat glands. Lacrimal glands are located in an upper palpebral area and are serous-type salivary glands. As a consequence of this complex structure, there are numerous pathological conditions that are useful to determine before therapy to preserve the functionality of the eyelid.

In practice, ophthalmologists often encounter inflammatory eyelid lesions caused by various microorganisms such as bacteria, viruses, fungal infections, parasites, or other conditions like allergic conjunctivitis. A common clinical entity is a hordeolum with an acute bacterial inflammatory abscess filled with pus, most often caused by obstruction of the meibomian duct and staphylococcal infection with acute inflammatory reaction. Chalazion or lipogranuloma is a common granulomatous reaction to the sebaceous material spilled into the surroundings from the obstructed meibomian gland ducts. Cytological sample shows inflammatory reaction with epithelioid macrophages, histiocytic aggregates, occasional multinucleated giant cells, and varying proportions of neutrophils and lymphoplasmacytic cells with dirty and lipid background. Malignant lesions such as basal cell carcinoma, squamous carcinoma, or sebaceous carcinoma can clinically be mistaken for chalazion and hordeolum, so a simple cytological examination can facilitate the diagnostic procedure.

Basal cell carcinoma (BCC) is the most common malignant tumor of the eyelid skin and accounts for 90% of all eyelid carcinomas [8]. They are slowly growing, locally invasive tumors that can cause extensive tissue destruction but rarely metastasize. Ulcerating lesions can be sampled by scarification, while FNA must be used for nodular lesions. Smears of the most common nodular type of BCC are typically high cellular with clusters of tightly packed basaloid cells with high N/C ratio, hyperchromatic nuclei with condensed, finely granular chromatin, and inconspicuous nucleoli (Fig. 23.1). The cytoplasm is very scant and ill-defined. Peripheral pallisading of nuclei at the edge of the cluster may be visible. In some cases, prominent spindle cell component or myxoid stroma may be present. All variants of BCC are strong Ber-EP4 positive, and this helps to differentiate them from other tumors with similar morphology [9].

Squamous cell carcinoma (SCC) is the second most common malignancy of the eyelid with invasive growth and the ability to produce metastases [10]. It accounts for 5–10% of all malignant eyelid tumors. Smears are usually cellular with clusters and dispersed malignant cells. The nuclei are enlarged, hyperchromatic, sometimes pyknotic, and spindle-shaped. In well-differentiated tumors, the cytoplasm is densely basophilic in MGG stain and orangephilic in the Papanicolaou stain as a sign of keratinization. The abundant necrotic background is often seen. In poorly differentiated tumors, the tumor cells have different degrees of polymorphism and loss of keratinization. ICC show positivity for epithelial membrane antigen (EMA), p63, and high molecular weight cytokeratin [11].

The periorbital region and eyelids contain the most concentration of sebaceous glands in the human body. *Sebaceous carcinoma* is a rare malig-

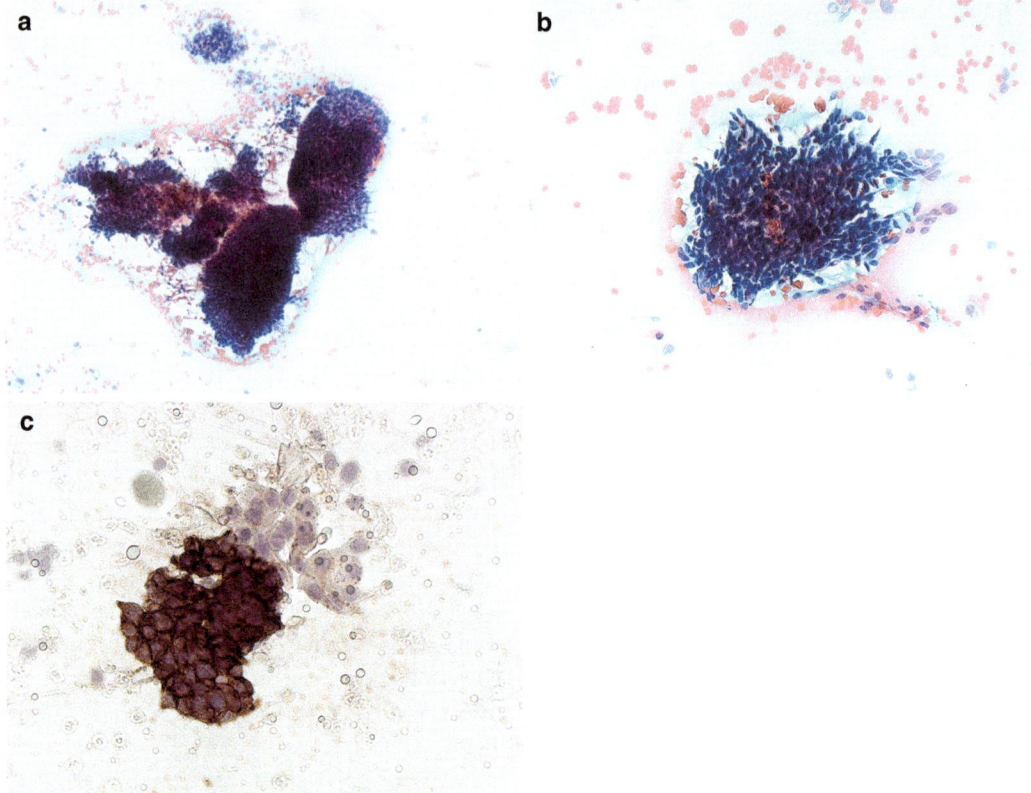

Fig. 23.1 Scarification of persistent ulcerated lesion of the lower eyelid margin, basal cell carcinoma. (**a**): Cellular smear with solid fragments of basaloid cells (Papanicolaou, 100X). (**b**): Tightly packed basaloid cells with high N/C ratio, hypercromasia, and scant cytoplasm (Papanicolaou, 400X). (**c**): ICC on alcohol-fixed smear stained Ber-EP4 strong positive (400X)

nant tumor of the sebaceous glands with the most common localization on the eyelid. The incidence varies from 1 to 5.5% of all malignant neoplasms of the eyelid [12]. It is an aggressive tumor that spreads locally, can metastasize to regional lymph nodes and distant organs, and can recur. It occurs more often in older people, and prior irradiation is an important risk factor [13]. Due to the low incidence and nonspecific clinical picture, it is often confused with inflammatory changes, like chalazion or persistent unilateral blepharitis or conjunctivitis, thus delaying appropriate treatment. For this reason, cytology can be an important tool in the diagnosis of sebaceous carcinoma and the differential diagnosis of other eyelid malignancies, mostly BCC and SCC. The samples are mostly cellular with clusters of larger malignant epithelial cells with moderate to scanty amount of cytoplasm, round to oval hyperchromatic nuclei, and prominent nucleoli. Well-differentiated carcinomas, as a result of lipid content, show foamy vacuolated cytoplasm or small vacuoles visible in smear background, best seen on MGG stain. Oil red O lipid staining is useful in establishing the diagnosis [11]. ICC show positivity for EMA, low molecular weight cytokeratins, androgen receptors, and adipophilin (Fig. 23.2).

Other less common malignant neoplasms that may be found on the eyelid include cutaneous melanoma of the eyelid, pleomorphic adenoma, adenoid cystic carcinoma, and mucoepidermoid carcinoma of the lacrimal gland.

Samples from the cornea and conjunctiva are most often direct smears obtained by scarifica-

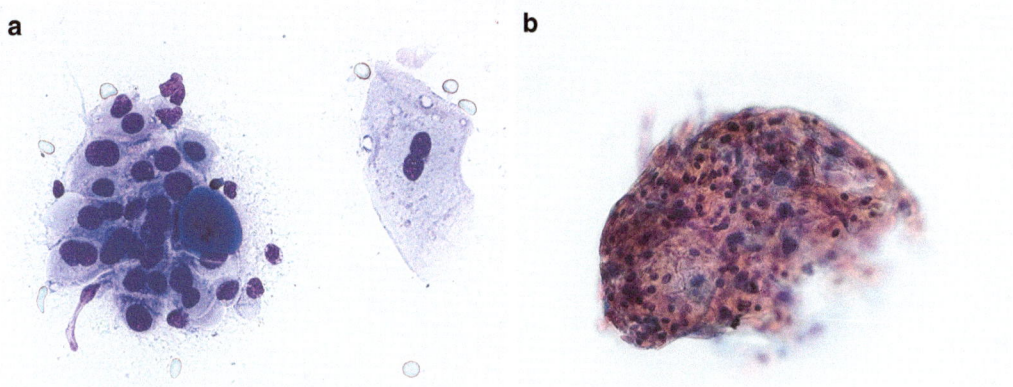

Fig. 23.2 Scarification of raised gelatinous mass at the ocular limbus, ocular surface squamous neoplasia. (**a**): Dysplastic cells with increased N/C ratio, hyperchroma-sia, and coarse chromatin (MGG, 400X). (**b**): Cluster of keratinized dysplastic cells with pycnotic nuclei (Papanicolaou, 400X)

tion or imprint cytology. The *conjunctiva* is composed of two to five layers of cuboidal to cylindrical cells with mucin-secreting goblet cells and lies on a loose connective tissue. Conjunctival scrapings are mostly cellular with clusters and single cuboidal to columnar cells, with single round to oval nuclei, finely granular chromatin, and occasional small inconspicuous nucleoli. Goblet cells are easily visible with clear vacuolated cytoplasm and eccentric nuclei. The epithelium of the *cornea* consists of five to six layers of three different types of cells: two to three layers of flattened superficial cells, two to three layers of wing cells, and a monolayer of smaller columnar basal cells with higher N/C ratios that adhere to the basement membrane overlying Bowman's layer. The smears from normal cornea demonstrate cohesive sheets of nonkeratinized squamous cells.

Ocular surface squamous neoplasia (OSSN) is the most common tumor of the ocular surface and includes a spectrum of diseases ranging from mild to severe conjunctival intraepithelial neoplasia (CIN), carcinoma in situ to invasive squamous cell carcinoma [14]. It is considered to be a premalignant lesion that can progress to invasive squamous cell carcinoma. The process arises at the corneoscleral junction (limbus) from corneal stem cells [15] and involves either or both conjunctiva and cornea. Risk factors for the development of these lesions are ultraviolet light

exposure, immunosuppression, HIV infection, HPV types 16 and 18 infections, and advanced age, among other factors [16]. Intraepithelial neoplasia and invasive squamous cell carcinoma are difficult to distinguish on clinical appearances alone, and they can mimic other benign and malignant conditions. Cytology is useful for diagnosing OSSN and also for monitoring treatment success and detecting disease recurrence that are relatively common. Cytology samples are cellular, often with abundant keratinization, making it difficult to obtain a sample from the deeper layers. Cell morphology can range from mildly atypical keratinized cells, cells with an increased nuclear to cytoplasmic ratio, or with prominent nucleoli to syncytial clusters of atypical cells with sparse cytoplasms (Fig. 23.3). The presence of keratinization in a smear from the cornea is an abnormal finding.

Vitreoretinal lymphoma (VRL) is a rare ocular malignancy with primary involvement of vitreous lymphoma cells. It usually involves the retina, the vitreous, or both structures, but in up to 50% of cases of intraocular findings, there is concomitant involvement of the central nervous system [17]. The majority of cases are CD20-positive B-cell lymphoma, but rare cases of T-cells VRL have been reported [18]. Early and accurate diagnosis is crucial to ensure appropriate treatment and reduce the high mortality associated with VRL. The main differential diagnosis includes

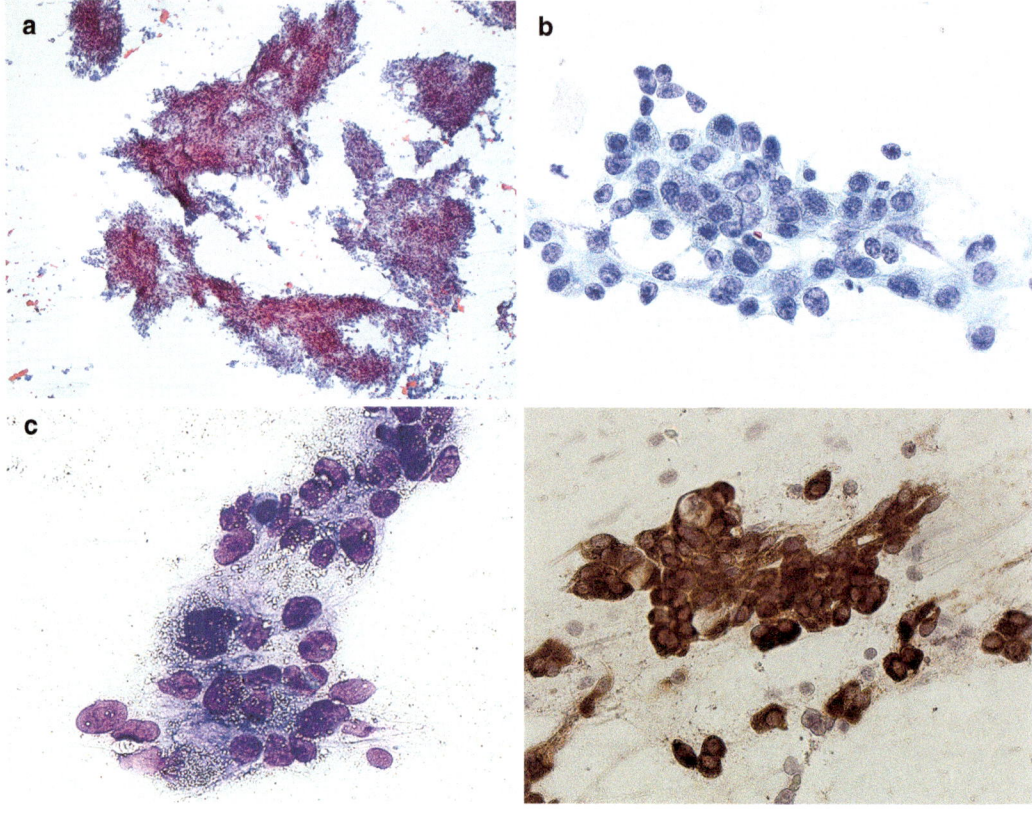

Fig. 23.3 Scarification of nodular tumor of the upper eyelid, sebaceous carcinoma. (**a**): Cellular smear with tumor cells arranged in clusters (Papanicolaou, 40X). (**b**): Cluster of cells with foamy vacuolated cytoplasm, rounded nuclei, and prominent nucleoli (Papanicolaou, 100X). (**c**): Cluster of cells with anisonucleosis and small vacuoles visible in cytoplasm and background (MGG, 400). (**d**): ICC on alcohol-fixed smear stained EMA strong positive (400X)

lymphocytic infiltration in chronic uveitis or sarcoidosis. Various methods must be used in diagnosis, including cytology, ICC, cytokine analysis (IL-10 to IL-6 ratio), flow cytometry (cell clonality), and molecular analysis [19]. Recently, studies have shown the value of testing for hotspot mutation of the myeloid differentiation primary response gene 88 (MYD88) in fluids from the anterior chamber and vitreous [20]. MYD88 mutation was detected in the aqueous humor of 75% of patients with cytologically proven vitreoretinal lymphoma. Clinically suspected VRL with cytology suspicious for lymphoproliferative disorder, abnormal flow cytometry result, a heavy-chain gene immunoglobulin rearrangement, or an MYD88 L265P mutation, can be diagnosed as VRL, which has the practical significance of early diagnoses and the start of chemotherapy treatment.

Samples used in diagnostics are anterior chamber and vitreous fluids; they are often with scant cellularity which makes the diagnosis difficult. The specimens should be handled rapidly because malignant cells are prone to degenerative changes. Typical preparations of undiluted material contain atypical, large lymphoid cells with convoluted nuclei, conspicuous nucleoli, scant basophilic cytoplasm, and are two to four times larger than normal lymphocytes. Small, reactive T lymphocytes and debris are usually present. A cell block preparation can be made for ICC testing including B and T-cell markers, Ki-67, and monoclonality [21].

Intraocular melanoma is the most common primary intraocular malignant tumor of adults and the most common noncutaneous melanoma [22]. It is a malignant neoplasm of melanocytes within the uveal tract that may arise from preexisting uveal nevi or de novo [23]. Most malignant melanomas are diagnosed clinically and treated with radiotherapy, while large tumors are treated by enucleation [24]. In the majority of cases of uveal melanoma, FNAC is performed to confirm the clinical diagnosis, to obtain material for molecular testing, or to rule out metastatic carcinoma, uveal nevi, and other lesions involving the uvea and retina. The specimen is processed for direct smears using standard staining, cytospin preparation, LBC method, and cell block preparation. FNAC material is used for cytogenetics testing for loss of chromosome 3 (monosomy 3), gain on 6p, loss on 6q, and gain on 8q [25]. Air-dried cytology slides can be used for fluorescence in situ hybridisation (FISH) analysis for the presence of monosomy 3. Long-term studies have shown a poorer prognosis in cases with monosomy 3, so this test is considered an important prognostic marker in patients with ocular melanoma [26]. Malignant melanomas can be classified by gene expression profiling using undiluted FNA samples placed in a special fixative provided by a collection kit (DecisionDx-UM; Castle Biosciences Incorporated) [27]. The gene expression profile test has been refined to a 15-gene assay performed on a microfluidc PCR platform that allows accurate and reproducible molecular classification of melanomas and prediction of high-risk patients. Uveal melanoma is usually characterized by point mutations in GNAQ and GNA11 genes that encode the G-protein alpha subunit. On the other hand, mutations in the BRCA1-associated protein-1 (BAP1) appear to occur later and demarcate a molecular brink beyond which metastasis becomes highly likely. BAP1 mutations can also occur in the germline, leading to a distinctive cancer predisposition syndrome. These muta-

tions appear to be key events that provide the potential for targeted therapy. The cytology of malignant melanoma shows atypical cells in solid clusters or singly with large epitheloid, polygonal cells, or spindle-shaped cells. The nuclei can be binucleated with prominent, centrally placed, red nucleoli. Sometimes pigment or intranuclear pseudoinclusions may be seen. The differential diagnosis includes uveal nevi that have the cytomorphology of spindle-shaped amelanotic or pigmented cells with bland nuclei, finely dispersed chromatin, and lacking nucleoli or mitoses [1].

The most common intraocular tumors in adults are *metastatic carcinomas*, and the choroid is the most common site of uveal metastases [28]. In women, most common metastatic tumors are breast and lung carcinoma and lung and gastrointestinal carcinomas in men. FNAC of ocular lesions suspected of a metastatic process enables a relatively simple diagnosis, while additional ICC enables immunophenotyping of the tumor in the case of an unknown primary malignancy. Intraocular metastases show the same cytomorphology as primary tumors.

Small blue round cell tumors mostly occur in children, and lesions included are retinoblastoma, rhabdomyosarcoma, and orbital lymphoid lesions. *Retinoblastoma* (RB) is the most common intraocular malignancy in childhood which forms when both RB1 alleles mutate in a susceptible retinal cell. Loss of the tumor suppressor functions of the retinoblastoma protein, pRB, leads to uncontrolled cell division and recurrent genomic changes during tumor progression [29]. RB is usually easily diagnosed clinically and radiologically, and on rare occasions, FNAC may be performed. There are controversies about the use of FNAC with concern for tumor seeding. FNAC can have a supportive role in the preoperative diagnosis of RB cases that pose a dilemma to the clinician [30]. Cytology of RB shows small, round, uniform tumor cells are seen in loose clusters, tightly packed clusters, or singly. The cells have rounded hyperchromatic nuclei, coarse, uniformly distributed chromatin, and scant cytoplasm, and the background is necrotic. Thigh cohesion and nuclear molding are distinct cytologic features. Cluster and rosette formation and PAS-positive granules can be seen [31]. The tumor cells are NSE, bcl-2, and synaptophysin positive [30].

The complex structure of the orbital region is the source of various other intraorbital tumors such as histiocytoma, leiomyosarcoma, teratoma, schwannoma, and meningeomas, as well as secondary orbital tumors.

Ocular cytology has an important role in the diagnosis of ocular lesions, clinical management, and patient monitoring after treatment. With the growth of knowledge about the nature of ocular lesions and in addition to standard cytomorphology, a small cell sample is suitable for ancillary molecular tests and thus follows the aim of applying personalized medicine.

23.3   Main Massage

- Ocular cytology is a relatively simple, noninvasive, safe, and accurate technique that helps establish a working diagnosis in case of neoplastic lesion, reduces the number of unnecessary biopsies in case of non-neoplastic findings, and is suitable for monitoring the treatment success.
- The obtained sample is usually scanty, so it is important to choose the optimal sampling method and appropriate specimen handling with the selection of the necessary additional analysis of a small cell sample.
- The scraping technique using the corneal dissector instrument gives very good results due to simple handling and easy transfer of the cellular sample onto the slides. It is necessary to make several passes to obtain adequate cellularity from deeper layers as well.
- Proper handling of the small volume of intraocular fluid is essential to perform the necessary ancillary tests according to the presumed diagnosis.
- Malignant lesions such as basal cell carcinoma, squamous carcinoma, or sebaceous carcinoma can clinically be mistaken for chalazion or hordeolum, and a simple cytological examination can facilitate the diagnostic procedure.

- Cytology is useful for diagnosing OSSN and also for monitoring treatment success and detecting disease recurrence that are relatively common.
- Ocular cytology suspicious for lymphoproliferative disorder, abnormal flow cytometry result, a heavy-chain gene immunoglobulin rearrangement, or an MYD88 L265P mutation can be diagnosed with vitreoretinal lymphoma which has the practical significance of early diagnoses and the start of chemotherapy treatment.
- In the case of uveal melanoma, FNAC is performed to confirm the clinical diagnosis, to obtain material for molecular testing, or to rule out metastatic carcinoma, uveal nevi, and other lesions involving the uvea and retina.
- Air-dried cytology slides can be used for FISH analysis for the presence of monosomy 3 in uveal melanoma.
- The most common intraocular tumors in adults are metastatic carcinomas. Intraocular metastases show the same cytomorphology as primary tumors. ICC from cytology specimens enables immunophenotyping of the tumor in the case of an unknown primary malignancy.

References

1. Laver NMV. Ocular cytopathology: a primer for the generalist. Semin Diagn Pathol. 2015;32(4):311–22.
2. Metha M, Laver NV. Ocular cytology. In: Xu H, Qian X, Wang H, editors. Practical cytopathology: frequently asked questions. Springer Nature Switzerland AG; 2020. p. 323–33.
3. Nolan GR, Hirst LW, Wright RG, Bancroft BJ. Application of impression cytology to the diagnosis of conjunctival neoplasms. Diagn Cytopathol. 1994;11(3):246–9.
4. Schyberg E. Fine needle biopsy of orbital tumors. Acta Ophtalmol Suppl. 1975;125:11.
5. Vemuganti GK, Murthy SI. A review of ophthalmic pathology techniques. Noida J Ophthalmol. 2005;2:5–15.
6. Font RL, Lauciricia R, Ramzy I. Cytological evaluation of tumours of the orbit and ocular adnexa: an analysis of 84 cases studied by the "squash technique". Diagn Cytopathol. 1994;10(2):135–42.
7. Laver NMV. Ocular cytology: diagnostic features and ongoing practices. Cancer Cytopathol.

2021;129(6):419–31.

8. Deprez M, Uffer S. Clinicopathological features of eyelid skin tumors. A retrospective study of 5504 cases and review of literature. Am J Dermatopathol. 2009;31(3):256–62.

9. Carr RA, Sanders DSA. Basaloid skin tumours: mimics of basal cell carcinoma. Curr Diagn Pathol. 2007;13(4):273–300.

10. Donaldson MJ, Sullivan TJ, Whitehead KJ, Williamson RM. Squamous cell carcinoma of theeye-lids. Br J Ophthalmol. 2002;86(10):1161–5.

11. Salomão D, Tóth J, Kennedy S. Eyelid pathology. In: Heegaard S, Grossniklaus H, editors. Eye pathology. Berlin/Heidelberg: Springer; 2015. p. 443–546.

12. Shields JA, Demirci H, Marr BP, Eagle RC Jr, Shields CL. Sebaceous carcinoma of the ocular region: a review. Surv Ophthalmol. 2005;50(2):103–22.

13. Howrey RP, Lipham WJ, Schultz WH, Buckley EG, Dutton JJ, Klintworth GK, Rosoff PM. Sebaceous gland carcinoma: a subtle second malignancy following radiation therapy in patients with bilateral retino-blastoma. Cancer. 1998;83(4):767–71.

14. Kiire CA, Stewart RMK, Srinivasan S, Heimann H, Kaye SB, Dhillon B. A prospective study of the incidence, associations and outcomes of ocular surface squamous neoplasia in the United Kingdom. Eye (Lond). 2019;33(2):283–94.

15. Schlötzer-Schrehardt U, Kruse FE. Identifi cation and characterization of limbal stem cells. Exp Eye Res. 2005;81(3):247–64.

16. Lee GA, Williams G, Hirst LW, Green AC. Risk factors in the development of ocular surface epithelial dysplasia. Ophthalmology. 1994;101(2):360–4.

17. Grossniklaus HE, Coupland SE. Primary choroidal lymphoma. In: Grossniklaus HE, Eberhart CG, Kivela TT, editors. WHO classification of tumours of the eye, WHO classification of tumours, vol. 12, 4th ed. Lyon: IARC Press; 2018. p. 98.

18. Coupland SE, Heimann H, Bechrakis NE. Primary intraocular lymphoma: a review of the clinical, histopathological and molecular biological features. Graefes Arch Clin Exp Ophthalmol. 2004;242(11):901–13.

19. Tan WJ, Wang MM, Ricciardi-Castagnoli P, Chan ASY, Lim TS. Cytologic and molecular diagnostics for vitreoretinal lymphoma: current approaches and emerging single-cell analyses. Front Mol Biosci. 2021;7:611017.

20. Miserocchi E, Ferreri AJM, Giuffrè C, Cangi MG, Francaviglia I, Calimeri T, Ponzoni M, Pecciarini L, Bandello FM, Modorati GM. Myd88 L265p mutation detection in the aqueous humor of patients with vitreoretinal lymphoma. Retina. 2019;39(4):679–84.

21. Kase S, Namba K, Iwata D, Mizuuchi K, Kitaichi N, Tagawa Y, et al. Diagnostic efficacy of cell block method for vitreoretinal lymphoma. Diagn Pathol. 2016;11:29.

22. PDQ Adult Treatment Editorial Board. Intraocular (Uveal) Melanoma Treatment (PDQ®): Health Professional Version. 2022 Oct 14. In: PDQ Cancer Information Summaries [Internet]. Bethesda: National Cancer Institute (US); 2002.

23. Shields CL, Furuta M, Berman EL, Zahler JD, Hoberman DM, Dinh DH, Mashayekhi A, Shields JA. Choroidal nevus transformation into melanoma: analysis of 2514 consecutive cases. Arch Ophthalmol. 2009;127(8):981–7.

24. Kath R, Hayungs J, Bornfeld N, Sauerwein W, Höffken K, Seeber S. Prognosis and treatment of disseminated uveal melanoma. Cancer. 1993;72(7):2219–23.

25. Maat W, Jordanova ES, van Zelderen-Bhola SL, et al. The heterogeneous distribution of monosomy 3 in uveal melanomas: implications for prognostication based on fine-needle aspiration biopsies. Arch Pathol Lab Med. 2007;131(1):91–6.

26. Harbour WJ, Chao DL. A molecular revolution in uveal melanoma: implications for patient care and targeted therapy. Ophthalmology. 2014;121(6):1281–8.

27. Harbour JW. The genetics of uveal melanoma: an emerging framework for targeted therapy. Pigment Cell Melanoma Res. 2012;25(2):171–81.

28. Ferry AP, Font RL. Carcinoma metastatic to the eye and orbit. I. A clinicopathologic study of 227 cases. Arch Ophthalmol. 1974;92(4):276–86.

29. Dimaras H, Corson TW, Cobrinik D, et al. Retinoblastoma. Nat Rev Dis Primers. 2015;1:15021.

30. Chawla B, Tomar A, Sen S, Bajaj MS, Kashyap S. Intraocular fine needle aspiration cytology as a diagnostic modality for retinoblastoma. Int J Ophthalmol. 2016;9(8):1233–5.

31. Garg V, Gupta A, Pruthi SK, Khare P. Retinoblastoma in an adult. J Cytol. 2018;35(2):120–4.

Damjana Versa Ostojic Clinical cytopathologist at Clinical Hospital Centre Rijeka, Croatia Area of interest include gynecological cytology, HPV detection, cervical biomarkers, ocular cytology and implementation of Quality Control/Quality Assurance in cytology. Member of Croatian Society of Clinical Cytology and Croatian Gynecological Oncology Society. Author of 13 articles in peer-reviewed journals, 4 book chapters, and over 50 abstracts.

Danijela Vrdoljak-Mozetic Assistant Professor at Faculty of Medicine, University of Rijeka, Croatia. Past president of Croatian Society for Clinical cytology. Secretary General of European Federation of Cytology Societies since 2021. Representative of EFCS in UEMS Section of pathology. Member of National committee for cervical screening and Working group for specialty training in pathology and cytology of Croatian Ministry of Health. Author of more than 50 papers in domestic and international medical journals and over 100 abstracts.

Conclusions

Wojciech Golusiński

This book is the result of an interdisciplinary collaboration between authorities from all over the world in their respective fields. Tumours of the head and neck are a unique group of cancers due to their particular location. The head and neck region is extraordinarily vascularised and innervated. All the sensory organs on which our quality of life depends are located here. Therefore, extensive diagnostics and interdisciplinary treatment are demanding and difficult.

There is a constant search for histopathological and cytological features that are universally accepted and that can be associated with prognosis, which in turn could influence the choice of therapy. There may be artefacts in the specimen collected for examination, especially paraffin-embedded specimens, related to the method of collection and the fixation and embedding process. These have a certain influence on the structure of nucleoproteins and other cell and tissue components, thus causing changes in the morphological picture. It is these facts that the histopathologist must consider when evaluating the slides and, in cases of doubt, inform the clinician. It is also important to bear in mind that it is not uncommon for the histological picture of the specimen taken before surgery to differ from that found in the surgical specimen. An important element of histopathological diagnosis is the way in which the tissue material is collected by the clinician—the head and neck surgeon. His or her experience cannot be overestimated. First and foremost, the material should be taken from the tumour. Some authors have highlighted the existence of differences in the nature of the tissue of the central and peripheral parts of carcinomas, which may explain the differences in histological findings [1].

Tissue diagnosis is mandatory before starting treatment for any malignant tumour. The diagnosis can be obtained by performing a biopsy or fine-needle biopsy of shallow tumours or a core-needle or open biopsy of the more deeply located tumours. If there is a clinically reasonable suspicion that the tumour is malignant and the first biopsy does not confirm this, a second biopsy is recommended. Fine-Needle Aspiration (FNA) with which we can obtain a cytological diagnosis can be performed under palpation or using ultrasound and CT imaging techniques. Currently, fine-needle biopsy is a highly effective and commonly used tool in obtaining a diagnosis for most head and neck cancers, but it is important to remember that a negative cytological diagnosis does not exclude the presence of a malignant tumour. If the FNA result is inconclusive, a core-needle or open biopsy should be performed. Both methods usually provide sufficient tissue material for an accurate histopathological diagnosis.

W. Golusiński (✉)
Department of Head and Neck Surgery, Poznan University of Medical Sciences, The Greater Poland Cancer Centre, Poznań, Poland
e-mail: wgolus@ump.edu.pl

In order to properly process and diagnose the tumour tissue, the pathologist must become familiar with all the relevant details of the patient's medical history. In addition, the collaboration between the head and neck surgeon and the pathologist is essential in order to formulate a proper diagnostic impression of the collected tumour tissue [2].

The complicated mechanism of tumour formation, on the one hand, and the poorly understood biology of tumours, on the other hand, result in a constant search for new research techniques that would enable the prediction of a patient's future and the selection of the optimal treatment method. Today, it is not possible to rely only on histopathological diagnosis and diagnostic methods that assess the size of the tumour and the degree of infiltration of the surrounding tissues. A number of diagnostic methods to determine cells in the proliferative phase have been known for a long time. A simple method for assessing division rates has found practical application. It is used to determine the degree of histological malignancy in tumours of epithelial and mesenchymal origin. As new research techniques were developed, flow cytometry was introduced to quantify cellular DNA. An important advance has been the introduction of immunohistochemical tests for the detection of P53 and P16 gene mutations and antigens of proteins supporting the synthesis of cell cycle enzymes. Today, modern histopathology has a wide range of techniques for chromosomal and molecular analysis, ranging from basic karyotyping to 24-colour spectral karyotyping and fluorescence in situ hybridisation of cloned deoxyribonucleic acid. Chromosomal translocation analysis by fluorescence in situ hybridisation has become the basis for the diagnosis of many head and neck tumours such as Ewing's sarcoma or rhabdomyosarcoma. The study of head and neck cancer genetics has been objectivised with the development of the human head and neck cancer genome and the advent of high-reliability genetic imaging tools. The success as well as the hopes associated with the identification of the epidermal growth factor, as well as many further breakthroughs in this field, means that the field of cancer genetics will

continue to grow and will certainly have a significant impact on treatment in the years to come [3].

Finding a well-selected biomarker in head and neck cancers continues to be a problem. This is due to the high histological and genetic heterogeneity of tumour tissue of one anatomical region with multiple anatomical locations and the influence of oncogenic viruses such as HPV and EBV on the development of head and neck cancers [4, 5].

I believe that the conclusion of this valuable study should be the realisation that only multidisciplinary collaboration between multiple specialists involved in the diagnosis and treatment of head and neck cancer can be successful. Such interdisciplinarity and the resulting personalisation of treatment should be inherent to all centres dedicated to the treatment of head and neck cancer.

References

1. Kumar V, Abbas AK, Aster JC, Perkins JA, Robbins SL. Robbins basic pathology. 10th ed. Elsevier—Health Sciences Division.
2. Wagner JM, Monfore N, McCullough AJ, Zhao L, Conrad RD, Krempl GA, Alleman AM. Ultrasound-guided fine-needle aspiration with optional core needle biopsy of head and neck lymph nodes and masses. J Ultrasound Med. 2018;9999:1–10.
3. René Leemans C, Braakhuis BJM, Brakenhoff RH. The molecular biology of head and neck cancer. Nat Rev Cancer. 2011;11:9–22.
4. Wondergem NE, Nijenhuis DNLM, Poell JB, Leemans CR, Brakenhoff RH, van de Ven R. At the crossroads of molecular biology and immunology: molecular pathways for immunological targeting of head and neck squamous cell carcinoma. Front Oral Health. 2:647980.
5. The Cancer Genome Atlas Network. Comprehensive genomic characterization of head and neck squamous cell carcinomas. Nature. 2015;517:576. https://doi.org/10.1038/nature14129.

Wojciech Golusiński, Professor of ENT and head and neck surgery at University of Medical Sciences at the Greater Poland Cancer Centre. Past president of the European Head and Neck Society (2018–2022). Co-author of European recommendations on diagnosis and treatment of head and neck cancer, prepared by members of three societies: EHNS, ESTRO and ESMO. Author of over 300 papers, reports and lectures. Author and organizer of the National Head and Neck Cancer Prevention Program in Poland.